Excellence in Dementia Care
Research into practice

SECOND EDITION

Edited by Murna Downs and Barbara Bowers

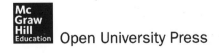
Open University Press

Open University Press
McGraw-Hill Education
McGraw-Hill House
Shoppenhangers Road
Maidenhead
Berkshire
England
SL6 2QL

email: enquiries@openup.co.uk
world wide web: www.openup.co.uk

and Two Penn Plaza, New York, NY 10121-2289, USA

First edition published 2010
First published in this second edition 2014

A catalogue record of this book is available from the British Library

ISBN-13: 978-0-335-24533-8
ISBN-10: 0-335-24533-1
eISBN: 978-0-335-24534-5

Library of Congress Cataloging-in-Publication Data
CIP data applied for

Typeset by Aptara®, Inc.

Fictitious names of companies, products, people, characters and/or data that may be used herein
(in case studies or in examples) are not intended to represent any real individual, company,
product or event.

Praise for this book

"Awareness of dementia is at its highest and this reflects the importance of the condition for individuals, their families, health and social care services and the wider community. While we have made significant advances in the care for people with dementia and their families, there is much work yet to be done. This book provides a fantastic framework in which to set our understanding of dementia and to take things forward."

Alistair Burns, Professor of Old Age Psychiatry, Faculty of Medical and Human Sciences, University of Manchester, UK

"This edition of Excellence in Dementia Care provides an important, new and comprehensive overview of the state of the art in caring for the diversity of people with dementia. The international authors and global focus have created a unique textbook that will help educators, students and the broader care community to better understand the challenges and opportunities related to dementia care. I am particularly excited about this new edition because it goes beyond the individual and the family by showcasing efforts to create dementia-friendly communities and adapt physical design, offers a critical perspective on how dementia is portrayed in the media, literature and the arts, tackles issues related to whole person assessment, care planning and care transitions, and addresses the unique concerns of living with young-onset dementia. This volume is a welcome addition to the dementia care toolbox and will prove valuable to a very diverse international audience."

Dr Robyn I. Stone, Senior VP for Research, LeadingAge, Washington DC, USA

"The depth and breadth of this book invites all involved in practice, research and policy to reconsider dementia as something other than a degenerative brain disease and to shift their perspective to the person. The voice of the individual living with dementia, their family, care partners and collaborating professionals are all reconsidered within the context of our current evidenced-based knowledge. This book deeply challenges the status quo of dementia care and sets an expectation for so much more."

Anna Ortigara, Organizational Change Consultant, PHI PolicyWorks, USA

"This text will meet the needs of registered and preregistered student nurses working with people with dementia. It skilfully discusses all aspects of dementia drawing on the work of a number of experts in the field. The book considers the biological, social and physiological impact of the condition. It presents a balanced discussion of current research and thinking on the treatment of the condition and the care of dementia sufferers and their families. New and updated chapters help ensure readers of this text gain a holistic understanding of contemporary issues around this distressing and life-limiting condition."

Nichola Barlow, Senior Lecturer Adult Nursing, University of Huddersfield, UK

"The first edition of this book was a vitally important and a key text in its field combining the talents of multiple experts in dementia and older people's care. It is pleasing to say that the second edition is equally as pivotal in gathering key expertise and providing the reader with the essential and important insight to provide forward-thinking care. The text takes forwards the concepts of dementia-friendly communities and explores the crucial topics of care in acute wards and end of life care. The text is a comprehensive book that would be useful to many health and social care professionals across a range of diverse organisations within the NHS, Voluntary Sector and other private and public health sector providers. Anyone working with older people and people with dementia and their carers should have access to a copy within their organization or I would strongly encourage individuals to purchase their own copy. I feel this is an essential text for anyone teaching health and social care courses from undergraduate to postgraduate students across a range of health and social care education settings. The sound evidence base to each chapter allows people working with individuals with dementia and their families to have access to the evidence quickly and easily, which is ultimately useful to practitioners and staff working on the ground. I feel this text is long overdue and of immense value to the field."

Donna Doherty, Senior Lecturer, Faculty of Health Sciences, Staffordshire University, UK

"Bravo to the authors of Excellence in Dementia Care! They have created a must read guidebook for those providing care to persons experiencing cognitive changes and their families. This collaborative effort focuses on successful provider strategies encompassing topics across the dementia journey and is filled with spot on, relevant, and timely information. Best of all, this work is loaded with real case studies to help translate knowledge to practice, making it a true resource for all practitioners."

Suzanne Bottum-Jones, MA, Wisconsin Alzheimer's Institute, School of Medicine & Public Health, University of Wisconsin-Madison, USA

We would like to dedicate this book to:

Sweens and her Tommy Tomkins for their inspiration
Christopher Robin for his generosity
And all people with dementia and their family members.

Contents

Contributors

Kate Allan has been working in the dementia field for about twenty years and has particular interests in communication and creativity. She co-authored *Communication and the Care of People with Dementia* with John Killick (Open University Press, 2001), and when working at the Dementia Services Development Centre at the University of Stirling carried out a project looking at ways of consulting people with dementia about their views of services. She is currently undertaking a PhD exploring experiences of well-being in persons with dementia at the University of Edinburgh, and is practising as a clinical psychologist.

Clive Baldwin is Canada Research Chair in Narrative Studies and Professor of Social Work at St. Thomas University, Fredericton, New Brunswick. He undertakes research and writing on the forms, uses, and influence of narrative in social and health care.

Jesse F. Ballenger is the author of *Self, Senility and Alzheimer's Disease in Modern America: A History* (Johns Hopkins University Press, 2006), and co-editor of *Concepts of Alzheimer Disease: Biological, Clinical and Cultural Perspectives* (Johns Hopkins University Press, 2000) and *Treating Dementia: Do We Have a Pill for It?* (Johns Hopkins University Press, 2009). He is a faculty member in the Bioethics Program and affiliated with the Rock Ethics Institute at Penn State University.

Linda Boise is Associate Professor of Neurology and Director of the Outreach, Recruitment, and Education Core for the Layton Aging and Alzheimer Disease Center at Oregon Health and Science University, Portland, Oregon. Over the past 22 years, she has provided education and conducted research related to chronic illness and dementia. She has carried out numerous studies on family caregiving and primary care physician practices related to dementia. Her research interests include the factors associated with delayed diagnosis of dementia, barriers to health care for persons from black and minority ethnic groups, interventions to improve primary care for persons with dementia, and community-based research that promotes and improves the health of diverse populations. She holds a Master of Public Health degree from the University of North Carolina at Chapel Hill and a PhD in Urban Studies from Portland State University, Portland, Oregon.

Barbara Bowers is a professor and Associate Dean for Research in the School of Nursing at the University of Wisconsin-Madison. She has a long history of conducting research in care homes, with a particular interest in workforce development and organizational influences on care practices. Barbara's recent research has focused on practice variations in culture change models and the influence of worker training and development. Her work includes consultation to state and federal government work groups on long-term care practices and models.

Carol Brayne is Professor of Public Health Medicine in the Department of Public Health and Primary Care at the University of Cambridge. She is a medically qualified epidemiologist and public health academic. After training in general medicine and gaining membership, she moved on to training in epidemiology with a Medical Research Council (MRC) Training Fellowship focusing on ageing and dementia. Her main research area has been longitudinal studies of older people following changes over time with a public health perspective. She is lead principal investigator in the group of MRC Cognitive Function and Ageing Study (CFA). Carol is Director of the Cambridge Institute of Public Health at the University of Cambridge.

Errollyn Bruce is a former lecturer in dementia studies with the Bradford Dementia Group at the University of Bradford. Following retirement she has a continuing interest in life-story work and creative reminiscence, working with Pam Schweitzer on European Reminiscence Network projects, and as a volunteer in local reminiscence groups.

Andrea Capstick is the postgraduate programme leader in Dementia Studies with Bradford Dementia Group at the University of Bradford. She holds a doctorate in Education for her work on the use of film and narrative in dementia education, and is a Fellow of the Higher Education Academy. She is co-author and editor of *Tom Kitwood on dementia: a reader and critical commentary.* Since 2009 she has been researching the use of participatory methods with people with dementia. Her work on participatory video in long-term care has been funded by the National Institute for Health Research's School for Social Care Research. Additional research interests are service user involvement, and the use of creative and arts-based methods in education and research.

Georgina Charlesworth is a consultant clinical psychologist in North East London NHS Foundation Trust and a lecturer in the Research Department of Clinical, Educational and Health Psychology at University College London. She has worked in NHS services for older people for over twenty years. Her research has been funded by the Alzheimer's Society, Economic and Social Research Council, and National Institute of Health Research, and includes evaluations of befriending, peer support, and cognitive behavioural therapy with family carers and people with dementia.

Habib Chaudhury is Professor in the Department of Gerontology at Simon Fraser University, Canada. He is also affiliated with the Centre for Research on Personhood in Dementia Care at the University of British Columbia. He has conducted extensive research in several areas within the field of environmental gerontology. These include physical environment for people with dementia in long-term care, memories of home and personhood in dementia, community planning and urban design for active ageing, and design in acute care settings. Published books include *Remembering Home: Rediscovering the Self in Dementia* (Johns Hopkins University Press, 2008) and the co-edited volume *Home and Identity in Later Life: International Perspectives* (Springer Publications, 2005). Organizations providing funding for his work include the Canadian Institutes of Health Research (CIHR), Social Science and Humanities Research Council (SSHRC), Canada Mortgage and Housing Corporation (CMHC), and Coalition of Health Environments Research.

Linda Clare is Professor of Clinical Psychology and Neuropsychology in the School of Psychology, Bangor University, UK, where she leads the Research in Ageing and Cognitive Health (REACH) group. The group's aim is to improve the lives of older people and people with dementia through research focused on promoting well-being, preventing or reducing age-related disability, and improving rehabilitation and care. She has pioneered the application of cognitive rehabilitation approaches for people with early-stage Alzheimer's disease. She has published over one hundred peer-reviewed journal articles and book chapters. Linda is a chartered clinical psychologist and clinical neuropsychologist, and in 2004 she received the May Davidson award from the British Psychological Society for her contribution to the development of clinical psychology in the UK. She serves as NISCHR Senior Faculty, and is a Fellow of the British Psychological Society and of the Gerontological Society of America. Linda is an editor for the Cochrane dementia group and for the journal *Neuropsychological Rehabilitation*. She currently chairs the professional interest area in psychosocial understanding and intervention for ISTAART within the US Alzheimer's Association.

Jiska Cohen-Mansfield is Professor at the Department of Health Promotion at the School of Public Health at Tel-Aviv University. She is the Director of the Minerva Center for the Interdisciplinary Study of End of Life and a member of the staff of the Herczeg Institute on Aging at Tel-Aviv University. Her work focuses on improving quality of life for persons with dementia by understanding the perspective of the person with dementia, on end-of-life decision-making, and on health and mental health promotion in older persons. Jiska has published extensively on the topic of agitation in persons with dementia, as well as addressing important issues for older persons such as sleep, religious beliefs, decisions regarding medical treatments, physical restraints, vision problems, depression, autonomy, and stress in nursing home caregivers. She has published over three hundred publications in scientific books and journals, and has developed a number of assessment tools, which have been translated and used internationally. Jiska is the recipient of several awards and is a highly cited researcher as listed by the ISI.

Heather Cooke has a Masters degree in Gerontology from Simon Fraser University, Canada, and is currently an interdisciplinary PhD candidate at the Center on Aging, at the University of Victoria, Canada. She has worked in the field of dementia care for almost twenty years, in both home and residential care settings. Her research interests include: quality of life and quality of care issues within long-term care; staff caregiving practices within long-term care; therapeutic design of environments for individuals with dementia; and long-term care policy. Her dissertation research, which is funded by the Alzheimer Society of Canada, seeks to examine how organizational and physical environmental features facilitate or hinder the provision of person-centred dementia care.

Karen Croucher is a research fellow at the Centre for Housing Policy (CHP) at the University of York. Her work focuses on the interface between housing, health, and well-being, and in particular on housing services and models that support older people to live independently. Recently completed and on-going work includes the provision of care and support to people with concurrent dementia and a visual impairment, and developing supportive communities in housing with care.

Anne Davis Basting is an artist, a teacher, and a scholar. She holds a PhD in Theatre and is Full Professor of Theatre at the University of Wisconsin Milwaukee's Peck School of the Arts. In 1998, she founded and continues to direct TimeSlips Creative Storytelling (timeslips.org), which is now an independent, non-profit programme offering training in creative engagement. She is author of two books, including *Forget Memory: Creating Better Lives for People with Dementia* (Johns Hopkins University Press, 2009). She is author of more than a dozen plays and public performances, including *Finding Penelope*, which was staged with Sojourn Theatre and the staff and residents of Luther Manor care community (thepenelopeproject.com). She is now at work on the Islands of Milwaukee, an effort to bring creative engagement to older adults living alone or under-connected to their communities (islandsofmilwaukee.com).

Murna Downs is Professor in Dementia Studies at the University of Bradford and Head of the Bradford Dementia Group, the academic Division of Dementia Studies within the School of Health Studies. Her research interests focus on promoting quality of life through the development and evaluation of care and services for people with dementia and their families. She has published on a variety of topics, including primary care and the end-of-life care for people with dementia.

Brandi Estey-Burtt is a doctoral student at Dalhousie University, Halifax, Nova Scotia. Her research interests include ethics, the philosophy of Emmanuel Levinas and the use of poetics in critical animal studies.

Simon Evans, PhD, is Head of Research with the Association for Dementia Studies at the University of Worcester. In this role, he manages a range of mixed methods projects that focus on contributing to the evidence base for improving quality of life for people with dementia, across a wide range of settings. Simon has published widely in the field of social gerontology, including *Community and Ageing* (The Policy Press, 2009), a book that explores quality of life in housing with care settings. His other work interests include research ethics and user involvement in research, and he is an associate editor of *Ageing and Society*.

Richard H. Fortinsky, PhD, is a professor at the University of Connecticut (UConn) School of Medicine, where he holds the Health Net, Inc., Endowed Chair in Geriatrics and Gerontology. Richard collaborates with researchers from a wide range of clinical and basic science disciplines to design and carry out studies with the goals of improving care and maximizing health and independent living for older adults and their families. He also teaches on ageing-related topics in the public health, medical, and dental school curricula at UConn. Richard received his doctoral degree in Sociology in 1984 from Brown University, specializing in medical sociology and gerontology.

Jane Fossey is an associate director of Psychological Services for Oxford Health NHS Foundation Trust and Honorary Senior Clinical Research Fellow in the Department of Psychiatry at the University of Oxford. She has specialized in clinical practice in working with older people, people with dementia, and with care homes for over twenty years. She has published a number of research studies into the quality of life in care homes. Jane's research interests include the effectiveness of psychosocial interventions on care practice and the therapeutic effects of animals for older people and people with mental health conditions.

Katherine Froggatt is a senior lecturer at the International Observatory on End of Life Care at Lancaster University. With a background in nursing she undertakes research focused on older people and palliative and supportive care. Her main interests are care provision in care homes, palliative care for people with dementia and awareness education for the general public about end-of-life issues.

Andrea Gilmore-Bykovskyi is a PhD candidate and National Hartford Centers of Gerontological Nursing Excellence Patricia G. Archbold Predoctoral Scholar at the University of Wisconsin-Madison School of Nursing. Her research examines health services and outcomes for persons with dementia in long-term care settings and during transitions in care with an emphasis on reducing social isolation and pain and behavioural symptom management.

Claire Goodman is a district nurse by background and Professor of Health Care Research at the Centre for Research in Primary and Community Care (CRIPACC) at the University of Hertfordshire. Her research focuses on the oldest old and how primary health care works with social care and long-term care providers to support this population. She leads a programme of nationally funded studies on health care provision to care homes that includes evaluations of interventions to support access to health care for residents and end-of-life care for older people with dementia. She is a founder member of the Enabling Research in Care Homes (ENRICH) project board that is run through the Dementia and Neurodegenerative Diseases Research Network (DeNDRoN). She has published widely and is the co-editor of the *Oxford Handbook of Primary Care and Community Nursing* (Oxford University Press, 2007).

Cathy Henwood leads on the Bradford Dementia Friendly Communities project. The project has developed tools to enable organizations to review their approach to people living with dementia and write action plans. She has recruited organizations ranging from a local pharmacy, branches of Lloyds Bank and the Co-operative Supermarket to community centres, churches and Gurdwaras to get involved in making their organizations dementia friendly. She is now developing a community-based approach, working with Bradford City Council and other organizations, to empower communities to be more accessible and inclusive to people living with dementia. Cathy is passionate about involving people with dementia in the process of making the aspiration of a dementia-friendly Bradford District a reality. Her work is jointly funded by the Joseph Rowntree Foundation and Bradford City Council.

Amy Illsley trained in medicine at the University of Leeds, graduating in 2007, and is now a trainee registrar in geriatric medicine in the Yorkshire and Humber Deanery.

John Killick has a background in teaching and writing. He began working with people with dementia in 1993, and since then has promoted communication through the arts generally. He has recently explored the potential of improvised drama with people with the condition. His most recent book is *Dementia Positive* (Luath Press, 2013), which is an exploration of communication and relationships for relatives and friends in a supporting role.

Amy Kind, MD, PhD is an assistant professor in the Department of Medicine, Division of Geriatrics in the University of Wisconsin School of Medicine and Public Health. Her research focuses on patient safety during transitions between health care settings, particularly for highly vulnerable older adult populations including those with dementia.

Pia Kontos is a senior research scientist at Toronto Rehabilitation Institute-University Health Network, and Associate Professor at the Dalla Lana School of Public Health, University of Toronto. Her training is in medical anthropology, gerontology, and public health sciences. Central to her programme of research is "embodied selfhood", a philosophy and approach to person-centred care that emphasizes the importance of the body for self-expression. Her research relies heavily on arts-based methodologies both as a strategy for implementing embodied selfhood into practice and for their creative and innovative potential to engage persons with dementia in meaningful ways. She has presented and published across multiple disciplines.

Rachael Litherland has worked with people with dementia since 2002. With a background in psychology and advocacy, she developed and managed the national "Living with Dementia" programme for the Alzheimer's Society (2000–2006). This included providing leadership on issues relating to the involvement and support of people with dementia and supporting people with dementia in service and information development, campaigning, and self-advocacy. Rachael is now a director with Innovations in Dementia CIC, a national community interest company. Innovations in Dementia works on a range of positive projects with people with dementia, including Shared Lives, circles of support, work on dementia-friendly communities, and the Dementia Engagement and Empowerment project (DEEP). The work of the organization is centred on the voices and experiences of people with dementia.

Michael L. Malone is the Medical Director of Aurora Senior Services and Aurora Visiting Nurse Association of Wisconsin. He is an adjunct clinical professor of medicine at the University of Wisconsin School of Medicine and Public Health. He leads clinical programmes to improve care of older patients in Aurora Health Care in Wisconsin. Michael and his colleagues have developed an electronic medical record software program, called ACE Tracker, which is used to identify the unique needs of vulnerable older patients in Aurora's 14 acute care hospitals.

Benjamin T. Mast, PhD, is an associate professor and Vice Chair in the Department of Psychological and Brain Sciences and an associate clinical professor in the Department of Family and Geriatric Medicine at the University of Louisville. He is the author of *Whole Person Dementia Assessment* (Health Professions Press, 2011), a guide for bringing person-centred principles and methods to the assessment and diagnosis of people with cognitive changes. He is also Co-Editor-in-Chief of the forthcoming American Psychological Association *Handbook of Clinical Geropsychology* (2015).

Kimberly Nolet is a researcher in the School of Nursing at the University of Wisconsin-Madison. She has been engaged in research related to the professional development of care staff in residential aged care and home care, and has investigated the implementation of new educational models and new models of care. Kimberly has worked with a variety of government agencies, private foundations, and care organizations in her work across long-term care settings.

Jan Oyebode is a clinical psychologist specializing in work with older people. She is Professor of Dementia Care with the Bradford Dementia Group at the University of Bradford. Her research interests concern people living with dementia in the community, especially in relation to young-onset dementia, fronto-temporal dementia, relationships in families and cultural influences.

Tonya Roberts is an advanced nurse fellow in the Geriatric Research, Education, and Clinical Center at the William S. Middleton Veteran Affairs Hospital in Madison, Wisconsin. The aim of her research programme is to change care delivery systems to improve the quality of life and quality of care for older adults needing long-term care. Her current studies focus on the relationship between person-centred care and psychosocial well-being. She has had extensive experience caring for older people and persons with dementia, holding both direct care and administrative positions in long-term care facilities prior to her graduate studies.

Steven R. Sabat is Professor of Psychology at Georgetown University in Washington, DC. The focus of his research, published in numerous scientific journal articles, has been on the intact cognitive and social abilities, and the subjective experience of people with moderate to severe dementia, as well as on how to enhance communication between people with dementia and their carers. He is also the author of *The Experience of Alzheimer's Disease: Life through a Tangled Veil* (Blackwell, 2001) and co-editor of *Dementia: Mind, Meaning, and the Person* (Oxford University Press, 2006).

Pam Schweitzer has many years' experience developing reminiscence work both in the UK and internationally. In 1983, she founded the Age Exchange Theatre Trust and Reminiscence Centre and remained its Artistic Director until 2005. For the last decade she has been actively developing reminiscence projects for people with dementia and their carers, including developing and coordinating a Europe-wide project, "Remembering Yesterday, Caring Today". In 2000, she was awarded an MBE for services to Reminiscence and she continues to direct the European Reminiscence Network. She is an Honorary Research Fellow of Greenwich University and continues to lecture, train, and write on all aspects of reminiscence.

Blossom Stephan completed her training in psychology and mathematical statistics at Sydney University in Australia. Her PhD was in the field of clinical neuropsychology, undertaken at the School of Psychology at Sydney University. She completed her postdoctoral training in epidemiology at Cambridge University, at the Institute of Public Health and Primary Care. Blossom was recently appointed as a lecturer within the Ageing, Health and Society Research Group at the Institute of Health and Society, at Newcastle University, UK. Her research focuses on issues related to risk prediction of neurodegenerative diseases. She is currently working with several large epidemiological studies conducted in the UK and internationally to integrate risk factor research across multiple disciplines (e.g. genetics, metabolic, nutrition, cardiovascular, and lifestyle) to identify not only those individuals at risk of cognitive decline and dementia, but to determine how different risk and protective factors interact to promote successful ageing.

Sarah Vallelly is Housing 21's intelligence manager. She has over ten years of research and policy experience in the older people's housing and care sector, having led a number of ground-breaking research projects on dementia, extra care housing, personalization, and end-of-life care. Housing 21 is a leading provider of care and housing services in England. As a not-for-profit organization that dates back to 1964, Housing 21 is recognized as a major provider of retirement housing and a driving force in the development of dementia services.

Carol J. Whitlatch, PhD, is Assistant Director of the Margaret Blenkner Research Institute of the Benjamin Rose Institute on Aging in Cleveland, Ohio. She holds adjunct faculty appointments at Case Western Reserve University in the Mandel School of Applied Social Sciences and in the Department of Sociology as an Adjunct Associate Professor. Carol is Associate Editor of *Dementia: The International Journal of Social Research and Practice*, and on the Editorial Board of *Aging and Mental Health*. Currently, she is involved in a variety of federally funded projects in the USA that develop and evaluate evidence-based dyadic interventions for persons with early-stage dementia and their family carers.

John Young has over 20 years' experience as a consultant geriatrician. He is Professor of Elderly Care, University of Leeds and Head of the Academic Unit of Elderly Care and Rehabilitation, Bradford Teaching Hospital Trust. His research interests focus on stroke rehabilitation, intermediate care services, frailty, dementia and delirium, and he has received major grant awards, predominantly from the National Institute for Health Research. He is National Clinical Director for Integration and the Frail Elderly.

Steven H. Zarit, PhD, is Distinguished Professor of Human Development and Family Studies at the Pennsylvania State University. He is a pioneer in the study of caregiver burden and stress. Steven's most recent work examines the role of adult day care in lowering stress and improving health for caregivers of people with dementia. He also studies family relationships across the life span and functioning and mental health in very old age.

Judy M. Zarit, PhD, was trained as a clinical psychologist with a specialty in ageing. In private practice for 30 years, seeing older adults as outpatients, Judy also worked in local retirement and nursing facilities. She had a special interest in working with caregivers and people with dementia. Judy retired in 2011, but she continues to do consultation and writing.

Hannah Zeilig is a senior research fellow at the University of the Arts, London and also a senior research associate at the University of East Anglia. Her work explores the intersections between literature, culture, and ageing. Hannah coordinates a multidisciplinary team comprising poets, artists, a psychiatrist, dementia care workers, and researchers in health care and the humanities to find ways of using the arts in educating and supporting the dementia care workforce. This project uses innovative methods (such as comics) to challenge some of the stigmas surrounding dementia and to encourage new ways of thinking about "dementia". She also curates an international event on representations of age(ing), "Mirror Mirror" at the London College of Fashion. She is currently critically reviewing the role of the arts in dementia care across the UK.

Foreword

Estimates suggest dementia affects nearly 36 million people worldwide, and the prevalence of dementia is expected to rise as those over 65 increase to 66 million by 2030 and over 115 million by 2050 (Alzheimer's Disease International 2010). Alzheimer's disease (AD) accounts for approximately 60–70% of all dementias and is the most common type of age-related dementia (Fratiglioni *et al*. 2000; Barker *et al*. 2002). In 2010, the global cost of dementia was estimated to be over US$600 billion, about 1% of the world's gross domestic product (Alzheimer's Disease International 2010). Care for the increasing number of people with dementia will strain world governments and public health systems. Dementia and related disorders signify a global public health crisis of indescribable proportions, and demand a massive integrated, multidisciplinary, and global response.

Over the past few years, there has been a most welcome commitment by individual nations to develop and implement dementia strategies or plans. These have provided a framework for discussion and action aimed at turning the tide on this challenge. Moves to create dementia-friendly communities, to build health and social care systems that are fit for purpose, and increase investment in cure and care research are a big step in the right direction. Though given the financial challenges that dementia and related disorders presents the community, there is now a clear need for a networked global response to this public health problem. In addition to re-evaluating assumptions, ideas, and approaches to evidence-based care and support, we must improve the process by which we communicate community needs and best practices across the globe. The field must articulate a unified and integrated vision recognizing that the *problem of dementia* is complex. No single entity or country has the capability, resources or knowledge to solve or mitigate the challenges we face today and in the future: the need for new multinational partnerships in care, support, and research is critical. The leadership shown by the G8 in holding a dementia summit in London in December 2013 has provided an exciting platform to stimulate a conversation around global solutions for this global problem, and it is one that we ought use to maximum effect.

Dementia is an illness that affects the brain and eventually causes a person to lose the ability to perform daily self-care. All areas of daily living are affected over the course of the disease. Over time, a person with dementia loses the ability to learn new information, make decisions, and plan the future. Communication with other people becomes difficult. People with dementia ultimately lose the ability to perform daily tasks and to recognize the world around them.

Dementia also affects family caregivers. Seventy per cent of persons with dementia live in the community, and family caregivers are largely responsible for helping them to remain at home. Family caregivers must be vigilant 24 hours a day to make sure that the person with dementia is safe and well. Providing constant, complicated care to a person with dementia takes a toll on family caregivers. Family members and other unpaid caregivers of people with dementia are more likely than non-caregivers to report that their health is fair or poor (Alzheimer's Association 2009).

This second edition of *Excellence in Dementia Care* addresses critically important social and interpersonal challenges experienced when facing dementia. The personal challenges that care partners and family members experience in many instances go beyond the financial to highly stressful and exhausting contributions of unpaid caregiving. These challenges exist not only due to the nature of the disorder itself but also in large part to a lack of national and global coordination of best practices in care planning, support, long-term care, education, and accessibility of information on resources. Research is key to driving innovation and improvements in dementia care and support, though it is of little value if it is not implemented in practice to reach the people that could benefit. This publication responds directly to this need for compilation and dissemination of best practices in dementia care and provides the type of blueprint that will put the international community on the path towards addressing the most significant health challenge facing our global ageing population, that of dementia.

Doug Brown and Maria Carrillo
November 2013

References

Alzheimer's Association (2009) *Alzheimer's Disease: Facts and Figures.* Chicago, IL: Alzheimer's Association [http://www.alz.org/national/documents/report_alzfactsfigures2009.pdf].

Alzheimer's Disease International (2010) *World Alzheimer Report 2010.* London: Alzheimer's Disease International [http://www.alz.co.uk/research/world-report-2010].

Barker, W.W., Luis, C.A., Kashuba, A., Luis, M., Harwood, D.G. et al. (2002) Relative frequencies of Alzheimer disease, Lewy body, vascular and frontotemporal dementia, and hippocampal sclerosis in the state of Florida brain bank, *Alzheimer Disease and Associated Disorders,* 16: 203–12.

Fratiglioni, L., Launer, L.J., Andersen, K., Breteler, M.M., Copeland, J.R. et al. (2000) Incidence of dementia and major subtypes in Europe: a collaborative study of population-based cohorts, Neurologic Diseases in the Elderly Research Group, *Neurology,* 54 (Suppl. 5): S10–S15.

Preface

Since the publication of the first edition of this book (in 2008), much has been written about dementia care and what should be done to improve it. I am honoured to be asked to write a preface to this second edition. My dementia, diagnosed very early, has thankfully not progressed very much. My involvement in projects, teaching, and discussions has however increased, and takes up a great deal of my spare time. I am sure that the many new developments and ideas since 2008 have informed much of the reformation of this valuable book.

As someone involved in the work to produce the Department of Health's "Living Well with Dementia: A National Dementia Strategy for England" (2009), I was so pleased that both carers and people with dementia were involved in reference groups to ensure that their ideas were included. Three years after the publication of the Strategy for England (and several other national strategies in the UK and Europe followed), the Prime Minister issued his Challenge on Dementia: "delivering major improvements in dementia care and research by 2015". As we move towards 2015, more work has been done and particular areas of concern and policy have been highlighted.

In this climate of moving on, there is an even greater need for this scholarly work to be updated. New ways of working and different expectations have led to a variety of initiatives and research projects in this changing situation. The sub-title "Research into Practice" points to the value of investigative work and the possibilities of continuing improvements in dementia care.

When I worked as a professional in assessing and – with the help of the team I worked with – improving the lives of those with dementia and their carers, I could not imagine such a growth in purpose as there is now. There is a long way to go but creating "dementia-friendly communities" is now a recognized way of increasing awareness and encouraging inclusion of those affected by dementia in the social framework of our daily lives. As those affected by dementia gain courage at speaking out, the acceptance of their problems and the development of ways of helping are improving the lives of those around us.

Dementia is not fussy in choosing victims. People in all walks of life and all ethnic groups develop dementia but their culture may have a different interpretation of what is happening and why. A chapter in the book provides help with these very important issues.

Chapter 5 looks at a very important issue – representation of people with dementia can affect perceptions and lead to increased stigma. There are still those in the community who have not knowingly met anyone with an early diagnosis. The idea that such a person can contribute to education, campaigning, and general understanding may be difficult to believe but can be a very powerful aid to banishing former prejudices.

One omission noted in the first edition was the fact that younger people with dementia were not specifically given much attention. This has been rectified by a special chapter on this group and how dementia may have a different effect on the lives of themselves and their families. Other omissions mentioned in the introduction to the first edition are dealt with in Part 2, "Conceptualizing dementia care". In Chapters 8 to 11, a bio-psycho-social approach offers a new way of looking at the capabilities of the person with dementia and at approaches in care that respect their individual personhood.

In Part 3, important areas also covered are new to many people's way of working. Best practice care recognizes that people with dementia need support and cognitive intervention. Important ways of working are outlined, including: life-history work that assists person-centred care; recognition that behaviour changes are a form of communication; health and well-being of the individual and its significance; and recognition of the importance of relationships between people with dementia and their families, who themselves need support.

Part 4 looks at care pathways in the person's journey with dementia. The stages and types of help appropriate are covered. An area of understanding of end-of-life issues is covered in Chapter 26. This is part of recent campaigns and hopefully people with dementia will get the best care available as others do at the end of life.

Altogether, this second edition breathes new life into the ways of achieving the admirable objectives of the various recent plans and strategies. Many of the challenges of care of people with dementia are experienced by people with other disabilities. Person-centred approaches are important to everyone.

A document published in the same year as the Dementia Strategy (but not as often quoted) by the Equality and Human Rights Commission is equally applicable to the overall objectives of this book. The Foreword, after quoting Eleanor Roosevelt, "Where, after all, do universal rights begin? In small places, close to home . . . ", goes on to say, "A decent quality of life where people are able to live with dignity and respect is a basic human right. For millions today and many millions more in the future, only effective care and support has the power to translate that right from an aspiration into an everyday reality" (*From Safety Net to Springboard: A New Approach to Care and Support for All Based on Equality and Human Rights*, 2009).

Daphne Wallace
September 2013

Preface

My mother lived and died with Alzheimer's disease and during the years that she lived with us, I learned a great deal about the disease, about health services, adult and social services, and the voluntary sector as we were necessarily involved with all of them. I discovered a parallel universe. At one point, we were in touch with over thirty professionals and others *simply* because my mother had Alzheimer's disease. During that time, I learned about the way people with dementia were seen and treated and particularly I learned much about people's attitudes, whether professionals, care workers or the general public. Thus this book has huge resonance with me.

During the years that I looked after my mother, I valued the consultation, the discussion, and feeling part of the team that cared for my mother, as in effect I had become my mother's memory and her voice. There were many positives and some negatives, but the positives far outweighed the negatives. Though my mother's memory was increasingly damaged by her condition, she was able to comment with insight on her situation, she was able to think and analyse. Her memory caused her to forget what she had said but at the time she said what she did it was important and pertinent. After a member of staff and a volunteer had come to see us about using the sitting service, she commented: "What a lot of good friends we have". On being reminded that it was the day she went to the day centre, she said: "I like going there, don't I?" and a comment, which continues to haunt me, towards the end of her life in an acute ward – "I don't like it here".

As I reflect on my mother's experience and that of our family, I believe that ultimately dementia can only be defeated by research but meantime there is an imperative to care for those with dementia as well as we possibly can, which is why I so love and approve the assertion in the title of the goal of this book – *Excellence in Dementia Care*.

Research into dementia means looking for the cause or causes of dementia, looking for a cure or cures, looking to prevent dementia, and *looking for the best ways of caring for those with dementia now*. Research into the care of those with dementia is vital but it is only a first step for both dissemination and implementation of the research is necessary to make a difference. Techniques of best practice that are evidence based need to be disseminated and implemented to make life better for those with dementia and their carers. They then need to be monitored and evaluated following their use. Perhaps routinely it should be asked: "What did we do well?" and "What could we do better?"

There has been increasing research into the best ways to care for people with dementia but there has been a shortfall in the implementation of such research findings. Evidence-based approaches for improving dementia care exist but who is implementing the findings and who should implement the findings? The contributors to this textbook (how dry that sounds for such an inspiring book) are well respected, highly regarded researchers in their fields with published peer-reviewed work who have shown that by putting into practice their findings, quality of life for people with dementia can be enhanced. The researchers are so obviously on the side of those with dementia. The book translates existing knowledge into practice in such a way that all those who work with people with dementia can be empowered.

Personally, I would like to see compulsory training for all staff who deal with the elderly, especially those with memory problems, whether in hospitals, care homes or in the community. Training, using this book alone, could mean that all such staff could be equipped with appropriate skills, knowledge, and improved attitudes. Many – I guess most – of those who work in the care field do want to do the best for those for whom they are caring but only with sufficient knowledge, appropriate skills, and training using well-researched evidence will the standards improve overall. This book is a distillation of so much proven good practice that really there is no excuse for people not to know how the most vulnerable people in society should be cared for. The translation of existing knowledge into practice could revolutionize the care sector (what a horrible phrase) and perhaps hopefully see an end to the seemingly endless scandals reported all too frequently in the media. The negatives I alluded to earlier could have been avoided had some of those my mother came into contact with had more understanding of the condition that is dementia. I cannot recommend this book highly enough.

Looking after my mother as I did, I know how important the right care and support is. I am grateful that all those who have contributed to this book have chosen to research in the field of dementia care and so have made it possible that those affected by dementia can have the very best care.

Barbara Woodward-Carlton
November 2013

Introduction

The aim of this textbook is to provide a contemporary and comprehensive overview of research to help us achieve *excellence in dementia care*. As with the first edition, our aim is to make excellence in dementia care an integral part of everyday care practice and services for people with dementia and their families. As before, we have sought to be inclusive of a wide range of disciplines and professionals. In this edition, we have made additional efforts to ensure that the perspectives and voices of people with dementia and their families are represented.

The key contexts in which this book has been written include:

- the unprecedented political commitment to dementia
- the public prominence of people with dementia
- recognition of the diversity of the experience of living with dementia

The unprecedented political commitment to dementia

Dementia has truly come of age since the first edition of this textbook was published in 2008. In 2012, The World Health Organisation called for dementia to be a public health priority and the British Prime Minister issued his "Challenge on Dementia Care" (Department of Health 2012). At the end of 2013, the British Prime Minister convened the first G8 summit on dementia, with plans for legacy events to be held in the USA, UK, Germany, and Japan. G8 ministers crafted and signed an unprecedented Declaration, committing their nations to work collaboratively, to improve dementia care and services, reduce the stigma and financial burden associated with dementia, increase investment in research (with the goal of finding a cure by 2025), and openly share promising innovations.

This unprecedented groundswell of high-level interest has arisen for a variety of reasons, including:

- the growing numbers of people affected by dementia
- the rising cost of (informal and formal) caring for people affected by dementia
- the widespread ignorance, fear, and stigma of this condition
- the relative and universal neglect of practice and service development in this area
- inadequate research investment, for both biomedical and social, care and services and public health research

Many countries have now made dementia a national priority. The focus and scope of these plans include:

- increasing public and professional awareness
- training and education to ensure an informed and effective workforce
- improved rates of diagnosis

- improved quality of care across the journey – home care, hospital care, residential and nursing home care, palliative care
- innovation, research, and development to improve supports and services
- partnership with people with dementia and their families
- measurement and monitoring of outcomes achieved

There are challenges ahead. Most countries with national plans are high to middle income, while the biggest growth in numbers of people with dementia will come from low-income countries. Furthermore, to date few plans have been subject to rigorous evaluation (Rosow et al. 2011). Nevertheless, this groundswell of political commitment offers us many opportunities to achieve excellence in dementia care and transform the nature of living with dementia.

The public prominence of people with dementia

Together with this high-level policy interest in dementia, people directly affected by dementia are coming centre-stage. In the past ten years, there has been an unprecedented growth in the number of people with dementia speaking out about their experience of living with the condition. The slogan from the disability rights movement, "nothing about us without us", is receiving widespread acceptance by the dementia community. There are several examples where people with dementia are contributing to policy and debate as experts by experience (see, for example, the Scottish Dementia Working Group; www.sdwg.org.uk). Most recently, in the UK the Dementia Engagement and Empowerment Project supports groups of people with dementia to influence services and policy (Williamson 2012).

In England, the Department of Health (2010) published the quality outcomes it sought to achieve through its national dementia strategy. Written as "I statements", these can be easily described as person centred (Downs 2013) and include:

- I can enjoy life.
- I understand so I make good decisions and provide for future decision-making.
- I am treated with dignity and respect.
- I am confident my end-of-life wishes will be respected and I can expect a good death.

Recognition of the diversity of the experience of living with dementia

More and more recognition is being given to the fact that people with dementia are not a homogenous whole. Of course, by definition, dementia is an umbrella term for a range of diseases. People with dementia also differ in terms of their age, ethnicity, gender, sexual orientation, socioeconomic group, religious group, cultural group and degree of acculturation, presence of co-morbid conditions, where they live and who they live with, and the level of care and support they receive.

This second edition draws on current research thinking, practice, and policy from the English-speaking western world, primarily the UK and the USA, to:

- provide comprehensive coverage of a range of evidence about quality dementia care, including user and family carer experience, practice wisdom, and research evidence

- synthesize the wide range and multidisciplinary nature of evidence to guide professional practice, care and services and further academic work in this area
- stimulate critical appraisal of existing systems, services, and supports with respect to the rights and diversity of needs of people with dementia and their families
- provide strategies for developing sustainable practices that actively promote health and well-being for people with dementia and their families

There is now a compelling argument for communities and care environments to accommodate to people's changed abilities, facilitate well-being, and support participation. Following the G8 dementia summit's call to work collaboratively and share best practice, it is now time to bring the wealth of evidence we have to bear on achieving excellence in dementia care. Expectations about what is possible for people with dementia are higher than ever. We have achieved improved awareness of, and understanding about, the potential for a quality life with dementia. Our new horizons are the challenge to ensure that we are developing and embracing ways to implement what we know. Competent and compassionate dementia care requires knowledge, skills, cooperation, and resources. It is essential that we provide the workforce with a portfolio of education and training opportunities drawing on the evidence of what works, both in terms of how we care for people with dementia and how we embed such care in mainstream practice. This requires that we turn our attention to effective approaches to practice development and culture change.

A note on language and culture

While we recognize the role of language in both reflecting and creating culture, we have accepted the language of our contributors.

New for the second edition

In this second edition, we have updated all chapters to reflect latest policies, and have introduced areas omitted in the first edition. The latter include:

- Chapter 2: *Dementia-friendly communities* – focuses on what can happen in communities, towns, and cities to support people to live well with dementia. This includes a focus on the transport, emergency, retail, and banking sectors.
- Chapter 6: *Representations of people with dementia in the media and in literature* – a critical perspective is brought to bear on the common imagery and language we use. This chapter challenges us to recognize the power of language to not only reflect but also construct culture.
- Chapter 7: *Living with young-onset dementia* – provides an overview of the unique circumstances of younger people with dementia and their families. It draws attention to the need for appropriate services and supports for this group.
- Chapter 9: *Selfhood and the body in dementia care* – provides an alternative perspective to the assumption that loss of self is inevitable. It demonstrates the many ways people with dementia continue to express themselves through their bodies.
- Chapter 10: *The arts in dementia care* – challenges us to reconsider what we mean by art and the potential it has for engaging with people with dementia. The chapter covers a range of arts-based approaches in dementia care.

- Chapter 11: *Design matters in dementia care: the role of the physical environment in dementia care settings* – provides an overview of the many ways we can design environments to support people with dementia.
- Chapter 12: *Understanding and enhancing the relationship between people with dementia and their family carers* – describes the differing perspectives people with dementia and their families may hold. It suggests ways we can directly address these discrepant perspectives.
- Chapter 20: *Whole person assessment and care planning* – describes an approach that is concerned with documenting the person's strengths and remaining abilities and aspirations. It argues for the need to conduct holistic assessment that provides suggestions for how people can live well with dementia.
- Chapter 27: *Supporting persons with dementia through transitions in care* – addresses a neglected concept in dementia care. Over time, many people with dementia and their families will need higher levels of support that may require relocation. How we facilitate these transitions is an essential part of quality of care.

Guide to the parts

Part 1, *The Context of Dementia Care*, sets the context for best practice in understanding and supporting people with dementia and their families. The section includes a discussion of prevalence of dementia (Stephan and Brayne), dementia-friendly communities (Henwood and Downs), ethnicity and dementia (Boise), ethics (Estey-Burtt and Baldwin), dementia as a public health issue (Ballenger), representations of people with dementia (Zeilig), and living with young-onset dementia (Oyebode).

Part 2, *Conceptualizing Dementia Care*, explores bio-psycho-social understanding of dementia (Sabat), selfhood and the body in dementia care (Kontos), the arts in dementia care (Basting), and design matters in dementia care (Chaudhury and Cooke).

Part 3, *Best Practice Dementia Care for the Person*, looks at the requisite knowledge and skills to provide effective and empathic support for people with dementia. We focus on the many ways we can improve quality of life for people with dementia. These include understanding and enhancing relationships between people with dementia and family carers (Whitlatch), supporting families coping with dementia (Zarit and Zarit), supporting cognitive abilities (Oyebode and Clare), working with life history (Bruce and Schweitzer), understanding behaviour (Cohen-Mansfield), communication and relationships (Allan and Killick), and supporting physical health and well-being (Young and Illsley).

Part 4, *Care Pathways*, highlights and discusses specific points of intersection with services and supports along a person's journey through the condition. People with dementia are cared for in a range of settings throughout their journey with dementia. This includes a discussion of how they first come to the attention of service systems (Fortinsky), appropriate whole person assessment (Mast), supports for living in one's own home (Charlesworth), acute care for people with dementia (Malone), the role of specialist housing (Evans), care homes (Fossey), and palliative care (Froggatt and Goodman), and grief and bereavement (Oyebode), and supporting people through transitions in care (Kind and Gilmore-Bykovskyi). Throughout, there is recognition that excellence in dementia care requires multidisciplinary and multiprofessional input. In this part, the full potential of an effective service system is elucidated.

The final part, *Making Sustainable Change Happen in Dementia Care*, examines the challenges of ensuring excellence in dementia care and outlines approaches to meeting them. The complex interrelationships between personal and organizational competencies and structures are discussed. This part of the book includes discussion of involving people with dementia (Litherland and Capstick), a trained and supported workforce (Bowers), and leadership in dementia care (Nolet and Roberts).

Who the book is for

This book is intended for practitioners, professionals, and academics working or volunteering in health and social care with people in dementia. It will serve as a core resource for those involved in training and education in dementia care and will be of use to undergraduate and postgraduate students in applied dementia studies and dementia care, gerontology, disability studies, medicine, nursing, occupational therapy, physiotherapy, psychiatry, psychology, and social work. It is also relevant to students of organizational behaviour and management with an interest in organizations and systems designed for service delivery, and to future public policy workers who wish to understand how policies affect the lives of individuals and systems. The book will also be of interest to people with dementia or their advocates, family members, charity and voluntary sector organizations, policy-makers, and those in senior positions in health and social care management.

Distinctive features of the book

The book adopts a modular structure so that each chapter can be read in sequence or in isolation from another. Each chapter has the same structure, including:

- learning objectives that let the reader know what to expect from each chapter
- text exercises that encourage readers to actively engage with the material presented
- debates and controversies in the field
- conclusion
- further information section highlighting organizations established for a purpose relevant to the chapter topics, and other resources
- references

The editors

Murna Downs is Professor in Dementia Studies at The University of Bradford and Head of the Bradford Dementia Group, the Division of Dementia Studies. Her research interests focus on quality of life and quality of care for people with dementia and their families. She has published on a variety of topics, including primary care and end-of-life care for people with dementia. The University of Bradford offers undergraduate and postgraduate degrees in dementia studies alongside a portfolio of short courses and consultancy in person-centred care.

Barbara Bowers is a professor and Associate Dean for Research in the School of Nursing at the University of Wisconsin-Madison. She has a long history of conducting research in care homes, with a particular interest in workforce development and organizational influences on care practices.

Her recent research focuses on practice variations in culture change models and the influence of worker training and development. Her work includes consultation to state and federal government work groups on long-term care practices and models.

The contributors

Excellence in dementia care requires input from people with dementia and their families and a range of disciplines and professionals. We are fortunate to have represented in this book contributions from the full range of professionals and disciplines concerned with the care of people with dementia. These include art, ethics, geriatric medicine, medical anthropology, neurology, nursing, philosophy, psychology, public health occupational therapy, old age psychiatry, social work, and sociology. In this book, we have embraced the diversity of language and terminology presented to us by contributing authors. Biographical sketches of each of the authors can be found above.

References

Department of Health (2010) *Quality Outcomes for People with Dementia: Building on the Work of the National Dementia Strategy*. London: Department of Health [https://www.gov.uk/government/uploads/system/uploads/attachment_data/file/213811/dh_119828.pdf].

Department of Health (2012) *Prime Minister's Challenge on Dementia*. London: Department of Health [https://www.gov.uk/government/uploads/system/uploads/attachment_data/file/215101/dh_133176.pdf].

Downs, M. (2013) Putting people – and compassion – first: the UK's approach to person-centred care for individuals with dementia, *Generations: The Journal of the American Society on Aging*, 37: 53–9.

Rosow, K., Holzapfel, A., Karlawish, J.H., Baumgart, M., Bain, L.J. *et al*. (2011) Countrywide strategic plans on Alzheimer's disease: developing the framework for the international battle against Alzheimer's disease, *Alzheimer's and Dementia*, 7: 615–21.

Williamson, T. (2012) *A Stronger Collective Voice for People with Dementia*. York: Joseph Rowntree Foundation.

World Health Organization and Alzheimer's Disease International (2012) *Dementia: A Public Health Priority*. Geneva: WHO.

The context of dementia care

Chapter contents

CHAPTER 1

Prevalence and projections of dementia

Blossom Stephan and Carol Brayne

66 If the world needed a wake-up call, it is on this global crisis. I do not see any alternative than to treat Alzheimer's with at least the attention we gave HIV/AIDs. 99

"The time to act is now by:

- promoting a dementia-friendly society globally;
- making dementia a national public health and social care priority worldwide;
- improving public and professional attitudes to, and understanding of, dementia;
- investing in health and social systems to improve care and services for people with dementia and their caregivers;
- increasing the priority given to dementia in the public health research agenda."

—Dr. Peter Piot

Learning objectives

By the end of this chapter, you will be able to:

- Explain the implications of an ageing population for the prevalence and incidence of dementia
- Describe the different types of dementia and the difficulty in distinguishing between them
- Summarize the incidence and prevalence of dementia, regionally, nationally, and worldwide
- Identify risk factors for the development of dementia
- Explain that dementia is associated with both disability and mortality

Introduction

In the next decades, large numbers of people will enter the ages when the incidence rates of dementia are highest. People aged 60 and over make up the most rapidly expanding segment of the population. Currently, it is estimated that there are approximately 841 million persons aged 60 years or over worldwide. This figure is projected to more than double to two billion by 2050 and rise to three billion by 2100 (United Nations 2013).

The change in population age structures will influence both the prevalence and incidence of age-related conditions such as dementia. In the United Kingdom alone, the proportion of people age 65+ is 17.2% and this is projected to increase to 22.4% in 2032 (Office for National Statistics 2011). It is estimated that of those individuals aged 65 and over, 6% will have dementia, with those in their eighties having more than a 30% chance (Peters 2001). Worldwide the proportion of very old people (85 years and above) is also projected to grow (Table 1.1). Developing regions,

Population	2000	2025	2050
65 and over (%)	6.9	10.5	16.2
80 and over (%)	1.1	1.9	4.4
TOTAL (millions)	6055	7823	8900

Source: United Nations (2007)

Table 1.1 Estimated changes in the world population age structure of the elderly

particularly China, India, and Latin America, which are set to dominate world ageing, will show the greatest increase (Alzheimer's Disease International 2009).

Identification of modifiable risk factors that prevent or delay dementia onset is a major public health priority. Over age 65 there is an increased risk of mortality for even moderate levels of cognitive impairment and at more severe levels the risk increases two-fold (Dewey and Saz 2001). In addition to an increased risk of mortality for even moderate levels of cognitive impairment (Dewey and Saz 2001), dementia is associated with increased dependence. The economic cost of dementia is already higher than that of heart disease and cancer combined.

Epidemiological studies of dementia have been carried out with three main aims: (1) to determine the frequency and distribution of dementia to inform health services planning and public health priorities; (2) to identify risk factors that can guide treatment and prevention; and (3) to assess the possible impact of protective action. It is assumed that the clinical expression of dementia is to some extent environmentally modifiable, so that its clinical manifestations can be delayed or prevented and its signs and symptoms alleviated.

Defining dementia and its subtypes

The term "dementia" defines a group of syndromes characterized by progressive decline in cognition of sufficient severity to interfere with social and/or occupational functioning, often associated with increasing age. Over 200 subtypes have been defined, each characterized by differences in course with subtle variations in pattern of expression and neuropathology. The main subtypes include Alzheimer's disease, vascular dementia, dementia with Lewy bodies, frontal lobe dementia, Pick's disease, and alcohol-related dementia (see Table 1.2).

Alzheimer's disease (AD) is the most prevalent subtype of dementia, accounting for approximately 70% of all cases (Barberger-Gateau and Fabrigoule 1997; Cowan et al. 2000; Nourhashemi et al. 2000). Alzheimer's disease is characterized by a steady and progressive loss of memory and cognitive faculties, including language deterioration, impaired visuospatial skills, poor judgement, and an attitude of indifference. Alzheimer's disease has a distinct neuropathological pattern of amyloid plaques and neurofibrillary tangles predominately in the neocortex, becoming more widespread with disease progression. The second most common cause of dementia is vascular dementia, accounting for 10–20% of all cases (Barberger-Gateau and Fabrigoule 1997; Ladislas 2000). Vascular dementia represents a group of conditions resulting from ischaemic, anoxic or hypoxic brain damage. Onset is progressive and life expectancy poor,

	Primary impairments/disability/symptoms	Pathology/causes
Alzheimer's disease	Memory, language, and functional disability	Neuritic plaques (consisting mainly of amyloid-beta peptide fragments) and neurofibrillary tangles (twisted fibres of a protein called tau)
Vascular dementia	Poor concentration and communication, together with physical symptoms such as paralysis or weakness in limbs	Problems with blood circulation to the brain – related to stroke, high blood pressure (hypertension), diabetes and heart problems
Dementia with Lewy bodies	Hallucinations, spatial disorientation, impaired recent memory, fluctuations in mental performance	Presence of Lewy bodies, abnormal structures within brain nerve cells
Frontal lobe dementia	Changes in personality and behaviour, emotional and language dysfunction. No dysfunction in memory	Frontal lobe degeneration
Pick's disease	Impairment in emotional and social functioning	Abnormalities in Pick's bodies. Focal damage in the frontal and temporal lobes
Alcohol-related dementia – Korsakoff's syndrome	Impaired memory, planning, organizing, judgement, social skills, and balance	Chronic/excessive alcohol intake

Table 1.2 Types of dementia

although the disease course can be highly variable. The exact prevalence of dementia with Lewy bodies is not known, although some estimates suggest that it may be as common as vascular dementia.

The risk of developing dementia increases with age. Indeed, results from the Medical Research Council Cognitive Function and Ageing Study (MRC CFAS) found that of those individuals aged 65–69 years at death, 6% had dementia, while for those aged 95 years and above at death, 58% had dementia. This pronounced increase in dementia with age has been interpreted as an increase in the rates of AD, as shown in Figure 1.1. In contrast, rates for clinically diagnosed vascular dementia remain relatively constant across age.

Considerable overlap in pathology of subtypes suggests that mixed forms may be more common (Peters 2001). Increased levels of amyloid plaques and neurofibrillary tangles characteristic of AD pathology have been found in hypertensive individuals *post mortem*, and it has been suggested that vascular pathology may play a role in the development of amyloid plaques (Peters 2001). Furthermore, AD and vascular dementia have similar risk factors (e.g. advancing age and poor cardiovascular health), overlapping clinical symptoms, and cerebro-microvascular pathology (Skoog 1998). Yet, a steady progressive decline is still considered characteristic of AD, whereas a stepwise deterioration characterized by periods of sharp decline alternating with plateaus or periods of minimal decline is characteristic of vascular dementia (Peters 2001). Diagnosis of dementia depends on the defining criteria and sampling method (Corrada *et al.*

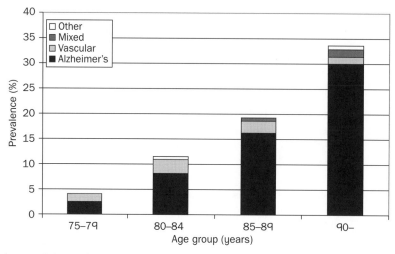

Figure 1.1: Prevalence of dementia subtypes
Source: The Cambridge City Over-75s Cohort Study (CC75C)

1995). Different diagnostic criteria can produce up to a ten-fold variation in prevalence (O'Connor *et al.* 1996). For example, the WHO International Classification of Diseases, 10th revision (ICD-10) sets a higher threshold for dementia diagnosis than the widely used Diagnostic and Statistical Manual of Mental Disorders (DSM-IV-TR) criteria. Dementia variation can also be related to culture or diagnostic applicability (e.g. views of ageing and validity of instruments). When applying criteria it is also necessary to distinguish dementia from poor physical health, depression, anxiety, sensory difficulties, language barriers, and level of education, all of which can reduce cognitive scores.

Prevalence and incidence of dementia

Variation in the incidence and prevalence of dementia across populations may provide insight into the aetiology and prevention of the disease (Table 1.3). Although there have been few large population-based studies of dementia internationally or in multi-ethnic communities, in general early studies reported lower prevalence and incidence in: (1) Asian nations than in Western Europe and North America; (2) rural than urban areas; and (3) developing rather than

| Prevalence | The total number of individuals with a disease in the population at a particular instant |
| Incidence | The rate of occurrence of new cases with a given disease during a specific period of time |

Table 1.3 Definitions of prevalence and incidence

developed countries (White 1992; White *et al.* 1996; see also Alzheimer's Disease International 2009). These differences have been linked to various factors, including diet, genetics, mortality, and the criteria for case selection. However, more recent projections suggest that over the next 20 years the proportional increase in the number of people with dementia will be steeper in developing than developed countries. This has been linked to population growth and demographic ageing trends that are currently seen in developing countries, in addition to changes in lifestyle and patterns of risk and protective factors in these countries. In the following section, we look at the challenges inherent in conducting research into the prevalence and incidence of dementia.

Methodological issues when studying prevalence and projections

Population-based studies of incident disease, where risk factors are identified before disease onset and individuals followed up longitudinally to document change, are powerful tools for the identification of risk factors and modifiable strategies. However, such studies are expensive, time-consuming, and are only now being conducted. Furthermore, differences in methodology and sample population lead to inconsistencies in findings, making comparisons difficult.

All epidemiological research depends on the definition of a "case" – that is, who is identified as having that particular condition. When evaluating dementia research, the following must be considered:

■ *Observation bias* – individuals with dementia often are unable to provide their own past medical and social histories and the information has to be supplied by surrogate informants who may have variable amounts of knowledge about these factors.
■ *Selection bias* – due to the choice of population source. The percentage of individuals with AD living in institutions, for example, varies widely from place to place but may exceed half of all cases with severe AD. Exclusion of institutionalized persons would result in an underestimation of prevalence rates.
■ *Response rate* – it is likely that response is affected by cognitive status, so that more impaired individuals are less likely to have complete data and typically refuse further testing. This affects prevalence estimates and it is hard to determine in what direction they may have been biased because non-response can cause over- as well as underestimation.

Exercise 1.1: Determining dementia prevalence in an area of interest

Katherine is an epidemiology student who is interested in determining the prevalence of dementia in the United Kingdom. She designs a questionnaire to capture dementia and using it she interviews all individuals aged 65 years and older that visited her local library in Cambridge in the last five months. Based on this she found that the number of people with dementia was quite low, leading her to conclude that dementia is not very common in the UK.

■ How might this conclusion be wrong?
■ How could Katherine go about determining the prevalence of dementia in the UK in order to obtain an accurate estimate of disease?

Prevalence of dementia

In 2009, the World Alzheimer Report estimated that worldwide there would be 36 million people living with dementia in 2010, increasing to 66 million by 2030 and 115 million by 2050 (Alzheimer's Disease International 2009). However, increases are not projected to be uniform across the world. As shown in Table 1.4, the greatest increase is likely to be in developing countries.

Subtype prevalence (Alzheimer's disease and vascular dementia) is also variable. In North America, AD accounts for approximately two-thirds of all cases. In Japan prior to 1990, vascular dementia was found to be more common than AD, although more recent data suggest AD is now nearly twice as prevalent as vascular dementia (Shigeta 2004). Similar changes have been observed in Seoul, Korea (Lee *et al.* 2002) and Taiwan (Liu *et al.* 1995; Liu *et al.* 1998) linked to urbanization, industrialization, and lifestyle changes (e.g. alcohol use). Reasons suggested for variations include: over-diagnosis of vascular dementia, differences in case definition, vascular risk, and relative number of the young-old and oldest-old (Ineichen 1998).

Cross-ethnic comparisons from the UK, the USA, and Canada have found differences in rates between ethnic groups sharing the same territory (Ineichen 1998). In the USA, vascular dementia is significantly more prevalent in individuals of African American and Hispanic origin (vs. Caucasian Americans) (Miles *et al.* 2001). In Washington and Hawaii, although individuals of Japanese origin were found to show similar AD estimates to those reported in European ancestry populations, prevalence was found to be lower when a Japanese diet was adhered to (White *et al.* 1996; Hatada *et al.* 1999). Furthermore, although the prevalence of vascular dementia was slightly lower in Japanese Americans than that reported in Japan, it was higher than that reported in European ancestry populations (White *et al.* 1996). However, there were differences in diagnostic approaches between countries that may have confounded this finding. In Canada, the prevalence of all dementias was found to be significantly lower in Cree Indians than Caucasians (0.5% vs. 3.5%, respectively) (Hendrie *et al.* 1993); while in the UK, vascular dementia has been found to be more

Region	Percent increase
Europe	40
North America	63
Southern Latin American cone	77
Developed Asia Pacific countries	89
South Asia	107
East Asia	117
North Africa and the Middle East	125
Rest of Latin America	134–146

Source: Alzheimer's Disease International (2009)

Table 1.4 Latest projections of the percent increase in the number of people with dementia across world regions (ordered lowest to highest)

prevalent than AD in individuals of African Caribbean origin versus British Caucasians (Richards *et al.* 2000; Livingston *et al.* 2001).

Prevalence studies indicate that dementia doubles approximately every five years after the age of 65 (Jorm *et al.* 1987). This increase is usually more marked for females for whom prevalence is higher in the old-old (e.g. persons aged 85 years and older) than males. In the old-old population, prevalence estimates remain controversial and range from 18% to 38% (Gardner *et al.* 2013). This could result from older individuals not living as long with dementia as younger individuals with dementia, or survivors into late old age being relatively resistant to developing dementia. Smaller sample sizes and decreased response rate in this age group may also influence findings.

Incidence of dementia

The incidence of dementia rises rapidly with age. Generally, in people younger than 65 years, dementia is rare: early-onset dementia (prior to the age of 65 years) between 40 and 50 years of age is generally linked to genetic risk factors (e.g. defect on chromosome 14 and Down's syndrome) (see Chapter 7 for more on younger people with dementia). The incidence of AD increases from approximately 0.2% of 60–69 year olds, to 1% for people who are 70 years old, 3% for people who are 80 years old, and approximately 8% for people who are older than 85 (Barberger-Gateau and Fabrigoule 1997; Patterson and Gass 2001). In contrast, the incidence of vascular dementia does not appear to show an age effect (Brayne *et al.* 1995).

The effects of gender on the incidence of dementia are controversial. Some studies suggest that the female sex is associated with increased risk (Hofman *et al.* 1991; Jorm and Jolley 1998; Dartigues *et al.* 2000; Black *et al.* 2001). However, another concluded that women had a higher risk of AD at older ages (above 80 years) and that men had a higher risk of vascular dementia at younger ages, but that age-specific incidence rate differences were small (Copeland *et al.* 1999). Cohort studies in the UK and the USA have consistently reported no gender differences in the incidence or prevalence of dementia or AD (Edland *et al.* 2002; Matthews and Brayne 2005). Increased longevity, increased survival with disease, and some increase in intrinsic vulnerability are considered to play a part in the predominance of females in some estimates.

In a study based in Rochester, Minnesota, incidence rates of AD and dementia were stable between 1960 and 1984, except for a slight increase in the very old (Kokmen *et al.* 1993; Rocca *et al.* 1998). In the Lundby Study in Sweden, incidence rates for multi-infarct dementia (caused by multiple strokes) and senile dementias (which typically consist of a group of diseases including AD and vascular dementia) remained stable from 1947 to 1972. However, more recent data suggest that rates of dementia in the USA increased from 1984/1990 to 1991/2000 and that this increase was more marked in persons with stroke compared with the stroke-free population (Ukraintseva *et al.* 2006).

Variation across regions

At present, it is difficult to establish to what extent findings are merely an artifact of methodology (e.g. sampling procedures and diagnostic criteria), differential exposure to risk factors (e.g. education, health care, cardiovascular disease), demographic changes (e.g. increased numbers of the old-old), cultural views on ageing (status of dementia as a "devastating disease"), response rates or survival trends (Fratiglioni *et al.* 1999), or whether differences reflect real geographical and ethnic variations. A marked geographical dissociation in Europe between the north and south, linked to differences in vascular risk factors has been proposed to account for the higher incidence rates in the old-old of north-western countries (Finland, Sweden, Denmark, the Netherlands, and the United Kingdom) compared with southern countries (France and Spain) (Fratiglioni *et al.* 2000).

Risk factors

The pathological origin and aetiology of dementia remain unknown. Treatment and prevention will largely depend on the level of understanding of the underlying biological and environmental factors associated with increased risk both in current and future cohorts of older people. Conclusions from previous studies have determined that dementia is a complex, multi-factorial process that is essentially under genetic control (Salib 2000). However, there is also compelling evidence for a predominantly acquired (environmental) form of AD. Indeed, Kumar *et al.* (1991) reported detailed neuroanatomical, neuropsychological, and neuropathological examination of three monozygous pairs of twins containing an individual with onset of AD disease between the ages of 50 and 60 years. All three twins remained well and each disease-free pair had been AD-free for over a decade. While this does not rule out the operation of genetic influences in the affected members of the pairs, this finding suggests that any such predisposition would have been exaggerated substantially by environmental variation between pairs of twins that accelerates disease onset.

Age

Age is the strongest risk factor for dementia. Beyond this, controversy remains as to whether dementia is an inevitable consequence of ageing or whether risks reach a plateau so that some individuals over a reasonable life span would never develop the disease (Goa *et al.* 1998; Matthews and Brayne 2005). Findings about age as a risk factor are complicated by the lack of consensus as to exactly what cognitive changes occur as a function of the normal ageing process and where the boundary between normal and pathological ageing lies. Furthermore, the extent to which age is responsible for disease, rather than serving as a proxy for as yet unidentified age-related factors that lead to disease, is unclear.

Family history and genetics

Dementia risk can increase two- to four-fold among individuals who have at least one first degree relative with dementia (van Duijn *et al.* 1991; Devi *et al.* 1999). This effect is stronger for those where a relative had early-onset dementia. However, while the familial occurrence of dementia may reflect shared environmental factors, there is strong evidence to support a genetic link (Black *et al.* 2001). In very rare cases (less than 5%), AD can be inherited in an autosomal dominant pattern. This occurs when a single abnormal gene on one of the first 22 non-sex chromosomes is inherited. Disease onset is typically in the beginning of middle age (Bird 1994). By the age of 40, almost all individuals with Down's syndrome have neuropathological changes consistent with AD (Prasher *et al.* 1997; Schupf *et al.* 1998). Individuals with Huntington's disease are also at risk of early-onset dementia.

The most studied genetic risk factor for late-onset dementia is the apolipoprotein E (ApoE) gene. The ApoE gene has three allelic variants (e2, e3, and e4) that combine to form five genotypes

(2–3, 3–3, 2–4, 3–4, and 4–4). Individuals carrying the e4 allele are found to be at increased risk of dementia, with the highest risk found in the 4-4 group (Farrer *et al.* 1997; Small *et al.* 2004). However, the molecular mechanism(s) underlying this association remains unclear. More recent studies have identified new risk variants for AD, including CR1, CLU, BIN1, MS4A, CD2AP, CD33, EPHA1, SORL1, and TREM2 (Harold *et al.* 2009; Hollingworth *et al.* 2011; Bettens *et al.* 2013; Guerreiro *et al.* 2013). These genes have been linked to: inflammation, lipid metabolism, endothelial function, immune function, exosomes, endocytosis, energy metabolism, and integrity of the blood–brain barrier. However, it is important to note that the clinical role of each of these genes has not been tested and therefore they are not recommended for routine testing in susceptible individuals (Patterson *et al.* 2001).

Lifestyle risk factors

Findings for alcohol and smoking as risk factors are not consistent. Alcohol has been found to have a protective effect in moderate drinkers with a five-fold increase in dementia in both abstainers and those who drink heavily (Orgogozo *et al.* 1997; Anttila *et al.* 2004). However, Orgogozo *et al.* (1997) found a link between increasing alcohol consumption and vascular dementia. With regard to smoking, after adjusting for age, ApoE, education, cardiovascular and respiratory factors, Tyas *et al.* (2003) found an increased risk of AD with medium and high levels of smoking, but not for very heavy smokers. Smoking is known to cause cardiovascular and respiratory diseases that are both risk factors for AD. For heavy smokers, it could be that they are not living long enough to develop dementia. In some studies, alcohol and smoking (never, past, and current) are neither strongly protective nor predictive (Doll *et al.* 2000), while in others both have been associated with an increase in the age-specific onset rate of AD (Brayne 2000). Conflicting results as to the direction of association between smoking and AD may be due to survival bias and methodological differences across studies. Yet, if smoking and drinking do confer increased risk of dementia, educational programmes on prevention and cessation ought to be public health priorities.

A healthy diet across the life span may have a protective effect. A role for dietary antioxidants (from foods containing vitamin E, especially vegetables, beta-carotene, omega-3, and vitamin C) in preventing or delaying dementia has been reported (Engelhart *et al.* 2002). Higher adherence to a Mediterranean diet (high in fruit and vegetables, grain, and unsaturated fats, and low in meat and dairy products) has been found to significantly lower the risk of developing AD, even after adjusting for age, gender, ethnicity, education, caloric intake, weight, smoking, and co-morbid conditions (Scarmeas *et al.* 2006). However, these findings have not been replicated, particularly in randomized controlled trials (the most rigorous form of clinical research to determine the impact of an intervention). Inconsistency in findings and questions regarding the accuracy of diet measurement suggests that no definitive evidence exists for dietary recommendations for the prevention of dementia beyond general exhortation of healthy diet and lifestyle to minimize vascular risk.

Exercise 1.2: I have the ApoE e4 allele – will I get dementia?

Adam is a 65-year-old male who is healthy with no evidence of cognitive problems. His mother had dementia and he heard on the news that the disease is hereditary. He therefore sent a saliva sample to a company he found online that offered to do a genetic health test. His results indicate that he is carrying the ApoE e4 allele (group 4-4). He thinks that any day he will develop dementia and is spending all of his time planning for a future with the disease. This has consumed his life.

■ Based on his genetic test results, will he inevitably develop dementia? Why?
■ What are three main risk factors for dementia?

Vascular factors

Vascular factors and conditions, including a history of stroke or transient ischaemic attack, diabetes mellitus, hypertension, congestive heart failure, and obesity are major risks for cognitive decline and dementia (Stephan and Brayne 2008). They work by accelerating Alzheimer-type changes in the brain. Indeed, vascular disease is thought to reduce blood flow to the brain and hypoperfusion (decreased blood flow through an organ) has been found to cause cognitive decline (de la Torre 2002). Imaging studies support the hypothesis that the clinical expression and severity of dementia (including AD and vascular dementia) are both mediated at least in part by the presence of cerebrovascular disease (Snowdon *et al.* 1997). Stroke and hypertension accelerate atrophy and degenerative changes resulting from neuronal shrinkage or loss (de la Torre 2002). The aggregation of risk factors is suggested to have a greater impact on the development of dementia than each factor independently. Attention to these modifiable risk factors will have important implications for reducing the incidence and prevalence of dementia.

Exercise 1.3: Can we prevent dementia?

Health promotion and prevention of chronic illness in later life are now common approaches in the government's approach to health care. Get hold of last week's newspaper and leaf through, looking for examples of health promotion in relation to chronic health conditions including dementia.

■ List all the examples that you find.
■ How many of the examples have to do with dementia?
■ What do you think is the reason for this?

Hypertension and anti-hypertensive medications

Hypertension (high blood pressure) has been associated with impaired cognitive function even in otherwise healthy individuals. It has been suggested that for every 10 mmHg rise in blood pressure, the risk of cognitive impairment rises by 7% (Peters 2001). While hypertension has traditionally been considered a contributor to vascular dementia, recent data suggest that vascular factors may also influence the clinical expression of AD (Bennett 2000). Although hypertensive treatment reduces the incidence of AD (Peters 2001), it is difficult to distinguish the effects of blood pressure reduction from the direct action of anti-hypertensives on preservation of cognitive function.

Mild cognitive impairment

Clinical criteria dictate that the onset of dementia is preceded by mild cognitive decline, and individuals with mild cognitive impairment (MCI) have been found to be at increased risk of dementia compared with unimpaired individuals (5–15% per year vs. 1–3%, respectively).

However, some individuals with MCI remain stable or even show improved cognitive functioning at follow-up (Portet *et al.* 2006; Matthews *et al.* 2008). Variability in rates may be due to population selection, threshold for impairment, and follow-up interval. Indeed, rates of conversion to dementia are generally highest among clinic-based samples and for definitions of MCI where memory impairment predominates (Matthews *et al.* 2008). Due to a lack of standardized diagnostic criteria, the prevalence of MCI in older populations has varied widely across studies (3–36%) with an incidence of 8–58% per thousand per year (Busse *et al.* 2003; Stephan *et al.* 2007). Furthermore, defining what distinguishes this condition from normal age-associated changes, early dementia, and dementia itself is unclear. As such, criteria for dementia and pre-dementia states are currently undergoing revision, with the borders shifting with regard to what is considered impaired versus not impaired (Dubois *et al.* 2010; Sperling et al. 2011). For example, MCI may no longer be considered at-risk, but as already AD, and encompassed in the new term "prodromal AD". This is defined as an early symptomatic stage pre-dementia where a patient shows evidence of memory impairment and positive ratings on pathophysiological and topographical markers of AD (Dubois *et al.* 2010; Jack *et al.* 2010). Individuals at high risk may instead be captured using terms to defined asymptomatic at-risk states such as pre-MCI. However, there are currently no criteria for defining pre-MCI and work needs to be undertaken on determining and validating operational criteria before being utilized in clinical practice and research studies.

Education

People who have less than six years of formal education are reported to have a higher risk of developing dementia, particularly AD (Black *et al.* 2001). Education as a protective factor has been linked to the ability to compensate for cognitive decline, thus delaying the diagnosis of dementia (Meng and D'Arcy 2012; Stern 2012). It has also been hypothesized that this effect may be mediated by brain reserve/size (Schofield *et al.* 1997). Whether it is education itself that makes a difference or other related factors such as occupational status and income level is unclear.

Head injury

Head trauma with loss of consciousness is a risk factor for dementia in some but not all studies (Bennett 2000; Salib 2000; Haan and Wallace 2004). Several hypotheses have been offered to explain the association, including neuronal damage, which reduces neuronal reserve and results in release of amyloid (Bennett 2000). An interaction between head injury and ApoE e4 has also been reported (Bennett 2000; Kukull and Ganguli 2000). The hypothesis of head trauma as a risk factor for AD comes from the observation of neurofibrillary tangles, indistinguishable from those seen in AD in the brains of boxers with dementia pugilistica (Breteler *et al.* 1992). However, the possibility that in some cases head trauma may be a consequence of an early stage of the dementia cannot be excluded.

Other risk factors

Other risk factors include brain tumour, kidney failure, liver disease, thyroid disease, vitamin deficiencies (B12, folic acid, thiamine), chronic inflammatory conditions (such as certain forms of arthritis), a history of episodes of clinical depression, stress, inadequate mental exercise, exposure to aluminium, pesticides and other toxins (for an overview, see van der Flier and Scheltens, 2005). The unique risk associated with each and the timing of their effect are yet to be determined.

Exercise 1.4: The use it or lose it hypothesis

Look at newspaper articles over the last year and list all the things that an individual is recommended to do to increase their cognitive reserve.

Summary of risk

A number of risk and protective factors for dementia, in particular AD, have been reported in the literature. The general conclusion is that the pathophysiology of dementia is very complex and may include genetic, physiological, psychological, as well as lifestyle elements, some of which may be linked. The heterogeneous genetic influences on dementia have probably contributed to difficulties in the detection of host or environmental factors associated with modified disease. These alleged linkages offer the basis for potential intervention for the prevention or the slowing down of those processes that lead to disease (Nourhashemi *et al.* 2000). Because of the number of people expected to be affected by dementia, even a small reduction in prevalence could have a huge impact on numbers and a substantial effect on health and social care costs depending on the extent to which survival is lengthened.

Studies that combine clinical and pathological assessment have a special role in the search for risk factors. A small number of ongoing longitudinal epidemiological studies include a *post mortem* brain donation programme [e.g. the Nun Study, the Religious Orders Study, the Baltimore Longitudinal Study on Aging, the Medical Research Council Cognitive Function and Ageing Study, the Cambridge City Over-75s Cohort Study (CC75C); the Vantaa 85+ Study, the Cache County Study]. This provides researchers with an opportunity to examine the neuropathology and molecular biology underlying the changes associated with dementia and link risk factors directly to brain pathology to understand how risk factors lead to clinical disease.

Disability and mortality associated with dementia

Disability

Dementia is one of the leading causes of non-fatal disability in the developed world, and by 2030 it is predicted that dementia will be the third leading cause of years of life lost due to death and disability in high-income countries (Mathers and Loncar 2006). In the WHO Global Burden of Disease Report (WHO 2003), it was estimated that the disability from dementia is higher than almost all conditions with the exception of spinal cord injury and terminal cancer. The WHO 2003 report estimated that among people aged 60 years and over dementia contributed 11.2% of all years lived with disability, while stroke contributed 9.5%, musculoskeletal disorders 8.9%, cardiovascular disease 5.0%, and all forms of cancer 2.4%. With increasing pressure on health care budgets, accurate estimations of the type and distribution of dementia in addition to the burden it causes are necessary to help quantify health and social care needs and highlight areas for future research into curative and preventative strategies.

Mortality

It is estimated that AD and other dementias are the seventh leading cause of death in high-income countries, accounting for 3.6% of total deaths. Studies from developed countries report a median survival time after the onset of dementia symptoms ranging from 5.0 to 9.3 years (Walsh *et al.*

1990), while in developing countries the reported median survival is 3.3 years for all individuals with dementia and 2.7 years for those with AD (Chandra *et al.* 1998). Overall, individuals with dementia have poorer survival and a shorter life expectancy than those without, with the risk of mortality greater the earlier the disease onset.

Debates and controversies

There are several areas of debate and controversy. These include mild cognitive impairment (MCI), diagnostic criteria for AD and vascular dementia, and applicability of risk factors internationally.

Debates regarding MCI include the extent to which classification concepts of MCI accurately capture those at risk of progressing to dementia. The clinical course is not always pathological: while in some studies impairment has been associated with increased risk of progression to AD, in others individuals remain stable or even show improved cognitive functioning at follow-up. The lack of consistency in definition may explain the resulting discrepancy in conversion rates.

The diagnostic criteria for AD and for vascular dementia are mutually exclusive. Yet mixed forms are common. Do we need accepted criteria for mixed dementia?

Should the same factors (e.g. life expectancy and diet) be taken into consideration when estimating prevalence of dementia across the developed and developing world? How accurate are our calculations and what assumptions are we making? Furthermore, we can ask what are the risk and protective factors for dementia? For example, what is the risk associated with exposure to aluminium and the role of genetic and environmental factors (e.g. alcohol, smoking, diet) in moderating risk.

Conclusion

Accurate estimates of both prevalence and incidence are necessary not only as a foundation for health and social policy but also to generate awareness. Of particular importance is the rapid demographic shift in developing countries. The global challenge to policy-makers is two-fold: (1) to implement immediate policy and infrastructure for the future provision and health and social care for the older population in all regions of the world; and (2) to develop strategies and treatment to delay disease onset and progression. Application of these measures is critical in less-developed countries, which have a shorter time frame to adjust to an ageing population. Opportunities missed by developing counties may have devastating economic and social consequences.

Further information

The Cognitive Function and Ageing Study (CFAS) is a large longitudinal multi-centre population-based study of cognitive decline and dementia in people aged 65 and over living in the UK [http://www.cfas.ac.uk/].

The World Health Organization is the directing and coordinating authority for health within the United Nations system [http://www.who.int/en/].

The Alzheimer Research Forum is an independent non-profit-making organization. Its website reports on the latest scientific findings, from basic research to clinical trials; creates and maintains public databases of essential research data and reagents; and produces discussion forums to promote debate, speed the dissemination of new ideas, and break down barriers across the numerous disciplines that can contribute to the global effort to cure Alzheimer's disease [http://www.alzforum.org/].

Alzheimer's Disease International is an umbrella organization of national Alzheimer associations around the world [http://www.alz.co.uk/].

Alzheimer's Research UK is a research charity for dementia in the UK. It is dedicated to funding scientific studies to find ways to treat, cure, and prevent Alzheimer's disease, vascular dementia, Lewy body disease, and fronto-temporal dementia [http://www.alzheimersresearchuk.org/].

The report of the United Nations Department of Economic and Social Affairs, Population Division, entitled *World Population Ageing 2000*, presents the current assessment of the status of the world's older population and prospects for the future. It provides a description of global trends in population ageing and includes key indicators of the ageing process for each of the major areas, regions, and countries of the world.

References

Alzheimer's Disease International (2009) *World Alzheimer Report*. London: Alzheimer's Disease International.

Anttila, T., Helkala, E., Viitanen, M., Kareholt, I., Fratiglioni, L. *et al.* (2004) Alcohol drinking in middle age and subsequent risk of mild cognitive impairment and dementia in old age: a prospective population based study, *British Medical Journal*, 329(7465): 539.

Barberger-Gateau, P. and Fabrigoule, C. (1997) Disability and cognitive impairment in the elderly, *Disability Rehabilitation*, 19: 175–93.

Bennett, D.A. (2000) Part I. Epidemiology and public health impact of Alzheimer's disease, *Disease-a-Month*, 46: 657–65.

Bettens, K., Sleegers, K. and Van Broeckhoven, C. (2013) Genetic insights in Alzheimer's disease, *Lancet Neurology*, 12(1): 92–104.

Bird, T.D. (1994) Clinical genetics of familial Alzheimer disease, in R.D Terry, R. Katzman and K.L. Bick (eds.) *Alzheimer Disease*. New York: Raven Press, pp. 65–74.

Black, S.E., Patterson, C. and Feightner, J. (2001) Preventing dementia, *Canadian Journal of Neurology Science*, 28 (Suppl. 1): S56–S66.

Brayne, C. (2000) Smoking and the brain, *British Medical Journal*, 320(7242): 1087–8.

Brayne, C., Gill, C., Huppert, F.A., Barkley, C., Gehlhaar, E. *et al.* (1995) Incidence of clinically diagnosed subtypes of dementia in an elderly population: Cambridge Project for Later Life, *British Journal of Psychiatry*, 167: 255–62.

Breteler, M.M., Claus, J.J., van Duijn, C.M., Launer, L.J. and Hofman, A. (1992) Epidemiology of Alzheimer's disease, *Epidemiologic Reviews*, 14: 59–89.

Busse, A., Bischkopf, J., Riedel-Heller, S.G. and Angermeyer, M.C. (2003) Mild cognitive impairment: 1. Prevalence and predictive validity according to current approaches, *Acta Neurologica Scandinavica*, 108: 71–81.

Chandra, V., Ganguli, M., Pandav, R., Johnston, J., Belle, S. *et al.* (1998) Prevalence of Alzheimer's disease and other dementias in rural India: the Indo-US study, *Neurology*, 51: 1000–8.

Copeland, J.R., McCracken, C.F., Dewey, M.E., Wilson, K.C., Doran, M. *et al.* (1999) Undifferentiated dementia, Alzheimer's disease and vascular dementia: age- and gender-related incidence in Liverpool. The MRC-ALPHA Study, *British Journal of Psychiatry*, 175: 433–8.

Corrada, M., Brookmeyer, R. and Kawas, C. (1995) Sources of variability in prevalence rates of Alzheimer's disease, *International Journal of Epidemiology*, 24: 1000–5.

Cowan, L.D., Leviton, A. and Dammann, O. (2000) New research directions in neuroepidemiology, *Epidemiology Review*, 22: 18–23.

Dartigues, J.F., Letenneur, L., Joly, P., Helmer, C., Orgogozo, J. *et al.* (2000) Age specific risk of dementia according to gender, education and wine consumption, *Neurobiology of Aging*, 21: 64.

de la Torre, J.C. (2002) Alzheimer disease as a vascular disorder: nosological evidence, *Stroke*, 33: 1152–62.

Devi, G., Ottman, R., Tang, M., Marder, K., Stern, Y. *et al.* (1999) Influence of ApoE genotype on familial aggregation of AD in an urban population, *Neurology*, 53: 789–94.

Dewey, M.E. and Saz, P. (2001) Dementia, cognitive impairment and mortality in persons aged 65 and over living in the community: a systematic review of the literature, *International Journal of Geriatric Epidemiology*, 16: 751–61.

Doll, R., Peto, R., Boreham, J. and Sutherland, I. (2000) Smoking and dementia in male British doctors: prospective study, *British Medical Journal*, 320: 1097–102.

Dubois, B., Feldman, H.H., Jacova, C., Cummings, J.L., Dekosky, S.T. *et al.* (2010) Revising the definition of Alzheimer's disease: a new lexicon, *Lancet Neurology*, 9: 1118–27.

Edland, S.D., Rocca, W.A., Petersen, R.C., Cha, R.H. and Kokmen, E. (2002) Dementia and Alzheimer disease incidence rates do not vary by sex in Rochester, Minn, *Archives of Neurology*, 59: 1589–93.

Engelhart, M.J., Geerlings, M.I., Ruitenberg, A., van Swieten, J.C., Hofman, A. *et al.* (2002) Diet and risk of dementia: does fat matter?, The Rotterdam Study, *Neurology*, 59: 1915–21.

Farrer, L.A., Cupples, L.A., Haines, J.L., Hyman, B., Kukull, W.A. *et al.* (1997) Effects of age, sex, and ethnicity on the association between apolipoprotein E genotype and Alzheimer disease: a meta-analysis. ApoE and Alzheimer Disease Meta Analysis Consortium, *Journal of the American Medical Association*, 278: 1349–56.

Fratiglioni, L., de Ronchi, D. and Aguero-Torres, H. (1999) Worldwide prevalence and incidence of dementia, *Drugs and Aging*, 15: 365–75.

Fratiglioni, L., Launer, L.J., Andersen, K., Breteler, M.M., Copeland, J.R. *et al.* (2000) Incidence of dementia and major subtypes in Europe: a collaborative study of population-based cohorts. Neurologic Diseases in the Elderly Research Group, *Neurology*, 54: S10–S15.

Gardner, R.C., Valcour, V. and Yaffe, K. (2013) Dementia in the oldest old: a multi-factorial and growing public health issue, *Alzheimer's Research and Therapy*, 5: 27.

Goa, S., Hendrie, H.C., Hall, K.S. and Hui, S. (1998) The relationships between age, sex, and the incidence of dementia and Alzheimer's disease: a meta-analysis, *Archives of General Psychiatry*, 55: 809–15.

Guerreiro, R., Wojtas, A., Bras, J., Carrasquillo, M., Rogaeva, E. *et al.* (2013) TREM2 variants in Alzheimer's disease, *New England Journal of Medicine*, 368: 117–27.

Haan, M.N. and Wallace, R. (2004) Can dementia be prevented? Brain aging in a population-based context, *Annual Review of Public Health*, 25: 1–24.

Harold, D., Abraham, R., Hollingworth, P., Sims, R., Gerrish, A. *et al.* (2009) Genome-wide association study identifies variants at CLU and PICALM associated with Alzheimer's disease, *Nature Genetics*, 41: 1088–93.

Hatada, K., Okazaki, Y., Yoshitake, K., Takada, K. and Nakane, Y. (1999) Further evidence of Westernization of dementia prevalence in Nagasaki, Japan, and family recognition, *International Psychogeriatrics*, 11: 123–38.

Hendrie, H.C., Hall, K.S., Pillay, N., Rodgers, D., Prince, C. *et al.* (1993) Alzheimer's disease is rare in Cree, *International Psychogeriatrics*, 5: 5–14.

Hofman, A., Rocca, W.A., Brayne, C., Breteler, M.M.B., Clarke, M. *et al.* (1991) The prevalence of dementia in Europe: a collaborative study of 1980–1990 findings, *International Journal of Epidemiology*, 20: 736–48.

Hollingworth, P., Harold, D., Sims, R., Gerrish, A., Lambert, J.C. *et al.* (2011) Common variants at ABCA7, MS4A6A/MS4A4E, EPHA1, CD33 and CD2AP are associated with Alzheimer's disease, *Nature Genetics*, 43: 429–35.

Ineichen, B. (1998) The geography of dementia: an approach through epidemiology, *Health and Place*, 4: 383–94.

Jack, C.R., Knopman, D.S., Jagust, W.J., Shaw, L.M., Aisen, P.S. *et al.* (2010) Hypothetical model of dynamic biomarkers of the Alzheimer's pathological cascade, *The Lancet Neurology*, 9(1):119.

Jorm, A.F. and Jolley, D. (1998) The incidence of dementia: a meta-analysis, *Neurology*, 51: 728–33.

Jorm, A.F., Korten, A.E. and Henderson, A.S. (1987) The prevalence of dementia: a quantitative integration of the literature, *Psychiatrica Scandinavica*, 76: 465–79.

Kokmen, E., Beard, C.M., O'Brien, P.C., Offord, K.P. and Kurland, L.T. (1993) Is the incidence of dementing illness changing? A 25-year time trend study in Rochester, Minnesota (1960–1984), *Neurology*, 43: 1887–92.

Kukull, W.A. and Ganguli, M. (2000) Epidemiology of dementia: concepts and overview, *Neurologic Clinics*, 18: 923–49.

Kumar, A., Schapiro, M.B., Grady, C.L., Matocha, M.F., Haxby, J.V. et al. (1991) Anatomic, metabolic, neuropsychological, and molecular genetic studies of three pairs of identical twins discordant for dementia of the Alzheimer's type, *Archives of Neurology*, 48: 160–8.

Ladislas, R. (2000) Cellular and molecular mechanisms of aging and age related diseases, *Pathology and Oncology Research*, 6: 3–9.

Lee, D.Y., Lee, J.H., Ju, Y.S., Lee, K.U., Kim, K.W. et al. (2002) The prevalence of dementia in older people in an urban population of Korea: the Seoul Study, *Journal of the American Geriatrics Society*, 50: 1233–9.

Liu, C.K., Lai, C.L., Tai, C.T., Lin, R.T., Yen, Y.Y. et al. (1998) Incidence and subtypes of dementia in southern Taiwan: impact of socio-demographic factors, *Neurology*, 50: 1572–9.

Liu, H.C., Lin, K.N., Teng, E.L., Wang, S.J., Fuh, J.L. et al. (1995) Prevalence and subtypes of dementia in Taiwan: a community survey of 5297 individuals, *Journal of the American Geriatrics Society*, 43: 144–9.

Livingston, G., Leavey, G., Kitchen, G., Manela, M., Sembhi, S. et al. (2001) Mental health of migrant elders: the Islington Study, *British Journal of Psychiatry*, 179: 361–6.

Mathers, C.D. and Loncar, D. (2006) Projections of global mortality and burden of disease from 2002 to 2030, *PLoS Medicine*, 3: e442.

Matthews, F. and Brayne, C. (2005) The incidence of dementia in England and Wales: findings from the five identical sites of the MRC CFA Study, *PLoS Medicine*, 2: e193.

Matthews, F.E., Stephan, B.C.M., McKeith, I.G., Bond, J. and Brayne, C. (2008) Two-year progression from mild cognitive impairment to dementia: to what extent do different definitions agree?, *Journal of the American Geriatrics Society*, 56: 1424–33.

Meng, X. and D'Arcy, C. (2012) Education and dementia in the context of the cognitive reserve hypothesis: a systematic review with meta-analyses and qualitative analyses, *PloS One*, 7: e38268.

Miles, T.P., Froehlich, T.E., Bogardus, S.T. and Inouye, S.K. (2001) Dementia and race: are there differences between African Americans and Caucasians?, *Journal of the American Geriatrics Society*, 49: 477–84.

Nourhashemi, F., Gillette-Guyonnet, S., Andrieu, S., Ghisolfi, A., Ousset, P.J. et al. (2000) Alzheimer disease: protective factors, *American Journal of Clinical Nutrition*, 71: 643S–649S.

O'Connor, D.W., Blessed, G., Cooper, B., Jonker, C., Morris, J.C. et al. (1996) Cross-national interrater reliability of dementia diagnosis in the elderly and factors associated with disagreement, *Neurology*, 47: 1194–9.

Office for National Statistics (ONS) (2011) *National Population Projections, 2010-based Projections* [http://www.ons.gov.uk/ons/rel/npp/national-population-projections/2010-based-projections/index.html, accessed 27 August 2013].

Orgogozo, J.M., Dartigues, J.F., Lafont, S., Letenneur, L., Commenges, D. et al. (1997) Wine consumption and dementia in the elderly: a prospective community study in the Bordeaux area, *Revue Neurologique (Paris)*, 153: 185–92.

Patterson, C. and Gass, D.A. (2001) Screening for cognitive impairment and dementia in the elderly, *Canadian Journal of Neurological Sciences*, 28: S42–S51.

Patterson, C., Grek, A., Gauthier, S., Bergman, H., Cohen, C. et al. (2001) The recognition, assessment and management of dementing disorders: conclusions from the Canadian Consensus Conference on Dementia, *Canadian Journal of Neurological Sciences*, 28: 3–16.

Peters, R. (2001) The prevention of dementia, *Journal of Cardiovascular Risk*, 8: 253–6.

Portet, F., Ousset, P.J., Visser, P.J., Frisoni, G.B., Nobili, J. et al. (2006) Mild cognitive impairment in medical practice: critical review of the concept and new diagnostic procedure. Report of the MCI Working Group of the European Consortium on Alzheimer's disease (EADC), *Journal of Neurology, Neurosurgery, and Psychiatry*, 77: 714–18.

Prasher, V.P., Chowdhury, T.A., Rowe, B.R. and Bain, S.C. (1997) ApoE genotype and Alzheimer's disease in adults with Down syndrome: metaanalysis, *American Journal of Mental Retardation*, 102: 103–10.

Richards, M., Brayne, C., Dening, T., Abas, M., Carter, J. et al. (2000) Cognitive function in UK community-dwelling African Caribbean and white elders: a pilot study, *International Journal of Geriatric Psychiatry*, 15: 621–30.

Rocca, W.A., Cha, R.H., Waring, S.C. and Kokmen, E. (1998) Incidence of dementia and Alzheimer's disease: Aa reanalysis of data from Rochester, Minnesota, 1975–1984, *American Journal of Epidemiology*, 148: 51–62.

Salib, E. (2000) Risk factors for Alzheimer's disease, *Elder Care*, 11: 12–15.

Scarmeas, N., Stern, Y., Tang, M.X., Mayeux, R. and Luchsinger, J.A. (2006) Mediterranean diet and risk for Alzheimer's disease, *Annals of Neurology*, 59: 912–21.

Schofield, P.W., Logroscino, G., Andrews, H.F., Albert, S. and Stern, Y. (1997) An association between head circumference and Alzheimer's disease in a population-based study of aging and dementia, *Neurology*, 49: 30–7.

Schupf, N., Kapell, D., Nightingale, B., Rodriguez, A., Tycko, B. *et al.* (1998) Earlier onset of Alzheimer's disease in men with Down syndrome, *Neurology*, 50: 991–5.

Shigeta, M. (2004) Epidemiology: rapid increase in Alzheimer's disease prevalence in Japan, *Psychogeriatrics*, 4: 117–19.

Skoog, I. (1998) Status of risk factors for vascular dementia, *Neuroepidemiology*, 17: 2–9.

Small, B.J., Rosnick, C.B., Fratiglioni, L. and Backman, L. (2004) Apolipoprotein E and cognitive performance: a meta-analysis, *Psychology and Aging*, 19: 592–600.

Snowdon, D.A., Greiner, L.H., Mortimer, J.A., Riley, K.P., Greiner, P.A. *et al.* (1997) Brain infarction and the clinical expression of Alzheimer disease: the Nun Study, *Journal of the American Medical Association*, 277: 813–17.

Sperling, R.A., Aisen, P.S., Beckett, L.A., Bennett, D.A., Craft, S. *et al.* (2011) Toward defining the preclinical stages of Alzheimer's disease: recommendations from the National Institute on Aging-Alzheimer's Association workgroups on diagnostic guidelines for Alzheimer's disease, *Alzheimer's and Dementia*, 7: 280–92.

Stephan, B.C. and Brayne, C. (2008) Vascular factors and prevention of dementia. *International Review of Psychiatry*, 20: 344–56.

Stephan, B.C.M., Matthews, F.E., McKeith, I., Bond, J., Brayne, C. *et al.* (2007) Early cognitive change in the general population: how do different definitions work?, *Journal of the American Geriatrics Society*, 55: 1534–40.

Stern, Y. (2012) Cognitive reserve in ageing and alzheimer's disease, *Lancet Neurology*, 11: 1006–12.

Tyas, S.L., White, L.R., Petrovitch, H., Webster Ross, G., Foley, D.J. *et al.* (2003) Mid-life smoking and late-life dementia: the Honolulu–Asia Aging Study, *Neurobiology of Aging*, 24: 589–96.

Ukraintseva, S., Sloan, F., Arbeev, K. and Yashin, A. (2006) Increasing rates of dementia at time of declining mortality from stroke, *Stroke*, 37(5): 1155–9.

United Nations Department of Economic and Social Affairs, Population Division (2007) *World Population Prospects*. New York: United Nations [http://esa.un.org/unpp, accessed 27 August 2013].

United Nations Department of Economic and Social Affairs, Population Division (2013) *World Population Prospects: The 2012 Revision, Vol. I: Comprehensive Tables* (ST/ESA/SER.A/336) [http://esa.un.org/unpd/wpp/Documentation/pdf/WPP2012_Volume-I_Comprehensive-Tables.pdf, accessed 27 August 2013].

van der Flier, W.M. and Scheltens, P. (2005) Epidemiology and risk factors of dementia, *Journal of Neurology, Neurosurgery, and Psychiatry*, 76: 2–7.

van Duijn, C.M., Hendriks, L., Cruts, M., Hardy, J.A., Hofman, A. *et al.* (1991) Amyloid precursor protein gene mutation in early-onset Alzheimer's disease, *Lancet*, 337: 978.

Walsh, J.S., Welch, H.G. and Larson, E.B. (1990) Survival of outpatients with Alzheimer-type dementia, *Annals of Internal Medicine*, 113: 429–34.

White, L.R. (1992) Towards a program of cross-cultural research on the epidemiology of Alzheimer's disease, *Current Science*, 63: 456–69.

White, L., Petrovitch, H., Ross, G.W., Masaki, K.H., Abbott, R.D. *et al.* (1996) Prevalence of dementia in older Japanese-American men in Hawaii: the Honolulu–Asia Aging Study, *Journal of the American Medical Association*, 276: 955–60.

World Health Organization (WHO) (2003) *Global Burden of Disease (GBD) Report*. Geneva: WHO.

CHAPTER 2

Dementia-friendly communities

Cathy Henwood and Murna Downs

> ❝Well I have very good neighbours . . . They know I have Alzheimer's. Some of my neighbours have a key. If there was a problem they would be there. When I was first diagnosed I kept losing my key. They just, you know, do you need anything but they're not in my face. But it's reciprocal too. I help them. They have two dogs and they work. So you know, they might ask me, do you mind letting somebody in while we're out, they both work. It's two ways.❞
>
> —Marlene Aveyard Yorkshire, UK

Learning objectives

By the end of this chapter, you will be able to:

- Define what we mean by dementia-friendly communities
- Describe the theory underlying dementia-friendly communities
- Know some examples of dementia-friendly communities
- Appreciate the key steps to becoming a dementia-friendly community

Introduction

A person with dementia said that "dementia" was by itself a very difficult and rather frightening word but "friendly" was "well – a friendly everyday word". He said that, for him, the juxtaposition of these two very different words was very powerful.

People with dementia have been described as being the most stigmatized and socially excluded members of society (Graham *et al.* 2003; Alzheimer's Disease International 2012; Alzheimer's Society 2013). The stigma and discrimination experienced by people with dementia pose a significant additional challenge to people already having to contend with cognitive and functional impairments (Katsuno 2005; Alzheimer's Disease International 2012). This experience of social exclusion can occur throughout the course of living with dementia, from diagnosis to death, both for the person with dementia and their family carers.

Case example 2.1: A person with dementia

I had a difficult incident at my bank that made me very angry because I was placed in a position where I was surprised about the way they treated me. I've not been in that position before. I have been a very capable person. I was shocked to be talked down to. They didn't listen to me. As a customer, I expected to be treated with respect, even if I don't remember my pin number. I was offended by the lack of respect.

In our work, we have found that what matters most to people living with dementia is other people's attitudes. These can either support people or undermine them. For the person with memory problems and those close to them, it can be hard; everyone they come into contact with – be it at the local shop, hairdresser, bank, church or mosque – can make living with dementia a little easier or a lot harder.

Families of people who have dementia experience what is termed 'courtesy stigma' and discrimination, and also become socially isolated (Werner and Heinik 2008). This can be because neighbours, friends, and extended family withdraw; families avoid public contact in order to protect their relative from embarrassment and exposure; and opportunities to engage socially become restricted because of caring responsibilities. As a result, families can be left with depleted support systems and social networks at a time when they are most needed (see Chapter 21).

People with dementia and their family members are first and foremost people, and members of their community (Bartlett and O'Connor 2007). It is now recognized that we will fail to fully uphold their rights to citizenship and ensure their well-being if we focus exclusively on health and social care reform. Without an equal emphasis on upholding citizenship and community participation, no amount of health and social care reform will lead to people living well with dementia.

Definition of dementia-friendly communities

Exercise 2.1: What is a dementia-friendly community?

Think for a moment about what you would want in order to live well with dementia.

- What businesses and everyday services would you want to be able to access?
- What sorts of support and services would support you to live your life the way you want to?
- What would give you a sense of fulfilment and fun in your life?

These questions form a starting place for thinking about what a dementia-friendly community might be. We will all have our own individual answers to these questions. Our responses make it personal to us all.

Case example 2.2: A dementia-friendly community

A carer told one of the Bradford Alzheimer's Society Dementia Support workers about how their family had been supported by their local corner shop. Their Mum lived alone; generally she was still managing well, and did most of her shopping in their local mini market. However, every time their Mum went shopping she would buy a tin or two of cat food. The stack of tins of cat food in the cupboard built up. She used to have a cat but it had died several years earlier. The family tried reminding their Mum that she didn't have a cat, but seeing the cat food in the shop seemed to act as a trigger for buying more food. Once the family explained the situation to the shop owner, the owner was happy to help. The family simply returned the food every week or so to the shop for a refund, and the money was put back in their Mum's purse.

The Alzheimer's Society (2013) published foundation criteria for communities that are participating in the dementia-friendly communities recognition process; this was based on the findings of a national consultation. Communities participating in the recognition process are seen as "working to become dementia-friendly" – as an acknowledgement that it is a journey that will take a number of years of work and because being fully dementia-friendly is more of an aspiration. There are likely to be aspects of any community that are not fully on board. In brief, the criteria are:

1. Make sure you have the right local structure in place to maintain a sustainable dementia-friendly community.
2. Identify a person to take responsibility for driving forward the work to support your community to become dementia-friendly.
3. Have a plan in place to raise awareness about dementia in key organizations and businesses within the community that support people with dementia.
4. Develop a strong voice for people with dementia living in your communities. This will give your plan credibility and will make sure it focuses on areas people with dementia feel are most important.
5. Raise the profile of your work to increase reach and awareness to different groups in the community.
6. Focus your plans on a number of key areas that have been identified locally.
7. Have a plan or system in place to update the progress of your community.

More details about the criteria can be found in "Guidance for communities registering for the recognition process for dementia-friendly communities" and "Foundation criteria for the dementia-friendly communities recognition process" (see http://www.alzheimers.org.uk/recognitionprocess). The guidelines are deliberately broad – the expectation for a small village would clearly need to be different from that for a major town or city. It is hoped that criteria such as these will give enough direction and challenge to encourage communities to take up the challenge of building their own local version of dementia-friendly communities.

Innovations in Dementia (2011) interviewed people with dementia and their supporters and identified the following as important aspects of community life:

- the physical environment
- local facilities
- support services
- social networks
- local groups

While there is no one definition of dementia-friendly communities, there is a broad agreement of the goal of such communities. Guidance on building dementia-friendly communities from the Alzheimer's Society (2013) includes:

- involvement of people with dementia
- challenge stigma and build understanding
- accessible community activities
- acknowledge potential
- ensure an early diagnosis
- practical support to ensure engagement in community life
- community-based solutions
- consistent and reliable travel options

- easy-to-navigate environments
- respectful and responsible businesses and services

Similarly, "Dementia Without Walls", York's dementia-friendly community research project funded by the Joseph Rowntree Foundation suggests there are four cornerstones to a dementia-friendly community – place, people, resources, and networks.

1. **Place** covers the person's home, their neighbourhood, and how easy or difficult it is for the person to get out and about.

   ❝Some of the negative effects of dementia can be reduced if attention is paid to the quality of a person's environment.❞

   —Joseph Rowntree Foundation (2012: 3)

2. **People** – be they partners, family, neighbours, everyday shops and services, health professionals, paid-for carers.

   ❝Increasing awareness of dementia and changing our attitude towards it can help to remove the stigma many people feel. This may help people to talk about their experience, to engage more in society and to ask for the help they need.❞

   —Joseph Rowntree Foundation (2012: 4)

3. **Resources** – these are not just the services provided directly for people with dementia linked with their care and health needs, but also include leisure and social activities, shops and services.

   ❝York is well placed to use its rich cultural and leisure facilities to engage and support people with dementia in the community.
   There is an opportunity with the NHS reforms and the City of York Council review of Elderly Persons' Homes to improve commissioning and delivery of services for dementia.❞

   —Joseph Rowntree Foundation (2012: 5)

4. **Networks** – how well linked up and accessible information and services are and how friendly a neighbourhood is are both important factors in helping a community to be dementia-friendly:

   ❝Strengthening and building networks of dementia champions at neighbourhood level will optimise the impact of resources for people with dementia in the community.❞

   —Joseph Rowntree Foundation (2012: 6)

Policy support for dementia-friendly communities

It is only recently that the potential for communities working alongside the voluntary, state, and private sectors to more effectively support people with dementia has been realized. People with dementia and their families are becoming actively involved with professionals, providers, and policy-makers in the planning of local services and supports. Through these dementia-friendly initiatives, the potential of local social networks and community organizations to support and connect people with dementia to mainstream opportunity is being realized.

Increasingly, national policies seek to ensure that people with dementia are afforded their rights and entitlements to participate to the extent they wish in community life. See, for example, Scotland's rights-based approach to standards of care (http://www.scotland.gov.uk/ Publications/2011/05/31085414/0), which includes:

■ I have the right to be as independent as possible and be included in my community.

In 2010, the Department of Health published outcomes of importance to people affected by dementia. In the National Dementia Declaration published in England in 2011, people with dementia and their family carers described seven outcomes they would like to see in their lives, of which two are (Dementia Action Alliance 2011):

■ I live in an enabling and supportive environment where I feel valued and understood.
■ I have a sense of belonging and of being a valued part of family, community and civic life.

National plans for England (Department of Health 2009) and Scotland (Scottish Government 2013) emphasize the need for community awareness and acceptance and promotion of social inclusion through community-based approaches. For example, in the Scottish plan emphasis is placed on:

> 66 People want to see better use being made of natural supports, peer support and wider community resources, to ensure that people with dementia are enabled to live well with dementia and remain part of their communities. 99

—p. 27

In these national plans, people with dementia are seen not exclusively as recipients of care but as parents, friends, and neighbours. In short, they are viewed as citizens – members of our communities. This directly addresses the fact that it is these roles and social networks that are threatened early on in the journey, both for people with dementia and their family carers.

The World Health Organization's *Dementia: A Public Health Priority* (WHO/ADI 2012), the *Prime Minister's Challenge on Dementia* (Department of Health 2012), and the Alzheimer's Society's (2012) *Dementia 2012* include a call for dementia-friendly communities:

> 66 We must work in partnership to improve quality of life, focusing on all outcomes that are important to people living with dementia, including developing dementia-friendly communities. This partnership must have people with dementia and carers at the heart and must include a range of partners from business, the public sector, civic and voluntary organisations, as well as the government, NHS and local authorities. 99

—Alzheimer's Society (2012: iv)

Paralleling this development, the Dementia Action Alliance (DAA) has established alliances at national, regional, and local level. The DAA brings together diverse organizations from the private, professional, statutory, and commercial sectors to assist with achieving person-centred outcomes for people with dementia (see http://www.dementiaaction.org.uk/).

Until recently, there had been a neglect of this commercial, community, and social responsibility in most policy documents, both nationally and internationally. For example, while Norway's National Plan (Ministry of Health and Care Services 2008) seeks "to help to give individuals the opportunity to live independently and to have an active and meaningful existence in community with others", there is little attention paid to the role of communities in ensuring this. Most of the attention in this plan is placed on health and social services.

Internationally, dementia-friendly communities are increasingly seen as a key route to ensuring a good life with dementia. Pioneered in Belgium (Bruges), Japan, and Germany (ACTION), they are being established all over the UK (e.g. Plymouth, Sheffield, York, Bradford). These community development and community engagement projects are increasingly recognized as the new horizon in dementia care (Downs, 2013).

Theory underlying dementia-friendly communities

Dementia-friendly communities have their roots in the public health approach of the World Health Organization's "Healthy Cities", with its emphasis on the interaction between the personal experience of health and social support and community participation. For people with dementia, such communities are perhaps most closely aligned with Kellehear's (2005, 2013) "Compassionate Cities", in which he sought to redress the exclusion from WHO's Healthy Cities of people who were dying. Most recently, he has turned his attention to people with dementia and has argued for a more public health approach to care of people with dementia, one which includes community engagement as well as direct care service provision (Kellehear 2009). While there are examples in palliative care where community development can enhance individual empowerment, such an approach is only now being explored in relation to ensuring people with dementia live well.

A focus on dementia-friendly communities is closely aligned to the social model of disability, which argues that impairments are not inherently disabling but become so because of the social, physical or economic environment in which the person lives (Oliver 1990). This literature recognizes the importance of using the perspective of people with impairments in order to design, develop, and evaluate services (Barnes and Shardlow 1996; Barnes and Walker 1996). Much of Kitwood's (1997) pioneering work on humanizing care for people with dementia is also consistent with a social model of disability. He argued that we need to move beyond the reductionism of the medical model to seeing a person living in relation to others – close family and friends and broader society – and recognizing the influence such relationships can have on their sense of value and well-being. For Kitwood, the greatest threat to living well with dementia was not living with cognitive and functional impairments *per se*, but rather with the depersonalizing and dehumanizing consequences of stigma (Downs 2013). Sabat (2003), also coming from a social psychological viewpoint, used the term "malignant social positioning" to explain the effects of demeaning interactions on people with dementia (see also Chapter 8).

Examples of dementia-friendly communities

Case example 2.3: Germany

This goal is to transform our villages, cities and communities into better places to live in for people with dementia . . . Raising awareness, putting dementia in the spotlight and finding ways to promote integration of people living with dementia are the main goals. In some cases posters and banners appear all over the city. But also specialised training for police, bank employees, shop owners, and others is involved, as well as the organisation of cultural and sports activities to promote integration of people living with dementia in the local community. A special initiative

(continued)

is to welcome people with dementia in bistros and restaurants. "We find it most important to build a civil social alliance in which the citizen with dementia is involved and not the 'sick' person. Therefore we need the actual inclusion of persons with dementia on the spot. We should let people with dementia speak for themselves and let them define what their needs are and where their place in society is. Of course, in all this, we have to be creative, because very often these local initiatives need to run without much financial support."

—Weissman 2009, cited by King Baudouin Foundation (2010)

Case example 2.4: Japan

In Japan dementia is no longer seen as "somebody else's business" but a big challenge for the whole nation. A person with dementia was once considered to be "someone who lost the ability to recognize anyone or anything," or "someone who did one strange thing after another," and was the target of social prejudice. There have been, however, more and more cases in which the patients themselves participate in symposiums or other events to talk about their own painful experiences and express their desire to stay involved in society in whatever way they can. Studies have shown that the peripheral symptoms of dementia are greatly affected by the attitudes of the surrounding people. This has contributed to a growing recognition in Japan that society should not leave the care of people with dementia to only medical staff or welfare service providers. It is now considered crucial that residents have a proper understanding of dementia, and can support people with this condition in the community in which they live.

Taking these social circumstances into account, the Ministry of Health, Labour and Welfare, together with organizations concerned with dementia, launched a 10-year nationwide public campaign in FY 2005. It is called the Campaign to Understand Dementia and Build Community Networks. The campaign has been promoted by an organization called 100-Member Committee to Create Safe and Comfortable Communities for People with Dementia (in short, 100-Member Committee), consisting of about 100 organizations and individuals.

—see http://www2f.biglobe.ne.jp/~boke/dementiajp1.htm

Case example 2.5: Bruges, Belgium

Bruges in Belgium is one of the European leaders in the Dementia-Friendly Communities movement. They have engaged with shops, theatres, colleges, the local communities, and the emergency services to support people to continue to live their lives to the full in as independent a way as possible, and to enable people to have a safe space to turn to if they are lost or confused.

A significant part of the work in Bruges is the attention that has been paid to supporting families in their individual journey to adapt their relationships to the changes dementia brings and ensure that people get supported to explore their needs and wishes. A large team of volunteers and family councillors support this process in people's own homes and in the Foton Centre (meaning quantum of light), which operates an open house in the city centre offering drop-in support in a peaceful, calm setting.

> ## Case example 2.6: Plymouth, UK
>
> Plymouth has developed an active Dementia Action Alliance (DAA) involving many local organizations, including the City Council, the health service, the university, the Royal Navy Base, and the local basketball team Plymouth Raiders and many other local organizations.
>
> The Navy realized that many of its employees were struggling with balancing their responsibilities as carers with their work role. They realized that if they could provide flexibility and understanding when possible, employees, those cared for, and themselves as employers would all benefit.
>
> As Plymouth is a tourist destination, Plymouth DAA is aiming to widen its reach to make Plymouth a great place to stay for holidaymakers with dementia as well as a good place to live for local residents living with dementia. Plymouth City Council is working closely with the health service to ensure that it provides the support and help people need. In addition, it is working with its libraries and schools to increase the understanding of dementia.

Steps to communities becoming dementia-friendly

There is no single way to become dementia-friendly; several different approaches have been used. There is guidance from the Local Government Association (2012). From our work in Bradford, we have learned that there are several important principles, including:

- involving people with dementia and their family members
- involving the public sector and local government
- involving the business community
- involving the voluntary sector and community groups
- involving the community and raising awareness about how they can help
- using different approaches in different communities
- setting up a project steering group
- ensuring a shared vision of what you are trying to achieve
- providing simple checklists and tools
- learning from others who have done this work
- staying positive
- starting small
- raising the profile
- sharing what you know with others

Involving people with dementia and their family members

People living with dementia need to be central to the process. We need to find out what gets in the way of people with dementia maintaining their independence and self-confidence, and continuing to have full and fulfilling lives. This can be done by talking to people about their experiences, whether in their own homes or by inviting people with dementia and their family carers to participate in focus groups. In the case of the latter, photos of shops, banks, community centres, and cafes along with expressive smile and sad or worried faces, and a limited number of questions written in simple language can be used to help those with dementia take a full part in the conversations and express their views about how they feel when out and about in the community. (For additional suggestions, see Chapter 28.)

Areas explored in focus groups might include discussions about stressful situations and how they could be made easier, and drawing up guidelines on how organizations could become more dementia-friendly. Our focus group in Bradford has also contributed to reviewing the consultation documents about the dementia-friendly recognition process. To do this, we needed to pick out the key points of this document to make it more accessible and break it up for discussion. We have also found mystery shopping trips to businesses a useful way to gain information.

Another key way people with dementia contribute to our dementia-friendly work is by speaking at events. Having a real person, someone people can relate to talking about their experiences and feelings about having dementia, is much more powerful than having a health professional or member of the Alzheimer's Society speaking about the condition. Involving people with dementia is very important to the progress and integrity of any dementia-friendly community work. It also gives people with dementia a role they can justifiably feel valued in: a role where they are the experts, when so many of their roles appear to be diminishing.

People with dementia and family carers can have differing perspectives (see Chapter 12). As such, it is important that we find ways to validate both perspectives. Some tips for doing this include: having some ground rules for carers about not putting down or correcting the person with dementia; ensuring carers have a chance outside the meeting to tell their story if they need to; and ensuring that the feelings and dignity of the person with dementia are validated. Where possible, it may be helpful to run two groups – one for people with dementia and one for carers.

> ## Case example 2.7: An example from Bradford's focus group
>
> The group was discussing their experiences of shopping in supermarkets. One of the members who has dementia said he had no problems with shopping and went to his local supermarket regularly, while his carer gently told him and the group that he hadn't been shopping on his own for the last six months or so.
>
> It was important to be positive about the "felt" experience of the person with dementia; he felt he was able to go shopping and therefore in his mind he did. It was important not to undermine his sense of competency and self. I acknowledged the carer's remarks with a nod, and asked the person with dementia what made that shop a good place to go, and what would make it better for someone who was struggling with their memory. This moved the conversation away from his abilities or lack of them and on to a place everyone could contribute.

Whatever the approach used, it is vital to have people living with dementia as a key part of any dementia-friendly work. It is vital for the following reasons:

- They know better than anyone else what it is to live with dementia.
- They know the sorts of problems they face and are able to research problems and possible solutions through mystery shopping trips and through walking round premises and test driving systems designed to help them.
- They can be a vital part of any awareness raising undertaken and help to break down stereotypes and prejudices.
- They give your work credibility and help you practise what you preach.
- Working with people with dementia to find ways of helping them engage with the work helps us learn so much ourselves.
- Last but by no means least, it gives people with dementia roles as experts.

Involving the public sector and local government

The Alzheimer's Society in the UK has succeeded in building cross-party support for dementia-friendly communities. Internationally understanding is building, that due to an ageing population and the subsequent rise in the numbers of people with dementia, it is important to develop new approaches to enable people to live well within their communities for as long as possible. Together with ethical arguments about the rights of people living with dementia to have the support to continue to live their lives in the way they want to, there is a creditable economic argument to be made. Where the state is involved in paying for health and social care, any action that helps to support people to live in the community for longer will result in substantial savings compared with paying for more hospital admissions and long-term residential care. In *Building Dementia-friendly Communities: A Priority for Everyone*, the Alzheimer's Society (2013) calculates that a well-supported person living with dementia in the community with a supportive community and an appropriate care package costs £11,000 per year less than that person living in residential care.

Education and awareness raising about the needs of families and individuals living with dementia in general and the potential cost savings are an important way to build support with local government, be it on a district or village level. Elected members and local government staff have the potential to make a big difference in building a dementia-friendly community through the provision of appropriate services, making sure public sector employees have awareness training, and ensuring services and facilities are accessible to people living with dementia.

The emergency services, police, and hospitals also have a big part to play and can make time and cost savings if staff have appropriate training and support is given to help people live well independently. For example, a fireman from Kent spoke at an event about the fire safety checks they made for elderly residents and how they had helped a gentleman who lived on his own with dementia buy a microwave. This simple action had already reduced the number of call outs to his house for kitchen fires (they had had three call outs in the last quarter).

Involving the business community

It is not always easy to get businesses on board – personal contacts really help. For example, in Bradford the bank manager of one of our focus group members got involved. Some businesses know they have customers with memory problems, and some managers and employees have personal experience of dementia from their friends or family.

Shops, pubs, hairdressing salons, and banks should be helped to identify what they need to do to be more accessible to those living with dementia. They should review themselves and through this process write action plans addressing the issues identified. Start with general conversations with organizations considered likely to be sympathetic to the idea of dementia-friendly communities. For example, in Bradford we worked with people in organizations known to us – the Co-operative group's membership officer, the local Anglican church, and a local pharmacist. Remember three key principles:

1. Understand that any business's primary aim will be to make money so any "ask" must not conflict with this too much, must not be too costly, time consuming or have a negative effect on sales.
2. Emphasize that being more accessible to people living with dementia and their carers will be good for business; and that by taking positive action they can encourage more customers and build their standing in the community.
3. Remind them of the Equalities Act 2010 and their legal obligation to make reasonable adjustments so that their business is accessible and not discriminating for people with disabilities – and that this includes people with dementia.

Exercise 2.2: Challenges in completing an everyday task

Think about a shopping trip to buy the food you need for the week ahead. Break down the task into individual steps.

- How many steps are there?
- What additional challenges might having dementia pose for you doing your shopping?
- What do you think you would feel if you where at the till, with a queue of people behind you and couldn't remember your pin number?
- What steps could the shops or supermarkets take to make themselves more user-friendly to those with dementia and their carers?
- How would the staff's attitude and understanding impact on the person with dementia?

Involving the voluntary sector and community groups

For example, in Bradford our pilot group of organizations included a local Sikh Gurdwara, the Anglican Diocese of Bradford, a healthy living project, and a community centre. This sector very readily saw that being accessible to people with dementia was important; however, many organizations also felt under-resourced in terms of time and money. There was sometimes a fear that people with dementia might have too many or too complex needs for the organization to deal with. Raising awareness about the range of needs and abilities of people with dementia was important. People with dementia want to be part of and contribute to their local community, and organizations need to consider each person's situation as unique rather than making over-generalized assumptions.

It is useful to work in partnership with existing local organizations in the community: churches, mosques, community centres, health projects, local council neighbourhood officers, and councillors. All of these groups have access to local networks and can encourage local people to engage.

Many of these organizations are short of money and are staffed by volunteers or paid workers who have many calls on their time. So keeping things simple and looking at low-cost solutions is important. Organizations can sometimes tap into knowledge and experience of their members and associates. For example, in Bradford one of our pilot organizations traded some free room hire for some staff awareness training from a local dementia expert. Sometimes organizations have old buildings that are difficult to make dementia-friendly, particularly if their budget is very tight, but with a little knowledge and awareness staff or volunteers can look out for and offer support to people who may be lost and confused. In some buildings, low-cost solutions like simple laminated paper signs can make a big difference to helping people with memory problems navigate round the building, especially to places such as the rest room and exit.

Faith organizations like our Sikh group saw it as their religious duty to be there for all the community. Once they started thinking about dementia, it was clear to them that these were people they should be reaching out to. Many community organizations have a clear remit to be inclusive and may even be able to tap into funding or free training if they need to make changes to help them be more dementia-friendly.

Involving the community and raising awareness about how it can help

Dementia is high on the agenda of many members of the public. Most people know someone directly affected by dementia through family or friends, if they are not themselves directly affected. To make a dementia-friendly community, it is essential for the community itself to be involved. In England and Wales, the Dementia Friends initiative seeks to create a network of dementia friends and advocates (see http://www.dementiafriends.org.uk/).

To involve your community, invite people to come along to public meetings, and use the time to start to raise awareness. Involving people with dementia and carers to talk about their experiences is an effective approach to raising awareness. Providing personal stories has a real impact. Ensure that you know and support your speakers; it is important to remain positive, and focus on practical things that people can start to change.

This can be coupled with some consultation to find out what people perceive as the key issues for their community, what makes their neighbourhood a good place to live, and what could make it better if you had dementia. Finally, include a call to action. In Bradford, we ask everyone at our events to commit to do something – however big or small.

Some people will willingly volunteer their time and skills to take an active role in making change in their community and take things forward, but small, good, neighbourly actions are also vital. Neighbours, friends, and passers-by all have a role to play. Provide information and awareness raising about what dementia is and how it affects people.

You should provide community members with suggestions about how best to support and enable people with dementia. For example, people with dementia in Bradford suggested the following:

> Slow down a little when you talk, to give me a chance to keep up.

> Treat me as me – I am still here, don't just talk to my wife or husband.

> Do offer to help if I look lost or confused.

> Remind me if you see I have forgotten to put the bin out, or bring my washing in – practical things like that really help.

And things that were hurtful included:

> Feeling people are irritated with me if I am struggling over my change in a shop.

> Crossing the road and avoiding talking to me – it really hurts when people do that.

> Being criticized for telling the same story over and again.

> Being talked down to, or talked about as though I wasn't there.

Make it clear that dementia affects everyone. Engage people in thinking about what they would want to support them to continue to live well with dementia. Identify what already works in their neighbourhood to support people and what could be improved. Encourage everyone in the community to participate, as any action – no matter how small – contributes to making a community dementia-friendly.

Exercise 2.3: How does community action start or develop?

Community action can take many forms – encouraging local organizations to become more dementia-friendly; making sure there is access to support and information for people with dementia; making sure people are safe and members of the community are willing to offer assistance to someone who is struggling, lost or confused. Action may be undertaken by volunteers or staff in formal groups, but just as important is a sense of good neighbourliness.

- What are the blocks to neighbours, friends or strangers on the street offering help and support?
- What might encourage and support people to make them more likely to step in and offer support?

Using different approaches in different communities

For example, in Bradford's South Asian community the national awareness-raising campaigns have had less impact, and there is still a significant stigma around dementia. A gentler approach involving building trust, reminiscing, and talking about memories and ageing is needed. We are aiming to ensure our South Asian colleagues from our dementia support team take part in our events and are working with partner organization Meri Yaadain to raise awareness in the South Asian community (see www.meriyaadain.co.uk).

Setting up a project steering group

Key stakeholders include the local council, local members of the voluntary sector, people living with dementia, and their family carers. The remit of the steering group is to define the direction of the project.

Ensuring a shared vision of what we are trying to achieve

This should be done in partnership with others; use your steering group to develop and share your vision. Listen to and take on board views from people you want to involve.

Providing simple checklists and tools

See, for example, *Developing Dementia-friendly Communities: Learning and Guidance for Local Authorities* (LGA 2012). These checklists where drawn up by "Innovations in Dementia", and form the backbone of the checklists used in Bradford. Checklists can include the physical environment, staff awareness and training, being a dementia-friendly employer, and encouraging more access. These tools can be developed over time with feedback from the organizations that use them.

Learning from others who have done this work

As dementia-friendly work spreads, there are more and more examples to find out about. Try to make direct contact with others if you can.

Staying positive

Some people think that anyone anyone with a diagnosis of dementia is best kept at home or in residential care and should never be out and about on their own. The experience of the dementia-friendly community work internationally and the contemporary emphasis of "living well with dementia" shows these views to be outdated. Like the rest of us, people with dementia do better when they have full, active, and engaged lives. They need our support and acceptance to help them achieve this.

Starting small

Start with a small pilot group before beginning to build a larger-scale movement. For example, Bradford's dementia-friendly work started life as an awareness-raising project with organizations in the business and community sector.

Raising the profile

Use local media, local businesses, leaflet drops, and targeted mail-outs. In Bradford, we have held community meetings and consultations.

Sharing what you know with others

You won't have all the answers. Each community is different and should find its own response. By sharing effective approaches, and learning from others both in the dementia field and wider disability rights campaigns, the momentum for this work will grow.

Debates and controversies

People have differing views as to whether or not we need a kite mark to recognize a dementia-friendly community setting. This would require rigorous standards and assessment processes. Many people are of the view that we should aim for a mass campaign and make it easy for organizations and communities to sign up. However, it is also critical that dementia-friendly actions lead to real and sustainable changes that result in improved outcomes for people living with dementia. Certainly, the process needs to be adaptable and easy enough to encourage people and organizations to get started but not end up being a "tick box" exercise that has no meaning and fails to support real change.

Conclusion

Dementia-friendly communities are in a state of rapid growth in many parts of the UK, with longer established examples elsewhere in Europe and Japan. Lots of different approaches are being used with some core common elements. We now have a good understanding of the core steps required to ensure communities work towards being dementia-friendly.

Further information

Konfetti im Kopf ("Confetti in the head") uses theatre and photography in Germany to raise awareness and build a positive image of living with dementia [www.konfetti-im-kopf.de].

EC Employment, Social Affairs and Inclusion, "Ten European projects win the the Living Well with Dementia 2012 EFID awards" [http://ec.europa.eu/social/main.jsp?langId=en&catId=89&newsId=1172&furtherNews=yes].

MinnPost, dementia-friendly Bruges and the start of work in Minnesota [http://www.minnpost.com/cityscape/2013/05/toward-making-twin-cities-dementia-friendly-community].

Joseph Rowntree Foundation's "Dementia Without Walls" programme in York [http://www.jrf.org.uk/work/workarea/dementia-without-walls].

Alzheimer's Disease International's (2012) *World Alzheimer Report 2012: Overcoming the Stigma of Dementia* has lots of examples of good practice [http://www.alz.co.uk/research/WorldAlzheimerReport2012.pdf].

The Alzheimer's Society's "Dementia-friendly Communities" programme [http://www.alzheimers.org.uk/site/scripts/documents_info.php?documentID=1843].

Plymouth University news centre, "Plymouth plays a key role in PM drive to create dementia friendly communities" [http://www.plymouth.ac.uk/pages/view.asp?page=39017].

The Alzheimer's Society's (2013) Dementia-friendly financial charter [http://www.alzheimers.org.uk/site/scripts/download_info.php?fileID=1983].

References

Alzheimer's Disease International (2012) *Overcoming the Stigma of Dementia*. London: Alzheimer's Disease International.

Alzheimer's Society (2012) *Dementia 2012: A National Challenge*. London: Alzheimer's Society [http://www.alzheimers.org.uk/dementia2012].

Alzheimer's Society (2013) *Building Dementia-friendly Communities: A Priority for Everyone*. London: Alzheimer's Society.

Alzheimer's Society (2013) *Foundation Criteria for the Dementia-friendly Communities Recognition Process*. London: Alzheimer's Society [www.alzheimers.org.uk/dementiafriendlycommunities, accessed 13 September 2013].

Barnes, M. and Shardlow, P. (1996) Effective consumers and active citizens' strategies for users' influence on services and beyond, *Research, Policy and Planning*, 14(1): 33–8.

Barnes, M. and Walker, A. (1996) Consumerism versus empowerment: a principled approach to the involvement of older service users, *Policy and Politics*, 24(4): 375–93.

Bartlett, R. and O'Connor, D. (2007). From personhood to citizenship: broadening the lens for dementia practice and research, *Journal of Aging Studies*, 21(2): 107–18.

Dementia Action Alliance (2011) *National Dementia Declaration*. London: Dementia Action Alliance [http://www.dementiaaction.org.uk/assets/0000/1157/National_Dementia_Declaration_for_England.pdf].

Department of Health (2009) *Living Well with Dementia: A National Dementia Strategy*. London: Department of Health.

Department of Health (2010) *Quality Outcomes for People with Dementia: Building on the Work of the National Dementia Strategy*. London: Department of Health.

Department of Health (2012) *The Prime Minister's Challenge on Dementia*. London: The Stationery Office.

Downs M. (2013) Putting people – and compassion – first: the UK's approach to person-centered care for individuals with dementia, *Generations*, 37(3): 53–9.

Graham, N., Lindesay, J., Katona, C., Bertolote, J.M., Camus, V. *et al.* (2003) Reducing stigma and discrimination against older people with mental disorders: a technical consensus statement, *International Journal of Geriatric Psychiatry*, 18: 670–8.

Innovations in Dementia (2011) *Dementia Capable Communities: The Views of People with Dementia and Their Supporters*. Exeter: Innovations in Dementia [www.innovationsindementia.org.uk, accessed 13 September 2013].

Joseph Rowntree Foundation (2012) *Creating a Dementia-friendly York*. York: Joseph Rowntree Foundation [http://www.jrf.org.uk/sites/files/jrf/dementia-communities-york-summary.pdf].

Katsuno, T. (2005) Dementia from the inside: how people with early-stage dementia evaluate their quality of life, *Ageing and Society*, 25(2): 197–214.

Kellehear, A. (2005) *Compassionate Cities: Public Health and End-of-Life Care.* London: Routledge.

Kellehear, A. (2009) Dementia and dying: the need for a systematic policy approach, *Critical Social Policy*, 29(1): 146–57.

Kellehear, A. (2013) Compassionate communities: end-of-life care as everyone's responsibility, *QJM: An International Journal of Medicine*, 106(12): 1071–5.

King Baudouin Foundation (2010) *Improving the Quality of Life of People with Dementia: A Challenge for European Society.* High-Level Conference on Dementia in the framework of the Belgian EU Presidency 2010.

Kitwood, T. (1997) *Dementia Reconsidered: The Person Comes First.* Buckingham: Open University Press.

Local Government Association (LGA) (2012) *Developing Dementia-friendly Communities: Learning and Guidance for Local Authorities.* London: LGA [http://www.local.gov.uk/c/document_library/get_file?uuid=b6401bb0-31a8-4d57-823b-1fde6a09290e&groupid=10180].

Ministry of Health and Care Services (2008) *Dementia Plan 2015.* Oslo: Ministry of Health and Care Services.

Oliver, M. (1990) *The Politics of Disablement.* Basingstoke: Palgrave Macmillan.

Sabat, S. (2003) Malignant positioning and the predicament of people with Alzheimer's disease, in R. Harré and F. Moghaddam (eds.) *The Self and Others.* Westport, CT: Greenwood.

Scottish Government (2013) *Scotland's National Dementia Strategy 2013–2016.* Edinburgh: The Scottish Government.

Werner, P. and Heinik, J. (2008) Stigma by association and Alzheimer's disease, *Aging and Mental Health*, 12(1): 92–9.

World Health Organisation and Alzhiemer's Disease International (WHO/ADI) (2012) *Dementia: A Public Health Priority.* Geneva: WHO.

CHAPTER 3

Ethnicity and dementia

Linda Boise

> 66 Like if she was there by herself all the time and there's no one there with her, then her illness gets worse. But, if she's there and her family is there with her, her whole family, and she gets to see them all day and all night, then she will get better quicker. Otherwise the patient won't heal. Americans don't like people to be there to bother the patient. But with us Hmong, if the elderly sees their family members all the time, like grandchildren and children, it makes them happier, and that makes them heal faster. 99
>
> —Cheng Yang Madison, Wisconsin, USA

Learning objectives

By the end of this chapter, you will be able to:

■ Describe characteristics of persons from diverse ethnic groups and how these characteristics may interact with ethnicity to influence how people with dementia and their families experience dementia

■ Understand barriers that keep people from black and minority ethnic communities from obtaining the help and support they need

■ Discuss the diverse ways people understand dementia and their beliefs about family caring and how these may affect help-seeking behavior

■ Apply your understanding of the diversity in knowledge and beliefs of black and minority ethnic groups to the provision of culturally competent dementia care

Introduction

Although each individual with dementia and his or her family experience dementia uniquely, ethnicity and culture provide a foundation for one's beliefs and values about dementia and dementia care. In this chapter, we consider the many factors that affect how black and minority ethnic individuals and their families experience dementia. We draw predominantly on research from the USA and UK. The chapter begins with a discussion of the growth of the number of people with dementia in black and minority ethnic communities in the USA and UK. It then discusses characteristics of minorities and their social environments, including: physical health; socioeconomic status; education and health literacy; and household and neighborhood structures that may affect how people from these communities experience dementia. We then consider the varying ways people think about and understand dementia, the responsibilities of caring for someone with dementia, and the use of medical and social services. The chapter concludes with suggestions for improving cultural competence in serving persons with dementia and their families.

Expanding minority ethnic communities in the USA and UK

In recent years, the number of black and minority ethnic groups in the USA and UK has increased dramatically. In 2010, over one million immigrants gained legal permanent residency in the USA, and there were over 92,000 refugees and 43,550 asylees. In our increasingly global world, migration from other countries will continue in the coming decades. Combined with the relatively high birth rates within minority families compared with Caucasian families, these populations will continue to grow in the USA and UK. In fact, it is projected that in both countries, whites will be in the minority compared with all other races by about 2050 (Lievesley 2010; Henry J. Kaiser Family Foundation 2013). As immigrants settle into their new neighborhoods and establish long-term residency, the average age of immigrant groups is also rising. Given that dementia increases with age (see Chapter 1), in the coming years more people in minority ethnic communities will be affected by dementia.

Factors that interact with ethnicity to affect the experience of dementia

Prevalence of dementia

Accurate statistics on dementia among persons from different ethnic groups are hard to come by, owing in large part to the lack of available and reliable data. Existing data indicate that African Americans and Hispanics in the USA have a higher prevalence of dementia than Caucasians (Chin *et al.* 2011), although the reasons for this are unclear. Some studies suggest that the higher prevalence of diabetes and cardiovascular risk factors are the cause (Froehlich *et al.* 2001; Fitzpatrick *et al.* 2004). Others have investigated whether the measures used to assess cognitive status are unfairly biased towards classifying individuals from minority groups as having dementia (Manly 2006). Yet others attribute these differences in dementia rates to the accumulation of stressful lifetime experiences (such as poverty, illnesses, economic and social stressors) that disproportionately affect black and minority ethnic populations (Manly and Espino 2004).

Physical health

Since most people who develop dementia are over the age of 65, physical health conditions often co-exist with dementia (Maslow 2004; Artaz *et al.* 2006). For people with dementia from diverse ethnic groups, the likelihood of co-existing physical illnesses may be even greater. African Americans have a higher prevalence of diabetes and hypertension than Caucasians, both of which are risk factors for stroke and cognitive impairment (Ritchie and Lovestone 2002; Schwartz *et al.* 2004). Hispanics also have disproportionately high rates of diabetes and cardiovascular conditions, including stroke and hypertension when compared with whites (Mensah *et al.* 2005). South Asian populations in the UK are reported to have as much as six times the prevalence of diabetes as the white population there (Khuntl *et al.* 2009). Current research on dementia is increasingly focusing on the role of the cardiovascular system on dementia (Luchsinger 2012), highlighting the differential effects of these conditions on elders from black and minority ethnic groups.

Socioeconomic status, health, and dementia

Socioeconomic status, defined as the combined characteristics of income, education, and occupational status, is a major source of health disparities, particularly for persons from minority ethnic groups in the USA and UK (Townsend and Davidson 1982; Nazroo 2003; Fiscella and

Williams 2004; Pew Research Center 2006). Specifically, low socioeconomic status is associated with higher prevalence of chronic illness, more limitations in activities of daily living, and greater prevalence and more rapid cognitive decline among older adults (Kington and Smith 1997; Melzer *et al.* 2001; Schwartz *et al.* 2004). Since carers are also generally in older age groups, chronic illnesses that affect persons with dementia may also affect their carers. Such conditions as arthritis, diabetes, and cardiovascular diseases in the carer are likely to exacerbate the challenges of caring for someone with dementia (Maslow 2004).

Statistics for both the USA and UK indicate that many people from black and minority ethnic groups have lower incomes than whites. In the USA in 2009, 67% of blacks and 62% of Hispanics had household incomes less than the median and 23.5% of blacks and 16.5% of Hispanics had household incomes less than $15,000 (US Census Bureau 2012b). A similar story is revealed in the UK, where 65% of Bangladeshis, 55% of Pakistanis, and 45% of black Africans live in poverty (Joseph Rowntree Foundation 2007). It is important to keep in mind, however, that while many minorities have lower average incomes than Caucasians, there are many ethnic groups that do not have high rates of poverty, such as only 30% of black Caribbeans and 25% of Indians, proportions similar to that of whites in the UK. Even within the groups that on average have low incomes, there are many individuals with middle and higher incomes. Relevant US Census data from 2009 (US Census Bureau 2012b) show that 33% of households headed by an African American and 38% of households headed by a Latino had incomes above the median for the USA as a whole. While these statistics illustrate the disadvantage African Americans and Hispanics face as a group, they also point to the substantial number of people from these ethnic groups with at least moderate incomes. Asian Americans have a higher average income than other ethnic groups, with 61% of households having incomes above the median. The proportion of Asians with higher than average incomes has led to the assumption that Asians are an economically comfortable population group. However, a number of studies have established that there is a bimodal pattern of socioeconomic and health characteristics of Asians in the USA. Thus, while many Asians have above-average incomes, a large proportion has low incomes (Chen and Hawks 1995; Tanjasiri *et al.* 1995). Of course, many people from the majority Caucasian population have incomes below average and face similar financial challenges as ethnic minorities (US Census Bureau 2012b).

During hard economic times, such as have occurred worldwide since 2008, incomes decline and hardships increase. As shown in Figure 3.1, the median incomes for each ethnic group, including Caucasians, reported by the US Census Bureau (2012c), declined between 2000 and 2009 (using constant 2009 dollars). These figures highlight the increased economic challenges for those in the lower income brackets, especially minorities.

Barriers to services

The limited financial resources available to many black and minority elders present a critical barrier to accessing services for persons with dementia. In the USA, where many services require either insurance or direct payment, carers with low incomes have fewer options for support services such as home care, medical care, rehabilitation services, and long-term care. African American and Hispanic carers have also been found to be more likely than white carers to reduce work hours to provide family care (Covinsky *et al.* 2001), which may compound their economic disadvantage.

Access to health services is not only affected by one's income but also by one's employment history, insurance coverage, and legal status. While most older adults in the USA are covered by health insurance through Medicare (a federal health insurance program for people over 65 and those with permanent disability), Medicare covers home care or nursing home costs only for a

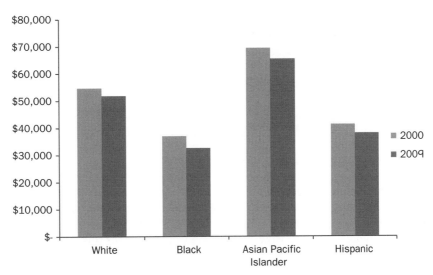

Figure 3.1: Change in median income between 2000 and 2009 (in constant dollars)
Source: US Census Bureau (2012c)

time-limited period following a hospital stay. For older immigrants, many of whom come to the USA late in life and have minimal or no work history in the USA, Medicare is often unavailable so access to health care is especially problematic. For persons under age 65, as some people with dementia and many carers are, health insurance is often unavailable. As shown in Figure 3.2, 19.5% of African Americans and 30.1% of Hispanics in the USA were uninsured in 2011 (US Census Bureau 2012d). Recent changes in the USA through the Patient Protection and Affordable Care Act passed in 2010 have improved access to health care for many Americans, especially those whose access to insurance has been limited due to pre-existing health conditions, being unemployed or underemployed, or other factors inhibiting their purchase of private insurance. The

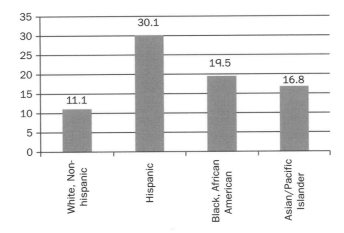

Figure 3.2: Percentage of adults uninsured in the USA by ethnic group
Source: US Census Bureau (2012d)

majority of reforms are scheduled to begin in 2014, assuming there are no repeals by Congress or pushbacks by the President or his administration.

Support services are even less accessible for people with limited means. States and regions within states vary substantially in the kinds and extent of services such as daycare, respite care, assisted living, home health, and homemaker services.

Exercise 3.1: Hard choices

Think of an older person you know who has limited income.

- What health problems do they have?
- Are there health services this person is unable to use because he or she cannot afford them?
- Are there resources that could help him or her to obtain these services at reduced cost? What is involved in applying for these? How challenging would it be for this person to apply for them given the level of literacy and knowledge about the community?
- Thinking about this person and others in similar situations, would you say your community is resource-rich or resource-poor for older persons with limited finances?

Education, literacy, and health literacy

Level of education, the ability to read and understand what one is reading (literacy), and knowledge about health and health resources (health literacy) are crucial foundations for addressing one's health needs.

Education and literacy

One's level of education is important for job attainment and is a strong predictor of income (US Bureau of Labor Statistics 2006) both during years of employment and in retirement. As shown in Figure 3.3, the proportion of US residents with college degrees varies substantially among ethnic groups. Within these broad categories are substantial variations among subgroups. For

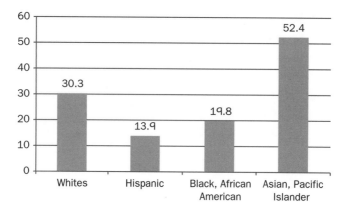

Figure 3.3: Percentage of US adults with college degree by ethnic group
Source: US Census Bureau (2012a)

example, among Hispanics, who have the greatest disadvantage with respect to education, there is substantial variation by country of origin in the proportions of college graduates: 10.6% for Mexicans, 17.5% for Puerto Ricans, and 26.2% for Cubans (US Census Bureau 2012a).

Literacy, the ability to understand verbal and written communication, is critical for functioning successfully in today's highly technical and impersonal society. While literacy is closely linked with education, the number of years of education does not fully explain how well one can read and communicate. Low education combined with a low level of English proficiency may exacerbate the difficulties of managing a serious chronic illness such as dementia, inhibiting effective communication with health and service providers, and jeopardizing the doctor–patient relationship. When one's preferred language is not the majority language, obtaining a clear medical understanding of dementia and its implications for treatment and care are that much more difficult. It is not just the ability to speak the language of the dominant culture that is important. Equally important is how comfortable one is in conversing in that language with others such as health providers. In 2011, 20.8% of US residents aged 5 or older spoke languages other than English at home. Among these, 41% spoke English less than "very well" (Migration Policy Institute, www.migrationinformation.org). In one study, members of African American, Latino, and Asian groups often felt that medical staff judged them unfairly based on how well they spoke English (Johnson *et al.* 2004).

Language and literacy may also affect the diagnosis of dementia. Manly, a neuropsychologist working in New York City, notes that one's level of education is used as a factor in determining the threshold for classifying individuals as demented or not demented on cognitive tests, such as the Mini-Mental State Examination (MMSE) (Folstein *et al.* 1975). She suggests that more sensitive measures such as degree of literacy may be more accurate for classifying one's true cognitive status, particularly for African Americans and other persons of color who grew up during segregation in the USA (Manly and Espino 2004).

Health literacy

Health literacy, the ability to read and understand health information, is a kind of literacy. As with literacy in general, there is no perfect correspondence between level of education and health literacy, and ethnicity may play a role in this. Roberts and colleagues at the University of Michigan found in an African American and Caucasian sample of mostly highly educated adults, that African Americans tended to have poorer knowledge of Alzheimer's disease (AD), fewer information sources, and a lower perceived threat of this illness (Roberts *et al.* 2003). In a study of blacks and whites with less than a high school education, the proportions with limited health literacy were substantially different: 80.7% of black men and 65.6% of black women had limited health literacy compared with 46.7% of white men and 32.9% of white women (Sudore *et al.* 2006). Ayalon and Areán (2004) found that African Americans and Asians had significantly lower scores on a knowledge test about Alzheimer's despite comparable years of education (Hispanics, who had lower levels of education, also had poor scores on AD knowledge). The reasons for these gaps in knowledge about dementia are unclear but they do suggest that greater effort is needed to deliver effective education for minority groups about dementia.

Household and neighborhood structures

People with dementia and their family carers live within a family, household, neighborhood, and community. These structures can have a profound effect on the quality of life of people affected by dementia. One source of diversity among people from different ethnic groups is household structure (Wilmoth 2001). Hispanic elders are especially likely to be cared for in multi-generational households (AARP 2001). African Americans are less likely than other ethnic groups to be married and more likely to be living in households headed by women (Stoller and Cutler 1992). Not surprisingly, African Americans with dementia are less likely to be cared for by a spouse than white sufferers and are more likely to be cared for by siblings, adult children, grandchildren, or other non-spousal family members (Peek et al. 2000; Kosberg et al. 2007).

In general, people from black and minority ethnic groups are more likely than Caucasians to live in close proximity to extended family members. Societal forces, however, may inhibit families from supporting their older members to the extent they need. Although new immigrants often move to communities and neighborhoods where others from their home country live, the mere presence of extended family members is no assurance that they or their carers will receive the support they need. In a study of several Asian subgroups of carers in Britain (Sikhs, Hindu, Bangladeshi, and Pakistani), Katbamna et al. (2004) found that although these carers lived in neighborhoods with other extended family members, they reported limited support from their social networks. The high rate of people of working age who are employed – often both husband and wife are working to make ends meet, while often caring for young children as well – is likely to inhibit younger relatives from taking an older relative with dementia into their home. An additional problem for immigrants is that when younger family members emigrate to western societies in search of jobs or education, their parents or other older relatives may remain in their home country, relegating the emigrating members to the challenges of long-distance caring.

A recent phenomenon of gentrification in traditionally ethnic inner-city neighborhoods has left many minority elders (especially African Americans) without neighborhood-based supports. The elders may be able to remain in homes they purchased many years previously, but their children are unable to purchase homes in these neighborhoods when home values rise beyond their means. Thus, the traditional neighborhood-based caring system is breaking down in many urban communities (Minnis 2011) and the complexion of people living in them makes for a less familiar and comfortable environment for older residents. Some communities are working together to ensure that people with dementia feel comfortable residing in and moving about in them. Such programs need to be broadly inclusive of the diverse populations living within the community. In Bradford, England, for example, community services, business and community members have launched a campaign to promote a dementia-friendly city (University of Bradford 2001).

Beliefs about dementia and caring

Understandings of dementia

The lens through which people view symptoms of dementia can affect whether they seek a medical diagnosis, community resources, and services. Dementia may be viewed as a disease, a consequence of old age, or as a mental illness (Henderson and Guitierrez-Mayka 1992; Jones et al. 2006; Downs et al. 2008). In some cultures, the symptoms of dementia may be thought to represent a religious or mystical experience (Downs et al. 2006; Mackenzie 2006). In others, dementia may be viewed as punishment for bad behavior (Mukadam et al. 2011). In a qualitative study with a multi-ethnic sample of African American, Latino, Asian-American, and Anglo family carers, Hinton et al. (2005) identified two distinct paradigms for understanding dementia, a "biomedical model" that views dementia as a disease with underlying brain pathology and a "folk model" that views the signs of dementia from a non-medical perspective, for example as "normal aging", forgetfulness", "difficult personality", or "crazy". They found that many people from all of these groups drew on explanations that combined folk and biomedical thinking, although carers from non-Caucasian ethnic groups and those with lower formal education were more likely to hold folk explanatory models of dementia or to combine both biomedical and folk models.

Beliefs about caring and service use

For most persons with dementia, families are a primary source of care. The severity of cognitive impairment, the extent to which the person with dementia exhibits troubling behaviors, and access to or unavailability of financial resources may affect families' need for and use of formal services, but values and beliefs about dementia and family responsibilities may overlay carers' response to the demands of caring. Family responsibilities about caring and/or feelings of shame and stigma about dementia may prevent them to seek help (Youn *et al.* 1999; Mukadam *et al.* 2011). In a systematic review of studies in the USA, UK, and Australia, Cooper *et al.* (2010) found substantial evidence that persons with dementia from minority and ethnic groups were often diagnosed later than whites and with more severe symptoms and were less likely to use anti-dementia medications and 24-hour care. In a study of older, recently hospitalized Medicaid recipients in Minnesota, Boult and Boult (1995) found that being Asian (in a sample that was 76% Hmong) was strongly associated with infrequent doctor visits.

In addition to the beliefs people have about dementia, expectations about family responsibility for care, structural factors that create barriers to access, one's prior experiences with health services or other providers or that of one's friends, can influence receptivity to seeking care. There is abundant evidence that people from black and minority ethnic communities have unsatisfactory experiences with health and social services more often than whites. African Americans often report physician disrespect (Mahoney *et al.* 2005) and both African Americans and Latinos have reported high levels of distrust of physicians (Armstrong *et al.* 2007). In a survey conducted in a US health care system, Johnson *et al.* (2004) reported that African American, Hispanic, and Asian adults were more likely than Caucasians to believe that they would receive better medical care if they belonged to a different race or ethnic group and to report having experienced racial bias in care they received.

Exercise 3.2: Talking with a new immigrant family in the community

Imagine that you meet an Indian family that has just moved into your neighborhood. When they find out you work in a health center, the daughter mentions to you that she is concerned about her father. He has been very forgetful and acting strangely. From what she tells you, it appears that he has signs of dementia. However, when you suggest that she take her father to the medical center for an evaluation, she changes the subject.

- Why might she be reluctant to talk with you about her concerns?
- What would you do? Drop the subject and wait for it to arise again? Talk with her at a later time about her concerns? How would you bring up the topic? What would you hope to achieve in talking with her?

Degree of acculturation

An important source of variation within ethnic groups is the degree of acculturation. Manly and Espino (2004: 100) define acculturation as "the level at which people participate in the values, language, and practices of their own ethnic community versus those of the dominant culture". The extent of acculturation often influences how people blend traditional beliefs about illness and caring with western medical perspectives and seeking of help. Mahoney *et al.* (2005) found that Latinos in the USA often expressed fears that acculturation would end family home care. Being less acculturated has been associated with a lack of knowledge of community resources, lower likelihood of seeking services (Otilingam and Gatz 2005), engaging in more risky health behaviors (Manly and Espino 2004), and higher risk of depression (Gonzalez *et al.* 2001). Acculturation has also been shown to affect the results of cognitive testing for blacks and Hispanics (Arnold *et al.* 1994; Artiola *et al.* 1998).

Case example 3.1: Kaltuun

Ahmed had been living in the USA for about 10 years, working as a home care aid, when his 70-year-old mother, Kaltuun, moved from their native country of Somalia to be with her son and his children. Ahmed's sister, Leyla, accompanied her mother on the long and tiring trip. As soon as they arrived, Ahmed noticed that things weren't right with his mother. She seemed very nervous, more than he would have expected. At first, he thought this was because of the exhausting trip and dramatic change between her new home and her native country, but, as time went by, he became more concerned. Even after several weeks, she seemed confused by her surroundings, unable to find her way from her bedroom to the kitchen, fearful about going outside, and forgetful of her grandchildren's names.

Ahmed asked his sister whether she was concerned, but she said it was just that their mother was old. Ahmed mentioned his concerns to his nurse supervisor who recommended that he bring her in to see one of the doctors who worked with the agency. When it was time for the appointment with the doctor, his mother refused to go. Ahmed's sister became angry with him, saying that it was shameful for him to subject his mother to such an intrusive examination. He understood that neither his sister nor his mother would be comfortable with western medicine, so Ahmed dropped the idea of a medical evaluation for the time being.

Soon after, Ahmed's sister returned home. Despite his sympathy with his mother's feelings, Ahmed felt that a medical evaluation was needed, not only for his mother's memory problems and unexplainable behaviors but also for her physical health. Ahmed knew that the doctor was a kind and trustworthy professional. The doctor addressed Kaltuun's general health, diabetes, and arthritis with the assistance of an interpreter but was unable to get a clear picture of Kaltuun's cognitive status. He suggested that Kaltuun return in six months. She was, however, visibly upset by the visit and didn't understand why the doctor was asking her so many questions. Ahmed wasn't sure if he should bring her in again.

Ahmed's mother continued to decline and, from his work with other elderly clients and his training in home care, it became clear to Ahmed that his mother was experiencing dementia. He began to worry about her being left alone when he had to work but he could not afford to hire a sitter or aide. Ahmed was well connected to the Somali community where he lived but his mother had not ventured outside much. Ahmed decided to invite some of the older women to his home for a visit with his mother, hoping that they might help out. Only one woman came. Ahmed was disappointed, but several days later, the woman returned with her daughter and a plate of traditional foods.
For a while, members of the community visited periodically, but these visits soon tapered off. Ahmed finally decided that his mother needed to be cared for in a nursing home, though he knew there would not be many, if any, Somali or other African residents there and that his mother would be very upset about being there. He felt terribly guilty but he did not know of any alternative.

Providing culturally competent care

Providing culturally competent dementia care is integral to excellence in dementia care (Mackenzie 2006). The goal should be to promote optimal wellness and to enhance families' efficacy within the conceptual framework of their understanding of the affected person's condition. The first step toward developing culturally competent care and support is to acknowledge that culture and ethnicity guide and affect expectations and behavior. Becoming aware of one's own cultural attitudes and beliefs can provide a basis for understanding how a person's life experiences may influence one's beliefs about dementia and caring. It is also valuable to consider the similarities as well as the differences in how people from diverse cultures experience dementia. For example, across diverse ethnic groups, early signs of dementia are often interpreted initially as normal aging. The explanations for why the person is forgetting or acting differently from how they previously behaved are likely to incorporate some elements of non-medical (folk/lay) reasoning. Also, families in every ethnic group have a sense of obligation and responsibility for caring for a relative with dementia, although how this plays out in specific families and communities may vary. Regardless of beliefs about the origin and causes of dementia, coping with day-to-day care requires knowledge, skill, and support. It is fair to assume that for most carers, of whatever ethnic or cultural background, caring for someone with Alzheimer's or other form of dementia is, at least at times, a stressful undertaking.

Providing care for persons with dementia from diverse ethnic groups should be approached from a perspective of discovery. Taking into consideration the many factors that can influence the experience of dementia, the provision of care for persons with dementia and their families requires an individualized and flexible approach that seeks to understand and accommodate the variety of experiences of carer and cared for. In response to the needs of diverse ethnic groups, many health systems now provide guidance in delivering services for persons from diverse cultural and language groups. As you gather information from a person with dementia and/or their family members, consider the following:

- Does he or she associate dementia symptoms with disease, with the inevitable progression of old age or other causes?
- Do the signs of dementia merit a clinical evaluation? Does the affected individual and members of that person's family and social network agree?
- Do they view behaviors associated with dementia as best kept hidden from neighbors, other family members, and friends?
- What are the strengths and abilities in the person with dementia?
- What decisions can the person with dementia participate in making?
- What kinds of formal help or assistance does the person with dementia and his or her family members desire and need?

Box 3.1 lists some questions to ask the person with cognition problems and/or the family when developing a culturally responsive dementia care plan (see also Chapter 20).

Box 3.1: Developing a culturally responsive dementia care plan

The goal is to determine a mutually acceptable plan for treatment, care, or support. The plan may incorporate community resources, family members and friends, and both traditional and western medical providers. It may include alternative treatments, spiritual or cultural practices.

(continued)

Questions to consider:

- What language do you prefer to speak when receiving medical care?
- In what language do you prefer to receive your written materials?
- What do you think has caused the dementia ("memory loss", "Alzheimer's disease" or other term as appropriate)?
- What kind of help ("treatment") are you seeking?
- What results do you hope to achieve?
- What have you done already to deal with this concern/problem?
- Have you sought advice from friends, alternative healers, or other practitioners?
- When you are sick, whom do you usually go to for help or treatment?
- Are you taking any treatments, medicines, or home remedies?
- Who from your family should we involve in the care plan?

Regardless of the primary language a person speaks or their ethnic group, clear communication between people and their health providers is essential. Communicating with patients and their families about dementia is more an art than a science (Boise and Connell 2005). When working with black and minority families, it is important to acknowledge the unique perspectives of the individual and his or her family and assist them in identifying their needs within their cultural frame. Be attentive to the varying levels of familiarity with the English language and acculturation to western society. Translation of complex medical information in ways that will helpfully guide families through the ever-unfolding path of dementia is needed. Professionals often warn against using a static stage-based approach to counseling families about the progression of dementia, but finding ways to communicate with families about the anticipated transitions the person will go through, acknowledging and preparing people for the inevitable uncertainty of what lies ahead, requires skill, sensitivity, and tact. Managers and supervisors must recognize that culturally responsive and sensitive care takes time and attention to the unique characteristics and needs of the individuals to be served.

An open and non-judgmental discussion with the person with dementia and with their family members or significant others about how their culture affects their understanding of dementia, their values related to care, and their needs provides the opportunity to ascertain how best to provide culturally appropriate care for this person and their family. Engaging in this conversation may, at times, be challenging and even awkward for the provider. Manly, a neuropsychologist at Columbia University, whose clinical practice and research often requires gathering detailed information about clients' cultural experiences and perspectives, offers helpful advice for interviewing clients or patients from diverse cultures:

> We have found that asking participants about their cultural and education experience can be weaved into a standard interview assessing demographic variables; however, the comfort level of the participant is largely determinant on the comfort level of the interviewers in discussing these issues. Like any other set of questions that are potentially sensitive, the interviewer must have had established good rapport with the interviewee, should spend time to provide sufficient explanation of why questions about educational history, literacy level, and cultural background are being asked, ensure the participant that their responses will remain confidential, and welcome any feedback the interviewee may have about the questions.

—Manly (2006)

Given the possibility that black and minority ethnic people and other minorities have had unsatisfactory experiences with services, providers should seek to build trust and respect when serving families from these ethnic groups. In recent years, a number of health and service providers have developed and adapted programs to better serve diverse ethnic groups. Not only should such programs be grounded in culture, language, and literacy, they should also allow for discussion of people's hesitations about receiving care and should encourage people to be open about their concerns about medical providers and other persons in authority. See examples in Box 3.2.

Box 3.2: Establishing positive relationships with doctors

A number of programs have been developed that promote positive communication and partnering relationships between doctors and patients. One program offered by the Alzheimer's Association is "Partnering with your Doctor". This program, which aims to empower patients and family members to effectively communicate their concerns and needs to health providers, may have particular application for persons from diverse ethnic groups and is available in English and Spanish (www.alz.org/we_can_help_partnering_with_your_doctor.asp). Other helpful online materials in English and Spanish can be found at www.njha.com/PFP/consumers.aspx (New Jersey Hospital Association) and www.nia.nih.gov/health/publication/talking-your-doctor-guide-older-people.

Many education materials are available in Spanish, Arabic, Chinese, Vietnamese, Korean, Russian, and other languages from the Alzheimer's Association (USA) and the Alzheimer's Society (UK). In the USA, federal laws require health care organizations to translate "vital" documents for patients with limited English proficiency. Health and service providers are expected to provide professional translation services for patients and their carers, but translation alone may not be enough to adequately address patients' and clients' need. Given the wide variations in educational levels, socioeconomic status, and comfort people have in group learning, Gallagher-Thompson *et al.* (1996) recommend that services be presented with a multi-modal approach consisting of oral, written, visual, and interactive elements.

Although worthwhile services are available for family carers and persons with dementia, many of these have not been adapted for use with specific ethnic or cultural groups. A helpful strategy is to work with representatives of the groups to be served to explore ways in which these programs can be adapted. Gonzalez and Lorig (1996: 160–1) offer valuable recommendations for working with community members, including using case examples that are specific and relevant for the cultural group being served, creating explanations or descriptions that fit people's understanding of the key concepts, and incorporating a group's cultural beliefs and practices into the program. Attention should also be devoted to how programs serving diverse ethnic groups are publicized. This needs to be sensitive to the words that best explain for the target group whom the program is intended for and the nature of the program. Many people, for example, will not respond to a program for "carers" (or the direct translation of that word in a language other than English), as they may view themselves as caring family members rather than as givers of care.

Providing culturally appropriate and responsive care for persons with dementia and their families is a responsibility that must be addressed at all levels of the social and health care system. The provision of care takes place within a complex system of individual, family, and neighborhood influences, and in health and social care systems supported by public and private sector resources. Training is needed to ensure that, regardless of the cultural attributes of patients and clients, providers will offer appropriate and sensitive care.

Training in culturally competent care is important but attention to the way health care is delivered and how resources are allocated in society are equally important. Western societies have yet to eliminate the disparities that exist among cultures. Even as we seek to redress these inequities, the values and needs of people from diverse cultural groups are likely to change continuously over time. Changes in immigration patterns, global economies, and governmental policies are constantly in flux. New immigrant groups arrive daily from regions of the world where health, health needs, and beliefs may be quite different from those of earlier immigrant groups. Subgroups within broad ethnic categories will have their own unique needs.

Debates and controversies

How best to ensure effective and responsive educational programs

One area of controversy is the extent to which simple translation of educational materials into the language of the minority ethnic group being served is desirable when resources are not available to develop culturally tailored materials. Government programs and policy sometimes imply that the provision of information in the language of a particular ethnic group is sufficient. Such an approach, however, fails to address the differences in how people from different ethnic groups may understand dementia care.

Understanding cultural differences means digging deeper into the habits, life patterns, relationships, and beliefs that are grounded in one's community and traditions. Such considerations have led some researchers to question whether the basic framework of self-efficacy that underlies some caregiver interventions developed for westernized cultures can be applied to other groups. These researchers describe the construct of "familism" found in Latino and Asian cultures (Gallagher-Thompson *et al.* 1996; Youn *et al.* 1999; Dilworth-Anderson and Gibson 2002; Gaugler *et al.* 2006). Luna *et al.* (1996: 267) define "familism" as "the perceived strength of family bonds and sense of loyalty to family", and point out that this conceptual frame "undoubtedly relates to family members' propensity to provide care to elder relatives". Although this has not been examined with scientific rigour, values based in familism may conflict with concepts of self-efficacy, which is a uniquely individualistic concept, and is an area worthy of further examination.

Ethnicity and stress

Another question asked by some researchers is whether caring for someone with dementia is more or less stressful for people from black and other ethnic minorities than for people from the majority white culture. In their review, Pinquart and Sorensen (2005) found that Hispanic and Asian American carers reported higher levels of depression than white carers. In contrast, Haley *et al.* (2004) reported lower stress for African American carers. Haley and colleagues also reported that African American carers rated memory and behavior problems of their family member with dementia as less distressing than Caucasian carers, and reported higher appraisals of the benefits of caring. Given the lower average incomes and high levels of morbidity among African Americans, these are surprising findings that not all experts would agree with. But if the findings are valid, it would be worth investigating how African Americans successfully cope with the demands of caring. Findings by Gitlin *et al.* (2007) and Dilworth-Anderson *et al.* (2002) suggest that internal resources, such as appraisal and religious coping, may protect African Americans from some of the negative consequences of caring.

Health reform

At the time of writing, a hotly debated issue that is relevant to this chapter is raging in the USA – what will be the shape of the US health care system? Will it essentially be a government-run program similar to the present US Medicare program for older adults and the disabled and the British health system, or will it be a program guided by the federal government but administered and managed by private health insurers? As in the UK, the cost of health care is a critical concern. The needs to ensure that the developing health system attends to the unique needs of all patients and that it emphasizes health promotion and prevention are of particular relevance for minorities. This evolving system offers the opportunity, with diligent activism both within the health care system and in communities, to tailor health services to the needs of all individuals, including those from diverse ethnic groups.

Conclusion

From this review of ethnicity and the experience of dementia, it should be clear that ethnicity plays an important role in beliefs about, and responses to, dementia. It should be equally apparent that regardless of one's ethnic identity, it is hard to pin down from a few demographic or cultural attributes what each person affected by dementia thinks about or needs. Individuals, whether from the majority or minority culture, are distinct in the combination of their understanding of dementia, education, literacy, economic resources, household composition, and community. A person's attitudes and beliefs, their family dynamics and perspectives, and the social networks they travel in can all influence how dementia is experienced. As a provider of services and care, thinking in terms of the multiplicity of factors rather than of a static concept of ethnicity may be a more fruitful approach to understanding the forces that shape how individuals from black and minority ethnic groups understand and cope with dementia.

Further information

The Family Caregiver Alliance is a community-based non-profit organization in the USA that addresses the needs of families and friends providing long-term care at home [https://www.caregiver.org/caregiver/jsp/home.jsp].

The Alzheimer's Disease Education and Referral (ADEAR) Center web site provides information and resources about Alzheimer's disease, and is run by the National Institute on Aging (NIA) in the USA [http://www.nia.nih.gov/alzheimers].

The Alzheimer's Association has a wealth of downloadable materials in English, Spanish, and Chinese and resources in all states in the USA [www.alz.org].

The Alzheimer's Society (UK) has a series of fact sheets on various aspects of Alzheimer's and caring, including "What is dementia?", "What is Alzheimer's disease?", and "How the GP can help", many of which are translated into French, Chinese, Arabic, and other languages [www.alzheimers.org.uk].

References

AARP (2001) *In the Middle: A Report on the Multicultural Boomers Coping with Family and Aging Issues.* A National Study Conducted for AARP, July.

Armstrong, K., Ravenell, K.L., McMurphy, S. and Putt, M. (2007) Racial/ethnic differences in physician distrust in the United States, *American Journal of Public Health*, 97: 1283–9.

Arnold, B.R., Montgomery, G.T., Castenada, I. and Longoria, R. (1994) Acculturation and performance of Hispanics on selected Halstead-Reitan neuropsychological tests, *Assessment*, 1: 239–48.

Artaz, M.A., Boddaert, J., Heriche-Taillandier, E., Dieudonne, B. and Verny, M. (2006) Medical comorbidity in Alzheimer's disease: baseline characteristics of the REAL.FR Cohort, *Revue de Medecine Interne*, 27(2): 91–7.

Artiola, I., Fortuny, L., Healton, R.K. and Hermosillo, D. (1998) Neuropsychological comparisons of Spanish-speaking participants from the US–Mexico border region versus Spain, *Journal of the International Neuropsychological Society*, 4: 363–79.

Ayalon, L. and Areán, P.A. (2004) Knowledge of Alzheimer's disease in four ethnic groups of older adults, *International Journal of Geriatric Psychiatry*, 19: 51–7.

Boise, L. and Connell, C.M. (2005) Diagnosing dementia: what to tell the patient and family, *Geriatrics and Aging*, 8(5): 48–51.

Boult, L. and Boult, C. (1995) Underuse of physician services by older Asian-Americans, *Journal of the American Geriatric Society*, 43: 408–11.

Chen, M.S. and Hawks, B.L. (1995) A debunking of the myth of healthy Asian Americans and Pacific Islanders, *American Journal of Health Promotion*, 9(4): 261–8.

Chin, A.L., Negash, S. and Hamilton. R. (2011) Diversity and disparity in dementia: the impact of ethnoracial differences in Alzheimer's disease, *Alzheimer's Disease and Associated Disorders*, 25(3): 187–95.

Cooper, C., Tandy, A.R., Balamurali, T.B.S. and Livingston, G. (2010) A systematic review and meta-analysis of ethnic differences in the use of dementia treatment, care, and research, *American Journal of Geriatric Psychiatry*, 18(3): 193–203.

Covinsky, K.E., Eng, C., Lui, L., Sand, L.P., Sehgal, A.R. *et al.* (2001) Reduced employment in caregivers of frail elders: impact of ethnicity, patient clinical characteristics, and carer characteristics, *Journals of Gerontology A: Biological Sciences and Medical Sciences*, 56(11): 707–13.

Dilworth-Anderson, P. and Gibson, B.E. (2002) The cultural influence of values, norms, meanings, and perceptions in understanding dementia in ethnic minorities, *Alzheimer's Disease and Associated Disorders*, 16 (Suppl. 2): S56–S63.

Dilworth-Anderson, P., Williams, I.C. and Gibson, B.E. (2002) Issues of race, ethnicity, and culture in caring research: a 20-year review (1980–2000), *The Gerontologist*, 42(2): 237–72.

Downs, M., Mackenzie, J. and Clare, L. (2006) Understandings of dementia: explanatory models and their implications for the person with dementia and therapeutic effort, in J.C. Hughes, S.J. Louw and S.R. Sabat (eds.) *Dementia: Mind, Meaning and Person.* Oxford: Oxford University Press, pp. 235–59.

Downs, M., Clare, L. and Anderson, E. (2008) Dementia as a bio-psychosocial condition: implications for practice and research, in R.T. Woods and L. Clare (eds.) *Handbook of the Clinical Psychology of Ageing* (2nd edn). Chichester: Wiley.

Fiscella, K. and Williams, D.R. (2004) Health disparities based on socioeconomic inequities: implications for urban health care, *Academic Medicine*, 79(12): 1139–47.

Fitzpatrick, A.L., Kuller, L.H. and Ives, D.G. (2004) Incidence and prevalence of dementia in the Cardiovascular Health Study, *Journal of the American Geriatric Society*, 52: 195–204.

Folstein, M.F., Folstein, S.E. and McHugh, P.R. (1975) 'Mini-mental state': a practical method for grading the cognitive state of patients for the clinician, *Journal of Psychiatric Research*, 12: 189–98.

Froehlich, T.E., Bogardus, S.T., Jr. and Inouye, S.K. (2001) Dementia and race: are there differences between African Americans and Caucasians?, *Journal of the American Geriatric Society*, 49: 477–84.

Gallagher-Thompson, D., Talamantes, M., Ramirez, R. and Valverde, I. (1996) Service delivery issues and recommendations for working with Mexican American family carers, in G. Yeo and D. Gallagher-Thompson (eds.) *Ethnicity and the Dementias.* Washington, DC: Taylor & Francis, pp. 137–52.

Gaugler, J.E., Kane, R.L., Kane, R.A. and Newcomer, R. (2006) Predictors of institutionalization in Latinos with dementia, *Journal of Cross Cultural Gerontology*, 21: 139–55.

Gitlin, L.N., Hauck, W.W., Dennis, M.P. and Schulz, R. (2007) Depressive symptoms in older African-American and white adults with functional difficulties: the role of control strategies, *Journal of the American Geriatric Society*, 55 (7): 1023–30.

Gonzalez, H.M., Haan, M.H. and Hinton, L. (2001) Acculturation and the prevalence of depression in older Mexican Americans: baseline results of the Sacramento area Latino Study on Aging, *Journal of the American Geriatric Society*, 49: 948–53.

Gonzalez, V.M. and Lorig, K. (1996) Working cross-culturally, in K. Lorig (ed.) *Patient Education: A Practical Approach*. Thousand Oaks, CA: Sage, pp. 151–71.

Haley, W.E., Gitlin, L.N., Wisniewski, S.R., Mahoney, D.F., Coon, D.W. *et al.* (2004) Well-being, appraisal, and coping in African American and Caucasian dementia carers: findings from the REACH study, *Aging and Mental Health*, 8 (4): 316–29.

Henderson, J.N. and Guitierrez-Mayka, M. (1992) Ethnocultural themes in caring to Alzheimer's disease patients in Hispanic families, *Clinical Gerontologist*, 11: 59–74.

Henry J. Kaiser Family Foundation (2013) *Health Coverage by Race and Ethnicity*. Washington, DC: Henry J. Kaiser Family Foundation

Hinton, L., Franz, C.E., Yeo, G. and Levkoff, S.E. (2005) Conceptions of dementia in a multiethnic sample of family carers, *Journal of the American Geriatric Society*, 53: 1405–10.

Johnson, R.L., Saha, S., Arbelaez, J.J., Beach, M.C. and Cooper, L.A. (2004) Racial and ethnic differences in patient perceptions of bias and cultural competence in health care, *Journal of General Internal Medicine*, 19: 101–10.

Jones, R.S., Chow, T.W. and Gatz, M. (2006) Asian Americans and Alzheimer's disease: assimilation, culture, and beliefs, *Journal of Aging Studies*, 20: 11–25.

Joseph Rountree Foundation (2007) *Poverty Rates among Ethnic Groups in Great Britain* [www.jrf.org.uk/publications/poverty-rates-among-ethnic-groups-great-britain, accessed 24 September 2013].

Katbamna, S., Ahmad, W., Bhakta, P., Baker, R. and Parker, G. (2004) Do they look after their own? Informal support for South Asian carers, *Health and Social Care in the Community*, 12(5): 398–406.

Khuntl, K., Kumar, S. and Brodie, J. (2009) *Diabetes UK and South Asian Health Foundation Recommendations on Diabetes Research Priorities for British South Asians*. London: Diabetes UK.

Kington, R.S. and Smith, J.P. (1997) Socioeconomic status and racial and ethnic differences in function status associated with chronic diseases, *American Journal of Public Health*, 87: 805–10.

Kosberg, J.I., Kaufman, A.V., Burgio, L.D., Leeper, J.D. and Sun, F. (2007) Family caring to those with dementia in rural Alabama: racial similarities and differences, *Journal of Aging and Health*, 19(1): 3–21.

Lievesley, N. (2010) *The Future Ageing of the Ethnic Minority Population of England and Wales*. London: Runnymede and the Center for the Policy on Ageing.

Luchsinger, J.A. (2012) Type 2 diabetes and cognitive impairment: linking mechanisms, *Journal of Alzheimer's Disease*, 30(Suppl. 2): S185–S198.

Luna, I., Torres de Ardon, E., Lim, Y.M., Cromwell, S.L., Phillips, L.R. *et al.* (1996) The relevance of familism in cross-cultural studies of family caring, *Western Journal of Nursing Research*, 18(3): 267–83.

Mackenzie, J. (2006) Stigma and dementia: South Asian and Eastern European family carers negotiating stigma in two cultures – dementia, *International Journal of Social Research and Practice*, 5: 233–48.

Mahoney, D.F., Cloutterbuck, J., Neary, S. and Zhan, L. (2005) African American, Chinese, and Latino family carers' impressions of the onset and diagnosis of dementia: cross-cultural similarities and differences, *The Gerontologist*, 45(6): 783–92.

Manly, J.J. (2006) Deconstructing race and ethnicity: implications for measurement of health outcomes, *Medical Care*, 44: S10–S16.

Manly, J.J. and Espino, D.V. (2004) Cultural influences on dementia recognition and management, *Clinics in Geriatric Medicine*, 20(1): 93–119.

Maslow, K. (2004) Dementia and serious co-existing medical conditions: a double whammy, *Nursing Clinics of North America*, 39(3): 561–79.

Melzer, D., Izmirlian, G., Leveille, S.G. and Guralnik, J.M. (2001) Educational differences in the prevalence of mobility disability in old age: the dynamics of incidence, mortality, and recovery, *Journals of Gerontology B: Social Sciences*, 56: S294–S301.

Mensah, G.A., Mokdad, A.H., Ford, E.S., Greenlund, K.J. and Croft, J.B. (2005) State of disparities in cardiovascular health in the United States, *Circulation*, 111(10): 1233–41.

Minnis, G. (2011) Gentrification pushing African Americans out of cities, *Black America Web* [www.blackamericaweb. com, accessed 12 September 2013].

Mukadam, N., Cooper, C. and Livingston, G. (2011) A systematic review of ethnicity and pathways to care in dementia, *International Journal of Geriatric Psychiatry*, 26: 12–20.

Nazroo, J.Y. (2003) The structuring of ethnic inequalities in health: economic position, racial discrimination, and racism, *American Journal of Public Health*, 93(2): 277–84.

Otilingam, P.G. and Gatz, M. (2005) Perceptions of dementia among Asian Indian Americans: does acculturation matter?, *The Gerontologist*, 45(Suppl.): 348.

Peek, M.K., Coward, R.T. and Peek, C.W. (2000) Race, aging and care: can differences in family and household structure account for race variations in family care?, *Research on Aging*, 22(2): 117–42.

Pew Research Center (2006) *2005 American Community Survey*. Washington, DC: Pew Research Center.

Pinquart, M. and Sorensen, S. (2005) Ethnic differences in stressors, resources, and psychological outcomes of family caring: a meta-analysis, *The Gerontologist*, 45(1): 90–106.

Ritchie, K. and Lovestone, S. (2002) The dementias, *The Lancet*, 360: 1759–66.

Roberts, J.S., Connell, C.M., Cisewski, D., Hipps, Y.G., Demissie, S. *et al.* (2003) Differences between African Americans and whites in their perceptions of Alzheimer's disease, *Alzheimer's Disease and Associated Disorders*, 17(1): 19–26.

Schwartz, B.S., Glass, T.A. and Bolla, K.I. (2004) Disparities in cognitive functioning by race/ethnicity in the Baltimore Memory Study, *Environmental Health Perspectives*, 12(4): 314–20.

Stoller, J. and Cutler, R. (1992) The impact of gender on configurations of care among married elderly couples, *Research on Aging*, 14: 313–30.

Sudore, R.L., Mehta, K.M., Simonsick, E.E., Harris, T.B., Newman, A.B. *et al.* (2006) Limited literacy in older people and disparities in health and healthcare access, *Journal of the American Geriatric Society*, 54: 770–6.

Tanjasiri, S.P., Wallace, S.P. and Shibata, K. (1995) Picture imperfect: hidden problems among Asian Pacific Islander elderly, *The Gerontologist*, 35(6): 753–60.

Townsend, P. and Davidson, N. (1982) *Inequalities in Health (the Black Report)*. Harmondsworth: Penguin.

US Census Bureau (2006) *Selected Characteristics of Native and Foreign-born Populations: 2006–2010 American Community Survey 5-Year Estimates*. Washington, DC: US Census Bureau.

US Census Bureau (2012a) *Statistical Abstract of the United States: 2012. Education Attainment by Race and Hispanic Origin: 1970 to 2010. Table 229*. Washington, DC: US Census Bureau.

US Census Bureau (2012b) *Statistical Abstract of the United States: 2012. Money Income of Households – Percent Distribution by Income Level, Race, and Hispanic Origin, in Constant (2009) Dollars: 1990–2009. Table 690*. Washington, DC: US Census Bureau.

US Census Bureau (2012c) *Statistical Abstract of the United States: 2012. Money Income of Households – Median Income by Race and Hispanic Origin, in Current and Constant (2009) Dollars: 1980–2009. Table 691*. Washington, DC: US Census Bureau.

US Census Bureau (2012d) *Overview of the Uninsured in the United States: A Summary of the 2012 Current Population Survey Report* Washington, DC: US Census Bureau. [http://aspe.hhs.gov/health/reports/2012/UninsuredInTheUS/ib.shtml, accessed 9 September 2013].

University of Bradford (2001) [www.bradford.ac.uk/mediacentre/news-releases/title-98670-en.php, accessed 11 September 2013].

Wilmoth, J.M. (2001) Living arrangements among older immigrants in the United States, *The Gerontologist*, 41(2): 228–38.

Youn, G., Knight, B.G., Jeong, H.-S. and Benton, D. (1999) Differences in familism values and caring outcomes among Korean, Korean American, and white American dementia carers, *Psychology and Aging*, 14: 355–64.

CHAPTER 4

Ethics in dementia care: storied lives, storied ethics

Brandi Estey-Burtt and Clive Baldwin

66 It's interesting that they ask you to tell them about the person, pages and pages of who they are and then they just ignore it. What happened to my mum? My mother, her mother didn't take her home from the maternity home. Just left her there. So her grandmother went to get her. That stayed with her all her life. So it was always really easy to make Mum feel unwanted or unliked. So when she runs into that (here), I can just imagine what that stirs up. It's all about that, feeling unwanted or unliked.

Sometimes she goes back to being a kid. When she didn't like being in a bed alone. So I asked them (staff) to put her in a room with others. They should have thought of that. They ask for pictures but then don't do anything with them, don't ask about them. When she is difficult, you could engage her in a discussion about the pictures, but they don't.

So it would have been good if the carers knew that that picture was the house where she lived with Gladys and Iola. When she wants to know where Iola is, they could say 'she went shopping.' Iola did the shopping. When she asked me 'where is Iola?' I said 'she went shopping' and she said 'why are you lying to me? She never shops on Monday. Monday was washing day. And it WAS Monday. 99

—Carolyn Worth Melbourne, Australia

66 When my Mum was in the EMI unit there was a gentleman who was quite demanding to handle. He had a shoe fetish and always wanted to look at and take off your shoes. One day a carer explained to me that he had had his own shoe mending business so shoes had very much been part of his life. With this explanation you become more understanding. 99

—Brenda Smith Yorkshire, UK

Learning objectives

By the end of this chapter, you will:

- Have an understanding of the strengths and limitations of different ethical frameworks to guide care for people with dementia
- Appreciate the particular strengths of story-based ethics in guiding care for people with dementia
- Have considered how we should think of a person as being understood through layers of stories
- Understand the relevance and applicability of a story-based ethics to dementia care practice

Introduction

Ethics is defined as both a framework of how we live with one another and a theory of moral values – that is, it covers the framework that guides us as well as the philosophical justification of that framework. There are many different possible frameworks, one of which is story-based, an ethics that centres on the stories of 'and that surround' an individual as the basis for ethical decision-making, and it is this framework or approach that we favour here. But given that we all tend to see ourselves as people of goodwill, why do we need to engage in specifically ethical reflection? And given the pressures and concerns of caring for people with dementia, reflecting on the ethics of what we do may seem like another burden, a distraction, or worse, a hindrance to providing care. Why should we take the time and trouble to reflect?

The answer is multi-faceted. First, if ethics is about how we live with one another, then reflection on the values and meanings behind our relationships can act as a way of keeping society together. Second, if there is a goal or purpose to human life, as Aristotle suggested, then living in a certain way may help us towards that goal. Ethics, in other words, helps us achieve the good life. Third, ethics provides practical support in guiding us when we face difficult situations, in protecting vulnerable people, and in promoting good practice. Finally, and perhaps most importantly, acting ethically contributes not only to the well-being of those receiving our care but our own also through establishing the right relationships.

Case example 4.1: Mr. and Mrs. Feldman

Mr. and Mrs. Feldman have been married for nearly 45 years. Mrs. Feldman, now 73, was diagnosed as having dementia four years ago. Before retirement, Mrs. Feldman owned and ran a manufacturing firm, employing twelve other staff. She was well known in the local community as being a firm but fair employer and was respected not only for her business sense but also as a role model and mentor for young women wanting to enter the world of business. She was frequently invited to speak to school students and other gatherings and the work experience placements she offered were highly sought after. Outside of work Mrs. Feldman was active in the local Rotary Club, especially in the economic and community development activities of the club. Mrs. Feldman enjoyed the attention and respect given to her.

Mr. Feldman, now 77, was happier with a quieter, more private life. He was a piano tuner by profession and also offered piano lessons to local children. He was happy to support his wife's endeavours but did not want to be part of the public image.

Although Mr. and Mrs. Feldman had mostly different interests, the one activity they shared, and enjoyed immensely, was rambling. They were members of the local Ramblers' Association and went on as many walks as Mrs. Feldman's busy schedule allowed. Every summer since they were married they had made sure to take at least one week for a long-distance walking holiday. At home, they "took an evening constitutional" around the local park most days.

With the onset and progression of dementia, Mrs. Feldman, while still physically active, started to get lost when out alone and had, on occasion, been found a few miles away, distressed at not knowing where she was. Her husband had then determined that he would go out with her when she wanted to go for a walk regardless of the time of day or the weather. This arrangement

(continued)

suited them both – Mrs. Feldman still enjoyed walking with her husband and Mr. Feldman felt less anxious about his wife.

Twelve months ago, however, Mr. Feldman slipped on ice and damaged his hip badly, requiring surgery. While now able to walk again, he cannot walk as fast as he did and he experiences a fair degree of pain if he walks too far. This has impacted his ability to take regular evening walks with his wife. Mrs. Feldman, however, still insists on going out. Out of concern for his wife's safety Mr. Feldman has tried to persuade her otherwise and this has resulted in a number of arguments. More recently, Mr. Feldman has taken to locking doors and windows at night and when he is unable to accompany his wife. When Mrs. Feldman wants to go out and finds the doors locked she becomes frustrated and further arguments ensue. At night, Mr. Feldman occasionally gives his wife a slightly increased dose of medication to "help her sleep through" so that she does not try to go for a walk in the middle of the night when he is asleep.

Furthermore, Mrs. Feldman still gets invited to a range of events to which she wants to go. Mr. Feldman, never one much for public engagements, had always found them trying at the best of times and now, with Mrs. Feldman having dementia, these events are becoming increasingly stressful. Where once Mrs. Feldman had a very keen sense of personal and social decorum, she has become less concerned about her appearance and somewhat less inhibited. This has resulted in occasional embarrassing moments for Mr. Feldman and some fairly unkind comments by Mrs. Feldman's erstwhile associates at the Rotary Club and other organizations who now really view the invitations as a courtesy only. For his part, Mr. Feldman is now very selective in telling his wife of the invitations she receives in part to protect her and in part as a means of "damage limitation".

Common ethical theories and their limitations for guiding dementia care

Three normative ethical theories frequently guide ethical decision-making: consequentialism, deontology, and principlism. None of these align with current understandings of person-centred care. Rather than embracing the richness, uniqueness, and history of each ethical encounter between the person with dementia and the carer, they limit their focus to one narrow facet of ethical choice. All three can roughly be called prescriptive or normative ethical frameworks, meaning that they have distinctive rules, principles or norms that guide decision-making. The following descriptions of these frameworks outline the central features and limitations of each.

Consequentialism

One of the most readily identifiable ethical theories, consequentialism stems from the work of philosophers Jeremy Bentham (1789) and John Stuart Mill (1861) and looks to the consequences of an action to determine if it is right or wrong. In other words, does an action bring about a harmful or beneficial outcome to the persons concerned? In the case above, Mr. Feldman's actions in locking doors and windows can be seen as an attempt to ensure his wife's safety – that is, preventing the potential harmful consequences of his wife leaving the house and becoming lost and distressed. Another frequent example of this dilemma occurs when a person with dementia is administered pills she or he may not wish to take. If the carers for that person feel that the outcome – the benefits the pills may give – is valuable, they might hide the pills in food against the person's wishes.

A crucial problem emerges for consequentialism if you refer only to the consequences of an action to establish its correctness. To rephrase slightly, does the end justify the means? By attending only to the outcome of an action, it becomes acceptable to ignore the action itself; for example, is it acceptable to justify deceiving a person with dementia into believing he is being taken for a day out in the country when in fact he is being taken to respite care, care which he has refused in the past? This is not to say that paying attention to the outcome of a choice is not important, but that a decision should be made on the basis of more than just the results of a certain situation.

Deontology

Although there are several forms of deontology, the most recognizable stems from philosopher Immanuel Kant (1785) and foregrounds duty as primary. Deontology in a sense inverts consequentialism to place importance on one's motives as the measure of ethical behaviour instead of on the consequences. However, unlike virtue ethics (another ethical theory), which emphasizes the character of the person carrying out an action, deontology simply asks whether or not a person has a duty in a particular situation or if they should be following a rule. For example, one might say Mr. Feldman has a duty to be honest and not to deceive his wife by surreptitiously increasing her medication. However, if he did not do so, Mrs. Feldman might leave the house while he was sleeping or Mr. Feldman would need to remain vigilant throughout the night, which, in the long term, might affect his ability to care for his wife. In this case, duty or rule takes precedence over potential consequences.

Similarly, the duty of care for others might result in one caring for persons with dementia regardless of the consequences to oneself, including significant contributions of time, effort, and emotional involvement.

The flaw in deontology can be seen as the opposite of that of consequentialism. In ensuring that duty is carried out, deontology disregards the consequences or effects of an action. While it is both valuable and practical to determine what one's responsibilities are or what right conduct is, deontology nevertheless imposes limits on what the motivating factor of ethical decision-making should be. Telling the truth – usually considered a fundamental duty – may result in unpleasant or harmful consequences. In dementia care, we might see examples of this in the insistence on repeatedly telling the truth to a person with dementia in response to, for example, the question, "Where's my mother?", although the answer, "She's dead" (even if not so bluntly stated), causes repeated distress. As with consequentialism, ethical decision-making involves more pieces of the puzzle than merely adhering to duty.

Principlism

Originating in medical ethics, principlism is the position that there are *a priori* principles that can (and should) be applied in health care decision-making. There are four foundational principles – autonomy, beneficence, non-maleficence, and justice – which highlight specific domains of ethical concern (Beauchamp and Childress 2008). Principlism has gained widespread approval in bioethics and other medical-related fields; consequently, the four principles are currently very influential in ethical decision-making. In making a decision about locking the doors and windows or administering increased medication, principlism would seek to weigh up the undermining of autonomy through restriction of liberty and covert administration against the benefits that such restrictions and the medication might achieve.

Although principlism has substantial support in medical ethics, a number of issues related to this theory have developed from the vantage point of person-centred dementia care. One of the most glaring weaknesses lies in principlism's lack of consideration for personhood or the narrative trajectory of a person's life (Baldwin and Estey-Burtt 2013). It makes no provision either for the uniqueness of the ethical encounter or for the communal nature of decision-making, as it places the greatest importance on individual choice (Wolpe 1998). Decisions regarding treatment for a person with dementia can potentially involve many different people at any one time, since family members, doctors, and the person with dementia her or himself all offer a perspective on what should be done. Such a scenario is not sufficiently spoken to by any of the four principles. Also, principlism incorporates a very western understanding of what each of the four principles means (Tan Alora and Lumitao 2001), thus limiting its application cross-culturally.

An alternative ethical framework – story-based ethics

If we want to ground our ethical reflections in the experience of the person with dementia, then we need to look beyond normative theories. To genuinely pursue person-centred care requires an understanding of what constitutes a person and how this relates to story. This leads to an approach to ethics that centres on the stories told by, and those surrounding, an individual as the basis for ethical decision-making – a narrative or "storied" ethics.

The individual self and narrative

The notion of the self or what it means to be a person has a long philosophical history. In the West, the Greek philosophers Pythagoras, Euripides, Socrates, Plato, and Aristotle all contended in some way with the philosophical issue of how to understand the self. In the third and fourth centuries, Augustine invented the self as a private "inner space" in which one could find God (Cary 2000). This notion of self became secularized during the Enlightenment with idealized traits of personhood coming to include "the continuity of identity, the coherence, unity and integration of the self, and the authentic, singular and progressive core self" (de Peuter 1998: 32). (There are also eastern philosophical traditions that address the notion of the self, but for the sake of brevity and focus we do not raise these here.)

In the 1980s, a number of authors began to reconceptualize the self in narrative terms: MacIntyre (1984) argued that an understanding of our selves requires an understanding of the narratives of which we are a part; Bruner (1987) argued that lives could best be understood in narrative terms; and Taylor (1989) explored what he termed "webs of interlocution", those relationships with conversation partners that help define our identity. Some authors later went further to argue that without narrative there could be no self:

> ❝The differences between the kind of life led by an individual with a totally non narrative self-conception and the kind of life led by the rest of us [a narrative self-conception] are so pronounced and important that it does not seem like an exaggeration to say that the individuals who live such lives are not persons. ❞

—Schechtman (1996: 101)

This version of the narrative self has been criticized (see Strawson 2004), but the notion that narrative and the self are, in some way, related has gained significant purchase. This relationship has been explored in the field of dementia by authors such as Mills (1998), Ryan et al. (2009), and Hydén (2010), and one need only look at the range of activities embedded within person-centred care (for example, life-history work, reminiscence, writing, storytelling, and narrative quilting) to sense the importance attributed in practice to understanding the stories of people living with dementia.

The social self and narrative

What many of the different approaches to the narrative self have in common is their incorporation of agency, relationships, and situated-ness into their understandings of how narrative and self relate to each other. In terms of agency, "In the modern Western world, being an autonomous agent seems almost quintessential" and "To be unable *to do* would, at least to a marginal degree, start to challenge our sense of ourselves as minded" (Hughes 2008: 127, emphasis in original). Thus, we would argue, the ability and opportunity to narrate one's own story is an important aspect of agency. Of course, as John Donne observed, none of us is an island and our agency is always situated within a network of relationships. There is much written about the relational or dialogical self, in which the self is seen as being significantly, if not solely, constituted by our relationships with others (see, for example, Hermans *et al.* 1992; de Peuter 1998). These relationships are, we think, captured in the stories that are told about us, our families, and our communities – stories that go a considerable way to framing our understandings of who we (and others) are. The stories within which we are framed by others can limit or expand who we might be or become. For example, in our case study, Mrs. Feldman is in danger of being framed primarily within stories of decline and problematic behaviour, whereas alternative stories might be fashioned in which she is still her self, wife, mother, friend, former business colleague, lover, and so on, retaining and even enhancing her sense of self.

Linked to this is the notion of situated-ness (see Hughes 2008) – the fact that we are situated within cultural, historical, moral, and legal contexts that shape our lives. In narrative terms, such situated-ness is embedded in the stories our families, communities, faith, culture, and society hold up as important and as encapsulating what it means to become and be part of this group and not another group. These wider webs of stories can, like our smaller or familial stories, also shape who we are and who we can become, and understanding these narratives is vitally important to understanding any individual.

Meta-narratives

In addition to the stories that situate us in time, place, and relationships, we live in webs of meta-narratives, which are prevalent stories found in all levels of society expressing dominant ideas about events, situations or groups of people (see Chapter 6). These meta-narratives exert considerable power over social resources, moral agency, and self-understanding, and are often linked to what is perceived as being "normal" or "given", configuring our understandings of how things should be. While they are not always negative (we could, for example, have a meta-narrative about social justice and the need to care for the disenfranchised in society), many displace or silence the stories of individuals or smaller groups, dictating the terms by which they should live (see Nelson 2001). Such societal or institutional narratives tend towards subsuming alternative stories, thus allaying potential threats and leaving little room for people to develop their own narrative trajectories outside that of the meta-narrative.

The medical narrative of dementia is one such meta-narrative, a narrative of deterioration in which persons with dementia are increasingly robbed of their cognitive and social abilities (see Chapter 5). Along this trajectory, communication becomes more difficult for persons with dementia and carers (and professionals) become more involved in decision-making, which often results in the silencing of the voice of the person with dementia, however unintended (see Chapter 12). Also, as Bryden (2005: 40) remarks, dementia is still perceived as shameful, and those diagnosed with it are increasingly isolated and cut off from society as the disease progresses (see Chapter 2). Combined with what Freeman (2000: 81) would call the "pre-scripted narratives of decline well in place" for ageing generally, such meta-narratives limit positive construction of narrative selfhood, identity, and personhood for those with dementia, replacing it with a therapeutic nihilism enfolded in a narrative of senescence.

Advantages of story-based ethics for dementia care

A story-based ethics has certain advantages over the three frameworks considered earlier:

1. It emerges from the situation and is thus rooted in the lived experiences of those affected by the decisions to be made. In other words, we move towards a person-centred ethic rather than an abstract, philosophical ethic.
2. It can accommodate the messiness, ambiguity, and indeterminacy of real-life situations that are not simply problems to be solved but are complex configurations of a person's values, wishes, needs, context, webs of relationships, situated-ness in terms of history and place, and their desired trajectory(ies) as well as being aware of the possible impact on self of emergent stories. In other words, a story-based ethics considers a person's narrative wholeness. Stories help us understand the richness and complexities of individual lives and lend themselves to acting as a basis for ethical reasoning.
3. There are good reasons for viewing narrative not only as a means of gathering information to aid decision-making as other frameworks seem to do (for example, McCarthy 2003), but as the basis of the decision-making process. In nursing, Keady et al. (2007) have argued for grounding clinical practice and decision-making in autobiographical narratives. In health care, Robinson (2002) has shown how narrative might set up particular possibilities and courses of action and close down others, while Baldwin (2009) has argued for the narrative framing of the decision-making process with regard to people living with dementia. For authors such as Walker (2003), story is the fundamental form of representation for moral problems and knowing something about how the situation arose says something about what is being attended to, the decisions to be made, and the actions to be taken and can thus "grasp some moral problems better than standard theoretical outlooks" (Paulsen 2011: 28).
4. It allows for the ethical decision-making itself to become part of the ongoing story. Rather than viewing the decision as divorced from the decision-maker, a story-based ethic recognizes that decisions made both reflect and constitute the person(s) making those decisions – in other words, there is a role for the development of character and virtue within a story-based ethics (see Hauerwas 1977).

Storied ethics in practice: a case study reflection

All of the above might appear somewhat academic – as interesting as the idea might be, how might this help us in our day-to-day thinking and practice when faced with the real-life issues of the real-life individual and her or his family whose vulnerability calls us to respond? Following a brief reflection on Mrs. Feldman's case illustrating how a storied approach can help identify key ethical areas, four possibilities for putting storied ethics into practice in dementia care are raised. The first, mapping the narrative landscape of an individual's life, forms the basis on which to move forward. The second, challenging meta-narratives of decline, seeks to locate these individual stories within a more positive, supportive, and constructive narrative environment. The third seeks to extend the notion of agency through the promotion of co-constructed stories within dementia care. The fourth places these ethical ideas within the wider communities of practice that can support the individual through the creation and maintenance of a web of narratives focused on person-centred care.

For the storied ethic, one of the major issues in the scenario is the disruption to the stories through which Mrs. Feldman has realized her personhood in the past is under assault in a number of ways. First, the variety and uniqueness of her stories as a strong, independent, capable businesswoman are being replaced by a narrative of dementia, which has become or is becoming the dominant story of Mr. and Mrs. Feldman's life together. Mrs. Feldman's behaviour is being constrained by those around her (the cognitively and physically intact) in ways that make no sense to her. The concern with Mrs. Feldman's safety is beginning to frame the situation as a problem to be resolved and Mrs. Feldman as someone whose behaviour must be managed. In so doing, this framing supplants the narratives that once upheld Mrs. Feldman's personhood and forecloses on the narrative possibilities within the situation.

Second, the shared narrative of Mr. and Mrs. Feldman that constructed their personhood together over many years is now being disrupted. Mr. Feldman is thinking and acting differently than he had previously – acting out of character. He has, by necessity in his mind, become more directive or even controlling than before, changing the overall narrative dynamics of the relationship and effectively constructing a different narrative. In this new narrative, Mrs. Feldman is cut adrift from the narratives that previously held her personhood in place – narratives of success, capability, independence, authority, and social status that are now displaced by what she cannot do and by Mr. Feldman's assumption of a more dominant role. The stories at stake are therefore more than simply how to keep Mrs. Feldman safe – they are intricately bound up in how Mr. Feldman's actions in restricting his wife's liberty and surreptitiously administering increased medication changes the family narrative and the characters and relationships of everyone involved. The previous narrative of a loving, faithful relationship slips into one of potential betrayal and deceit, framed by the perceived need to 'manage' Mrs. Feldman (in her own best interests, of course). And it is precisely because of this potential that it is vitally important to understand the underlying stories and narrative dynamics so as to facilitate the best possible narrative in the circumstances.

Third, the narratives that shaped Mr. and Mrs. Feldman's life together (in Taylor's words, the webs of interlocutions) have shifted. Mr. Feldman is now playing a far more controlling role in the relationship than he did previously and Mrs. Feldman experiences this as an inexplicable change in her husband. By focusing on stories of behaviour and dementia, attention is deflected from the changes in the relationship and support for the changing narrative dynamics are relegated to subsidiary features, consequently damaging the ethical reflection and communication.

Finally, Mrs. Feldman's moral development is linked to the stance he takes with regard to how to relate to his wife: the kind of decisions we confront – indeed the very way we describe the situation – is a function of the kind of character we have (Hauerwas 1977: 20). What sort of person is Mr. Feldman becoming in restricting his wife physically and chemically? While such actions might be given some ethical justification, other ethical frameworks do not address the effect of such actions on the actor. Character, according to Hauerwas, is forged not through adherence to abstract principles or theories but by the stories of which we were a part and that form the milieu within which we live our lives – that is, in our situatedness. These stories tie together the contingencies that make up our lives and set the context for our moral judgement.

Mapping the narrative landscape of an individual's life

A narrative approach to understanding an individual is not simply about listening to the stories that that person tells or the stories that others tell about that person. Stories, like people, are not islands; stories, like people, relate to and interact with others. So to understand an individual, we must not only listen to their stories but come to appreciate where stories are located in relation to each other. Some stories – which we might call signature stories – are central to understanding a person because they help shape or articulate something important about that person. Other stories, such as recounting a routine breakfast conversation, are more ephemeral. Some stories are connected to many other stories, while others are connected to only a few; some stories are bright, colourful, and exuberant, others less or not so at all. The metaphor we use for understanding a person through the stories of that person's life (past, present, and future) is an exploration of a narrative landscape – as we move around the landscape, we get different perspectives on what is around us, other things come into view and others recede. Some we can see from a long way off (the signature type stories), others are hidden away and are only found by careful and sensitive exploration. Mapping this landscape is the precursor to any well-developed story-based ethic.

Challenging the meta-narratives of decline

Although meta-narratives are often deeply entrenched in our everyday lives, it is possible to challenge them through what Nelson (2001: 6) identifies as counterstories: "a counterstory – a story that resists an oppressive identity and attempts to replace it with one that commands respect". Counterstories reclaim narrative agency from the meta-narratives that seek to control it; at the same time, they resist being called deviant for not following the dominant narrative, carving out their own narrative space free of such damaging labels.

Counterstories for dementia work by engaging both persons with dementia and the people surrounding them. This involves active re-storying of the negativity associated with dementia by those who are experiencing it, as well as efforts by carers and dementia organizations to reconceive the pathway of dementia as not one wholly of deterioration. Bryden (2005) offers one such potential counterstory in her vigorous support for an understanding of the possibilities of living well with dementia, insisting on the uniqueness of her own situation and story which cannot and should not be subsumed into the standardized medical narrative of decline. Using her own experience of dementia, Bryden challenges the medical and social focus on the lack of ability and capacity that dementia brings, preferring to concentrate on the things persons with dementia can still accomplish and groups and social functions in which they can still participate. Bryden therefore argues that people can live hopefully with dementia as she has learned to do: "I choose a new identity as a survivor. I want to learn to dance with dementia. I want to live positively each day, in a vital relationship of trust with my care-partners alongside me" (Bryden 2005: 170).

Carers – or what Bryden calls care-partners – are integral to this process, as they share in the daily renegotiation of the meanings of dementia along with those who have been diagnosed. The task of renegotiation of meaning also falls to dementia organizations such as the national or regional offices of the Alzheimer's Society, as they are crucial in educating people about understanding dementia. As Bryden demonstrates, an effective counterstory can be forged that works against the negative meta-narratives of society and medicine, recovering narrative agency for persons with dementia.

Exercise 4.1: Using narratives with a family

Think about the differing strands that make up Mr. (and Mrs.) Feldman's life – family, work, activities, and so on – and how the onset and progression of dementia has introduced the meta-narrative of dementia into the family's story.

■ What elements of the meta-narrative of dementia are at play in the case of the Feldman family?

■ In what ways might these be resisted?

■ What narratives are possible, from what you know of the family, that would serve to maintain Mrs. Feldman's personhood, and on which one might build, rather than undermine it?

Extending agency, co-constructing stories

As carers and persons with dementia are both crucial to the re-storying of dementia, so both are necessary for the co-construction of stories within a care setting. Stories do not exist in a vacuum, and tellers and hearers do a lot of work together in making them thrive. Following Keady and Williams (2005), we can call this element of narrative the "co-construction of stories", in which narrative space is shared so as to maintain the narrative agency of those for whom it might be compromised, such as persons with dementia. This suggests a highly participatory view of narrative wherein co-construction relies on relationality and openness to the other.

Co-construction implies a familiarity and a willingness to be involved in the texture of a person's narrative as well as to be influenced by that narrative. This requires not only being open to the fact that persons with dementia still have a story, but that this story increasingly becomes linked with the story of those active in a caring role. This ties into the idea that every story has what Newton, expanding on Levinas, calls a Said and a Saying, wherein the Said is the actual content and the Saying is the performance or process of telling. Neither should be privileged over the other, though it is necessary to recognize that "Narrative, as participatory act, is part 'Said' . . . and part 'Saying,' the latter – the level of intersubjective relation – being the site of surplus, of the unforeseen, of self-exposure" (Newton 1995: 3). This means that we are drawn into each other's stories as active participants and contributors, which entails the realization that others affect our stories as much as we affect theirs.

In practical terms, carers and/or care practitioners work with the person with dementia to change routines, identify possibilities, and be involved in the details of everyday life. It is not a simple relationship of do everything for the person with dementia, assuming that their story is over, but of allowing oneself to be pulled into their new ways of Saying their stories and being shaped in turn. This offers an opportunity to build a new story together that appreciates the vulnerability and self-exposure of each person involved in the relationship (see, for example, Alemán and Helfrich 2010).

Exercise 4.2: Participation in creating a narrative

The co-construction of narratives requires that the final narrative works for all parties involved. What possibilities are there in this case for constructing a mutually acceptable narrative on which to proceed? In thinking about this, you may want to consider the following:

■ How do we enable Mr. Feldman to participate in the co-construction of a meaningful narrative for him and his wife?

- How can narrative solidarity be expressed with Mrs. Feldman in the face of dementia?
- How do we support Mr. Feldman in maintaining narrative probity in changing – and possibly frightening – circumstances?
- What roles might be required of each of the participants in the narrative?

Drawing on communities of practice

Storied ethics affects the small aspects of life as well as big decisions like those concerning end-of-life care. It therefore extends into daily routines and influences how care is given – for example, how people are fed and washed, if their spiritual and emotional needs are given thought and consideration (paying attention to things as simple as providing music or touch), and how they are engaged in activities. Consequently, ethical decisions frequently do not seem all that weighty or drawn out, and people make them fairly quickly and practically. Indeed, practicality often becomes a key component of decision-making after an ethical concern has been identified.

Communities of practice connect to this, framing the countless decisions we make on a regular basis and how we feel about each one of them. All ethical choices, no matter how large or slight, are made within these communities, which act as reference points for our morality and guide our sense of what is acceptable and what is not. Moreover, there are a multitude of communities in which we are simultaneously immersed, including moral, legal, spiritual, religious, social, political, and cultural ones among others. As we incorporate aspects of each smaller community into our overall decision-making, we ultimately need some coherence between patterns of practice for them to make sense.

Such communities, however, are liable to criticism and misuse, and it is necessary to note that patterns of practice encouraged by these communities are usually public and require education, training, and experience. They can be changed, but changes need to uphold values of care, fitting into wider patterns of practice that deem them to be morally sound. That is, they must be informed by other communities of practice and be open to correction.

Ethical practice is always at some level eclectic – we constantly draw from a number of sources and influences, rather than a single moral theory, to make our decisions. This is not to say that we follow an "anything goes" or "this is what I like" approach. Instead, our decisions respond to the concrete situation while implicating wider communities of practice that both educate and correct us, therefore enabling us to maintain practicality in our decision-making as well as accountability.

Debates and controversies

Story-based ethics considers personal narratives, located within the narrative web of individual, familial, community, and social life, to be of crucial importance and therefore does not rely on abstract rules or principles. A number of authors have commented on the problems with such an approach. Strawson (2004) questions the two narrativist claims that (1) people experience their lives narratively and (2) that the well-lived life or personhood depends upon such narratives. While we do not agree with Strawson, even if it were the case that personhood is not narratively constituted, our argument for a storied ethic does not necessarily fall. One does not have to subscribe to the strong sense of the storied self to recognize the importance and influence of stories in people's lives, in their attempts to make meaning, understand, and communicate with others and to inform decision-making. The degree to which we might rely on stories might vary depending on where we stand in this debate, but it is not possible, we think, to do away with stories altogether.

Because of this, Arras (1997) asks how storied ethics can give satisfactory moral justification and point to ethical truths – it seems that there is nothing either to prevent people from relativism or ensure professional responsibility if ethics is based on the uniqueness of narratives. In other words, Arras wonders whether the narrative metaphor might be overextending itself.

While story-based ethics does not rely on professional codes or rule-based philosophies to act as safeguards for conduct, it does emphasize greater personal responsibility than can be dictated by such codes, which often function to protect a practitioner from legal issues rather than give adequate consideration to the vulnerable. The communities of practice within which all stories are rooted also offer influential guidelines for how personal behaviour can respect the stories of those around us, promote individual responsibility, and maintain ethical accountability.

Conclusion

Ethics offers an opportunity to reflect on our daily decision-making so that we can ensure we are contributing to the care and well-being of those around us. In particular, story-based ethics emphasizes the fact that people living with dementia are still living their own stories – their narrative(s) are not finished because of the disease (the meta-narrative of decline) but are simply moving in different directions. As a result of this insight, carers can participate in the co-construction of these stories, allowing themselves to be drawn into new possibilities for agency, participation, and relationship. Story-based ethics thus provides a way to respect the personhood of those with dementia and honour their narrative trajectories while responding to the ethical matters of the moment.

Major ethical theories such as consequentialism, deontology, and principlism lack the philosophical and practical wherewithal to account for the richness of an individual's story and take it into consideration when making ethical decisions. Story-based ethics can help us in the day-to-day by acknowledging the layers of story in which the person living with dementia is enfolded: it highlights the importance of personal responsibility while checking action against the input of established communities of practice. In this way, storied ethics promotes individual and social well-being for persons living with dementia as well as their carers, exemplifying a responsible yet textured approach to ethical decision-making.

Further information

Available from Alzheimer's Australia, "Ethical Issues and Decision-Making in Dementia Care" is a recording of a lecture and panel discussion addressing the complex ethical issues in policy and service delivery with regard to dementia care [http://www.fightdementia.org.au/common/files/VIC/Ethical_issues_dvd_orderform.pdf, accessed 3 December 2013].

EthicsWeb.ca is a web-portal providing links to many ethics institutes across the globe [http://www.ethicsweb.ca/resources/bioethics/institutes.html, accessed 3 December 2013].

Healthtalkonline.org provides information on a range of illnesses and conditions, including dementia, and videos, audio recordings, and texts of personal experiences of health and illness [http://healthtalkonline.org/, accessed 3 December 2013].

References

Alemán, M.W. and Helfrich, K.W. (2010) Inheriting the narratives of dementia: a collaborative tale of a daughter and mother, *Journal of Family Communication*, 10(1): 7–23.

Arras, J. (1997) Nice story, but so what? Narrative and justification in ethics, in H.L. Nelson (ed.) *Stories and Their Limits: Narrative Approaches to Bioethics*. New York: Routledge, pp. 64–88.

Baldwin, C. (2009) Narrative and decision-making, in D. O'Connor and B. Purves (eds.) *Decision-making, Personhood and Dementia: Exploring the Interface.* London: Jessica Kingsley, pp. 25–36.

Baldwin, C. and Estey-Burtt, B. (2013) Narrative and the reconfiguration of social work ethics. *Narrative Works,* 2 (2) [http://w3.stu.ca/stu/sites/cirn/narrative_works.aspx, accessed April 2013].

Beauchamp, T.L. and Childress, J.F. (2008) *Principles of Biomedical Ethics* (5th edn.). Oxford: Oxford University Press.

Bentham, J. (1789/1996) *An Introduction to the Principles of Morals and Legislation* (J.H. Burns and H.L.A. Hart, eds.). Oxford: Oxford University Press.

Bruner, J. (1987) Life as narrative, *Social Research*, 54(1): 11–32.

Bryden, C. (2005) *Dancing with Dementia: My Story of Living Positively with Dementia.* London: Jessica Kingsley.

Cary, P. (2000) *Augustine's Invention of the Inner Self: The Legacy of a Christian Platonist.* Oxford: Oxford University Press.

de Peuter, J. (1998) The dialogics of narrative identity, in M.M. Bell and M. Gardiner (eds.) *Bakhtin and the Human Sciences*. London: Sage, pp. 30–48.

Freeman, M. (2000) When the story's over: narrative foreclosure and the possibility of self-renewal, in M. Andrews, S. Sclater, C. Squire and A. Treacher (eds.) *Lines of Narrative: Psychosocial Perspectives*. London: Routledge, pp. 81–91.

Hauerwas, S. (1977) *Truthfulness and Tragedy: Further Investigations into Christian Ethics*. Notre Dame, IN: University of Notre Dame Press.

Hermans, H.J.M., Kempen, H.J.G. and van Loon, R.J.P. (1992) The dialogical self: beyond individualism and rationalism, *American Psychologist*, 47(1): 23–33.

Hughes, J.C. (2008) Being minded in dementia: persons and human beings, in M. Downs and B. Bowers (eds.) *Excellence in Dementia Care: Research into Practice*. Maidenhead: Open University Press, pp. 119–32.

Hydén, L.C. (2010) Identity, self, narrative, in M. Hyvärinen, L.C. Hyden, M. Saarenheimo and M. Tamboukou (eds.) *Beyond Narrative Coherence*. Amsterdam: John Benjamins, pp. 33–48.

Kant, I. (1785/1964) *Groundwork of the Metaphysic of Morals* (H.J. Paton, trans.). New York: Harper & Row.

Keady, J. and Williams, S. (2005) Co-constructed inquiry: a new approach to the generation of shared knowledge in chronic illness. Paper presented at the RCN International Research Conference, Belfast.

Keady, J., Ashcroft-Simpson, S., Halligan, K. and Williams, S. (2007) Admiral nursing and the family care of a parent with dementia: using autobiographical narrative as grounding for negotiated clinical practice and decision-making, *Scandinavian Journal of Caring Sciences*, 21(3): 345–53.

MacIntyre, A. (1984) *After Virtue: A Study in Moral Theory*. Notre Dame, IN: University of Notre Dame Press.

McCarthy, J. (2003) Principlism or narrative ethics: must we choose between them?, *Journal of Medical Humanities*, 29(2): 65–71.

Mill, J.S. (1861/1998) *Utilitarianism* (R. Crisp, ed.). Oxford: Oxford University Press.

Mills, M.A. (1998) *Narrative Identity and Dementia: A Study of Autobiographical Memories and Emotions*. Aldershot: Ashgate.

Nelson, H.L. (2001) *Damaged Identities, Narrative Repair*. Ithaca, NY: Cornell University Press.

Newton, A.Z. (1995) *Narrative Ethics*. Cambridge, MA: Harvard University Press.

Paulsen, J.E. (2011) A narrative ethics of care, *Health Care Analysis*, 19(1): 28–40.

Robinson, W.M. (2002) The narrative of rescue in pediatric practice, in R. Charon and M. Montello (eds.) *Stories Matter: The Role of Narrative in Medical Ethics*. New York: Routledge, pp. 100–11.

Ryan, E.B., Bannister, K.A. and Anas, A.P. (2009) The dementia narrative: writing to reclaim social identity, *Journal of Aging Studies*, 23(2): 145–57.

Schechtman, M. (1996) *The Constitution of Selves*. Ithaca, NY: Cornell University Press.

Strawson, G. (2004) Against narrativity, *Ratio*, XVII (4): 428–52.

Tan Alora, A. and Lumitao, J.M. (eds.) (2001) *Beyond a Western Bioethics: Voices from the Developing World*. Washington, DC: Georgetown University Press.

Taylor, C. (1989) *Sources of the Self*. Cambridge: Cambridge University Press.

Walker, M.U. (2003) *Moral Contexts*. Lanham, MD: Rowman & Littlefield.

Wolpe, P.R. (1998) The triumph of autonomy in American bioethics: a sociological view, in R. DeVries and J. Subedi (eds.) *Bioethics and Society: Constructing the Ethical Enterprise*. Upper Saddle River, NJ: Prentice-Hall, pp. 38–59.

CHAPTER 5

Dementia as a public health issue: research or services?

Jesse F. Ballenger

❝Alzheimer's disease burdens an increasing number of our nation's elders and their families, and it is essential that we confront the challenge it poses to our public health.❞

—President Barack Obama

❝If we are to beat dementia, we must also work globally, with nations, business and scientists from all over the world working together as we did with cancer, and with HIV and Aids.❞

—David Cameron

❝In the declaration and communiqué resulting from the summit, the G8 ministers agreed to:

■ set an ambition to identify a cure, or a disease-modifying therapy, for dementia by 2025
■ significantly increase the amount spent on dementia research
■ increase the number of people involved in clinical trials and studies on dementia
■ establish a new global envoy for dementia innovation, following in the footsteps of global envoys on HIV and Aids and on Climate Change
■ develop an international action plan for research
■ share information and data from dementia research studies across the G8 countries to work together and get the best return on investment in research
■ encourage open access to all publicly-funded dementia research to make data and results available for further research as quickly as possible.❞

Learning objectives

By the end of this chapter, you will understand:

■ The historical development of dementia as a public health issue
■ How history has shaped politics and policy
■ Public policy and debate related to dementia

Introduction

Politics and policy for dementia have revolved around two imperatives: funding for research into prevention or cure, and funding for services to support professional and family caregivers of people with dementia. On the face of it, these two imperatives would not seem inevitably to conflict. However, policy discourse, at least in the USA, has typically pitted these two imperatives against each other. The result has been that research on prevention and cure has generally enjoyed significantly more public funding than services or innovations to support care.

This chapter examines the history of advocacy efforts for Alzheimer's disease (AD) in the USA to help explain why public funding for cure has trumped funding for services, and considers what would be necessary to shift the balance. The USA, like other developed countries, spends enormous sums on care for people with dementia. Health care costs for people with dementia are high because such individuals are more likely to require hospitalization and treatment of concurrent illnesses (see Chapters 18 and 22). In the USA, the Alzheimer's Association estimated that Medicare costs for older people with dementia were three times higher, and Medicaid costs nineteen times higher, than for seniors without dementia. The Association estimated that the total cost of caring for people with dementia in the USA was $203 billion in 2013, including $142 billion from Medicare and Medicaid. With the ageing of the baby boom generation, costs were projected to reach $1.2 trillion in 2050 (in current dollars), including a 500% increase in combined costs to Medicare and Medicaid (Alzheimer's Association 2013). In the UK, estimates suggest the cost of dementia to be in the region of £23 billion annually.

By all accounts, spending in the USA is inadequate to meet the needs of people with dementia and those who care for them. Publicly funded services in the USA require that patients (and their spouses) spend down their savings to poverty levels before receiving government assistance for residential care, and many dementia-associated expenses are not covered. More importantly, health funding in the USA is structured around meeting the needs of people with acute illnesses and is less likely to cover many services needed by people with dementia and their families. Family members shouldering the physical and emotional burdens of caregiving find it difficult to access services, and struggle to piece together the fabric of care (see Chapters 13 and 21).

The US Government spends relatively little on services specifically designed for dementia. Of the $448 million the National Institutes of Health (NIH) targeted to Alzheimer's disease research in 2011, 54% was devoted to molecular pathogenesis and physiology, 22% to diagnosis, assessment, and disease monitoring, 14% to translational research and clinical interventions, 7% to epidemiology, and only 3% to care support and health economics (ADEAR Center 2012). The first National Plan to Address Alzheimer's Disease in the USA was released in 2012, and included as major goals enhancement of care quality and support for family caregivers. It is not yet clear, however, whether this will have an impact on priorities within the NIH's Alzheimer's budget (US Department of Health and Human Services 2013). This is in contrast to the UK where relatively limited investment has been made in research on dementia compared with other conditions such as cancer and heart disease (Alzheimer's Research UK, undated), despite it having had a national plan for dementia since 2009 (Department of Health 2009).

It is becoming increasingly clear that we cannot expect potential breakthroughs in biomedical treatment to solve the problems people with dementia and their families face. Policies that support caregivers and enrich the environment for people with dementia can have a dramatic impact on their quality of life (see the chapters in Parts 3 and 4). It is now essential that we redress the imbalances in the way the two policy imperatives are approached. This will require re-framing the problem in a way that does not pit policies against each other. It is encouraging that the recent G8 dementia summit, hosted in London, called for an international, collaborative response to dementia, both in terms of research and care.

Framing dementia in history

The politics and policy of dementia have been dominated by the emergence of AD, its most prevalent form, as a major public issue since around 1980. The seemingly rapid rise of AD

Period	Frame
1900–1929	Alzheimer, Kraepelin, and the foundations of Alzheimer's disease *Frame: AD as a prototypical brain disease*
1930–1969	American psychiatry, social gerontology, and the fight against senility *Frame: Dementia as a problem of ageing*
1970–present	Emergence of Alzheimer's disease as a public issue *Frame: AD as the dread disease afflicting an ageing society*

Table 5.1 Three periods in the modern history of dementia

from an obscure entity known only to specialists to a household word and object of a massive research programme is typically represented as a result of scientific progress. But the emergence of AD involved much more. The basic biological, clinical, and epidemiological facts of AD had been established and widely accepted since the early twentieth century: neuritic plaques and neurofibrillary tangles associated with memory loss and cognitive deterioration, occurring sometimes in people in their fifties and early sixties but much more often in older people. Certainly, there has been significant scientific progress in understanding age-associated progressive dementia between Alois Alzheimer's first description of AD in 1906 and the present. But these basic facts did not change in the 1980s, nor have they changed since. What has changed – significantly – is the cultural framing of dementia.

Frames are the concepts and metaphors that allow human beings to understand reality, transforming the indecipherable complexity of raw experience into a comprehensible pattern that we can recognize. Frames shape what counts as common sense, and as a result they shape our goals, plans, and actions for reaching them. In politics, frames shape social policy and the social institutions we form to implement policy (Lakoff 2004).

In the late 1970s, a group of neuroscientists, family members, and policy-makers successfully reframed age-associated, chronic, progressive dementia as the product of discrete disease processes rather than an outcome of ageing. By 1980, as we shall see, AD, as the most common and devastating of these, came to dominate the politics and policy of dementia, driving an emphasis on biomedical research over caregiving.

Of course, this was only the latest of several major re-framings of dementia that occurred over the past century. It is useful to divide the modern history of dementia into three periods, as indicated in Table 5.1. In the first period, the basic clinical, biological, and epidemiological facts of AD were established. Subsequent historical periods involved less a dramatic change in our understanding of those facts than a change in the way those facts have been framed – how researchers, policy-makers, and the general public thought dementia was related to ageing, and why it was important to pay attention to dementia. Table 5.1 shows the successive reframing of age-associated progressive dementia since Alzheimer and Kraepelin established its basic clinical and pathological features at the beginning of the last century.

The next three sections discuss the development and framing of dementia in each historical period.

Exercise 5.1: Don't think of an elephant

Try the following simple thought experiment: Don't think of an elephant! Whatever else you do, do not think of an elephant. Of course, it is impossible to meet this challenge, for the word *elephant* itself evokes the image of an elephant. Cognitive linguist George Lakoff uses this example to explain the power of cognitive frames: "Every word, like *elephant*, evokes a frame, which can be an image or other kinds of knowledge: Elephants are large, have floppy ears and a trunk, are associated with circuses, and so on. The word is defined relative to that frame. When we negate a frame, we evoke the frame" (Lakoff 2004: 3).

- What does this thought experiment say about the power of frames, and what are the implications for the politics and policy of dementia?

Alzheimer, Kraepelin, and the foundations of Alzheimer's disease

German psychiatrist Alois Alzheimer and his mentor Emil Kraepelin are generally held to have established the foundations of AD as a diagnostic category, 100 years ago, after Alzheimer's brief report of the case of a 51-year-old woman who developed progressive dementia. On post-mortem, her brain was found to contain numerous senile plaques and neurofibrillary tangles, which were made visible to microscopic observation through a newly developed silver-staining technique. In 1910, on the basis of this case and a handful of others, Alzheimer's mentor and boss Emil Kraepelin bestowed the eponym in the eighth edition of his influential psychiatric book, providing a unified description of the clinical symptoms of AD and the essential pathological features that remains the basis of AD (Ballenger 2000).

From our vantage point today, what perhaps seems most surprising about the early history of AD was that it seemed relatively insignificant to Alzheimer, Kraepelin, and their contemporaries. Alzheimer's initial report drew no enthusiastic reaction from the audience of psychiatrists who heard him give it, nor did its publication in 1907 draw any significant attention (Maurer and Maurer 2003). Kraepelin himself devoted only a few pages of a massive book to it. After Alzheimer's death in 1915, almost none of the many tributes to him written by his colleagues even mentioned AD. Alzheimer was remembered by his contemporaries, including Kraepelin, for his clinical and histopathological acumen and intensive work ethic, not for having discovered the "disease of the century" and for which his name is a household word today (Maurer and Maurer 2003).

Alzheimer's disease did not seem significant to Alzheimer, Kraepelin, and their contemporaries because they framed it in terms of the problems psychiatry faced at the time. At the turn of the twentieth century, the feeling was widespread that clinical psychiatry was far behind other fields of medicine that were increasingly able to identify the pathogenesis and aetiology of discrete disease entities through bacteriological and pathological research (Rosenberg 1992). Psychiatry, by contrast, appeared only able to explain mental illness in terminology that seemed more metaphysical than scientific. Kraepelin and Alzheimer were interested in AD because it seemed like a major mental disorder for which a clear pathological basis had been established. The problem was that it could not be disentangled from ageing. Although they recognized that the clinical and pathological features were virtually the same whatever the age of onset, Kraepelin created the entity "Alzheimer's disease" to distinguish the relatively rare cases in which dementia developed before the age of 65 (pre-senile dementia) from the common occurrence of dementia in more advanced ages (senile dementia). In this framework, the pathological processes of old age that produced senile dementia were understood to be on the extreme end of "normal", while dementia occurring at earlier ages, even though associated with the same brain pathology, seemed to suggest a disease (Ballenger 2006a). As many historians have pointed out, this assumption that mental and physical deterioration were normal in old age has been deeply embedded in medicine and western culture more broadly (Haber 1983; Katz 1996), possibly the reason that psychiatric literature maintained this distinction throughout the 1970s, despite the fact that researchers were well aware of and puzzled by its apparent similarity to senile dementia (Holstein 1997, 2000).

Framing dementia as a problem of ageing in mid-century American psychiatry

The first challenge to this framing of dementia within medicine was the work of American psychiatrists in the 1930s, whose interest was precisely because of its strong association with ageing. For American psychiatrists in the 1930s, age-associated progressive dementia posed a daunting problem. In the late nineteenth century, reforms in public policy made care of the mentally ill the responsibility of states rather than local governments. An unintended result of this was that local welfare officials were given a strong financial incentive to regard old people who could no longer live independently as insane, so that they would be institutionalized in the state mental hospitals at the expense of state governments. As a result, both the absolute and proportional number of aged patients admitted to the state hospitals increased dramatically (Grob 1983, 1986). Because psychiatry regarded senile dementia as incurable, its rising prevalence in the state mental hospital patient population undermined the therapeutic environment that state hospitals were supposed to provide. Because the population in society as a whole was ageing, the problem was regarded by many as an impending crisis – a demographic avalanche that would bury the state hospital as a viable institution, and the professional legitimacy of psychiatry along with it (Ballenger 2000).

American psychiatrists reacted to this problem in two ways. Some argued that since senile dementia was not a proper psychiatric condition, alternative care arrangements ought to be found for patients with dementia who were clogging the state hospital system. This was accomplished in 1965 through legislation making the federal government responsible for funding nursing home care, shifting many thousands of older patients out of mental hospitals and into nursing homes (Grob 1991).

Another group, led by David Rothschild, developed a new theory of dementia emphasizing psychosocial factors over brain pathology in the aetiology – thus bringing the age-associated dementias into the mainstream psychiatry of the time. The basis of this re-conceptualization was the imperfect correlation between dementia and brain pathology; in some cases, senile plaques and neurofibrillary tangles found in the brains of dementia patients were also found in the brains of patients who had shown no sign of dementia in life. In other cases, the brains of patients who died with severe dementia were found at autopsy to be relatively intact. For Rothschild and his followers, this lack of correlation between clinical and pathological data was the most interesting aspect of dementia because it suggested that individuals possessed differing abilities to compensate for organic lesions. Seen this way, age-associated dementia was more than the simple and inevitable outcome of a brain that was deteriorating. Rather, dementia was a dialectical process between the brain and the psychosocial context in which the ageing person was situated, a view shared by Kitwood (1997) in the UK. Factors such as pre-morbid personality structure, emotional trauma, disruptions of family support, and social isolation were regarded as equally important in explaining dementia (Ballenger 2000). For psychodynamically oriented psychiatrists and psychologists, the psychodynamic approach was a more satisfying theory of dementia, providing a basis for meaningful therapeutic interventions, and resulting in a surge of interest in age-associated dementias (Ballenger 2000).

But the psychodynamic model offered more than a rationale for the therapeutic efforts of desperate psychiatrists in the state hospitals. It also seemed to provide insight into the entire experience of ageing in post Second World War America. In the 1940s and 1950s, virtually all American psychiatrists working on senile dementia stopped investigating brain pathology. Nor did they attempt to delineate various disease entities based on pathological lesions, but folded Alzheimer-type dementia, cerebral arteriosclerosis, and functional mental disorders into a broad concept of senile mental deterioration, whose pathological hallmarks were not brain deterioration but modern social relations. The locus of senile mental deterioration was no longer the ageing brain, but a society which, through mandatory retirement, social isolation, and the disintegration of traditional family ties, stripped older people of their role in life. Bereft of any meaningful social role and suffering the effects of intense social stigma, it was not surprising that the mind of older people began to deteriorate. This thinking resonated with social constructionist, structure and agency sociological theorists and critical gerontologists in the UK (e.g. Gilleard 1992).

By bringing together cultural anxieties about the isolation, emptiness, and stigma of ageing in modern society with the frightening symptoms of dementia, the psychodynamic approach to senile mental deterioration contributed to a broad re-framing, seeking to make retirement a meaningful and desirable stage of life, financially secure, and emotionally satisfying. To the emerging field of social gerontology in both the USA and UK, the high prevalence of senile mental deterioration was an indictment of society's failure to meet the needs of the elderly (Ballenger 2006b).

"Adjustment" of the individual to ageing was the key concept for social gerontologists in the 1940s and 1950s. Adjustment could be negative, resulting in senile mental deterioration, or positive, resulting in the preservation of mental health (Ballenger 2000). Although adjustment to old age was ultimately a personal matter, prominent gerontologists argued that "in modern America the community must carry the responsibility of creating conditions that make it possible for the great majority of older people to lead the independent and emotionally satisfying lives of which they are capable" (Havighurst 1952: 17). The community's responsibility went beyond altruism, for if their needs were not met, the burgeoning ageing population would result in a catastrophic increase in senility.

The solution was to provide older people with meaningful activities. Broadly construed, this was the programme of social gerontology for reconstructing old age. And whatever the scientific merits of this model of the social production of 'senility' as an account of the pathogenesis of dementia, those who framed dementia this way were generally successful in winning a series of significant policy changes, transforming the experience of ageing in America. A similar transformation took place in the UK (Laslett 1989). The material circumstances of old age had been markedly improved (though not to an equal extent for all older people); significant legal protections had been won against age discrimination; negative stereotypes in popular and professional discourse were increasingly challenged; and older people had organized for effective political advocacy (Haber and Gratton 1994). In this context, the problem of age-associated dementia became more visible and tragic. After 1965, de-institutionalization increased the burden that dementia posed to communities and families, while heightened expectations for old age made senile dementia an even more devastating prospect (Ballenger 2006b).

Reframing senility as Alzheimer's disease

This framing of dementia as part of a broad category of senility began to seem inappropriate for the new era of ageing taking shape in the 1960s and 1970s. Ageism, a term coined by Robert Butler in the late 1960s to describe stereotyping and discrimination against the elderly, became the key term in social gerontology for a more aggressive and politicized generation. Butler and other gerontologists argued that virtually all of the physical and mental deterioration commonly attributed to old age was largely the product of disease processes distinct from ageing. "Senility", in the view, was not a medical diagnosis, but a "wastebasket term" applied to any person over 60 with a problem that rationalized neglect by assuming it was inevitable and irreversible.

> 66 Some of what is called senile is the result of brain damage. But anxiety and depression are also frequently lumped within the same category of senility, even though they are treatable and often reversible. [Because both doctors and the public found it so] convenient to dismiss all these manifestations by lumping them together under an improper and inaccurate diagnostic label, the elderly often did not receive the benefits of decent diagnosis and treatment. 99

—Butler (1975: 9–10)

Butler did not discount the reality of irreversible brain damage, as had an earlier generation of psychiatrists. Rather, he argued that the refusal to systematically distinguish various physical and mental disease processes from each other and from ageing was a manifestation of ageism that kept society from taking the problems of older people seriously. In this context, a group of clinical neurologists and psychiatrists, neuropathologists, and biochemists worked to re-frame age-associated dementia in old age as a number of disease entities distinct from ageing.

These researchers produced significant gains in scientific knowledge about dementia in the 1960s and 1970s. But scientific progress alone was not sufficient to resolve the central question of whether AD and other dementias were connected to the ageing process. A reasonable case could – and still can – be made either way. On the one hand, no pathological, biochemical or clinical markers existed or yet exist which qualitatively differentiate AD from an extreme form of normal ageing. If AD were a distinct disease entity, one would expect a number of these markers to be distributed in a bimodal pattern throughout the ageing population, differentiating the diseased from the normal. But every potential marker for AD more closely follows a linear distribution ascending with age, suggesting that AD is the end point of a continuum. There are also problems in viewing AD as an extreme point on the continuum of ageing. From the continuum model, it would follow that everyone who lived long enough would develop AD, making it possible to establish an age limit beyond which all survivors are demented. While the prevalence of AD clearly climbs with age, there are many well-established cases of people living well past a hundred years with little cognitive impairment. One could suppose that individuals age at different rates, but this would lead back towards viewing those who aged "prematurely" as suffering from a distinct disease (Huppert and Brayne 1994).

Although conclusive evidence was lacking, the question was too important to be ignored since many researchers seemed to feel that the issue called into question the value of their enterprise. Research on AD had to be about more than an investigation into one of the many effects of ageing; to ascribe an aetiological role to ageing, it seemed, was to associate research with a fanciful pursuit of the fountain of youth. Alzheimer's disease was re-framed by Katzman (1976) in an editorial in the *Archives of Neurology* where he argued for dropping the distinction between AD and senile dementia, since they were identical both clinically and pathologically. This dramatically increased the number of cases of AD. Katzman estimated that there were as many as 1.2 million cases of AD in the USA in 1976, and 60,000–90,000 deaths a year – making it the fourth or fifth leading cause of death in the USA (Katzman 1976). An essential outcome of Katzman's editorial and a subsequent National Institutes of Health supported conference, was consensus that AD and senile dementia were a unified entity – senile dementia of the Alzheimer type – and not part of the normal ageing process. Rather, it was a disease whose mechanisms could be unravelled through basic research leading eventually to effective treatments and ultimately prevention (Katzman and Bick 2000).

Exercise 5.2: Cultural framing and the experience of dementia

We have examined the historical shifts in the framing of dementia. Such shifts in frame probably had an impact on the direct experience of dementia for both caregivers and people with dementia. For example, a different framing of dementia may make the condition more or less stigmatizing. An interesting source for further exploration of this issue is autobiographies. As AD emerged as a major public issue, autobiographical accounts by caregivers became a popular resource for better understanding the experience of dementia. Notable caregiver accounts include Shanks (1999), Bayley (1999), and Levine (2004) – though many have appeared. More interesting still, perhaps, a number of autobiographies have been published by people with dementia (for example, Henderson 1998; DeBaggio 2002; Taylor 2006). It is difficult to compare the experiences described in these books to the experience of dementia in earlier historical periods because such memoirs simply did not appear prior to the emergence of AD as a major public issue. But, reading these autobiographical accounts, the struggle with stigma and fear are certainly dominant themes.

■ In what ways might the different historical frames described in this chapter have affected the experience of dementia for caregivers and people with dementia?

Framing cure versus care in Alzheimer's disease advocacy

The re-framing of AD was politically powerful, allowing researchers, ageing advocates, and policy-makers committed to AD research to make a convincing case that public resources should be allocated for such research. Perhaps the most prominent advocate for AD research was Robert Butler, who was appointed the first director of the National Institute on Aging (NIA) when it was established in 1974. Butler made AD the focal point of the fledgling institute. Butler knew it would be much easier to sell to Congress the need for research on a dread disease than on the basic science of ageing (Fox 1989). Butler's strategy was highly successful; by the end of the 1980s, the NIA budget for AD research had increased more than 800%. Federal funding for AD research has continued to grow, even in an era characterized by budgetary constraints, reaching a plateau of over $600 million by the first decade of the twenty-first century.

But the re-framing of dementia as AD and the disease-specific lobbying strategy built around it have had negative albeit unintended consequences for advocacy efforts to win support for caregivers, an imperative that most involved in the AD field recognize and endorse. This can be seen in the early history of the Alzheimer's Association, the leading advocacy organization for age-associated progressive dementia in the USA, whose commitment to support of caregivers cannot be questioned. Yet the association's exclusive focus on AD meant it would be a much more effective advocate for research than for caregiver support. Services that helped AD victims and their families would help victims and caregivers struggling with the effects of any type of brain impairment, and some policies dearly sought by AD families, such as long-term care insurance, would benefit those struggling with virtually any chronic disabling illness. If increasing support for caregivers had been the primary goal of the association, the logical course would have been to create a broader constituency of people affected by the many diseases that would have benefited from the same policies.

The marginalization of care can also be seen in the rhetoric of AD advocates which frequently posited a trade-off – albeit usually implicitly – between support for research and support for caregiving. Advocates of AD ostensibly endorsed with equal vigour an increase in federal money to support both research and caregiving. But in describing the "disease of the century", they forged a link between the costs of caregiving and the need for research that undermined the plausibility of arguments that could be made for major social policy initiatives to address the problems of caregivers. In making the case for research funding, AD advocates emphasized the tremendous economic burden the disease placed on society for items like nursing home care – costs that would dramatically increase if a treatment or cure for the disease were not found. In so doing, they also underscored the extent to which policy changes that would substantially benefit caregivers would be prohibitively expensive. For example, in the mid-1980s, the Alzheimer's Disease and Related Disorders Association's (ADRDA) first president Jerome Stone frequently decried what he saw as the imbalance between the amount of money spent on research and the amount of money spent on care. The ADRDA's first annual report (1984) noted that "our nation still spends 800 times more to care for our nearly three million Alzheimer's victims than it allocates for research. Federal and private insurance programmes still pay little or none of the staggering costs of Alzheimer's patient care" (ADRDA 1984: 2). Stone is not trying to marginalize the need for caregiver support here, but that is the effect. In such formulations, these two policy goals stand in an uneasy relationship. Caregiving is positioned as an unfortunate and unnecessary burden – the price we pay for our failure to commit enough resources to find a cure. The unintentional marginalization of caregiving in the rhetoric of AD advocates is perhaps most explicit in the frequent comparisons made between AD and polio, thus invoking one of the triumphal moments of modern medical science. For example, when ADRDA board member Lonnie Wollin was asked in his 1985 testimony before Congress to prioritize funding for caregiving versus funding for research, he found it difficult to choose. "There are people calling our office who are frightened. They need respite and care," he noted. "On the other hand, if you don't fund substantial research, you will have this problem for a long time. The only analogy would be polio. Had the money gone into treatment, we would have a magnificent portable iron lung, but no cure for the disease. I think the dollars that are available have to be spread out between the immediate respite care and research" (House of Representatives, Select Committee on Aging 1986: 24). The polio analogy was a rhetorical trump card, making funding for biomedical research a moral imperative in its ability to relieve suffering, and the most sensible fiscal policy because it would dramatically lower the costs of caring for disease victims. If polio was indeed the "only analogy", then, whether Wollin explicitly said so or not, research had to be the number one priority.

Exercise 5.3: Reframing dementia

To win broader support for innovative public programmes to support care for people with dementia, it will be necessary to re-frame dementia as something other than a degenerative brain disease.

■ What concepts, images, and metaphors would allow this kind of re-framing of dementia?

Debates and controversies

There are many reasons why it has been difficult to win support for dementia caregiving in the USA, but its marginalization within AD advocacy discourse has surely not helped. To move the politics and policy of dementia care forward, we will need to create new meanings and possibilities for dementia care. In part, this will require setting aside the logic of the disease-specific strategy to forge alliances between larger constituencies for policies that would aid caregivers for all sorts of chronic disorders. It will also require creating a new language for caregiver that lifts it free from an association with the goal of finding a cure for or prevention of dementia that inevitably marginalizes care. These meanings have begun to emerge through innovative approaches like the Timeslips storytelling project, which utilizes storytelling to transform the relationship between people with dementia and professional caregivers. The values embodied in these programmes must be translated into the language of advocacy, so that dementia care can begin to be seen as a good in itself rather than simply a burden that we must shoulder in the absence of medical breakthroughs. Finally, some in the AD field argue that we may need to challenge the framing of dementia as a medical entity itself and adopt a less rigid understanding of the experience of dementia that accepts not only the obvious losses, but recognizes the possibilities for meaning and enjoyment that can remain and perhaps even be enhanced (Whitehouse and George 2008).

Conclusion

In the USA, funding for research into prevention and cure of dementia has received significant government support, with evidence suggesting that this support is increasing. Far less has been expended on research or the development of services to support family and professional caregivers who provide the bulk of care for people with dementia. This trend in funding is compounded by the ongoing discrepancy in government health funding for acute versus chronic care. That is, funding for acute care is considerably greater than funding for chronic conditions. As a chronic condition, dementia care services fall into this less supported care category. One consequence is that family members who have long shouldered the burdens of caregiving are finding it difficult to access services that would help them continue to provide care. This chapter has outlined the history of developments in the USA that have led to these funding differences and the efforts to shift more dollars in the direction of developing care programmes for people with dementia and their caregivers.

Further information

The Timeslips Storytelling Project is actively engaged in re-framing dementia by emphasizing the creativity and imagination that remain in people with dementia through a creative storytelling method designed for people with dementia and their caregivers [http://www.timeslips.org/].

Anne Basting, the creator of the Timeslips Project, has a blog called "Forget Memory" that is broadly aimed at "imagining a better life for people with memory loss".

The Rockridge Institute was a non-profit, non-partisan think tank devoted to deepening and broadening public understanding of the worldviews, values, and ideas that drive the political process. Rockridge's approach was rooted in the theory of cognitive frames that informs this chapter [http://www.cognitivepolicyworks.com/resource-center/rockridge-institute/].

The Alzheimer's Association is the leading health care voluntary association in the USA advocating for public policy related to AD and related forms of dementia [http://www.alz.org/].

Alzheimer's Disease International (ADI) is a federation leading health voluntary associations from 77 different nations advocating for public policy related to AD and related forms of dementia [http://www.alz.co.uk/].

References

ADEAR Center (2012) *Alzheimer's Research Enters a New Era* [http://www.nia.nih.gov/alzheimers/publication/2011-2012-alzheimers-disease-progress-report/alzheimers-research-enters-new#.Um3x1nBwqSo, accessed 28 October 2013].

ADRDA (Alzheimer's Disease and Related Disorders Association) (1984) *ADRDA 1984 Annual Report*. Chicago, IL: ADRDA.

Alzheimer's Association (2013) *Alzheimer's Disease: Facts and Figures*. Chicago, IL: Alzheimer's Association.

Alzheimer's Research UK (undated) *Dementia Statistics*. Cambridge: Alzheimer's Research UK.

Ballenger, J.F. (2000) Beyond the characteristic plaques and tangles: midtwentieth century US psychiatry and the fight against senility, in P. Whitehouse, K. Maurer and J.F. Ballenger (eds.) *Concepts of Alzheimer Disease: Biological, Clinical and Cultural Perspectives*. Baltimore, MD: Johns Hopkins University Press, pp. 83–103.

Ballenger, J.F. (2006a) Progress in the history of Alzheimer's disease: the importance of context, *Journal of Alzheimer's Disease*, 9: 1–9.

Ballenger, J.F. (2006b) *Self, Senility and Alzheimer's Disease in Modern America*. Baltimore, MD: Johns Hopkins University Press.

Bayley, J. (1999) *Elegy for Iris*. New York: St. Martin's Press.

Butler, R.N. (1975) *Why Survive? Being Old in America*. New York: Harper & Row.

Department of Health (2009) *Living Well with Dementia: A National Strategy for Dementia*. London: DH Publications.

DeBaggio, T. (2002) *Losing My Mind: An Intimate Look at Life with Alzheimer's*. New York: Free Press.

Fox, P. (1989) From senility to Alzheimer's disease: the rise of the Alzheimer's disease movement, *Milbank Quarterly*, 67(1): 58–102.

Gilleard, C. (1992) Losing one's mind and losing one's place: a psychosocial model of dementia, in K. Morgan (ed.) *Gerontology: Responding to an Aging Society*. London: Jessica Kingsley.

Grob, G. (1983) *Mental Illness and American Society, 1875–1940*. Princeton, NJ: Princeton University Press.

Grob, G. (1986) Explaining old age history: the need for empiricism, in D.D. Van Tassel and P.N. Stearns (eds.) *Old Age in a Bureaucratic Society*. New York: Greenwood Press.

Grob, G. (1991) *From Asylum to Community: Mental Health Policy in Modern America*. Princeton, NJ: Princeton University Press.

Haber, C. (1983) *Beyond Sixty-five: The Dilemma of Old Age in America's Past*. Cambridge: Cambridge University Press.

Haber, C. and Gratton, B. (1994) *Old Age and the Search for Security: An American Social History*. Bloomington, IN: Indiana University Press.

Havighurst, R. (1952) Social and psychological needs of the aging, *Annals of the American Academy of Political and Social Science*, 279: 11–17.

Henderson, C.S. (1998) *Partial View: An Alzheimer's Journal*. Dallas, TX: Southern Methodist University Press.

Holstein, M. (1997) Alzheimer's disease and senile dementia, 1885–1920: an interpretive history of disease negotiation, *Journal of Aging Studies*, 11(1): 1–13.

Holstein, M. (2000) Aging, culture, and the framing of Alzheimer disease, in P.J. Whitehouse, K. Maurer and J.F. Ballenger (eds.) *Concepts of Alzheimer Disease: Biological, Clinical and Cultural Perspectives*. Baltimore, MD: Johns Hopkins University Press, pp. 158–80.

House of Representatives, Select Committee on Aging (1986) 99th Congress, *Alzheimer's Disease: Burdens and Problems for Victims and their Families*. Washington, DC: US Government Printer.

Huppert, F. and Brayne, C. (1994) What is the relationship between dementia and normal aging?, in F.A. Huppert, C. Brayne and D. O'Connor (eds.) *Dementia and Normal Aging*. New York: Cambridge University Press, pp. 3–14.

Katz, S. (1996) *Disciplining Old Age: The Formation of Gerontological Knowledge*. Charlottesville, VA: University Press of Virginia.

Katzman, R. (1976) Editorial: The prevalence and malignancy of Alzheimer disease – a major killer, *Archives of Neurology*, 33(4): 217–18.

Katzman, R. and Bick, K.L. (2000) The rediscovery of Alzheimer disease during the 1960s and 1970s, in P.J. Whitehouse, K. Maurer and J.F. Ballenger (eds.) *Concepts of Alzheimer Disease: Biological, Clinical and Cultural Perspectives*. Baltimore, MD: Johns Hopkins University Press, pp. 104–14.

Kitwood, T. (1997) *Dementia Reconsidered: The Person Comes First*. Buckingham: Open University Press

Lakoff, G. (2004) *Don't Think of an Elephant: Know Your Values and Frame the Debate*. White River Junction, VT: Chelsea Green.

Laslett, P. (1989) *A Fresh Map of Life: The Emergence of the Third Age*. London: Weidenfeld & Nicolson.

Levine, J. (2004) *Do You Remember Me? A Father, a Daughter, and a Search for the Self*. New York: Free Press.

Maurer, K. and Maurer, U. (2003) *Alzheimer: The Life of a Physician and the Career of a Disease*. New York: Columbia University Press.

Rosenberg, C.E. (1992) *The Crisis in Psychiatric Legitimacy: Reflections on Psychiatry, Medicine, and Public Policy. Exploring Epidemics and Other Essays in the History of Medicine*. New York: Cambridge University Press.

Shanks, L.K. (1999) *Your Name is Hughes Hannibal Shanks: A Caregiver's Guide to Alzheimer's*. New York: Penguin.

Taylor, R. (2006) *Alzheimer's from the Inside Out*. Baltimore, MD: Health Professions Press.

US Department of Health and Human Services (USDHHS) (2013) *National Plan to Address Alzheimer's Disease: 2013 Update*. Washington, DC: USDHHS.

Whitehouse, P.J. and George, D. (2008) *The Myth of Alzheimer's: What You aren't Being Told about Today's Most Dreaded Diagnosis*. New York: St. Martins Press.

CHAPTER 6

Representations of people with dementia in the media and in literature

Hannah Zeilig

> ❝I don't think people understand. They need re-educating about dementia. They just think of people, frail people in nursing homes. They don't see that you can live independently. ❞

—Marlene Aveyard Yorkshire, UK

Learning objectives

By the end of this chapter, you will have a clearer understanding of:

- Why it is important to understand "dementia" and Alzheimer's disease in terms of cultural context
- Why we should challenge the language that is often used to describe people living with a dementia
- Some of the prevailing representations of "dementia" in the media
- Alternative stories about dementia and people living with a dementia
- How representations of people with dementia can affect our perceptions of "dementia" and contribute to stigma
- The power of some representations of people with dementia to encourage understanding and empathy

Introduction

"Dementia" is not simply a biomedical category but is also a socially and culturally constructed condition (Kitwood 1997; Kontos and Naglie 2007; Basting 2009). Kitwood's (1997) seminal work pioneered the sense that dementia is a psychosocial condition, and has encouraged clinicians, practitioners, and academics to reconsider their narrow medical conceptions of dementia. One way to challenge the "malignant social psychology" (Kitwood 1997) that surrounds dementia and Alzheimer's disease (AD) is to question some of the cultural narratives that influence how we think about these conditions. These narratives are inscribed in the stories reflected by the media, in films, and in literature.

Although the words "Alzheimer's disease" and "dementia" are used frequently in the media, their exact meaning is unclear to most people. In the popular press, the terms are often confounded and are mostly associated with older people. It is worth noting that the word dementia (which comes from the Latin: *de mentis* – out of the mind) did not originally refer to an age-related condition (Zeilig 2013). Even today, the word "demented" is common slang for deviant behaviour regardless of age.

Both dementia and Alzheimer's have been subject to subtly changing psychiatric, biomedical, and social/cultural stories. An exploration of recurring media and literary representations of dementia reveals the historical and cultural forces that shape and structure this condition and affect the lives of people who have dementia. This chapter will consider: (1) the influence of cultural context on our understanding of AD and dementia; (2) the language that is often associated with these conditions; (3) a range of media representations (as these have appeared in the UK press, in recent political speeches, and in documentary TV programs); and (4) a number of literary representations (novels, poems, and memoirs).

Dementia: the influence of cultural context

The importance of exploring representations of dementia is increasingly recognized in academic circles. When these representations are scrutinized, they can help to uncover truths about how a society imagines, and most importantly, how it engages with the people who live with a dementia. Indeed, the pioneering field of "Medical Humanities" stresses the importance of the arts as a means of facilitating the re-engagement of the practitioner with the subjective world of the patient (Oyebode 2009). An analysis of how dementia and AD are culturally represented is also a "temperature gauge" – a means of exploring what we, collectively, consider dementia to be. There is an ever-increasing supply of these representations in film, television, novels, plays, memoirs, newspaper stories, poetry, and even opera (Zeilig 2012).

Equally, people with a dementia are starting to speak, without mediation, and so are representing (and advocating for) themselves (see Chapter 28). In the UK, the science fantasy writer Terry Pratchett is the best-known figure living with a form of dementia. He has been open about living with AD, which he famously described as an "embuggeration" (Russell 2009, 2011). The studied irreverence of this term is interesting, as it demonstrates Pratchett's refusal to dramatize the condition or to pose as a victim who requires our pity. On the contrary, Pratchett continues to make regular TV appearances and to produce his "discworld" novels and thus provides a persistent challenge to notions that people with dementia face an inevitable and swift decline. In a relatively recent interview with *The Telegraph* newspaper, he defiantly stated that his condition had given him a "new lease of life" (Grice 2012).

There are also vociferous campaigners such as Richard Taylor in the USA [see http://www.richardtaylorphd.com/] and Christine Bryden in Australia [see http://www.christinebryden.com/index.html] who are finding ways of countering societal prejudices about what people living with dementia are and therefore what dementia represents. The use of blogs and websites provide interesting outlets for the self-expression, recreation, and representation of individuals who live with a dementia.

The ways in which particular individuals attempt to oppose and even subvert existing views of dementia must, however, be understood against the backdrop of wider cultural imperatives and ideologies. These tend to dominate everyday apprehensions of what a person with dementia is like or what dementia might be. After all, the stories that we tell about these conditions are inextricably connected with contemporary societal and political mores. The UK and other European nations as well as the USA have in the early twenty-first century faced a number of crises – primarily economic, but also environmental. These crises have contributed to a widespread sense of anxiety at individual levels (there are concerns about the future of personal security as pension funds dissolve and in the USA the mortgage market exploded) and at societal level, as many European countries face an erosion of political power. In August 2011 credit ratings were downgraded in the USA (Port 2012), and in April 2013 the UK was stripped of its AAA status and downgraded to AA+. Thus, the economic credibility of both erstwhile superpowers is dubious and questions have arisen about the future solvency and the viability of major institutions in these countries.

As has been eloquently articulated by Cynthia Port in her essay on ageing, temporality, history, and reverse chronologies, it is against this backdrop of widespread decline that we have to understand the ways in which our culture represents age, ageing, and dementia. This assumes a particular urgency as the world in the twenty-first century is characterized by a demographic transition and unprecedented ageing populations. For the most part, ageing and dementia (these very separate concepts have become almost synonymous for many) are opposed to youth in a simplistic binary.

Youth is associated with positive progress and ageing with disintegration, memory loss, and decline. There are many problems with this binary. As Gullette recently pointed out, the young are also struggling with brain injury (accompanied by memory loss and aggression), due to the consequences of the Iraq and Afghanistan wars: ". . . but the growing terror of memory loss – even mild memory loss – is connected to old people" (Gullette 2012: 6).

Our reactions to dementia are shaped, in part, by a social and political narrative of declining economies and general crisis. Dementia and AD have become inextricably bound up with fears about the general decline of empires. The stories we are told and we tell about these conditions are necessarily shaped by these wider narratives. Data and discourses are not neutral – they come loaded with feelings and politics. Similarly, the representations of people who live with a dementia and their carers are influenced by this context (George and Whitehouse 2014).

The language of dementia

There is an intimate relationship between the words commonly used to describe AD and dementia and the representation of these conditions. A recent UK study (University of East Anglia) revealed that people with a dementia are often described as "doolally", as "nutters" or "fruit cakes", as having "lost their marbles", and that dementia care staff are known as "bum wipers" (Zeilig et al. 2012–2013).

This lexicon is wholly negative. It not only affects those who live with a dementia but also has negative implications for those who provide their care. People living with AD or dementia are described by pejorative adjectives. Crucially, they are what they have lost. Their carers are connected with the most demeaning of tasks. This language is also indicative of the regard that society has for people living with a dementia who are reduced to a collection of symptoms. Even references by scientists to amyloid plaques and tau tangles fuel the perception of dementia as a knotty problem. The language of medicine and science is not neutral – it, too, is replete with descriptions likening dementia to a plague (Mandell and Green 2011; Lees 2012) and outlining the dementia "crisis" (Zeilig 2013).

Debates and controversies

There is an ongoing debate about what constitutes personhood. Personhood concerns the status of being a person and is a controversial topic in philosophy, law, ethics, and health care. The notion of personhood is closely related to conceptions of the self. People living with a dementia often face stigma and discrimination that is related to an underlying questioning of their personhood and selfhood. The western representation of personhood emphasizes the achievement and maintenance of self-worth through the display of cognitive or intellectual abilities (Basting 2003, 2009; Kontos 2003). A core cultural belief about the "self" involves autonomy, productivity, self-control, and cleanliness (Herskovits 1995). Dementias, which involve the erosion of cognitive abilities as well as increasing dependency, are therefore particularly threatening to western conceptions of personhood and selfhood. As Kontos (2012) has cogently explained, when Alzheimer's disease (in particular) is analysed in terms of the cognitive dysfunction it produces, our notions of what constitutes the self are challenged at a fundamental level.

There is controversy about the ways in which society refers to people living with a dementia. As is clearly described by Julie Goyder (2001), the language often used by staff in care homes "abjects" people living with a dementia. This is also true of the language commonly found in newspaper reports and even in some advertisements by organizations that are working for people with a dementia. Language is powerful and political (as has been long appreciated by the civil rights movement and by feminists). Negative terminology creates and intensifies prejudice and should be challenged. Similarly, positive terminology can help to change the way we think about people and situations. The civil rights movement in the USA used language to help fight for equality for black Americans. For instance, in 1966 Jesse Jackson asserted: "I am black and I am beautiful! I am – Somebody!" The combination of black with beautiful was challenging for the white hegemony. The persistent association of dementia and AD with suffering and victim status has been questioned. In a recent play about living with a dementia, the protagonist rejects the notion of "suffering" (Smith 2010). The words that are commonly and casually linked with people who are living with a dementia help to separate "us" from "them" (where them = people who are living with AD or dementia).

Despite the rash of information that surrounds the conditions, both dementia and AD are currently shrouded in mystery. After all, information is not the same as knowledge. Dementia and AD are concepts that retreat from meaning. The term " Alzheimer's disease" is so imprecise that the scientific world is beginning to discard it (Gullette 2012; Zeilig 2013) on the basis that it does not provide a "differential diagnosis that can distinguish one malady from another in the pursuit of causes and remedies" (Gullette 2012). The uncertain evolution of AD and dementia as diagnostic labels is exemplified by changes to the new clinical and research guidelines – the *Diagnostic and Statistical Manual of Mental Disorders (DSM) V* (May 2013). These guidelines indicate that AD is a heterogeneous set of conditions rather than a single event (George *et al.* 2013). This profound lack of clarity about what dementia or AD might be arouses what Sontag (1991) aptly named "old fashioned" kinds of dread. As Sontag lucidly demonstrates, any disease or condition whose causality is murky, and for which medical treatment is ineffectual, excites particular horror. The disease then becomes a metaphor (Zeilig 2013) and is also used as an adjective to describe all that is morally or socially pernicious. "First the subjects of deepest dread (corruption, decay, pollution, anomie, weakness) are identified with the disease. The disease itself becomes a metaphor" (Sontag 1991: 60). In this context, a metaphor refers to a linguistic device whereby implicit comparison is made between two unlike things. We all use metaphors all the time: we talk about the journey of life or the tapestry of life, blue sky thinking, the black dog of depression, and so on. Thus "dementia" has become a metaphor for the ills associated with old age. Ironically, it is precisely because "dementia" is a hollow label (Gullette 2012) that it has become so replete with significance.

Exercise 6.1: Thinking about language

■ Why is it relevant to think about the language used to describe dementia and AD and those who live with these conditions?

■ Ask the people who are in your immediate vicinity the words that they would use to describe people who live with dementia. Are these similar to the words that you would use?

■ Think about an older person that you know well. What words would you use to describe him or her?

■ What language would you use to describe a dementia care worker? Why?

■ What do you think (or know) are the main tasks of dementia care workers?

■ When you look at the words that you have written down (to describe older people and dementia care workers), what sort of images come to mind?

Dementia and AD in the media and in politics

Water, tides, and flooding

Dementia has long been portrayed in newspapers and political speeches as a "rising tide" (this is imagery that recalls Shakespeare's political play *Julius Caesar* – "There is a tide in the affairs of men"). As long ago as 1978, *The Times* newspaper noted: "This epidemic of mental impairment in old age is creeping upon society with the quiet certainty of a rising tide" (Zeilig 2013: 3). Here, the conflation of a fast spreading infection (an epidemic) with rising water is particularly striking. Rising tides in relation to dementia appeared very recently in David Cameron's speeches about dementia: "the rising tide of people suffering with dementia" (O'Grady 2012), and echo the same watery imagery that Margaret Thatcher used in her speeches about mental impairment among the elderly. Indeed, *The Rising Tide – Developing Services for Mental Illness in Old Age* (Dick 1982) was the title of a Health Advisory report on the development of demonstration districts for old age psychiatry. More recently, a report analysing the impact of dementia on Canadian society was called *Rising Tide* (Alzheimer Society Canada 2010) and stresses the "urgent" need for "immediate action" on dementia from all Canadians. The image of a rising tide linked with dementia associates the condition with natural disaster. Water is particularly hard to contain; it changes shape, and is associated with apocalyptic catastrophe. The associative link with the way in which dementia may affect society – a disease that will swamp us all and which cannot be contained – has an insidious effect on the ways in which discourses of dementia are constructed.

As noted elsewhere (Zeilig 2013), the "silent tsunami" of dementia has also been a dominant watery image in many news stories. This image is an oxymoron, but it is arresting and it echoes imagery of the silver tsunami of ageing (Charise 2012). It neatly fuses fears about environmental disaster (the storms that recently ravaged America's east coast, the tsunamis in Japan and Indonesia) with terror about dementia. This barely conscious figurative language (Charise 2012) compares the catastrophic destruction of cities, food, and water supplies entailed by a tsunami with the effects of dementia on society. The imagery of rising tides and the disastrous flooding of tsunamis must be understood in the context of the alarmist or apocalyptic demography that characterizes much of the rhetoric about ageing in general and dementia in particular (Katz 1996; Cruikshank 2009). As is so amply demonstrated by Gullette (2004, 2012), we are always aged by culture and similarly illness is framed by our culture. This is particularly true of any illness that baffles medics and scientists and which has an unclear aetiology.

The image of infection also implies that the condition is virulent and might be catching. This sense that dementia might be caught informs some of our most emotive reactions to the condition. The impression that dementia might be caught echoes Sontag's analysis of mysterious diseases, mentioned earlier. Although Sontag is describing cancer, her acute observations are equally relevant to AD and dementia:

> Any disease that is treated as a mystery and acutely enough feared will be felt to be morally, if not literally, contagious. Thus a surprisingly large number of people with cancer find themselves being shunned by relatives and friends . . .

—Sontag (1991: 6)

Case example 6.1: A plague doctor

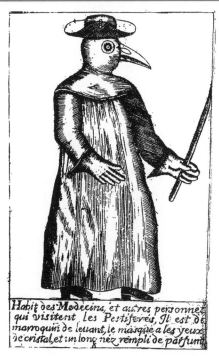

Figure 6.1: A plague doctor

Source: Jean-Jacques Manget, Traité de la peste: recueilli des meilleurs auteurs anciens et modernes, et enrichi de remarques et observations théoriques et pratiques: avec une table très ample des matières (1721)

This is an image of a "plague doctor" from the Middle Ages (c. 1340s), a physician hired by towns that had a great number of plague victims. The beak they had was a filter for what they believed to be bad, infected air. Plague doctors were rarities, as the work was so risky.

In the twenty-first century, we pride ourselves on our enlightened evidence-based medical practice. However, it is remarkable the extent to which our representations of dementia and AD and our treatment of people living with these conditions remains rooted in the "old fashioned dread" that Susan Sontag so convincingly reveals.

Dread

In the Middle Ages, the Black Death encapsulated all society's fears. Cancer and AIDS in the 1970s and 1980s/1990s, respectively, occupied centre-stage as the most deadly and feared of diseases. In the early twenty-first century, these have both been trumped by AD and dementia.

Dementia, as it is represented in the popular press, has a paradoxical nature. It is both a horribly active disease, a "killer", and yet one that simultaneously renders its "victims" passive and inert. Similarly, "we" – society, medics, and scientists – are rendered powerless in the face of its inevitable and insidious approach.

In his keynote speech, Prime Minister Cameron talked about "the quiet crisis, one that steals at lives and tears at the heart of families" (Prime Minister's Office 2012). Here, the image of dementia as a vigorous force is evident. This echoes descriptions of Grendel in the Anglo Saxon poem "Beowulf", who attacks warriors as they sleep and is shrouded in darkness. Grendel is a "killer of souls" (l.177) (Heaney 1999). Whether or not you also think of Grendel, the language used by David Cameron indisputably conjures up a monster or bogeyman. This monster has roots deep within our shared cultural fears of such creatures, which attack at night, are massive in size, and bent on destruction. It is mythic. Cameron also emphasizes silence, a "quiet crisis". This is curious because in the last five years or so, dementia has been the topic of fevered debate and attention; it nonetheless remains linked with silence. The impression is that dementia is a silent, stealthy invader, something that creeps up on people and steals them from themselves.

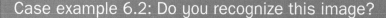

Case example 6.2: Do you recognize this image?

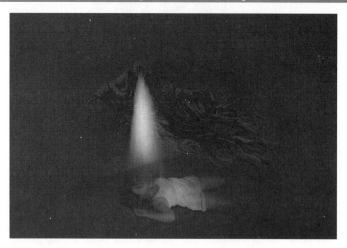

Figure 6.2: Dementor image
© Andrea Peipe

This is an impression of the dementors that are featured in the fifth and sixth Harry Potter novels and that most school children have heard of. These are vividly described as foul creatures that suck happy memories from their victims leaving them with memories only of the most miserable kind.

- Why do you think J.K. Rowling called these monsters "dementors"?
- To what extent do you think the dementors reflect the other monster imagery associated with dementia and AD?

War and military language

If dementia is a killer monster, we have to wage war against it. Thus another recurring linguistic device in the cultural framing of dementia is the reliance on military and war-like metaphors. So David Cameron proclaimed (*The Guardian*, March 2012): "We need an all-out fight-back against this disease; one that cuts across society" (Prime Minister's Office 2012). Dementia is pictured as something that requires a fight back. Britain's dementia "time bomb" crops up frequently (this is a phrase that was also coined in 1984 by Margaret Thatcher when discussing the need to finance old age welfare). The most common use of time bombs has been in politically motivated terrorism. The association of dementia and later life with terrorist tactics may have something to do with the sense of a threat that is in our midst. Thus dementia and war – perhaps above all the nebulous war on terror – are yoked together (George and Whitehouse 2014). It follows that people with dementia are depicted as "victims" and that dementia is indissolubly linked with death, or more precisely a living death.

So on the one hand, AD and dementia are represented as of mythic or biblical proportions, monsters that we must take arms against but that render us powerless. There are other metaphorical devices for describing AD or dementia. These include images of darkness and shadow. Darkness is often contrasted with light – the light of possible medical advances, for example. Language around "burden" and "weight" (usually in connection with the carers of those with AD or dementia) also recurs, as does the term "crisis" – and this is most often associated with financial imperatives. Indeed, the economics of dementia are confusing. In the UK, the Coalition government pledged vast sums (£54 million) as part of the Prime Minister's "Challenge" on dementia. Yet, in keeping with neoliberal agendas there is a continual emphasis on individual responsibility, on becoming a "dementia champion", and creating "dementia-friendly communities". These latter initiatives rely on the work of volunteers. The implicit message is that dementia is a private concern. (It is worth noting that the words "challenge" and "champion" recall competition and battle.)

On the other hand, the press and television documentaries abound in "personal" stories about dementia and in tales of cures that are imminent or preventative measures that can be taken to ward it off. These include reports on the preventative powers of Ginkgo Biloba and vitamin B and the possible causal links between such diverse factors as obesity or copper pipes and dementia (NHS Choices 2011). These reports are prolific. They serve to position dementia in our imaginations as forever mutating and utterly beyond the grasp of science. Dementia and AD therefore become phenomena that are almost paranormal.

For the most part, the UK media represents dementia and AD as conditions to be looked at in a forensic, even a mawkish fashion. For example, *The Express* newspaper reported on a husband's brutal "knifing" of his wife who had dementia (Twomey 2011). These stories contribute to society's ghoulish interest with the extremities to which dementia can lead. Dementia is thus framed as a particularly freakish condition. All of these accounts of dementia present us with an outside view. We – the audience – are in the position of witnesses (even judges) to something that is totally alien (a bit like the guided tours around lunatic asylums in the Victorian era). Thus although we seem to be connecting with individual stories about dementia in the press and documentary reports, to be united in our disgust of the maltreatment of those with dementia, the net effect is to create an even greater sense of distance between "us" and "them". Moreover, we are consistently presented with "dementia" as a vast natural force in the face of which we are helpless. Dementia and AD therefore provoke both distance (at an individual level) and apathy. These are both profoundly dangerous reactions that limit our abilities to interact humanely with people living with a dementia and cloud our ability to think rationally about the condition.

Exercise 6.2: Analysing media depictions of people with dementia

Think of three recent stories about dementia or AD from the media (a national or local newspaper, TV or radio programme, on-line blog) and consider:

■ The language used to depict AD or dementia: is it medical? What kinds of metaphors are used? What sorts of images recur?
■ The ways in which people living with AD or dementia are described: are they "sufferers", are they passive "victims", are they active members of the community?
■ The way in which AD or dementia is described in relation to wider society: is it a financial drain? A crisis? What is a "dementia friend"? What are "dementia-friendly communities"?
■ How do people living with a dementia talk about the condition?

Alternative stories about dementia

Until the late 1980s, there was a widespread cultural silence about dementia and AD. As outlined by others (Segers 2007), stories about dementia were avoided because they involved older people and sickness. The cultural landscape has radically altered in the last decade. A small number of these recent literary representations are discussed below.

The memoir

The memoir is a literary form with a long history (Yagoda 2009). Memoirs are representations of memory, reflexive recollections. There is a peculiar aptness when the form is used to represent a condition that affects the memory.

There are a number of delicately written memoirs that enable readers to engage imaginatively with some of the experiences dementia can entail. These are necessarily partial accounts (written from a carer's perspective) but several manage to communicate important insights. Above all, they enable the reader to see beyond a diagnosis to a person.

In *The House on Beartown Road* (2003), we are invited deep into Cohen's chaotic life. A string of events lead to Cohen becoming a single, working parent, caring for a father with AD. Cohen acutely notes how her father, who is slowly growing more confused, and her baby, who is learning to walk and talk, are actually travelling in parallel:

> Learning and forgetting are not so different, really. There is a pattern to the way they happen. In both there is powerful emotion, the sense of recognition, the sense of loss.
>
> —Cohen (2003: 30)

Indeed, the relationship between her ageing, sick father and her daughter is healing. At times, her father and daughter are so close that she feels excluded:

> They often laugh together. She has a plastic alligator . . . She likes to put her finger in its mouth and say 'Oh no!' It cracks them up.
>
> —Cohen (2003: 59)

Cohen does not gloss over the gruelling details of providing care. We learn about her struggles, the accidents in the toilet. The pain of watching a much-loved parent die is not avoided. This is not an idealistic or dreamy account. However, Cohen does provide an affirmation of life, even when life is steadily unravelling. Despite the distinct possibility that things will fall apart, there is no disintegration. On the contrary, her love for her father (who is known throughout the memoir as "Daddy", a close and personal epithet) is healing. The character that is "Daddy" is preserved as a sentient and dignified person.

Similarly, in *Strange Relation* (2011), Rachel Hadas sensitively honours her husband (George) while also exposing the searing pain of living with his silence. George and Hadas once shared a lively intellectual life:

> 66 The silence was the worst. Silence not as in solitude or concentration, but as in living with, eating with, waking up next to someone who has nothing to say to you. 99

—Hadas (2011: 1)

For Hadas, dreaming and the act of writing poetry provide portals into subliminal levels of consciousness where truths are often located. Throughout this memoir, Hadas emphasizes the comfort she was able to take from literature (from Greek tragedy to nineteenth-century novels). Reading helps to alleviate her loneliness. The memoir provides concrete examples of why and how literature can provide comfort: "Yes, I thought when I read this, yes . . ." (Hadas 2011: 18). As Hadas points out, fiction helps us to see through the confusions that cloud our judgements and to pay attention to the details of life.

Both Cohen's and Hadas's sensitive recollections provide a welcome contrast to the dizzying number of media stories that blunt our ability to empathize with people living with a dementia.

Exercise 6.3: Engaging with the experience of a person with dementia

- Have you read any memoirs about dementia or AD? Did they surprise you? If so, why? If not, why not?
- How can other people's experiences help us learn?
- Have you seen any films about AD or dementia? Did they help you imagine what it might feel like to live with this condition?
- If you were writing an imaginative account of AD or dementia, where would you begin? What genre would you chose – memoir, novel, play, poem, and why?
- Write a 500-word story about an experience you once had with dementia or AD.

The poem

"The Mother of the Muses" by Tony Harrison (1992) has dementia at its dramatic core and uses dementia as a metaphor. At one point in this quite long meditation, the poet asks:

> 66 If we are what we remember, what are they
> who don't have memories as we have ours . . . 99

The poem uses dementia as a starting point for a philosophical reflection on the nature of identity and its relationship to memory.

"Mother of the Muses" has at its centre a visit to the care home near Toronto where the poet's father-in-law (who died of AD) lived out his final days. The poem explores memory – both individual and collective. Indeed, the title invokes MNEMOSYNE. She is the Titan Goddess of memory and remembrance and the inventress of language and words. It is interesting that MNEMOSYNE is connected not simply with memory but also with language – her symbolic relevance for both poetry and dementia is evident. The poem begins and ends with the poet struggling and failing to recall lines from Prometheus, he is:

66 anxious to prove my memory's not ossified. 99

The image of a poet trying to remember is juxtaposed with vignettes of Harrison's father-in-law and eight other residents with Alzheimer's disease – nine in all, in ironic reference, perhaps, to the nine daughters of Memory. Each resident is carefully depicted: they share a sense of displacement and also the loss of their memories, "the mists" of Alzheimer's.

The poem explores the nature of memory at a collective level: as shaped by historical and political forces. Thus the background to the poem is the catastrophes of the twentieth century: the Second World War (the bombing of Dresden is an image of fire that connects with the poet's urge to remember lines from Prometheus). On the one hand, there is a desire to forget these horrors and on the other a duty to remember lest they be repeated – this tension is captured in the description of Ernst Zundel:

66 . . . who denies the Jews were gassed,

and academics are supporting his denial,

restoring pride by doctoring the past,

and not just Germans but those people who

can't bear to think such things could ever be,

and by disbelieving horrors to be true

hope to put back hope in history. 99

—Stanza 29

Harrison is concerned with the collective amnesia in which we all participate – to some extent at a cultural level we all have to forget in order to carry on, and yet we must also learn how to remember.

In the final lines of the poem, the poet is content to admit defeat in his own attempts to recall ancient Greek, but achieves a certain affirmation of life and love:

66 . . . Damn! I forget,

but remembering your dad, I'm celebrating

being in love, not too forgetful, yet. 99

Dementia, then, is a conceit (or extended metaphor) for considering the importance of historical memory, the place that creativity has in a world that has been blighted by the tragedies of Dresden and the Holocaust and the need to continue living and loving.

Conclusion

A critical examination of some of the representations of dementia has demonstrated the problematic consequences of popular discursive practices that associate dementia with disaster. Even medical and scientific texts tend to conflate dementia with crisis. Analysing the cultural scripts that feature dementia and AD helps to reveal the underlying assumptions that infuse the political, social, and medical narratives that are told about these conditions. A close analysis of these stories may also help to educate the dementia care workforce by encouraging questions about the dominant stereotypes of people living with a dementia. The role of stories is an integral part of a flagship study at the University of East Anglia (Zeilig *et al.* 2012–2013) that educates the dementia care workforce using the arts. Understanding the wider social stories that condition our responses towards those with a dementia is a key way of ensuring that negative attitudes and practices are questioned rather than accepted.

The chapter has also highlighted several alternative representations of "dementia". Individual memoirs have helped contribute to new perspectives on what the experience of living with a dementia may entail. Equally, Harrison's poetry locates the personal experience of AD within a wide historical framework and raises questions about memory at a collective level.

Finally, this chapter has explored the extent to which our (western) understanding of dementia and AD is connected with the conditions of postmodern capitalist life. Dementia and AD are terms that have been mystified – they are emotionally charged semiotic concepts. In semiotics, words such as dementia and AD can be understood as "signs" that carry meaning that is representative of cultural values. Just as cancer is no longer inextricably linked with fatality, so it is likely that in the decades to come, when dementia and AD are more fully understood, that they will no longer be the locus of and repository for all society's fears.

References

Basting, A.D. (2003) Looking back from loss: views of the self in Alzheimer's disease, *Journal of Aging Studies*, 17(1): 87–99.

Basting, A.D. (2009) *Forget Memory: Creating Better Lives for People with Dementia*. Baltimore, MD: Johns Hopkins University Press.

Alzheimer Society Canada (2010) *Rising Tide: The Impact of Dementia on Canadian Society*. Toronto, ONT: Alzheimer Society Canada.

Charise, A. (2012) Let the reader think of the burden: old age and the crisis of capacity, *Occasion: Interdisciplinary Studies in the Humanities*, 4 [http://arcade.stanford.edu/sites/default/files/article_pdfs/OCCASION_v04_Charise_053112_0.pdf].

Cohen, E. (2003) *The House on Beartown Road: A Memoir of Learning and Forgetting*. New York: Random House.

Cruikshank, M. (2009) *Learning to be Old: Gender, Culture and Ageing*. Plymouth: Rowman & Littlefield.

Dick, D. (1982) *The Rising Tide – Developing Services for Mental Illness in Old Age*. London: NHS Health Advisory Centre.

George, D. and Whitehouse, P.J. (2014) The war (on terror) on Alzheimer's, *Dementia*, 13(1): 120–30.

George, D.R., Qualls, S.H., Cameron, C.J. and Whitehouse, P.J. (2013) Renovating Alzheimer's: 'constructive' reflections on the new clinical and research diagnostic guidelines, *The Gerontologist*, 53 (3): 378–87.

Goyder, J. (2001) *We'll be Married in Fremantle*. Fremantle, WA: Fremantle Arts Centre Press.

Grice, E. (2012) Sir Terry Pratchett: 'I thought my Alzheimer's would be a lot worse than this by now', *The Telegraph*, 10 September.

Gullette, M.M. (2004) *Aged by Culture*. Chicago, IL: University of Chicago Press.

Gullette, M.M. (2012) *Wisdom and/or Dementia – is that the Choice American Society is Mired In?* Waltham, MA: Brandeis University.

Hadas, R. (2011) *Strange Relation: A Memoir of Marriage, Dementia and Poetry*. Philadelphia, PA: Paul Dry Books.

Harrison, T. (1992) *The Gaze of The Gorgon*. Newcastle Upon Tyne: Bloodaxe Books.

Heaney, S. (1999) *Beowulf*. London: Faber & Faber.

Herskovits, E. (1995) Struggling over subjectivity: debates about the 'self' and Alzheimer's disease, *Medical Anthropological Quarterly*, 9: 146–64.

Katz, S. (1996) *Disciplining Old Age: The Formation of Gerontological Knowledge*. Charlottesville, VA: University Press of Virginia.

Kitwood, T. (1997) *Dementia Reconsidered: The Person Comes First*. Maidenhead: Open University Press.

Kontos, P.C. (2003) 'The painterly hand': Embodied consciousness and Alzheimer's disease, *Journal of Aging Studies*, 17: 151–70.

Kontos, P.C. (2012) *The Painterly Hand: Rethinking Creativity, Selfhood, and Memory in Dementia*. London: King's College.

Kontos, P.C. and Naglie, G. (2007) Expressions of personhood in Alzheimer's disease: an evaluation of research-based theatre as a pedagogical tool, *Qualitative Health Research*, 17: 799–811.

Lees, A. (2012) *Alzheimer's: The Silent Plague*. London: Penguin.

Mandell, A.M. and Green, R.C. (2011) Alzheimer's disease, in A.E. Budson and N.W. Kowall (eds.) *The Handbook of Alzheimer's Disease and Other Dementias*. Chichester: Wiley-Blackwell, pp. 3–91.

NHS Choices (2011) *Alzheimer's in the News: Fear and Fascination*. A Behind the Headlines special report. London: NHS [http://www.nhs.uk/news/2011/08August/Documents/Alzheimer's%20in%20the%20press.pdf].

O'Grady, S. (2012) David Cameron: We need to do more to tackle dementia, *Daily Express*, 26 May.

Oyebode, F. (2009) The humanities in postgraduate medical education, *Advances in Psychiatric Treatment*, 15: 224–9.

Port, C. (2012) No future? Aging, temporality, history and reverse chronologies, *Occasion: Interdisciplinary Studies in the Humanities*, 4 [http://arcade.stanford.edu/sites/default/files/article_pdfs/OCCASION_v04_Port_053112_0.pdf].

Prime Minister's Office (2012) 'Dementia challenge' launched, 26 March [https://www.gov.uk/government/news/dementia-challenge-launched].

Russell, C. (2009) *Terry Pratchett: Living with Alzheimer's*. London: BBC Television, 4 February.

Russell, C. (2011) *Terry Pratchett: Choosing to Die*. London: BBC Television, 9 June.

Segers, K. (2007) Degenerative dementias and their medical care in the movies, *Alzheimer Disease and Associated Disorders*, 21: 55–9.

Smith, T. (2010) *An Evening with Dementia* (theatrical performance).

Sontag, S. (1991) *Illness as Metaphor, Aids and Its Metaphors*. London: Penguin Books.

TheGuardian.com (2012) David Cameron promises dementia funding boost [http://www.theguardian.com/society/2012/mar/26/david-cameron-dementia-funding-boost, accessed 31 January 2014].

Twomey, J. (2011) Half-brother of TV host killed wife, *The Express*, 8 October.

Yagoda, B. (2009) *Memoir: A History*. New York: Riverhead Books.

Zeilig, H. (2012) Gaps and spaces: representations of dementia in contemporary British poetry, *Dementia* [DOI: 10.1177/1471301212456276].

Zeilig, H. (2013) Dementia as a cultural metaphor, *The Gerontologist* [DOI: 10.1093/geront/gns203].

Zeilig, H., Poland, F., Fox, C. and Killick, J. (2012–2013) *Using the Arts in the Education of the Dementia Care Workforce*. Norwich: University of East Anglia.

CHAPTER 7

Living with young-onset dementia

Jan Oyebode

> "After the diagnosis the neurologist who we had been seeing said how sorry he was and that unfortunately there was nothing he could offer in the way of support as the limited services that were available were all geared up for the elderly."
>
> —Gillian Watson Yorkshire, UK

Learning objectives

By the end of this chapter, you will:

- Know about the prevalence of young-onset dementia, the types that are most common, and the ways these may present
- Know about the distinctive aspects of living with dementia in middle age
- Understand issues around behavioural variant fronto-temporal dementia and primary progressive aphasia
- Understand some of the issues for people with Down syndrome and dementia

Introduction

Significant numbers of people experience dementia under the age of 65 years. These people and their families, by definition, have an atypical experience. The changes they experience are not readily recognized as signs of dementia, whether by themselves, relatives or professionals, and this can delay the process of diagnosis. Once a diagnosis is made, people with young-onset dementia (YOD) and their families face a range of challenges that differ from those faced by people experiencing dementia in old age. Due to the relative rarity of YOD, however, staff may not feel confident to meet the needs of younger adults, and dedicated services and facilities are not always available. For these reasons, this is a distinctive area of dementia experience that demands our attention so that we can better support those who are affected.

This chapter is divided into three main sections. The first is on YOD in general, the second focuses on behavioural variant fronto-temporal dementia and primary progressive aphasia, and the third is about the care needs of people with Down syndrome and dementia.

Young-onset dementia: prevalence and life-stage issues

Young-onset dementia, also referred to as early-onset dementia or working-age dementia, has an onset before the age of 65 years. Although this is a cut-off point of convenience, there are differences in the profile and prognosis of YOD compared with late-onset dementia, and the needs of people with YOD and their families differ because of the stage of life at which the condition occurs. These include its impact on employment and hence family finances, the changes it provokes in intimate relationships, the realignment it causes in family roles, and the conflict this may engender (Rosness *et al.* 2008; van Vliet *et al.* 2010). These factors are briefly reviewed in Chapter 13.

Box 7.1 provides some basic facts about YOD, and the exercise that follows encourages you to think through some age comparisons to understand the impact of YOD compared with that of late-onset dementia.

Box 7.1: Some facts about young onset dementia

- Only 2% of people with dementia are under 65 years of age
- Alzheimer's disease (AD) accounts for 80% of late-onset dementias but only 34% of YOD
- In a famous study, Harvey and colleagues (2003) reported that:
    - 30% of YOD is AD
    - 15% is vascular dementia
    - 13% is due to fronto-temporal lobar degeneration
    - 12% is alcohol-related
    - 29% is rarer dementias
- YOD is more common in black and minority ethnic (BME) populations in the UK (6% of dementias in BME groups) than in the "white" population, partly linked to a high incidence of diabetes and cardiovascular problems
- Only 1 in 1000 people with AD has a known genetic cause but young-onset AD is more likely to run in the family than late-onset AD
- 1 in 3 people with dementia due to fronto-temporal lobar degeneration have had relatives with a similar illness

Source: Sampson *et al.* (2004), Moriarty *et al.* (2011)

Exercise 7.1: Differences between developing dementia at the ages of 53 and 78 years

Marie and her partner Gary are in their fifties. Marie has two daughters, Sonia and Marsha, aged 15 and 20, who both live at home. Her dad, Desmond, in his seventies, lives just around the corner. Gary and Marie have been together for five years and he is like a father to the girls. Marie has supported her dad for many years, since he separated from her mum.

About two years ago, Desmond had a blackout while at his social club and seemed a bit confused. He did not recover fully and started to have trouble managing his diabetic diet. The diabetes nurse asked the doctor to check him over and he was diagnosed with vascular dementia. He has lost interest in his garden and seems to spend a lot of time in his flat, watching TV and sleeping. When he goes out, he sometimes takes ages to come back and Marie thinks he is having trouble finding his way home.

Meanwhile, Gary has had business problems. He has become disorganized and has failed to keep appointments. Marie thought he might be depressed and insisted he go to the doctor. He was prescribed anti-depressants but they made no difference. Some months later, the household bills began getting into arrears. Marie and Gary are falling out, as he resists her attempts to get him to sort matters out, and Marsha has moved out to live with her friend, saying that the constant arguments get on her nerves. Marie has persuaded Gary to go back to see the doctor, who this time has referred him to the local memory assessment service, where they have made a diagnosis of young-onset dementia.

- Thinking about Desmond: How was the dementia detected? How has it affected his daily life, his income, his household, and his relationships? What do you think he needs and how could his family, community or local services meet his needs?
- Thinking about Gary: How was the dementia detected? How has it affected his daily life, his income, his household, and his relationships? What do you think he needs and how could his family, community or local services meet his needs?
- What do you conclude from this comparison of Desmond and Gary? Is dementia worse at one age or the other? How do the services available to the two age groups compare?

Impact of young-onset dementia on the wider family, including children and adolescents

Young-onset dementia also has an impact on other members of the family, who may include elderly parents and children or young people. In one survey, 75% of parents in families in which one parent had YOD reported their children suffered psychological/emotional problems, had problems at school, conflict with the person with YOD, and experienced stigma, shame, and bewilderment (Passant *et al.* 2005). Allen and Oyebode (2009) interviewed 12 individuals aged 13–23 years whose father had YOD. These young people feared for both parents, the father who had dementia and the mother who was "well" but under strain. They often withdrew from friendships, took on extra responsibilities at home, gave up ideas of moving away, and did not feel free to develop relationships with boyfriends or girlfriends. They showed maturity beyond their years but were also under stress. A follow up of seven of these participants 4 years later (Lord 2010) found that they were often still stressed but were also now grieving. Some felt they had experienced personal growth as a result of their experiences, becoming more empathic and aware as human beings, as illustrated by one young man, who said:

> 66 There are some things that I, ah, actually think are good like that . . . maturing more . . . I think it's made me a nicer person because I can understand if other people go through something similar. I think that I could understand more. 99

Exercise 7.2: Meeting the needs of families with young-onset dementia

- What do you think the needs of these children/young people are?
- How well do current services meet those needs?
- What sort of services could you design to meet their needs?
- Who is best placed to provide these services?

Two non-Alzheimer's young-onset dementias: behavioural variant fronto-temporal dementia and primary progressive aphasia

Definitions and characteristics

This section concentrates on the characteristics of behavioural variant fronto-temporal dementia (bvFTD) and primary progressive aphasia (PPA), clinical dementias that arise from underlying degeneration in the fronto-temporal lobes (i.e. fronto-temporal lobar degeneration or FTLD). The area is confusing, as terminology is changing rapidly in response to advancing research and understanding. However, rather than consider the underlying pathology, the focus here is on the needs that arise from these dementias and possible ways of providing support and care. Both bvFTD and PPA have a usual age of onset below 65 years, with most people seeking help aged 45–65 years. Together they are the second most common types of dementia in people under 65 and the fourth most common in those over 65 years. A brief outline of their nature is given in Table 7.1, and a fuller description can be found in the scientific papers referenced. They all have a gradual onset, become progressively worse, and affect more functions over time, but none of them affect memory in the early stages.

Meeting the needs of people with bvFTD and primary progressive aphasia

These dementias remain little understood, thus it can take a long time for people to receive an accurate diagnosis, highlighting the need to raise awareness not only with the public but also with professionals. Good information is available on the web sites of the national charities concerned with FTD in the UK and the USA (see "Further information" section). Joanne Douglas, a former lecturer and researcher into gene therapies, spoke of the value of early diagnosis in an interview with the journalist Alice Walton. An extract from her interview is quoted below:

> " My life is not the way I would have chosen, but I can choose what I can make of it now. Not everyone is at this exact point where I am; there may not always be strategies to intervene. But for others, there are. And earlier diagnosis means that we can have more for the future, and get the most from the time we do have. "

—Walton (2012)

Meeting the needs of people with bvFTD

There has been little work on what it is like for someone with bvFTD to live with the condition. People with bvFTD can usually say that they have been given a diagnosis and can describe at least some of the changes that have occurred in their lives, but they do not seem to have an emotional "lived" experience that allows them to grasp its impact on themselves and their ability to live independently. They cannot understand why others treat them differently (e.g. why they have lost their job or have freedoms restricted) because they do not experience themselves as having changed. This means that they may live with some degree of puzzlement about their situation or may simply seem unconcerned (Griffin 2013).

There are no evidence-based, tailored interventions but some of the ways family carers report maintaining their relative's quality of life (Oyebode et al. 2013) include:

- finding places where the person can be active without being at risk of offending others
- embedding opportunities for some compulsive behaviour, especially walking, into daily routines

Area of brain affected	Brief description
Behavioural variant FTD (bvFTD)	
Both frontal lobes	■ Progressive behavioural and/or cognitive changes, including at least three of: ■ impairment in executive functions (e.g. in forward planning and attention, or in starting actions) ■ disinhibited behaviour (e.g. lack of usual control over swearing, sexual behaviour, making personal remarks) ■ lack of empathy ■ apathy ■ stereotypical or compulsive behaviour (e.g. pacing, walking, rocking) ■ hyper-orality (i.e. excessive eating and putting inedible things in the mouth)
Primary progressive aphasia (PPA)	
Varied location in the three variants	Very gradual onset of progressive problems in expressive language (i.e. in speaking), in finding the name of objects, in producing grammatical sentences or in understanding words, which cause impairment in activities of daily living that involve language The language problems vary in the three sub-types
PPA – non-fluent agrammatic variant	
Left posterior fronto-insular region	Dominated by one or both of: ■ Problems in producing grammatical speech (e.g. "This is apple" rather than "This is an apple") ■ Problems producing speech sounds, resulting in distorted, slow, halting speech
Semantic dementia (also called semantic variant PPA – svPPA)	
Anterior temporal lobes on both sides but often more on one side than the other	Problems in understanding the meaning of single words, especially less frequently used ones (e.g. tortoise) and in recognizing faces or objects Speech is fluent but content may not make sense
Logopenic variant PPA	
Left temporal-parietal junction	Problems finding single words when speaking or when trying to name an object Problems repeating sentences.

Source: Rascovsky *et al.* (2007), Gorno-Tempini *et al.* (2011)

Table 7.1 Brief descriptions of bvFTD and PPA

■ using humour with the person with bvFTD to defuse tension when embarrassing mistakes are made
■ explaining on behalf of the person with bvFTD to members of the public when embarrassing situations occur
■ being assertive with care providers to access appropriate services

> ### Box 7.2: Caring for a man with bvFTD
>
> Hall and colleagues (2013) describe care from a treatment team over time for Jeff, a man with bvFTD. Their account shows how a responsive care team can support a person with bvFTD as his or her needs change over time. Initially, the care team's efforts were directed to helping Jeff to remain at home and to be able to go out without his family worrying about him getting lost. Later, the team focused on finding ways to manage more basic needs around self-care and personal hygiene, and finally, following Jeff's move into a care home, the team worked to find strategies that would divert Jeff from disinhibited behaviour, such as pulling female staff members onto the bed, and prevent him injuring himself through compulsive picking of his nails. Care needs change over time for all types of dementia. However, Hall and colleagues' description includes aspects that are typical of bvFTD: compulsive behaviour (walking and nail-picking), inability to initiate self-care, lack of self-control in relation to social convention and sexual behaviour (pulling nurses onto the bed). It shows how, even when it is not possible to restore awareness or previous levels of ability, it is possible, with creativity and sensitivity, to find solutions that maintain some dignity, activity, and quality of life.

Meeting the needs of carers of people with bvFTD

Carers of people with bvFTD have high levels of distress compared with carers of people with Alzheimer's. Stress arises from loss of empathy in the person with bvFTD, which can make the carer feel that they have lost the two-way relationship they used to have. One gentleman with bvFTD, for example, had been a loving husband. His wife now had cancer and was undergoing radiotherapy, but he did not ask after her welfare or express any concern for her well-being. Stress also comes from disinhibited behaviour that leads people with bfFTD into embarrassing or risky situations. In one study Oyebode et al. (2013) report that a woman had been arrested by store detectives for taking goods from a shop, while a man with bvFTD almost got into a fight with a customer he had let down and his wife had to step in and intervene. Others may find themselves involved with the police or adult or child protection agencies due to their disinhibited behaviours.

There are a very small number of published studies on providing education and support for FTD carers (Nunnemann et al. 2012). None has been rigorously evaluated, although Mioshi et al. (2013) recently conducted a small-scale study of a stress-appraisal coping intervention to produce some promising outcomes. Carers, who attended 2-hour sessions on a weekly basis for 15 weeks, focused on understanding and analysing stressful situations (appraisal) and considering how best to cope.

Meeting the needs of people with primary progressive aphasia

The main problem in early PPA is the need for assistance in communication. The effort that it takes people with semantic variant to communicate is graphically described by Joanne Douglas:

> **"** I can tell that my speech is changing over time. It's so exhausting to speak now. I put a lot of energy into being able to compensate for the losses. It sometimes takes a very long time to pull the right words forward through my brain. **"**

—Walton (2012)

The different types of language impairment are likely to benefit from specialized therapy from a speech and language therapist (SALT, aka Speech and Language Pathologist). This may help to slow deterioration and assist re-learning. SALT staff are rare in mental health services, but to get the best possible services for people with PPA, such individuals should be referred where possible. Sometimes simple language-based exercises may help. One study showed that four people with semantic variant PPA (svPPA) were able to gain improvements in speech and recognition of objects through home-based rehearsal of word–picture pairs (Savage *et al.* 2013). Some leaflets giving tips on communication for people with svPPA and for those communicating with them are available on the American Fronto-Temporal Association web site (see "Further information" section).

Most people with early PPA, especially svPPA, have insight into their condition, a good memory, and a good sense of self. They are often able to continue to care for themselves for some years after diagnosis. It may be this clear awareness, as well as the sense of isolation from being unable to use language, that leads to a high risk of suicide in this group (Sabodash *et al.* 2013). This shows that it is vital to find ways of helping people with this type of dementia to maintain a sense of self-worth and engagement with the world and their own lives. Despite severe language impairment, it may be possible to find ways of using preserved, non-language-based abilities to advantage. Victoria Jones, wife of Nick who has svPPA, gives an inspiring account of making the best of life (Jones 2010). She describes Nick's severe inability to understand what objects are:

> **66** He doesn't know whether something is for him to eat or use. If I put a dead mouse in the bread bin, he really would eat it for breakfast. **99**

But she recounts how, with support and encouragement, he has learnt to draw very skilfully, how he can solve "killer Sudoku", can still play chess well, and can enjoy swimming and walking.

Later in PPA when difficulties have progressed further, finding a way of enabling the person to relate to others may be a particularly powerful means of meeting needs, given the communication problems. One recent report tells of a 58-year-old woman with advanced FTD dominated by communication problems. She was being cared for in a nursing home for people with dementia but staff found her to be agitated, depressed, constantly on the move, and making noises. Music therapy, involving one-to-one interaction, using percussion instruments and voice, resulted in a dramatic reduction in her distressed and restless behaviour (Raglio *et al.* 2012).

Exercise 7.3: Meeting needs for activity and engagement in people with primary progressive aphasia

List as many activities as possible that you could use to encourage someone to keep busy and engaged with life in the face of language problems, given intact cognition in other areas.

Young-onset dementia in Down syndrome

Prevalence of dementia in people with Down syndrome

People with Down syndrome (DS) are more likely to develop dementia than the general population, and at a much earlier age (see Box 7.3). This is not the case for people with learning disabilities due to other causes, where the rates are comparable with the general population.

Box 7.3: Key facts about prevalence of dementia in Down syndrome

Risk of dementia is much higher in people with Down syndrome than those who are "neuro-typical" (i.e. those without learning disabilities). Of those with DS:

- about 9% aged 45–49 years have dementia
- about 18% aged 50–54 years have dementia
- about 33% aged 55–59 years have dementia

Those with DS and dementia have six times the risk of mortality than those without dementia.

Source: Nieuwenhuis-Mark (2009), Coppus *et al.* (2006), Coppus *et al.* (2008)

Nature of dementia in people with Down syndrome

It is hard to discern whether someone with DS is developing dementia because of their lifelong different level of cognitive and everyday abilities. A non-learning-disabled person, for example, may get lost or may repeatedly lose belongings, but many people with DS are not expected to go to unfamiliar environments or manage their belongings on their own. Cognitive limitations also mean that the neuropsychological tests that are used with people without learning disabilities are not generally suitable.

The first signs of dementia are usually noticed by relatives or support staff who know the person well and see changes in their functioning. They include loss of skills, withdrawal from activity or social contact, changes in personality, forgetfulness, and sleep problems (Janicki *et al.* 2005; McLaughlin and Jones 2011). Some questionnaires that can be used to gather information from carers of people with learning disabilities about possible changes are listed at the end of this chapter.

Supporting care for people with Down syndrome at home

Many people with DS are very attached to their familiar daily routine and find change difficult, so supporting people "in place" is usually preferable to them moving to a special facility. Their closest relatives are usually either ageing parents, with whom the person with DS has lived all their lives, or siblings with whom the person has moved to live after the death of their parents. Some of the issues caregiving relatives face are common to dementia carers generally, but there are also distinctive aspects (see Case example 7.1).

Case example 7.1: Harry, Joyce, and Laura

Harry and Joyce, now in their late seventies, have provided support to their daughter Laura all her life and she still lives with them now. When Laura was born, doctors painted a bleak picture of the future, telling them that she was not likely to have a very long life span. They nurtured her over the years, and were very proud that she learnt to speak quite well and had become an outstanding swimmer. Their mantelpiece was crowded with trophies she had won. Joyce said:

> "That's . . . how well she done for a Downs, you know, like. She achieved such a lot . . . I mean, it was hard work for the first few years and that, but it was very rewarding. Yeah, very rewarding. What she'd done."

They were enormously grateful that, against the odds, she had lived into her fifties, although they had expected to outlive her, so this was also a source of worry for them too. When they found out she had dementia, they felt it like a "body blow". Harry felt it was unfair:

> "She's been, we've been faced with this problem since birth and why is she still being punished and why are we being punished? And I'm thinking has she not suffered enough, have we not suffered enough?"

They found it hard work to provide the level of care she had come to need and were particularly worried that the day care she received might be cut, feeling this would jeopardize their ability to continue to care for her at home. Harry said:

> "All our plans, our hopes, our dreams have all changed dramatically. And er, er, what we planned for will not happen, so we just make the, we do the best with what we got and hope for the best."

Source: Based on research by Angela Foster for her Clinical Psychology Doctorate thesis, University of Birmingham, 2012

Surveys show that family carers, with a relative at home or in care, want more information, to be fully involved with their relative's health and social care, and to be invited to be present at appointments and review meetings and to have a chance to meet other carers and other people with dementia (McLaughlin and Jones 2011; Furniss *et al.* 2012).

Supporting care for people with Down syndrome in residential settings

Most people with DS in their fifties live in small-scale supported living or residential care. A survey of 10 UK and US homes for people with learning disabilities found that staff took 8.4 hours per day on average to care for residents with dementia compared with 5.4 hours for the most disabled person in the home who did not have dementia (Janicki *et al.* 2005). Staff spent just over 2.5 hours per day in "behaviour management", and they reported finding many changes in behaviour to be challenging, including screaming, verbal outbursts, physical aggression, and refusal by the person to comply with requests. Since challenging behaviour of this sort is often triggered by environmental demands, unmet needs or distress, this implies that attention to the environment and to the delivery of sensitive, person-centred responses would be helpful. Dementia Care Mapping can be a valuable tool for assessing and prompting enhancement of quality of care (Finnamore and Lord 2007).

Janicki *et al.* (2005) found that the key factors in keeping people in place were having flexibly minded staff who were willing to adapt programmes of care, having funding to ensure adequate staffing, and making physical adaptations to the care setting (see Box 7.4). Also important is attending to the understanding and comfort of co-residents who do not have dementia. These residents may resent the extra time staff have to spend with them and dislike some of the adaptations made to their homes (Forbat and Wilkinson 2008). A group intervention has been found to be promising in promoting residents' awareness and understanding of dementia (Lynggaard and Alexander 2004).

> ## Box 7.4: Adaptations in residential settings to help people with Down syndrome (Mahendiran and Dodd 2009)
>
> *Goals of adaptation*
>
> To make the environment:
>
> - calm and stress-free
> - predictable and easy to understand
> - familiar
> - suitably stimulating
> - safe
>
> *Possible adaptations*
>
> - To support reduced mobility, e.g. wider doorways to allow wheelchair access
> - To adapt for impaired hearing and attention, e.g. reducing unnecessary noise
> - To help with developing memory problems, e.g. graphics for bedroom doors
> - To adjust for diminishing 3D perception, e.g. flooring same colour throughout
> - To adjust for changes in colour perception, e.g. fewer patterns on wallpaper
> - To accommodate "wandering", e.g. circular garden paths, exit alert alarms

Staff needs also have to be considered. Most staff caring for people with DS and dementia know about meeting the needs of people with learning disabilities but know much less about dementia. Unlike mainstream dementia service staff, learning disability staff have often had a long and quite personal relationship with those they support. In our own study, we found those who were more recent to their job experienced feelings of loss but felt quite guilty about this. One young woman said, "You're not supposed to get attached to people you work with", whereas more experienced staff spoke of having to learn to cut off in order to cope.

Exercise 7.4: Sharing expertise between dementia and learning disability services

Janet, manager of a local group home for people with learning disabilities, contacts you asking for advice on how to meet the needs of Joan, a person with DS aged 46 years who she thinks may be developing dementia. What are three steps you would take in response to her request?

Implications for practice, policy, and further research

As a smaller population than people with late-onset dementia, individuals with YOD carry less weight when it comes to their needs being focused upon by service providers, researchers, pharmaceutical companies or interventionists. They also suffer from having needs that straddle the boundaries between working age and older people's services and between physical and mental health services. We need greater recognition of the particular needs of people with YOD, more research into effective interventions, and a more widespread implementation of good practice in holistic, family-oriented service provision.

Debates and controversies

There are lots of controversies relating to this area. One issue is whether people with YOD need to be seen in a dedicated service or whether they can receive adequate assessment and support from staff in an age-inclusive service. Discrimination on the grounds of age alone does not fit well with a person-centred approach to dementia care, as it implies that a person's identity and needs are dominated by their age to the exclusion of other influences. On the other hand, this chapter has highlighted some distinctive aspects of living with dementia at a younger than usual age. Some of these special needs demand competencies from staff that are additional to those required for work with people with late-onset dementia. When someone with YOD is coming to services for assessment and support at an early stage, staff need knowledge of social services and financial benefits for those of working age as well as expertise related to working with families at a different stage of development from those typical in later life. In addition, individuals with YOD and their families stress the need for opportunities to mix with others of their own generation when attending day care or social events, and to be offered age-appropriate activities and environments, both there and in nursing or residential care settings. Thus on the basis of the skills and knowledge required by staff, it would seem there is a good argument for distinct services.

Conclusion

Greater awareness and knowledge about the distinctive needs that arise when dementia occurs in middle age is essential. In addition, it is very important to appreciate the differences in the nature of young-onset dementias. For those with YOD, greater heritability is a key consideration prompting us to offer counselling to families as required. Where YOD is associated with DS, we need to combine the best understanding from learning disability-related knowledge and practice with that from dementia-related knowledge and practice. In relation to bvFTD and PPA, raised awareness, improved competence, and greater confidence are required to enable us to respond effectively to loss of empathy, apathy, and disinhibition in bvFTD and to communication difficulties and distress in PPA. With these specifics in mind, we will be better equipped to provide excellent care to people who develop dementia at a younger age.

Further information

Information on heritability
- Genetics of dementia: http://www.alzheimers.org.uk/factsheet/405
- Understanding the genetics of FTD: http://www.theaftd.org/wp-content/uploads/2009/02/Final-FTD-Genetics-Brochure-with-Cover-8-2-2012.pdf

Information on fronto-temporal dementia

- The Frontotemporal Disease Support Group: http://www.ftdsg.org/
- The Association for Frontotemporal Degeneration (AFTD): http://www.theaftd.org/
- Video about having PPA – "Nick's misericords": http://www.innovationsindementia.org.uk/videos_misericords.htm

■ Article by Nick's wife about PPA: http://www.alzheimers.org.uk/site/scripts/documents_info.php?documentID=1358

Information on Down syndrome and dementia

■ Kalsy, S. and Oliver, C. (2005) The assessment of dementia in people with intellectual disabilities: key assessment instruments, in J. Hogg and A. Langa (eds.) *Assessing Adults with Intellectual Disabilities: A Service Provider's Guide.* Malden, MA: Blackwell Publishing, pp. 207–19.

■ Llewellyn, P. (2011) The needs of people with learning disabilities who develop dementia: a literature review, *Dementia,* 10 (2): 235–47.

■ Parrott, M. (2011) Learning disabilities and dementia: a nursing student's A to Z guide, *Learning Disability Practice,* 14 (5): 35–8.

References

Allen, J. and Oyebode, J.R. (2009) Having a father with young onset dementia: the impact on well-being of young people, *Dementia,* 8(4), 455–80.

Coppus, A., Evenhuis, H., Verberne, G., Visser, F., van Gool, P. *et al.* (2006) Dementia and mortality in persons with Down's syndrome, *Journal of Intellectual Disability Research,* 50 (Part 10): 768–77.

Coppus, A.M.W., Evenhuis, H.M., Verberne, G., Visser, F.E., Oostra, B.A. *et al.* (2008) Survival in elderly persons with Down syndrome, *Journal of the American Geriatrics Society,* 56(12): 2311–16.

Finnamore, T. and Lord, S. (2007) The use of Dementia Care Mapping in people with a learning disability and dementia, *Journal of Intellectual Disabilities,* 11(2): 157–65.

Forbat, L. and Wilkinson, H. (2008) Where should people with dementia live? Using the views of service users to inform models of care, *British Journal of Learning Disabilities,* 36(1): 6–12.

Furniss, K.A., Loverseed, A., Lippold, T. and Dodd, K. (2012) The views of people who care for adults with Down's syndrome and dementia: a service evaluation, *British Journal of Learning Disabilities,* 40(4): 318–27.

Gorno-Tempini, M.L., Hillis, A.E., Weintraub, S., Kertesz, A., Mendez, M. *et al.* (2011) Classification of primary progressive aphasia and its variants, *Neurology,* 76(11): 1006–14.

Griffin, J. (2013) Living with a diagnosis of behavioural-variant frontotemporal dementia: the person's experience. ClinPsyD thesis, University of Birmingham [http://etheses.bham.ac.uk/4054/].

Hall, G.R., Shapira, J., Gallagher, M. and Denny, S.S. (2013) Managing differences: care of the person with frontotemporal degeneration, *Journal of Gerontological Nursing,* 39(3): 10–14.

Harvey, R.J., Skelton-Robinson, M. and Rosser, M.N. (2003) The prevalence and causes of dementia in people under the age of 65 years, *Journal of Neurology, Neurosurgery and Pshychiatry,* 74(9): 1206–9.

Janicki, M.P., Dalton, A.J., McCallion, P., Baxley, D.D. and Zendell, A. (2005) Group home care for adults with intellectual disabilities and Alzheimer's disease, *Dementia,* 4(3): 361–85.

Jones, V. (2010) A sense of self, *Living with Dementia Magazine,* May [http://www.alzheimers.org.uk/site/scripts/documents_info.php?documentID=1358, accessed 6 August 2013].

Lord, N.D. (2010) The continued impact of young onset dementia on dependent children as they make their make the transition to adulthood. ClinPsyD thesis, University of Birmingham [http://etheses.bham.ac.uk/3558/, accessed 25 May 2014]

Lynggaard, H. and Alexander, N. (2004) 'Why are my friends changing?' Explaining dementia to people with learning disabilities, *British Journal of Learning Disabilities,* 32(1): 30–4.

Mahendiran, S. and Dodd, K. (2009) Dementia-friendly care homes. *Learning Disability Practice,* 12(2): 14–17.

McLaughlin, K. and Jones, A. (2011) 'It's all changed': carers' experiences of caring for adults who have Down's syndrome and dementia, *British Journal of Learning Disabilities,* 39(1): 57–63.

Mioshi, E., McKinnon, C., Savage, S., O'Connor, C.M. and Hodges, J.R. (2013) Improving burden and coping skills in frontotemporal dementia caregivers: a pilot study, *Alzheimer Disease and Associated Disorders,* 27(1): 84–6.

Moriarty, J., Sharif, N. and Robinson, J. (2011) Black and minority ethnic people with dementia and their access to support and services, *Research Briefing 35.* London: Social Care Institute for Excellence [http://www.scie.org.uk/publications/briefings/files/briefing35.pdf, accessed 6 August 2013].

Nieuwenhuis-Mark, R.E. (2009) Diagnosing Alzheimer's dementia in Down syndrome: problems and possible solutions, *Research in Developmental Disabilities*, 30(5): 827–38.

Nunnemann, S., Kurz, A., Leucht, S. and Diehl-Schmid, J. (2012) Caregivers of patients with frontotemporal lobar degeneration: a review of burden, problems, needs, and interventions, *International Psychogeriatrics*, 24(9): 1368–86.

Oyebode, J.R., Bradley, P. and Allen, J.L. (2013) Relatives' experiences of frontal-variant frontotemporal dementia, *Qualitative Health Research*, 23(2), 156–66.

Passant, U., Elfgren, C., Englund, E. and Gustafson, L. (2005) Psychiatric symptoms and their psychosocial consequences in frontotemporal dementia, *Alzheimer Disease and Associated Disorders*, 19 (Suppl. 1): S15–S18.

Raglio, A., Bellandi, D., Baiardi, P., Gianotti, M., Ubezio, M.C. *et al.* (2012) Music therapy in frontal temporal dementia: a case report, *Journal of the American Geriatrics Society*, 60(8): 1578–9.

Rascovsky, K., Hodges, J.R., Kipps, C.M., Johnson, J.K., Seeley, W.W. *et al.* (2007) Diagnostic criteria for the behavioral variant of frontotemporal dementia (bvFTD): current limitations and future directions, *Alzheimer Disease and Associated Disorders*, 21(4): S14–S18.

Rosness, T.A., Haugen, P.K. and Engedal, K. (2008) Support to family carers of patients with frontotemporal dementia, *Aging and Mental Health*, 12(4): 462–6.

Sabodash, V., Mendez, M.F., Fong, S. and Hsiao, J.J. (2013) Suicidal behavior in dementia: a special risk in semantic dementia, *American Journal of Alzheimer's Disease and Other Dementias*, 28(6): 592–9.

Sampson, E.L., Warren, J.D. and Rossor, M.N. (2004) Young onset dementia, *Postgraduate Medical Journal*, 80(941): 125–39.

Savage, S.A., Ballard, K.J., Piguet, O. and Hodges, J.R. (2013) Bringing words back to mind: improving word production in semantic dementia, *Cortex*, 49(7): 1823–32.

van Vliet, D., de Vugt, M.E., Bakker, C., Koopmans, R.T.C.M. and Verhey, F.R.J. (2010) Impact of early onset dementia on caregivers: a review, *International Journal of Geriatric Psychiatry*, 25(11): 1091–100.

Walton, A.G. (2012) When words fail: a rare brain disease causes a professor to lose her powers of speech. *Pharma and Healthcare* [http://www.forbes.com/sites/alicegwalton/2012/06/01/when-words-fail-a-rare-brain-disease-causes-a-professor-to-lose-her-power-of-speech/, accessed 6 August 2013].

PART 2

Conceptualizing dementia care

Chapter contents

CHAPTER 8

A bio-psycho-social approach to dementia

Steven R. Sabat

    “I'm still me, even though I've been diagnosed.”

—Marlene Aveyard Yorkshire, UK

    “One of the 'gifts' that I do have and enjoy is singing and playing folk music on guitar or mandolin, depending on the tune. I try to organise a session of half a dozen songs which I perform at a weekly 'Alzheimer's café' in Bermondsey.”

—Doug Jenks London, UK

    “My Mum was always smartly dressed and had been used to a good social life and enjoyed the company of men. She was a very pretty lady. One day she had been to a coffee morning at the church next door (to the residential care home). When I went to visit she said what a lovely time she'd had and that she had talked for a long time to this nice gentleman. She said she had felt like a real person again.”

—Brenda Smith Yorkshire, UK

    “I learnt a great deal from caring for my mother and was supported by family, friends and professionals. I continue to learn and try to keep an open mind. Environmental factors, medication, the way we engage with people with dementia will determine the quality of that person's life.”

—Sue Tucker Yorkshire, UK

Learning objectives

By the end of this chapter, you will learn that people with dementia:

- Are capable of learning new things
- Can be sad about and embarrassed by their condition
- Retain their selfhood
- Can be powerfully affected by how they are treated by others

Introduction

In the coming decades, barring medical interventions that can prevent or reverse the occurrence of dementia, the numbers of people affected directly and indirectly will reach into the tens of millions and the financial costs required to care for such people will be significant (ADRDA 2000;

see also Chapter 1). It is of paramount importance in the absence of such interventions that we understand the effects of dementia in order to develop more effective means of supporting and sustaining those living with the condition. If we assume that everything a person with dementia does or feels is the outcome of brain damage and is "abnormal" in one way or another (such as anxiety, agitation, anger, etc.), we are then left with the job of "managing the patient" so as to make him or her more and more comfortable and compliant and less and less of a burden on caregivers. At its most extreme, such management relies on tranquillizing drugs such as anti-psychotics but can also include anti-anxiety and hypnotic medication.

For example, consider the case of Mr. U, a retired Army General diagnosed with dementia, who resides in a nursing home (Sabat and Lee 2012). Early in the morning, an aide tells him that it is time to take a shower. Mr. U does not want to take a shower at that time and refuses. The aide persists, and tries to pull Mr. U out of bed but Mr. U resists and hits the aide. The aide reports Mr. U as being "irrationally hostile, aggressive, and uncooperative" and Mr. U is given Seroquel that renders him zombie-like. Even though the manufacturer of the drug notes on its web site that Seroquel is not to be given to people with dementia, it is, nonetheless, given to Mr. U. The aide interpreted Mr. U's behaviour to be caused by dementia. Alternatively, we could recognize that the retired General was a person unaccustomed to taking orders from anyone "beneath his rank", did not want to take a shower, was physically accosted, and fought back. One could say that it was, in fact, the aide who was being "uncooperative" and "aggressive". This search for pharmaceutical solutions to the "problem" of dementia can also be seen in the search for drugs that may enhance synaptic transmission between neurons in the brain and thereby improve aspects of memory, such as the ability to recall recent events (see Chapter 14).

There is a very important assumption in the above paragraph: many, if not all, of the "symptoms" of dementia are, in one way or another, the direct outcome of the neuropathology caused by the disease process. This assumption is the foundation of the purely biomedical approach that dominated our understanding of dementia for decades (Katzman *et al.* 1978). In the past two decades, Kitwood (1997, 1998) called attention to significant problems with a strictly biomedical approach and, increasingly, research has shown that a broader understanding of people with dementia is required, for the behaviour of such people is affected by at least four factors (Snyder 1999; Killick and Allan 2001; Sabat 2001; Harris 2002; Wilkinson 2002):

- brain damage
- the person's reaction to the effects of the brain damage
- the ways in which the person is treated by healthy others
- the reactions of the diagnosed person to the ways in which he or she is treated by others

Kitwood (1990) captured some of these factors in the following formula:

$$SD = NI + MSP$$

where SD is senile dementia, NI is neurological impairment, and MSP is malignant social psychology.

"Malignant social psychology" was Kitwood's term for a style of interaction and relationship that had the effect of diminishing a person's personhood such as is seen in the depersonalizing treatment given to persons with dementia. In the quest for ways to sustain and care for people with dementia so as to enhance their quality of life as much as possible, it is important to examine closely each of the different factors so as to understand what people with dementia can and cannot do and under what conditions their abilities are facilitated and flourish as opposed to being inhibited. It is important, in other words, to identify correctly what constitutes a symptom of neuropathology as opposed to an appropriate emotional reaction and behavioural response to an extremely undesirable situation or to dysfunctional social treatment. This chapter examines the biological, psychological, and social domains so as to develop a clear picture of a bio-psycho-social approach. I will discuss research conducted in the USA and other countries.

The biological domain

As described in Chapter 1, the biological and clinical aspect is different in the different types of dementia. Depletion of certain transmitter substances occurs in Alzheimer's disease (AD), but not necessarily in vascular dementia. A person with a vascular dementia might not have damage to the hippocampus, but people with AD do have that damage. In addition, people with multi-infarct dementia have had several small strokes, but people with AD have not. As described in Chapter 1, AD is a type of dementia said to involve a depletion of a variety of neurotransmitters as well as the purported development of senile plaques and neurofibrillary tangles (Gaines and Whitehouse 2006). Regardless of the type of dementia, over the course of the illness there is a significant loss of neurons in the brain. This section will focus on the relationship between damage to particular areas of the brain (damage includes the loss of neurons) and losses in particular cognitive abilities and skills associated with AD.

Memory

Dementia involves brain damage that can affect a variety of cognitive abilities. Dementia of different types can affect different parts of the brain. One of the first areas of the brain that is affected by AD is the hippocampus, and the effects of damage here involve defects in what is known as "explicit" memory. Among the ways in which information can be retrieved from memory are explicit and implicit forms of retrieval (Squire 1994). *Explicit* memory involves the ability to recall consciously or to recognize specific pieces of information on demand. So, when we ask someone what today's date is, or what month it is, we are asking the person to recall in a conscious way a specific piece of information. Thus, when a person with AD asks a question and we answer it but then, five minutes later, the person asks the same question again as if it were the first time he or she was asking, we are witnessing a failure of recall. If we then ask the person, "What did I just tell you five minutes ago?", the person might say, "I don't know", and that would be another example of the failure to retrieve information via recall.

In some instances, one may change the format of the question from "What day of the week is it today?" (to which the person with AD replies, "I don't know") to a multiple-choice format ("Is it Tuesday?", "Is it Friday?", etc.), and with this format the person might identify the day correctly. This can happen because recall is much more difficult than recognition, which is the method of retrieval being used with a multiple-choice format, and this phenomenon is seen in many people with AD. Therefore, one should not assume that a person's failure to recall information means that the person cannot remember that information. Recall and remembering are not the same things. Recall is one way to remember, but there are other ways to do so, including recognition (Sabat 2001).

Another form of memory, apparently involving mechanisms of retrieval that are different than those used with explicit memory, is *implicit* memory, and this is defined as a change in behaviour that can occur as a result of an experience that the person is not consciously aware of having had (Grosse *et al.* 1990; Roedigger 1990; Howard 1991; Russo and Spinnler 1994; McDermott, 1997; Golby *et al.* 2005).

Case example 8.1: A person with memory dysfunction

In what is called a word-stem completion task, a person with a memory dysfunction, such as AD, is presented with a list of words including the word "defend". The person's memory of the words on the list can be tested in different ways. In one format, testing explicit memory, the person can be given the word-stem "def—", and then asked to complete the blank so as to make a word that he or she studied on the list presented earlier. In a different format, testing implicit memory, the person would be asked to complete the blank so as to form the first word that comes to mind. Note that with this latter format, there is no mention of the list of words presented previously. When employing the first format, using explicit memory, it is common for the person being tested to respond by saying, "What list?" By asking that question, the person with AD exhibits a dysfunction in explicit memory, specifically recall. The same person who appears to have no memory of having studied the list of words will complete the word-stem correctly if asked to complete the blank so as to make the first word that comes to mind. Note that there is a plethora of words that begin with "def—", so that one could not be "lucky" in guessing correctly simply because there are so few words that could be made by filling in the blank.

Such findings have been shown in people with AD in the mild to moderate stages (Russo and Spinnler 1994; Randolph *et al.* 1995). Thus, although the ability of a person with AD to recall information may be compromised, his or her ability to recognize the same information may be less compromised, and the ability to learn new information can be intact, even if the person does not recall having learned that information.

A specific version of the problem with recall is observed in what are called "word-finding" problems. The person with AD, while speaking, has difficulty in finding the word or words that he or she wants to use. Again, however, although the person may have a severe problem recalling the words in question, it is often possible for him or her to recognize the sought-after words if the healthy partner in conversation provides some possibilities. Similar findings using event-related fMRI have been reported (Schott *et al.* 2005).

Case example 8.2: A person with dementia

Person with dementia: "I went to see the uh, the, the, person who takes care of me when I'm not well physically."

Respondent: "Do you mean the dentist?"

Person with dementia: "Well, it could be, but not in this case."

Respondent: "Do you mean a physician?"

Person with dementia: "Yes."

—Sabat (2001)

Organization of movement

The cerebral cortex of the brain is comprised of four lobes, each associated with different cognitive functions – the frontal, parietal, occipital. and temporal lobes. Damage to the parietal lobe of the brain may result in "apraxia", or the inability to organize in the correct order a sequence of movements. Thus, although not paralysed, a person might not be able to:

- tie her shoelaces
- button his shirt
- sign her name
- use eating utensils correctly

It is important in each case to establish that the person can identify correctly the object in question (the eating utensils, the shirt, the shoes and laces), because if he or she cannot identify the object, it would be incorrect to say that the person's inability to use the object was due to a problem with the organization of movement. Another form of apraxia may, from the point of view of Brown (1972), be seen in instances of speech sounds that are misplaced so that the order of the sounds is incorrect, interfering with the communicative process. Brown proposed that some fluent aphasias might be considered apraxias of speech production. An aphasia is a dysfunction in the production or understanding of language, such that a person with "fluent aphasia" is able to speak with normal rhythm and intonation, but many of the spoken words themselves may not make sense to the listener, or the coherently spoken words may not seem to add up to something clearly understandable.

Visual identification of objects

Following damage to the occipital lobe of the brain, a person may see objects clearly but may be unable to identify them by name. This problem is known as "visual agnosia". A specific instance of this problem is "prosopagnosia", or the inability to identify another person by sight, by looking at the person's face. Thus, a person might be able to see and even acknowledge all the details – or features – of an object, but will be unable to organize those features into a coherent whole and name the object or person as the case may be.

Exercise 8.1: Different ways of interpreting behaviour

You are a staff member at a day centre that serves people including those diagnosed with dementia. You enter a room with a wardrobe containing participants' coats, and you see one of the participants who is diagnosed with dementia reaching into the pockets of one coat, looking at the contents, putting them back, and repeating this process with the next coat and the next.

- What do you assume about this behaviour and what do you do?
- How might our different views of what influences behaviour affect how we interpret this behaviour?

If the staff member's understanding of individuals with AD is one that emphasizes such individuals' defects, the staff member might well view this behaviour as a socially inappropriate "symptom" and proceed to stop the person from continuing.

Imagine you did not choose to intervene but simply watched the participant move from coat to coat, looking at the contents of the pockets of each before replacing them, until he came to one particular coat. When he looked at the contents of this particular coat's pockets, he replaced the contents but then took the coat off the hanger and put the coat on. And, most significantly, it was his coat. It is true that going through the pockets of coats that belong to others is inappropriate.

It is the case, however, that the intention of the person with AD in this example was not to act inappropriately, to invade the property of others or violate their privacy. Rather, the man was simply trying to find his coat, which he could not recognize by sight, perhaps not recalling which coat he wore that day. He did know that his coat pockets contained his property and he knew, consciously or unconsciously, that he would recognize his belongings when he saw them. Thus, his behaviour was not simply some species of "social disinhibition" resulting from brain damage caused by AD, but an adaptation to the effects of AD.

- How might it feel for a person not to be able to recognize his own coat by sight, or not to be able to put on a shirt or a pair of trousers or to sign his or her name?

This is very much a psychological issue and it is to such matters that we now turn.

The psychological domain

Together with significant advances in our understanding of the neurobiology of cognition, we have seen an unprecedented research interest in understanding the person's perspective on living with dementia. Understanding what dementia does to a person psychologically requires more than simply observing his or her behaviour from afar or examining standard neuropsychological test results. Indeed, it requires that we engage that person as a person so as to understand what he or she is experiencing (Laing 1965). To assume that a person would not have any reactions to the loss of his or her ability to use eating utensils, to tie shoelaces, sign his or her name, recall what happened moments ago, spell simple words, would be to assume that the person in question was quite dysfunctional. To assume that depression, anxiety, agitation, so-called "wandering", and the like are symptoms of AD in the same way that fever is a symptom of malaria, is to depersonalize the individual in question (Kitwood and Bredin 1992; Bender and Cheston 1997; Kitwood 1997; Sabat 2001; Harris 2002). What do we discover when we engage people with AD as people, even as partners in research?

Early research by Snyder (1999), in which she interviewed people recently diagnosed with probable AD, revealed much about their reactions to the symptoms, the diagnosis, and the ways in which others treated them. Some people reacted strongly and negatively to the treatment they received from the medical personnel involved in arriving at and communicating the diagnosis. For example, Bea described the neurologist who interviewed her:

> He was very indifferent and said it was just going to get worse . . . If he had just shown a little compassion. He was there to diagnose my problem, but he wasn't there to understand my feelings. He had no feelings for me whatsoever. I've hated him ever since. Health care professionals need to be compassionate.

—Snyder (1999: 18)

Another of Snyder's interviewees, Betty, a retired social worker and former faculty member at San Diego State University, discussed health care professionals whom she encountered during the process of being diagnosed:

> They're busy wanting to climb up to the next rung on the ladder. That's very human. I don't blame them. But they don't really accept the significance of illness for people. They know the diagnosis, but they don't take time to find out what it truly means for that person. This casualness with which professionals deal with Alzheimer's is so painful to

see . . . You have to really be willing to be present with the person who has Alzheimer's. But there are some people who don't want to learn, and it's the looking down on and being demeaning of people with Alzheimer's that is hard to watch. **"**

—Snyder (1999: 123–4)

Connell *et al.* (2004) have found these experiences to be similar in many ways to those reported by family caregivers.

Both Bea and Betty felt depersonalized by the health care professionals who informed them of their diagnosis, and who seemed to lack any interest in exploring with them what the diagnosis meant to them, how they felt, or in extending to them any human compassion or caring. Still, one should not assume that the professionals in question were callous, uncaring people. So why did they behave as they did? Among the possible reasons is how the professionals positioned Bea and Betty as well as how they positioned themselves (Harré and van Langenhove 1991). That is, the professionals understood their roles as being limited to communicating the facts of the diagnosis and nothing more. They did not think that there was any reason to discuss anything further with their patients, perhaps because there was nothing they could do to stop the disease from progressing towards its eventual conclusion. In a subtle way, though, they may have been incorrectly positioning Bea and Betty negatively as people who, because of their illness, would either have no particular reaction to the news, given that they have a form of dementia, or lack the ability to engage in any kind of discussion about what the news meant to them. (For discussion of sharing the diagnosis, see Chapter 19.)

It would be incorrect to assume that interactions of this type occur in each and every situation between health care professionals and their patients, but it surely was true in these cases, as well as in the case of Dr. B (Sabat 2001), whose doctor commented that "treating a person with Alzheimer's is like doing veterinary medicine". Under these conditions, the person with Alzheimer's disease feels ignored, unworthy of being treated as a human being, and someone who is defined to a great extent, if not completely, by his or her diagnosis. Betty said, "A person with Alzheimer's disease is many more things than just their diagnosis. Each person is a whole human being" (Snyder 1999: 123–4).

Once persons are positioned socially as nothing more than instantiations of a diagnostic category, their essential humanity, including their intellectual and emotional characteristics, needs, and their social personae beyond that of "demented, burdensome patient" become more and more invisible and can ultimately be erased. When viewed in this way, the extent to which such people can enjoy any semblance of a good quality of life is correspondingly reduced and this, in turn, will require increased resources in order to "manage the patients" instead of interacting with them as persons in ways that would not lead to conflict, disparagement, and the resulting need for "management". The case of Mr. U, discussed in the Introduction, is another example of this phenomenon. For a review of research on the experience of living with dementia, from the perspective of people with dementia, see Bunn *et al.* (2012). See also Manthorpe *et al.* (2011), who noted that few people in their study could call their experiences of memory assessment "patient-centred" and that they were in need of more understanding and support from professionals.

Although Bea commented that she often felt "nearly invisible" in social situations, she did perceive others' apparent discomfort about her diagnosis and her problems with aspects of memory as well as with organizing and directing bodily movements such as shaking hands. Others in her social milieu seemed to position her negatively as being far more disabled than she actually was, and treated her as if the negative positioning was actually valid, thereby creating a dramatic constriction of her social world to the point of her being isolated and increasingly dependent upon her husband. She was well aware of this entire dynamic: "I'm isolating him as well as myself and I'm not being fair to him" (Snyder 1999: 24) (see also Chapter 2). Feelings such as these, that arise from being negatively positioned by others and then treated in socially malignant ways such as being ostracized and banished (Kitwood 1998) create internal conflict within the person with dementia and diminish the person's sense of self-worth.

It may seem strange that the two women who were quoted verbatim above could be treated as they were, given that they expressed themselves clearly, cogently, and with grace. Nothing in what they said or how they said it could suggest that they were cognitively compromised, yet they were still treated by healthy others in ways that could be described as "dysfunctional" and "malignant". It is precisely this confluence of facts that underscores how powerful an influence a diagnosis can be. What is the foundation of this sort of treatment? Two possibilities spring to mind:

1. There is a stereotypic view, promoted by professionals, the public press, entertainment media, and the like, that focuses on the defects that dementia can ultimately cause, and simultaneously ignores the person's remaining intact abilities (see Chapter 6).
2. There is the tendency for diagnostic overshadowing to occur such that all reported "defects" in people thus diagnosed are due to the disease alone and not to the ways in which the people thus diagnosed are treated by others.

There is, however, the testimony of people in the moderate to severe stages of dementia, who express appropriate anger, frustration, sadness, and embarrassment regarding the losses that they have experienced. Dr. M was very clear about this when she spoke about writing and typing, things that she once did with great facility: "Now it is so miserable a chore that I avoid it as much as possible. And all these things take ridiculous amounts of time . . . as to how my symptoms affect me, do not think I am just being frivolous if I say they drive me crazy" (Sabat 2001: 115).

Add to this the fact that others see the person with dementia principally in terms of what he or she cannot do and is it any wonder that such a person would feel depressed? Indeed, for a person not to feel depressed in such circumstances would be "inappropriate" and worthy of being described as "having no insight" into, or being "blissfully unaware" of, one's problems. We could easily say that feeling all of the above negative emotions in reaction to the effects of dementia and to the ensuing dysfunctional social treatment is, itself, deeply significant. Indeed, it is evidence that the person is a "semiotic subject" – one whose behaviour is driven by the meaning that situations hold for him or her (Sabat and Harré 1994).

To summarize, negative positioning of people diagnosed with dementia is based on a medical view that every instance of seemingly "abnormal" behaviour seen in the person diagnosed is due to brain damage, and that such people are immune to being treated in dysfunctional ways by others. So, for example, if a person with a diagnosis of probable AD is treated in a way that would be humiliating and embarrassing to any reasonable, healthy person, and if the person with AD reacts with anger or grief or by pulling away from others or avoiding them completely, the anger, grief, and social isolation are viewed as symptoms of AD instead of symptoms of dysfunctional social treatment, so as to validate the original malignant positioning of the person.

Exercise 8.2: The importance of knowing the full context

(a) You are a staff member at a day centre that serves people including those diagnosed with dementia. The spouse of one of the participants tells you about his wife: "Her Alzheimer's is getting worse; yesterday, after I picked her up from the day centre, she became irrationally hostile towards me, wouldn't speak to me or look at me at all during the evening."

- What do you say?
- What do you think?

Consider what you might think if you also knew the larger context of the scenario: when the husband arrived to pick up his wife, she was standing in the hallway conversing with others, including staff members. The husband joined in the conversation but, as his wife was talking, he began to tuck her turtleneck top into her trousers (she was wearing it outside of her trousers and it looked fine). As he did this in front of others, thinking (incorrectly) that she'd forgotten to do so herself, she was clearly humiliated, her eyes bulging out of their sockets, so to speak, but this went unnoticed by her husband. She reacted towards him later with anger, but the anger was anything but "irrational". Indeed, one could quite easily refer to her reaction as "righteous indignation" instead of "irrational hostility".

(b) The primary carer of a woman diagnosed with AD tells you, "My mother has a problem with the concept of time."

- What do you say?
- Do you say that this is another symptom of the disease?

Consider what you might say if you knew why she thought this to be true: her mother was "worrying" about buying a dress for a wedding to which they were going in two months' time. Now, one could say quite reasonably that Mrs. E was engaging in higher-order executive (frontal lobe based) functioning in that she was displaying the appropriate ability to plan ahead. Given past experience in finding attire for a special occasion, Mrs. E was not content to wait until, what was for her, "the last minute". After all, one must first find a dress and then the dress might require alterations, both of which could take a long time, so that wanting to take action well in advance could be interpreted as being not only logical, but also as a sign of intact higher-order cognitive functioning. As a result of malignant positioning, this example of what might be viewed as being appropriate and healthy behaviour was explained in dysfunctional terms – that Mrs. E "had a problem with the concept of time".

The message in these cases is clear: it is of tremendous importance to understand the larger social context in which a person acts, and not to assume that because a person with dementia reacts in a way that is not immediately understandable to the caregiver, the behaviour in question is "irrational" and a product of brain damage as opposed to dysfunctional social treatment.

People with dementia live in a social world with others much of the time and it is to the social domain that we now turn.

The social domain

Case example 8.3: Mrs. R

Mrs. R attended an adult day centre and, according to standard assessments, was in the moderate to severe stages of dementia. Her husband commented that she did nothing around the house, save for watching television and walking around "aimlessly", that she did not help with the household chores, that he did everything. At the day centre, however, Mrs. R helped set tables prior to the

(continued)

lunch meal, acted almost as a volunteer (according to the staff members) by helping participants in wheelchairs navigate through doorways, by comforting others who were recovering from illness and by calling staff's attention to participants who needed a level of help that she could not provide (Sabat 2001). Although it is true that brain damage can result in increased variability in the performance of many tasks, there was no variability in Mrs. R's behaviour: at home she did nothing, but at the day centre, she did a great deal, much of which she could have done at home as well, such as setting the table. Thus, one must look beyond the biological level to find an explanation for this striking difference in her behaviour. In the past, Mrs. R served as a volunteer in a variety of ways, from working in hospitals to caring for abandoned children in developing countries. Being of service to others was an abiding aspect of her personality.

We can examine this as well as Mrs. R's situation at home and at the day centre by using the three-part social constructionist theory (Harré 1991). From moment to moment, from day to day, we feel a continuity of ourselves – that each of us is one and the same individual person (Self 1) to whom we refer as "I' and "me", for example. Another way that we define ourselves is through our mental and physical attributes, past and present. So, one's eye pigmentation, facility with languages, college degree, sense of humour, these are all part of this aspect of selfhood (called Self 2). Also part of Self 2 are one's beliefs (political, religious, etc.) and one's beliefs about one's attributes: one can take pride in some of one's attributes, while viewing other attributes with disdain, even antipathy. Even in the moderate to severe stage of the disease, people with dementia have made it clear that they view their losses as embarrassing, frustrating, even maddening. Also part of the selfhood of an individual is the multiple social personae (Self 3) that he or she constructs with the cooperation of others. Each of one's social personae is marked by a unique pattern of behaviour, so that the behaviour connected with being a loving spouse is quite different from that connected with being a devoted parent, a demanding supervisor at work, and a loyal friend, to name a few. We can examine Mrs. R's situation at home as opposed to the day centre by examining the social dynamics required for the construction of the social personae of Self 3.

Recall that it is necessary to have the cooperation of at least one other person to construct (jointly) a particular social persona.

Case example 8.3: Mrs. R (continued)

It would be impossible to behave as a loving spouse if one's husband or wife did not recognize you as being a spouse. One cannot construct the persona of the devoted parent if one's child does not recognize you as being his or her mother or father. Mrs. R could not construct the social persona of "helpful spouse" at home because her husband did not allow her to engage in helping him with household chores. He indicated his concern that she would fail to do what he would ask of her and so, according to him, he "protected" her by doing everything himself. In contrast, at the day centre, the staff cooperated with Mrs. R, allowing her to be of help to participants as well as to other staff members, thereby helping her in constructing the social persona of "helpful participant/quasi volunteer".

Similar examples have been reported (Sabat 2003; Sabat *et al*. 2004). In many cases, it appears, the person with dementia is prevented from constructing a valued social persona due to: (a) the lack of cooperation from healthy others in the social milieu, and (b) the intimately related tendency of others to view the person with dementia increasingly in terms of his or her deficits. By viewing the person in question mainly in terms of his or her diagnosis and all the losses it entails, healthy others thereby ignore more and more the attributes in which the person in question takes pride. This dynamic serves to restrict the social persona of the individual with dementia to something that the person with dementia finds abhorrent, embarrassing, humiliating – the "burdensome patient" or "defective patient" – because others do not provide the necessary cooperation for the person to construct a worthy social persona. In this way, the person with AD is confined to a social persona that is constituted of everything that is defective and embarrassing. Is it any wonder that Dr. M, a retired university professor in the moderate to severe stage, commented about Alzheimer's: "Is it even more embarrassing than a sexual disease?" (Sabat 2001: 115).

Interestingly, other people with dementia may provide each other with the kind of cooperation that is required for positive social relations to be created (Sabat and Lee 2012). One example involves two participants at an adult day centre, Mrs. E and Mrs. M, who appeared to gravitate towards and empathize with one another. It appeared that each had an awareness of the other's needs and a mutual understanding of their circumstances. On one occasion, Mrs. M was asked what she had done over the previous weekend. Mrs. M tried to reply but had difficulty finding the words she sought. After a few minutes, she shrugged her shoulders, laughed, and replied, "I can't remember". After a few moments, Mrs. E leaned toward Mrs. M, affectionately touched her arm and said, "You're just like me. You go in and out too." In so doing, Mrs. E acted not only to help Mrs. M save face in the situation, but simultaneously created a bond or alliance of sorts, by indicating that Mrs. M was not alone in being unable to recount the weekend's events, but rather that she was in "good company". Rather than focusing on her friend's dysfunction, Mrs. E supported her friend, minimizing Mrs. M's inability to respond, thereby giving Mrs. M some measure of comfort and helping her to construct the persona of "valued friend".

Exercise 8.3: How a person can be positioned malignantly by language

You make a visit to the home of a married couple. The husband has been diagnosed with dementia. You are greeted by the wife who then introduces you to her husband by saying, "This is my husband; he's the patient."

- Do you have a private reaction to this introduction, and if so, what is it?

Here we see a perfectly loving, devoted, respectful wife introducing her husband as "the patient". Of course, her husband had many other attributes that could have been used as part of an introduction, and it was clear that some of those attributes were positive and worthy of honour and respect. Yet, the wife focused on an attribute that he found abhorrent.

It is common to hear people described as "patients". Still, the plain fact is that people are patients only in relation to their physicians, nurses, dentists, and other health professionals. In other social relationships, people can be many things, but they cannot be patients in the true sense of the social situations at hand. Why, then, are people with AD seen as being "patients" regardless of the social situation of which they happen to be a part? In a sense, the restriction of a person's social persona to an attribute that the person loathes and is embarrassed by is a form of what Kitwood (1998) called "malignant social psychology", because this type of treatment depersonalizes the individual and constitutes an assault on the person's sense of self-worth.

It is clear that even in the moderate to severe stage of the disease, people with AD can construct worthy social personae when given the necessary cooperation. It is clear also that those who live in residential settings for people with dementia can still enjoy and experience meaningful social interactions (Hubbard *et al.* 2003). It is extremely important to note, however, that such people are far more dependent on there being supportive environments and venues within which they can have the opportunities to engage in these kinds of interactions. Hence, people with AD or other forms of dementia are far more vulnerable than they were during the balance of their adult lives because it is much more difficult for them to gain the cooperation they need to construct valued social identities. There is reason to emphasize strongly, therefore, that the measurement tools that are used to assess the so-called cognitive abilities of people with dementia, do not predict or assess a person's capacity to enjoy meaningful social interactions with others. In other words, practitioners (a) should not assume anything at all about the social identity or potential social identity of a person with dementia on the basis of his or her standard test scores because (b) such tests make little, if any, contact with the combination of cognitive abilities that is required for a person to be a semiotic subject who can enjoy valued social relationships with others.

Case example 8.4: A person with AD

A man to whom I was about to administer a battery of neuropsychological tests made what seemed to be a completely unsolicited (by me) comment: "Doc, ya gotta find a way to give us purpose again." Although he was in the moderate to severe stage of AD, he possessed the ability (and the requisite functional brain systems) to discern the importance of having a purpose in life, that he lacked a meaningful purpose, and that he needed help from someone else in his quest to regain what he so strongly desired. A bio-psycho-social approach allows us to understand that:

1. Some of the losses he sustained had their roots in biological terms, but also simultaneously.
2. He was able to experience and articulate a completely appropriate reaction to those losses.
3. He understood what those losses meant to him personally and socially.
4. There are non-pharmaceutical ways to enhance his quality of life.

Debates and controversies

There continues to be debate and controversy over the relative weight of contribution of the various biological, psychological, and social elements. Similarly, different professions and disciplinary groups may hold divergent views as to which avenue holds the most promise for helping people to live well with dementia. These differences of opinion influence the way resources are distributed. For example, if research funders see most potential in drugs that support cognition, they may be less inclined to support research on engaging staff in communicating effectively with people with dementia. While family carers have had a voice, the voice of people with dementia themselves is only now joining this debate. As such, different people may answer the following questions differently:

- Does a purely biomedical approach to dementia provide a complete understanding of the person diagnosed?

- Are pharmaceutical treatments (drugs) all that are required to treat the person?
- Is it practical to try to understand and treat each person in the light of his or her unique history when each person is different? Is this possible in residential homes?
- What is the difference between understanding the disease a person has and the person who has the disease?

Conclusion

The behavioural and emotional reactions observed in people with dementia were, for decades, attributed solely to brain damage. More recently, it has become clear that, in addition to the effects of brain injury, people with dementia also have psychological reactions to their brain injuries, and these reactions affect what they say and do in relation to others. Furthermore, people with dementia are affected by the ways in which they are treated by healthy others in social situations. Although biological explanations are appropriate in explaining certain aspects of dementia, such as the relationship between damage to the hippocampus and defects in explicit memory, there are other effects that are not explainable in purely biological terms. Specifically, people with dementia are embarrassed by, angry about, and sometimes depressed about the problems caused by brain injury and they seek to avoid embarrassment and humiliation. Furthermore, they can retain aspects of selfhood, including worthy social personae, but the latter depends upon how they are treated by others. A bio-psycho-social approach is required for understanding people with dementia and for the further evolution of good practice in supporting people to live well with dementia. Spector and Orrell (2010) have written persuasively that a psychosocial perspective is of value to researchers and clinicians, and Harris (2010) has argued that sociologists, who have long been concerned with social justice and exclusion, can play a valuable part in improving care for people with dementia. Teaching young people about a bio-psycho-social approach has been shown, in one four-month study (Sabat 2012), to have had remarkably positive effects on their understanding of the remaining strengths of people with dementia, so there is some reason to believe that similar types of education may be of value to older adults as well.

Further information

MedlinePlus provides information online about health conditions, including dementia. It brings together information from NLM, the National Institutes of Health (NIH), and other US government agencies and health-related organizations [http://www.nlm.nih.gov/medlineplus/].

The Merck Manual of Geriatrics is available online and provides information about the care of older people.

The National Institute of Neurological Disorders and Stroke is part of the US National Institutes of Health. It has web pages devoted to dementia [http://www.ninds.nih.gov/].

The University of California at San Francisco Memory and Aging Center has a web site with useful information about dementia [http://memory.ucsf.edu/].

References

Alzheimer's Disease and Related Disorders Association (ADRDA) (2000) *A Race Against Time*. Chicago, IL: ADRDA.

Bender, M.P. and Cheston, R. (1997) Inhabitants of a lost kingdom: a model of the subjective experiences of dementia, *Ageing and Society*, 17(5): 513–32.

Brown, J.W. (1972) *Aphasia, Apraxia, and Agnosia: Clinical and Theoretical Aspects*. Springfield, IL: C.C. Thomas.

Bunn, F., Goodman, C., Sworn, K., Rait, G., Brayne, C. et al. (2012) Psychosocial factors that shape patient and carer experiences of dementia diagnosis and treatment: a systematic review of qualitative studies, *PLoS Medicine*, 9 (10): e1001331.

Connell, C.M., Boise, L., Stuckey, J.C., Holmes, S.B. and Hudson, M.L. (2004) Attitudes toward the diagnosis and disclosure of dementia among family caregivers and primary care physicians, *The Gerontologist*, 44(4): 500–7.

Gaines, A.D. and Whitehouse, P.J. (2006) Building a mystery: Alzheimer's disease, mild cognitive impairment, and beyond, *Philosophy, Psychiatry and Psychology*, 13(1): 61–74.

Golby, A., Silverberg, G., Race, E., Gabrieli, S., O'Shea, J. et al. (2005) Memory encoding in Alzheimer's disease: an fMRI study of explicit and implicit memory, *Brain*, 128(4): 773–87.

Grosse, D.A., Wilson, R.S. and Fox, J.H. (1990) Preserved word stem completion priming of semantically encoded information in Alzheimer's disease, *Psychology and Aging*, 5(2): 304–6.

Harré, R. (1991) The discursive production of selves, *Theory and Psychology*, 1(1): 51–63.

Harré, R. and van Langenhove, L. (1991) Varieties of positioning, *Journal for the Theory of Social Behavior*, 21(4): 393–408.

Harris, P.B. (ed.) (2002) *The Person with Alzheimer's Disease: Pathways to Understanding the Experience*. Baltimore, MD: Johns Hopkins University Press.

Harris, P.B. (2010) Dementia and dementia care: the contributions of a psychosocial perpective, *Sociology Compass*, 4(4): 249–62.

Howard, D.V. (1991) Implicit memory: an expanding picture of cognitive aging, in K.W. Schaie (ed.) *Annual Review of Gerontology and Geriatrics* (Vol. 11). New York: Springer-Verlag, pp. 1–22.

Hubbard, G., Tester, S. and Downs, M.G. (2003) Meaningful social interactions between older people in institutional care settings, *Ageing and Society*, 23(1): 99–114.

Katzman, R., Terry, R.D. and Bick, K.L. (eds.) (1978) *Alzheimer's Disease: Senile Dementia and Related Disorders*. New York: Raven Press.

Killick, J. and Allan, K. (2001) *Communication and the Care of People with Dementia*. Buckingham: Open University Press.

Kitwood, T. (1990) The dialectics of dementia: with particular reference to Alzheimer's disease, *Ageing and Society*, 10(2): 177–96.

Kitwood, T. (1997) *Dementia Reconsidered: The Person Comes First*. Buckingham: Open University Press.

Kitwood, T. (1998) Toward a theory of dementia care: ethics and interaction, *Journal of Clinical Ethics*, 9(1): 23–34.

Kitwood, T. and Bredin, K. (1992) Towards a theory of dementia care: personhood and well-being, *Ageing and Society*, 12(1): 269–87.

Laing, R.D. (1965) *The Divided Self*. Baltimore, MD: Penguin Books.

Manthorpe, J., Samsi, K., Campbell, S., Abley, C., Keady, J. et al. (2011) *Transition from Cognitive Impairment to Dementia: Older People's Experiences*. Final report. NIHR Service Delivery and Organisation Programme [http://www.kcl.ac.uk/sspp/kpi/scwru/pubs/2011/manthorpeetal2011transitionfinalreport.pdf].

McDermott, K. (1997) Priming on perceptual implicit memory tests can be achieved through presentation of associates, *Psychonomic Bulletin and Review*, 4(4): 582–6.

Randolph, C., Tierney, M.C. and Chase, T.N. (1995) Implicit memory in Alzheimer's disease, *Journal of Clinical and Experimental Neuropsychology*, 17(3): 343–51.

Roediger, H.L. (1990) Retention without remembering, *American Psychologist*, 45(9): 1043–56.

Russo, R. and Spinnler, H. (1994) Implicit verbal memory in Alzheimer's disease, *Cortex*, 30(3): 359–75.

Sabat, S.R. (2001) *The Experience of Alzheimer's Disease: Life Through a Tangled Veil*. Oxford: Blackwell.

Sabat, S.R. (2003) Some potential benefits of creating research partnerships with people with Alzheimer's disease, *Research Policy and Planning*, 21(2): 5–12.

Sabat, S.R. (2012) A bio-psycho-social model enhances young adults' understanding of and beliefs about people with Alzheimer's disease: a case study, *Dementia*, 11: 95–112.

Sabat, S.R. and Harré, R. (1994) The Alzheimer's disease sufferer as a semiotic subject, *Philosophy, Psychiatry, and Psychology*, 1(1): 145–60.

Sabat, S.R. and Lee, J.M. (2012) Relatedness among people diagnosed with dementia: social cognition and the possibility of friendship, *Dementia*, 11: 311–23.

Sabat, S.R., Napolitano, L. and Fath, H. (2004) Barriers to the construction of a valued social identity: a case study of Alzheimer's disease, *American Journal of Alzheimer's Disease and Other Dementias*, 19(3): 177–85.

Schott, B.H., Henson, R.N., Richardson-Klavehn, A., Becker, C., Thoma, V. *et al.* (2005) Redefining implicit and explicit memory: the functional neuroanatomy of priming, remembering, and control of retrieval, *Proceedings of the National Academy of Sciences USA*, 102(4): 1257–62.

Snyder, L. (1999) *Speaking Our Minds: Personal Reflections from Individuals with Alzheimer's*. New York: Freeman.

Spector, A. and Orrell, M. (2010) Using a biopsychosocial model of dementia as a tool to guide clinical practice, *International Psychogeriatrics*, 22(Special Issue 06): 957–65.

Squire, L.R. (1994) Declarative and nondeclarative memory: multiple brain systems supporting learning and memory, in D.L. Schacter and E. Tulving (eds.) *Memory Systems*. Cambridge, MA: MIT Press, pp. 203–32.

Wilkinson, H. (ed.) (2002) *The Perspectives of People with Dementia*. London: Jessica Kingsley.

CHAPTER 9

Selfhood and the body in dementia care

Pia C. Kontos

❝I don't know if he recognizes me. If he knows me at all. No idea. He hasn't used my name. Hasn't said anything recognizable. Just things that don't seem to make a lot of sense. . . . We were both scouts in our youth, not together but we discovered we had both been scouts that it meant a lot to both of us. We shared that. After he found out we had both been scouts he always gave me that left handed hand shake. That's the scout hand shake. Still, now, when I visit him, he sticks out his left hand to me. Never misses it. That scout hand shake.❞

—Frank Webber Melbourne, Australia

❝My Dad was a professional footballer in his youth and he retained relatively exceptional physical fitness until the last three months of his life. He was always proud of that fitness and my brother and I used to groan whenever Dad challenged us to 'race him over 50 yards'. How delighted were we when the nursing staff at his care home confided to us that, on quiet evenings when most people had gone to bed but my Dad was still roaming the corridors – he was never still for long – someone would go and find the lightweight football that they had bought especially for him and gently pass the ball to him up and down the corridors. He won't have had to think, or work at it, he'll just have been able to relax and enjoy doing one of the things he was so good at before he became ill no doubt 'showing off' a little at the same time. The nursing staff's care on those occasions for an individual's happiness and fulfilment could be said to be above and beyond the line of duty, but those evenings made a world of difference to my Dad, and I will always be grateful.❞

—Fiona Hardy Yorkshire, UK

❝I remember taking nana out in her wheelchair from the care home, she was always so happy to get out and into the fresh air. Although she didn't know exactly who I was and she was long past remembering names at this point, her body language spoke volumes. She would light up when she saw me because she knew that I was someone who would take her out and allow her some freedom from the care home. She genuinely appeared at peace in those walks on the seafront like a weight had been lifted. We would drink hot chocolate and I would hold her hand and we would smile at each other, I could see that in those moments she would have a sparkle in her eye and seemed happy just to be.❞

—Shelley Angelique Cooper Yorkshire, UK

Learning objectives

By the end of this chapter, you will:

- Learn that the body is fundamental to self-expression
- Understand that people with dementia retain their embodied dimensions of selfhood, which are expressed through bodily habits, gestures, and movements

- Appreciate there is a breadth of meaning that can be conveyed by the body
- Understand the importance of recognizing and supporting embodied selfhood in dementia care

Introduction

Much of the literature on Alzheimer's promotes the view that individuals with dementia experience a steady erosion of selfhood to the point at which no person remains – described as a "death in slow motion" (Cooney 2003), and a "splintering of the sedimented layers of Being . . . until there is nothing left" (Davis 2004: 375). Richard Taylor, who writes of his own dementia, reflects on public perception:

> ❝ I think that, for most people, Alzheimer's disease means certain death before your 'natural time,' preceded by a period of time during which you have been stripped of your personality and your memories and have become someone you cannot imagine. You have no dignity and no sense of self, and eventually you just sit around waiting for your body to forget how to keep itself alive. ❞

—Taylor (2007: 114)

Thus, while Alzheimer's disease and other dementias are usually described in terms of the cognitive dysfunction they produce, there is also an assumed existential loss. In increasing numbers, social scientists and health-science scholars are examining the loss of self that is so widely associated with the cognitive deficiencies lying at the core of dementia (Kitwood 1997; Hughes *et al.* 2006; Behuniak 2011). These scholars challenge the notion that the personal deterioration associated with dementia comes about exclusively as the result of a neurological process that has its own autonomous dynamic (see Chapter 8). Much of this work is premised on a notion of personhood defined as "a standing or status that is bestowed upon one human being by others, in the context of relationship and social being" (Kitwood 1997: 8). However, to maintain that it is the socio-interactive environment alone that constitutes selfhood in dementia is to miss the significance of "embodied selfhood" (Kontos 2004, 2005, 2012) – the idea that bodily habits, gestures, and actions support and convey humanness and individuality.

This chapter presents an alternative to the presumed loss of selfhood in Alzheimer's disease, one that captures the ways selfhood continues to be expressed, even in severe stages of the illness, through bodily actions. This alternative view, what I term "embodied selfhood", is first presented in relation to its theoretical bearings: Merleau-Ponty's (1962) reconceptualization of perception, and Bourdieu's notion of *habitus* (1977, 1990). Examples of embodied selfhood are provided, capturing the richness of the social world of dementia and the importance of the body in expressing that richness. Emphasizing the importance of the body for self-expression is not merely a theoretical exercise; it has important practical implications. Thus the final part of this chapter is devoted to current research on the implications of embodied selfhood for person-centred dementia care (Kontos *et al.* 2010), research that involves the use of drama as an innovative method for translating this theoretical perspective to front-line dementia care practitioners (Kontos and Naglie 2006, 2007).

Embodied selfhood

Central to Merleau-Ponty's philosophy is a radical reconceptualization of perception not as cognitive consciousness but rather as embodied consciousness. Embodied consciousness, or basic intentionality, is the body's concrete, spatial, and pre-reflective directedness towards the lived world. It refers to a kind of inner map of movements the body naturally "knows" how to perform without having to reflect upon such movements (Merleau-Ponty 1964). In Merleau-Ponty's words (1964: 5), "a system of possible movements ... radiates from us to our environment", giving us at every moment a practical and implicit hold on our body. In this "system of possible movements", the body possesses, according to Merleau-Ponty, a coordinating capacity that does not rely on explicit awareness. Hence, as Merleau-Ponty notes, in their first attempts at reaching for an object, children look not at their hand but at the object, the implication being that the various parts of the body are known to us through their functionality without their coordination ever having to be learnt (Merleau-Ponty 1962: 149). In other words, the pre-reflective body is intentional in that it is directed towards the world without the need to understand how it is directed (Merleau-Ponty 1964). This capacity provides the foundation for selfhood, with selfhood emanating from the natural expressiveness of the body.

Bourdieu (1977, 1990) argues that the conditioning associated with membership in a particular social class tends to instil in the individual dispositions for being and perceiving. Bodily expressions (e.g. the way we walk or the way we eat) reflect the effects of socialization that result from cumulative exposure to certain social conditions associated with membership in a particular social class. Bourdieu defines a disposition as "a *way of being*, a *habitual state* . . . a *tendency, propensity,* or *inclination*" (1977: 214, note 1, original emphasis). In practice, these dispositions materialize as postures, gestures, and movements (Bourdieu 1977).

Of paramount importance is the notion that an individual's actions are the product of a *modus operandi* of which the individual is not the producer and, for the most part, has no conscious mastery (Bourdieu 1977). The body is understood as having a "generative, creative capacity to understand" – a kind of bodily awareness. Consequently, selfhood can be understood to reside in these dispositions, manifesting in socio-culturally specific ways of being-in-the-world.

The perspective on embodiment advanced here will provide the framework to explore the richness and complexity of selfhood as manifesting creativity, conversation, and social norms and customs.

Exercise 9.1: Developing an understanding of embodied knowing

Think about the diverse ways in which you move your body in the context of social, cultural, and leisure activities. Identify the movements, gestures, and actions you use in those contexts that were learned without having to think about what you were doing, and that you now perform without thought.

In engaging with this exercise, you are identifying examples of basic intentionality and/or socio-cultural practices, both of which are expressions of embodied selfhood.

Exploring the social world of dementia: Alzheimer expressions or expressions despite Alzheimer's?

The painterly hand

In research exploring selfhood in dementia, literature has become a vital source of ideas about Alzheimer's disease and individual experiences. Michael Ignatieff's novel, *Scar Tissue* (1993), is a story about a woman living with Alzheimer's, recounted by her son. The son describes his mother's passion for painting as she would spend much of her time, before becoming ill, working at her easel. Following the death of his father and the further progression of his mother's Alzheimer's disease, the son had no other option but to admit his mother into a nursing home. He recounts that shortly after his mother's admission to the nursing home, she became unable to feed herself and would spend most of her time staring out of the window; the advancing illness allowed her only a small margin of manoeuvre. The son would visit his mother daily, observing with admirable but painful honesty her decline while asking himself crucial questions about science, genetics, art, and personhood. One afternoon, while in the nursing home day room together, the son asks his mother to sketch him.

> **❝** I put the charcoal into her left hand and I put a fresh sheet of paper down, and I sat there holding her right hand, posing so that she would understand what was wanted of her. For a moment, she remained motionless, not looking at the pencil or the paper, just smiling faintly. Then, as if the pencil placed between her fingers and my expectant face triggered a forgotten power and a forgotten scene, she began to draw. The first charcoal line appeared. Her eyes rose to take in the fall of my eyebrows, my jaw and the shape of my head. She brought her free hand up towards my face, as if to estimate distance and proportion and shape. Then just as quietly as she began, my mother stopped. The charcoal remained in her hand, poised above the last line, but it would move no further. Such connection as had been made was now broken and my mother stared off once again into space. **❞**

—Ignatieff (1993: 152)

At the time that this incident takes place, the son indicates that the mother had reached the stage of Alzheimer's disease where she needed assistance with washing, dressing, toileting, and feeding. From a biomedical perspective, her ability to draw at this late stage of her illness would be accounted for, if at all, in terminology that would deny it agency. This incident, given the severity of his mother's cognitive impairment, leads the son to ponder a number of questions about the self and creativity: Did he witness in the nursing home day room an unleashing of a spontaneous and subconscious source of creative energy? Does art come from the intentional self or from the primal self?

Exercise 9.2: Selfhood and creativity

Willem de Kooning is regarded as one of the great painters of the twentieth century. His paintings from the 1980s represent a distinguishable period because he produced these paintings while living with Alzheimer's disease, and because this substantial body of work departed radically from anything he had done before. De Kooning's achievements, given what is known about the artist's mental decline during these years, have proved deeply troubling to art critics, as well as to experts of neuroscience.

- How can a man continue to make a significant artistic contribution without the powers of organization or judgement?
- Where does creativity reside?
- What is the relationship between memory and creativity?
- In what ways do you think that de Kooning's embodied selfhood served as a source of creativity that enabled de Kooning to continue to express himself through painting?

Immutable gentilities

In her book *Making an Exit* (2005), Elinor Fuchs, Professor at the Yale School of Drama, writes of her mother's experience with Alzheimer's disease. Not long after Fuchs moved her mother into a special care unit, she telephoned her mother, a conversation she recounts (2005: 179–80):

"How are you mother?" I begin.

"Oh, in a fast muff," she says briskly. "Getting out of the wet ditches."

"Wet ditches, well, that's interesting."

She's off and running. "Oh, I'm in a dedeford. There they're having a befurz. I mean, they're having a cressit. And would be considered hajardi. Would be picking dependent stuff." Her tone of authority is undiminished.

"Well," I ask, "are you recovered now from your fall where you had to have stitches in your forehead?" I always gave her the words she might need to flip back a response . . .

"We basent had any consedery other than a bull," she chats on, "which we're not getting. They've got the meat in the vettery, so they feel things aren't by any means all wet". . .

"Do you have some friends there?" I ask.

She is dismissive. "Oh, they have the thogs here with the wolfit beef. But they're still rather concerned about the westerd stuff being westered. They feel rather patz to that."

"Uh-huh. And how's the Professor, that nice man in the wheelchair?"

"Oh, the one in the fossilic? He's in habalik."

In this exchange, Fuchs allows us to witness the disease "performed", what is missing from most autobiographical and biographical accounts of living with dementia (Basting 2003). Most accounts "write *about*, and not *from within*, dementia", which is generally seen as the only way to address readers. This, in turn, results in descriptions of personhood, which are characterized by "normalcy" (Leibing 2006: 253). In contrast, Fuchs breaks from this tradition and permits meaning to emerge *from incoherence* evidenced by her observation that her mother's tone of authority is undiminished. There is also meaning in the notable exchange of speaking turns in that her mother does not interrupt Fuchs when they are speaking. In addition, the nature of the dialogue allows one to sense the intonation changes, the rise and fall of pitch level, and pauses, all of which are so full of life.

Even where speech is incoherent and completely void of linguistic meaning, there is still a smooth and appropriate alternating pattern of vocalizing back and forth as well as gesticulating back and forth (see Chapter 17). Take, for example, case example 9.1, drawn from an ethnographic study of an Alzheimer's support unit (Kontos 2004: 836; Kontos 2012: 337–8) – where only "Bah", "Shah", "BRRRRRR", and "Bupalupah" are uttered, Anna and Abe are able to communicate without any recourse to intellectual interpretation (Kontos 2012).

Case example 9.1: Abe

Abe sat down in the dining room and shouted "Bupalupah". Anna twisted around in her chair so that she could see Abe (his table was behind hers). Abe's face opened up. His eyes grew wider, his mouth eased into a broad smile, and he shouted "BRRRRRR!" with a rising and then falling pitch. Anna imitated him, shouting back "BRRRRRR!" following the same change in pitch. Abe then shouted "Bah" and paused while looking at Anna. Anna shouted "Shah" and then waited for Abe's response. Abe shouted "Bah!" and Anna "Shah", establishing a repetitious pattern of exchange.

Because of Abe's speech impairment and Anna mimicking him in jest, the force of their speech derived not from their semantic content but rather from the meanings that their bodies directly indexed.

These examples demonstrate how social history, acquired through the process of socialization, is expressed through the body. Practices of storytelling and conversation remain intact because dispositions and forms of know-how are internalized, function below the threshold of cognition, and are enacted as practical sense at a pre-reflective level.

The socio-cultural style or content of bodily movements and gestures is further evidenced by the regularity of social practices, such as adherence to proper etiquette. Observations on an Alzheimer support unit (Kontos 2012) illustrate that manners prescribed by social convention for interaction with others were, for the most part, observed by the residents. For example, when Florence compliments Edna on her pink beaded necklace and string of pearls, Edna replies "thank you". Bertha, with severe cognitive impairment, always says "thank you" when her private sitter wipes food from her mouth or chin. Dody routinely will say "good morning" when she sits down at the dining table for breakfast, to which Florence will in turn say "good morning", while Molly smiles and acknowledges Dody with a nod. "Bless you" can always be heard after a resident sneezes. When Molly uses a paper tissue, she softly wipes the tip of her nose. Covering one's mouth when yawning, coughing or belching is common. Frances always holds her napkin over her mouth while she attempts to remove a stubborn piece of food from her back dentures. Florence will never leave the dining table without first pushing in her chair.

Such adherence to politeness is similarly captured by Alan Bennett in *Untold Stories* (2005), an anthology of autobiographical sketches in which he writes of his mother, Mam, who has cognitive impairment and resides in a nursing home.

> 66 Words pour out of her as they always have and with the same vivacity and hunger for your attention. But to listen to they are utterly bewildering, following the sense like trying to track a particular ripple in a pelting torrent of talk. Still despite this formless spate of loquacity she remains recognizably herself, discernible in the flood those immutable gentilities and components of her talk which have always characterized her . . . So that now, with no story to tell (or half a dozen), she must needs still tell it as genteelly as she has ever done but at five times the speed, her old worn politeness detached from any narrative but still whole and hers, bobbing about in a ceaseless flood of unmeaning; demented, as she herself might have said, but very nicely spoken. 99

—Bennett (2005: 87)

Awareness of, and respect for, such conventions can also be inferred from the strong reaction of residents to those who lack manners. Case example 9.2 is noteworthy (Kontos 2004: 833; Kontos 2012: 336).

Case example 9.2: Molly

Molly took a bite of her buttered bread, and, as she chewed, she looked up at Dody, who sat directly across from her. Dody was using her napkin to clean her nostrils – twisting the corner of the napkin and inserting it into her nostril, turning it several times and then pulling it out. As Dody inspected the napkin after pulling it from her nose, Molly frowned and abruptly put her bread down on the table. She looked at the personal support worker with a scrunched up nose, the corners of her lips curved downwards, and furrowed brows. It was an expression of disgust.

Put simply, behaviour is negatively sanctioned when it offends the sensibility of one's selfhood.

Practice implications

Care practitioners need to develop ways of both interpreting and supporting embodied selfhood of persons with Alzheimer's. While there is some attention to body language in educational programmes for dementia care practitioners, non-verbal expression is most often understood either in terms of emotion (Magai *et al.* 2002; Ruckdeschel and Haitsma 2004) or physical discomfort and pain (Williams *et al.* 2005). However, as illustrated above, creativity, conversation, and social etiquette are also visibly manifest in how the body moves and behaves. Approaches to person-centred care that do not address the breadth of bodily movements and gestures for self-expression may contribute to the misreading of behaviour as symptomatic of dementia and the consequent introduction of medication to manage behaviour.

Exercise 9.3: Seeing "behaviour" through a different lens

A male resident in a long-term care facility who has lost the ability to speak seems to randomly strike others during meals. Upon closer observation you notice he removes his hat before entering the dining room and then strikes those at his table who are wearing a hat.

If the staff member assumes the resident's behaviour is symptomatic of dementia, she or he will likely choose a pharmacological intervention or some other form of restraint.

With the understanding that his "aggressive behaviour" is related to the etiquette of men removing hats before dining, how might the perception that the resident's behaviour is a meaningful expression inform an alternative intervention?

The notion of embodied selfhood has begun to make a significant contribution to the personhood movement (Twigg 2010; Hendriks 2012; Downs 2013) and has further influenced person-centred dementia care (Kontos 2005; Kontos and Naglie 2009; Kontos *et al.* 2010; Downs 2013). It has broadened interpretations of behaviour beyond a strictly psychosocial framework. Grounding selfhood in the body has significantly informed critiques of treatment and management approaches to "behavioural problems", which traditionally have been mandated by institutional policies of control and containment (i.e. combinations of environmental, mechanical, or pharmacological restraint). In contrast to pathologizing behaviour, understanding bodily movements and gestures as manifestations of embodied selfhood underscores their possible meaning in terms of skills, hobbies, and other important aspects of life histories, the immediate physical and social environment, organizational policies and health practitioner approaches to care practice, and social discourses. This is consistent with the call for a "responsive behavior discourse" (Dupuis *et al.* 2012) that moves away from viewing behaviour as a "problem" to be controlled towards understanding the breadth of meaning underpinning self-expression in dementia. Case example 9.3 exemplifies the positive practice outcomes that result from understanding embodied selfhood and using this understanding to tailor care.

Case example 9.3: A war veteran

A physical therapist recounts: "There are a lot of war veterans who live here and I'll never forget this one resident who I worked with. I had a hell of a time getting him to stand up from his wheelchair so we could work on his walking . . . He refused. One day I was thinking

(continued)

about who this man was, and what his life experiences were, and started singing the national anthem. Well you wouldn't believe it but he stood up from his wheelchair and saluted me! So from then on we began our physio sessions with the national anthem."

—Kontos and Naglie (2009: 697)

The introduction of an embodied selfhood approach to person-centred care has been shown to improve the quality of dementia care. An evaluation of a 12-week inter-professional arts-informed educational programme to improve person-centred dementia care premised on the importance of embodied selfhood (Kontos *et al.* 2010) demonstrated its effectiveness in teaching the embodied selfhood approach to care, and in facilitating the positive relational outcomes that resulted from its implementation. When embodied selfhood is a vital source of caring practice, significant outcomes result: health practitioners understand that behaviour may be indicative of meaningful self-expression; family is engaged to help decipher meaning and significance of behaviour that was previously unrecognized or deemed symptomatic of dementia; and health practitioners slow down during care activities, which reduces residents' agitation and resistance to care, and improves the time efficiency of practice in the absence of pharmacotherapies and other forms of restraint.

Recognizing the significant impact of dementia on families and communities, Alzheimer and other seniors' associations around the world have identified dementia as an international health and social priority, advocating for governments to take direct steps to begin planning how to better address the needs of persons with Alzheimer's and their families, and to ensure support staff working in dementia care have the knowledge and skills required to meet the complex needs of persons with dementia (World Health Organization 2012). Given the significance of bodily expressions of selfhood, particularly when cognitive faculties are impaired, their recognition and support should be part of the culture change initiatives that are emerging in response to these calls for action (Doty *et al.* 2008; Bowers *et al.* 2009). Not only is the support of bodily expressions of selfhood crucial to the achievement of person-centred care, but in the context of fiscal constraints and the restructuring of health care, it also has the potential to improve the quality of dementia care for patients and caregivers, and is thus worthy of further study and evaluation.

Debates and controversies

Embodied selfhood introduces an important challenge to the presumed loss of personhood in Alzheimer's, but it also challenges Western philosophy's tendency to split mind from body, and to position the former as superior to the latter. This tendency to assign the body the subordinate role is difficult to transcend. Some maintain that meaningful expressions – such as creativity – in the later stages of dementia are to be explained by the sparing of a crucial area of mental capacity. Because intention is presumed to be dependent solely upon cognition, this denies that the body itself could be a source of intention that persists despite cognitive impairment. Scholars and professionals of different disciplinary and clinical backgrounds thus still engage in debates around the issues of mind/body dualism and the nature of selfhood:

- Should cognition be granted such supreme value in conceptions of selfhood?
- Can we know whether an expression derives its meaning from cognitive knowing or embodied knowing?
- When cognition is intact, what is the relationship between reflective and pre-reflective intentionality?

Conclusion

While we eagerly await a "cure" for Alzheimer's disease, there is another approach besides scientifically informed paths to prevention we can use now to improve the lives of people with dementia. That is, we must take part in the creation of a new ethic of dementia care that respects individuals with Alzheimer's as embodied beings deserving of dignity and worth. This entails a shift in the current preoccupation with treating selfhood exclusively as a product of reflective thought, to treating the body as itself having creative and intentional capacity. It is a shift that not only broadens the discourse on selfhood in Alzheimer's disease, but also has enormous potential to foster humanistic and quality-enhancing dementia care practices.

Acknowledgements

I am presently supported by a New Investigator Award (MSH-87726, 2009–2014), Canadian Institutes of Health Research (CIHR), which facilitated the writing of this chapter. I also acknowledge the support of the Toronto Rehabilitation Institute-University Health Network, which receives funding under the Provincial Rehabilitation Research Program from the Ministry of Health and Long-Term Care in Ontario. The views expressed do not necessarily reflect those of CIHR or the Ministry.

Further information

The Registered Nurses' Association of Ontario [http://rnao.ca/] offers an e-learning course on client-centred care that includes dramatized vignettes as a novel pedagogical approach to facilitate understanding of embodied selfhood. This is a four-module e-learning course that is a complement to the Registered Nurses' Association of Ontario Nursing Best Practice Guideline for Client Centred Care. For additional information about the vignettes, see Kontos et al. (2010) and Kontos and Naglie (2007).

The Centre of Excellence in Movement, Dance and Dementia is a National Health Service (UK) based site offering important online resources and information for people living with dementia and their family care-partners. It also is an important resource for dancers, dance movement therapists, health professionals, and others working in dementia care who currently use, or are interested in developing the use of movement and dance in their practice [www.dancedementiahub.co.uk].

The Bitove Wellness Academy provides service to persons with dementia, their families and care-partners that is focused on relationships and human expression of self through movement and art [http://www.dotsabitove.com/].

References

Basting, A. (2003) Looking back from loss: views of the self in Alzheimer's disease, *Journal of Aging Studies*, 17: 87–99.
Behuniak, S.M. (2011) The living dead? The construction of people with Alzheimer's disease, *Ageing and Society*, 31(1): 70–92.

Bennett, A. (2005) *Untold Stories*. London: Faber & Faber.

Bourdieu, P. (1977) *Outline of a Theory of Practice*. Cambridge: Cambridge University Press.

Bourdieu, P. (1990) *The Logic of Practice*. Cambridge: Polity Press.

Bowers, B., Nolet, K., Roberts, T. and Esmond, S. (2009) *Implementing Change in Long-term Care: A Practical Guide to Transformation* [http://www.pioneernetwork.net/Data/Documents/Implementation_Manual_ChangeInLongTerm Care%5B1%5D.pdf, accessed 25 May 2014].

Cooney, E. (2003) *Death in Slow Motion: A Memoir of a Daughter, Her Mother, and the Beast Called Alzheimer's*. New York: HarperCollins.

Davis, D. (2004) Dementia: sociological and philosophical constructions, *Social Science and Medicine*, 58 (2): 369–78.

Doty, M.M., Koren, M.J. and Sturla, E.L. (2008) *Culture Change in Nursing Homes: How Far have We Come? Findings from the Commonwealth Fund 2007 National Survey of Nursing Homes* [http://www.commonwealthfund.org/Pub-lications/Fund-Reports/2008/May/Culture-Change-in-Nursing-Homes--How-Far-Have-We-Come--Findings-From-The-Commonwealth-Fund-2007-Nati.aspx, accessed 25 May 2014].

Downs, M. (2013) Embodiment: the implications for living well with dementia, *Dementia*, 12(3): 368–74.

Dupuis, S.L., Wiersma, E. and Loiselle, L. (2012) Pathologizing behavior: meanings of behaviors in dementia care, *Journal of Aging Studies*, 26: 162–73.

Fuchs, E. (2005) *Making an Exit*. New York: Metropolitan Books.

Hendriks, R. (2012) Tackling indifference – clowning, dementia, and the articulation of a sensitive body, *Medical Anthropology: Cross-Cultural Studies in Health and Illness*, 31(6): 459–76.

Hughes, J.C., Louw, S.J. and Sabat, S.R. (eds.) (2006) *Dementia: Mind, Meaning, and the Person*. New York: Oxford University Press.

Ignatieff, M. (1993) *Scar Tissue*. London: Penguin Books.

Kitwood, T. (1997) *Dementia Reconsidered: The Person Comes First*. Buckingham: Open University Press.

Kontos, P. (2004) Ethnographic reflections on selfhood, embodiment and Alzheimer's disease, *Ageing and Society*, 24: 829–49.

Kontos, P. (2005) Embodied selfhood in Alzheimer's disease: rethinking person-centred care, *Dementia*, 4(4): 553–70.

Kontos, P.C. (2012) Rethinking sociability in long-term care: an embodied dimension of selfhood, *Dementia*, 11(3): 329–46.

Kontos, P. and Naglie, G. (2006) 'Expressions of personhood in Alzheimer's': moving from ethnographic text to per-forming ethnography, *Qualitative Research*, 6(3): 301–17.

Kontos, P. and Naglie, G. (2007) 'Expressions of personhood in Alzheimer's disease': an evaluation of research-based theatre as a pedagogical tool, *Qualitative Health Research*, 17(6): 799–811.

Kontos, P. and Naglie, G. (2009) Tacit knowledge of caring and embodied selfhood, *Sociology of Health and Illness*, 31(5): 688–704.

Kontos, P., Mitchell, G.J., Mistry, B. and Ballon, B. (2010) Using drama to improve person-centred dementia care, *International Journal of Older People Nursing*, 5: 159–68.

Leibing, A. (2006) Divided gazes, in A. Leibing and L. Cohen (eds.) *Thinking about Dementia: Culture, Loss and the Anthropology of Senility*. New Brunswick, NJ: Rutgers University Press, pp. 240–68.

Magai, C., Cohen, C.I. and Gomberg, D. (2002) Impact of training dementia caregivers in sensitivity to nonverbal emotion signals, *International Psychogeriatrics*, 14(1): 25–38.

Merleau-Ponty, M. (1962) *Phenomenology of Perception*. London: Routledge & Kegan Paul.

Merleau-Ponty, M. (1964) An unpublished text by Maurice Merleau-Ponty: a prospectus of his work, in J. Edie (ed.) *The Primacy of Perception*. Evanston, IL: Northwestern University Press, pp. 3–11.

Ruckdeschel, K. and Haitsma, K.V. (2004) A workshop for nursing home staff: recognizing and responding to their own and residents' emotions, *Gerontology and Geriatrics Education*, 24(3): 39–51.

Taylor, R. (2007) *Alzheimer's from the Inside Oout*. Baltimore, MD: Health Professions Press.

Twigg, J. (2010) Clothing and dementia: a neglected dimension?, *Journal of Aging Studies*, 24(4): 223–30.

Williams, C.L., Hyer, K., Kelly, A., Leger-Krall, S. and Tappen, R.M. (2005) Development of nurse competencies to improve dementia care, *Geriatric Nursing*, 26(2): 98–105.

World Health Organization (WHO) (2012) *Dementia: A Public Health Priority* [http://www.alzheimer.ca/en/Get-involved/Raise-your-voice/~/media/Files/national/External/WHO_ADI_dementia_report_final.ashx, accessed 25 May 2014].

CHAPTER 10

The arts in dementia care

Anne Davis Basting

> ❝Mum also enjoyed watching the 7-year-old grand daughter of one of the other residents dancing – 'oh look she's dancing!'. It was lovely to see Mum taking an interest in something. She was so appreciative that the little girl would make a bee line for us to show off her latest dance.
>
> Mum has always been a radio listener, although mainly speech radio, so I made sure she had a radio with her and tuned to classic in the hope she would recognize and enjoy some of her favorite music. We took the radio and added a cd player when she moved to a new nursing home and here a cd of Viennese music became a favorite – she really responded to music. ❞
>
> —Anne Warburton Yorkshire, UK

Learning objectives

By the end of this chapter, you will be able to:

- Describe the key characteristics of the arts
- Describe the benefits of the arts for a range of stakeholders
- Describe the types of arts programs
- Describe the various locations where arts practices can take place
- Discuss who is best prepared to conduct which arts approaches

Introduction

The last decade has seen a significant expansion internationally of the use of the arts in dementia care. Since Kate Allan and John Killick addressed the arts in the last volume of this book, the field has seen a series of think tanks, conferences, organizations, publications, awards, and funding streams dedicated to it. Several studies have called for more research to assess the impact of the arts in dementia care, which remains largely experiential. Those who are practicing, engaging in, and/or witnessing creative interventions in dementia care can attest to their power. But thus far there are very few studies large enough to – or designed in ways that – convince the scientific community of the value of the arts for people with dementia.

This flowering of arts programs coincides with several other trends in the field of dementia care. While there is no cause/effect relationship, they complement each other. With the aging of global populations, arts and cultural institutions are realizing that as their membership ages, their members are also encountering dementia. To serve their constituents and to grow the number of people they serve, many are beginning to offer educational programs for families with dementia. The Museum of Modern Art in New York, the Louvre in Paris, the Ufizzi Gallery in Florence, and the Museum of Fine Arts in Murcia, Spain – to name just a few – all offer discussion and/or art-making programs for families with dementia.

Another shift in the field is toward person-centered and relationship-centered care and away from institutional models focused on the efficiency of the system over the care of the individual. This shift supports a growing focus on the arts as a way to engage with and draw out people who have difficulty with rational written or spoken language. In the USA, arts programming is often featured in promotional materials seeking to entice new residents/customers. The arts are seen as synonymous with attention to resident quality of life.

With the considerable growth of the field of arts in dementia care, this chapter seeks to provide an introduction to the value and role of the arts in dementia care by attention to the following aspects: (1) define what we mean by arts programs; (2) key continua in arts approaches; (3) potential benefits for the varied stakeholders; (4) where arts programs commonly take place; and (5) who provides them.

Thinking about what "art" means

The first step toward understanding the value and role of the arts in dementia care is to stretch our understanding of what "art" means. Most people have a different explanation of "art".

Exercise 10.1: How do you define art?

Ask the next three people you meet, "what is art?" You will likely hear words like painting, drawing, photography, dance, music, poetry. In fact, you might hear a different explanation of "art" from each person you ask.

- Consider what "art" means to you.
- Consider where your perception of what "art" means might come from.

I offer three brief stories here to identify some of the key characteristics of the arts and to broaden our understanding of traditional boundaries of art.

Case example 10.1: Expanding what we think of as art, Part I

In 2009, artist Steve Lambert worked with Andy Bichlbaum to write and print a completely fictitious issue of the *New York Times*. Lambert's NYT bore the headline "Iraq War Ends". The rest of the paper also featured fictitious ads and articles that inspired people to dream of a moment when their hopes became reported as reality. Lambert and Bichlbaum not only printed the paper, but also organized an extensive network of people to distribute and make it public – from handing it out on street corners in Los Angeles, to reading it on the subways in New York. This was Lambert's art.

Case example 10.2: Expanding what we think of as art, Part II

As part of an arts fellowship, Milwaukee artist Sara Luther created a rolling cart on which she put flowers and seeds. Over the course of several months, Luther rolled her cart to different neighborhoods and invited residents to plant seeds. Luther herself drew pictures of these neighborhoods and made postcards that she would also feature on her cart, showing one neighborhood to another as her visits progressed.

The examples above of Lambert and Bichlbaum and of Luther illustrate how art inspires people to imagine, grow, and see the world around them differently.

Case example 10.3: How art resonates in dementia care

Mamie came to a care center with a mixed diagnosis that included dementia. Mamie spent her life playing and teaching piano to children in a small town. Her confusion and depression kept her from playing the piano in her new home. Yet Mamie became very attached to the creative discussion groups that were part of The Penelope Project – a year-long effort to explore Homer's *Odyssey* from the perspective of the heroine who never left home. When her niece (who also worked at the care center) talked with her one day, Mamie was very confused – unsure of who or where she was. But when her niece asked about Penelope, Mamie became very clear. "Oh, let me tell you," she said, "what we're doing with Penelope is so important."

The above case example illustrates how art can provide meaning, purpose, and value to people with dementia.

As these illustrations show, I use a broad definition of "art" that draws on Langer's (1966) classic definition of the cultural arts as "the practice of creating perceptible forms expressive of human feeling" (p. 6). Langer distinguishes between "'perceptible' rather than 'sensuous' forms because some works of art are given to imagination rather than to the outward senses" (p. 6). Imagination is indeed a common element in the wide array of interventions that hold promise in dementia care, including music, poetry, storytelling, dance, and the visual arts.

Benefits of the arts for a range of stakeholders

The role of perspective

The potential and perceived benefits of the arts vary depending on the perspective from which they are viewed. For example, a doctor or a nurse will likely view an arts program for people with dementia differently than an artist, a teacher supervising a student volunteer, a family member, or a long-term care ombudsman/advocate.

Framework	Desired outcome
Medical	Improvements in physical and mental health conditions
Arts	Creation of a new, valued work of art
Educational	Growth of skills and knowledge
Social justice	Achievement of human rights
Community-building	Increased social capital of a given community
Spiritual	Healing families, individuals, and communities

Of course, in reality these perspectives may overlap. For example, a theatre improvisation group of older adults with symptoms of early memory loss may be seen from multiple perspectives. A physician might recommend the group to a "patient" because she sees it as a way to increase cognitive reserve. The participant may relish the improvisation sessions because he feels like he belongs to a group that understands and supports him. The theatre professional who facilitates the group may be primarily focused on building the skills of the participants and building a scene that can be used in a performance at a local theatre company.

Researching the benefits

Two recent reports demonstrate the increasing interest and urgency in understanding the impact of the arts on people with dementia. These reports address the arts across a spectrum of abilities and disabilities among older adults. *An Evidence Review of the Impact of Participatory Arts on Older People* (Mental Health Foundation 2011) focuses on the body of evidence for engaged arts practices with older adults. *The Arts and Aging: Building the Science* (National Endowment for the Arts 2013) is a summary of the National Academies Workshop, "Research Gaps and Opportunities for Exploring the Relationship of the Arts to Health and Well-Being in Older Adults".

Both reports suggest that there is significant potential for the arts to improve quality of life of older adults with dementia, but also point to similar challenges. There are very few studies of the impact of the arts in caring for people with dementia of the scale and design that satisfy researchers used to pharmaceutical research designs. Studies of arts interventions are commonly excluded from systematic reviews because of weaknesses in study design such as the small number of people studied, poor descriptions of the intervention used. Arts-based interventions commonly invite and are adjustable to individual participants' varying tastes and abilities. This is the very reason they are powerful tools for modeling person-centered dementia care. This is also the reason that it is difficult to conduct large-scale studies on their benefits.

It makes little sense to hold arts-based programs to the same randomized control trial (RCT) standards as pharmaceutical studies. As my colleague Katherine de Medeiros and I wrote recently, arts-based interventions, and some of the psychosocial interventions, tap into and develop individual potential and social meaning systems to achieve a transformative experience. Pharmacologic interventions do not (De Medeiros and Basting 2013).

Researchers are still trying to articulate the "mechanisms" behind the benefits of the arts for people with dementia. When arts programs work, what exactly is happening and how? Researchers are actively pursuing answers to these questions, and the answers will depend on the framework they choose to see the arts (medical, education, social justice, etc.). The following is a list of potential mechanisms that show promise. Some items here are followed by citations, while others show general promise for dementia care by studies done with healthy older adults or other populations.

Arts programming can:

- build a sense of self through creation, pride/value (social capital), facilitating growth, and reducing stigma (Cohen *et al.* 2006)
- build community (social networks) through collaboration and increased communication
- improve mood and affect, in turn reducing behaviors that care partners might consider to be disruptive (Phillips *et al.* 2010; van Dijk *et al.* 2012)
- improve attitudes of carers toward their care partners with dementia (Fritsch *et al.* 2009)
- build a sense of meaning and purpose by creating feelings of connection to the world beyond the self and the care setting (Boyle *et al.* 2010; Savundranayagam *et al.* 2011)
- build a rich, complex environment to improve quality of life (Rodriguez *et al.* 2011)
- build a sense of play/pleasure in an environment without much of it (Killick 2012)

In addition to benefits to the immediate care partners, the arts also offer potential positive outcomes for the general public and to our care systems.

Arts projects can be used to deepen public understanding of dementia by relaying the visual and narrative imagination of those with the condition. For students, arts projects provide a positive first engagement with people with dementia, and can both dissolve misconceptions and build the understanding that all behavior is a form of communication (George *et al.* 2012). For care systems, embedding the arts has the potential to help shift the organizational structure from one that is based on a rigid hierarchy to one that is more horizontal, team-based, and collaborative in nature (Mello 2012). There is enormous potential in the use of the arts as a tool in facilitating organizational change in long-term care by introducing collaborative, ensemble creation of arts programming.

Compared with pharmaceutical treatments for dementia, arts-based programs have several advantages. They are considerably less expensive and have few if any harmful side-effects. They also foster social connectedness, which can begin to alleviate many of the iatrogenic symptoms of dementia, or those symptoms that are caused by the way in which we treat or provide care (De Medeiros and Basting 2013).

New directions in practice and research in the arts in dementia care should embrace these strengths. Rather than isolate individual "modes" of arts ("Is music better than painting?", "Is storytelling better than dancing?"), artists and researchers can work together to identify the common elements that unite their approaches in order to better evaluate and bring the programming to more people.

Exercise 10.2: Using imaginative expression

Too often we imagine various kinds of artistic expressions as discrete types of activities when they share common roots.

- Think of a **movement** that symbolizes your personality.
- Think of a **sound** that symbolizes your personality.
- Ask a friend to do the same.
- **Teach** your sound and movement to your friend, and **learn** your friend's as well.
- Try some combinations of the sounds and movements together. If it feels silly – good!

This is an exercise that demonstrates the power of imagination to carers and that can also be facilitated with people with dementia.

Kinds of arts approaches

A rts approaches differ. They can be thought of as existing along a continuum at either end of which are extreme positions. These include: passive to participatory; offering limited or offering plentiful opportunities for individual expression; reminiscence or imagining; and from less to more meaningful for the person.

Passive to participatory

There are several categories of arts practice in dementia care. The clearest division is between those practices that involve people with dementia in the *creation* of the work, and those practices in which people with dementia are *passive recipients*. Passive arts practices might involve playing background music or having artwork or soothing colors on the walls. Passive arts more commonly are done *for* people with dementia, rather than *with* them. In passive activities, staff, facilitators, or visitors *entertain* rather than *engage*.

Passive	Active
do for	do with
entertain	engage

In collaborative, participatory arts programs, people with dementia are invited to participate as creators and exercise individual choice in shaping the outcomes of the various projects. Research suggests that background music, soothing colors, and murals can be effective in reducing anxiety that can emerge in certain living conditions for those experiencing dementia. While passive art is important, participatory expression through art-making has significant potential to improve the living conditions of families with dementia by benefiting care partners at all levels, people with dementia, family members, and extended community members.

Limited opportunities for individual expression to plentiful opportunities for individual expression

Within the category of participatory art-making, there are programs that offer limited opportunities for individual expression, and those that are guided almost completely by people with dementia themselves. As an example, consider the difference between "paint by numbers" or coloring book pages that have a clearly defined way to complete the project, and a blank piece of paper with collage materials set out on the table. The latter offers considerably more opportunities for personal choice and expression.

Reminiscence to imagination

The subject matter of participatory art-making also varies along a continuum. Some art-making activities focus primarily on retrieving stories or memories of one's past. These "reminiscence"-based arts projects commonly aim to unite care staff with people with dementia by sharing stories of their lives, or helping a person with dementia feel comforted by invigorating their memories. Some examples of these approaches are provided in Chapter 15.

Other art-making endeavors shift focus away from memory to inspiring the imagination of people with dementia and their care partners. Playing, imagining, and creating a new world together can bring people with dementia and their care partners together in a new relationship, one that operates in a new, shared language and moment, and one in which both are right. Working with imagination, there is no risk of stigmatizing people with dementia for not being able to access memories, and no hierarchy created between those with and those without access to chronological memory.

Less meaningful for an individual to more meaningful for an individual

Finally, some art-making programs enable people with dementia to create something that is personally *meaningful* to them. "Meaningfulness" can be defined in several ways. I prefer a combination of elements that include:

- connected to an individual's past and/or present
- pleasurable
- connected to the larger community or the future (a legacy)
- builds skill (learning)

Exercise 10.3: Purpose and art

"Art" can be made out of seemingly mundane activity by linking it to:

- purpose beyond yourself
- individual expression/choice
- skill-building
- fun

For example: looking at magazines can be a meaningless task to occupy time.
OR . . .
A group might tell stories about the advertisement in the magazines. They can make up stories, or tell stories from their own lives. They can write down the stories on separate pieces of paper – perhaps creating/decorating their own paper. The group can select a nearby shop and take a trip there. Together, they can find the product and tape the advertisement and the story to the product – and then quietly sneak away, leaving a gift for the next shopper.
Can you make a meaningful art activity out of

- matching socks?
- raking leaves?
- sorting silverware?

Exercise 10.4: An arts activity

The arts can invite us to create meaning through metaphor (equating one thing with another). This can often help us see each other differently. Here is an arts activity you can do either on your own or with a group.
Answer the following questions:

- What kind of animal are you? I am a . . .
- What kind of food? I am a . . .
- What kind of moving vehicle? I am a . . .

What have you learned about yourself from this exercise? What have you learned about your colleague/friend?

Location of arts programs

The location of arts programming for people with dementia also varies and includes: care settings, people's own homes, and cultural institutions.

Care settings

Arts programming is most often conducted in congregate care settings (day programs, nursing homes, or assisted living care homes) where staff can prepare the conditions for an arts activity, and where economies of scale enable the artists to be paid for training or conducting programming.

People's own homes

It has been more challenging to bring arts programming to people living in their own private homes with family or other supportive care. This is a crucial area of much needed development, as more and more older adults across the world will strive to stay in their own homes through their journey into dementia, and many will become isolated and without stimulation other than the television. Several training programs are being developed to train homecare workers and family members to use the arts as a way to engage with people with symptoms of dementia in one-on-one settings.

The National Center for Creative Aging in the USA is working to create a family caregiver arts toolkit. This kit will be advised by, and feature elements from, leading arts organizations in the USA, including the Alzheimer's Poetry Project, TimeSlips Creative Storytelling, Kairos Alive (dance and movement focused), and Songwriting Works.

The TimeSlips Creative Storytelling interactive web site (timeslips.org) and online training is also used by family caregivers to open pathways for positive emotional connection in what can be a challenging blur between love and stressful labor.

Cultural institutions and memory cafes

There has been tremendous growth in the field because cultural institutions have begun to recognize that their longstanding visitors now have cognitive disabilities and that they can and should continue to serve them. Families with dementia are also experiencing arts programming at cultural institutions and memory cafes.

In New York State, Lifetime Arts offers art-making programs for people with dementia at public libraries. The effort to bring art-making opportunities to families with dementia outside of the traditional "medical" framework can help normalize the experience of dementia as a disability to be managed, rather than a disease that demands a uniquely separate care system that can inadvertently sever ties to friendship networks.

In Wisconsin, ten cultural institutions (and growing) have formed the Spark Alliance, which brings cultural programming to families with memory loss. Members of the Alliance share training, logos, calendars, and promotion to reach families. While inspired by the Museum of Modern Art's Meet Me at MOMA program, Alliance members quickly realized that their much smaller institutions (often with an educational staff of one) would demand a new approach. Now the Racine Cultural Heritage

Museum and the Madison Children's Museum are among the valued support networks for families supporting their members with dementia.

In summary, while arts programming for people with dementia commonly takes place in congregate care settings, it is expanding to cultural (non-medical) settings and in-home use.

Who provides arts programs?

In some instances, the arts are used to achieve specific therapeutic and medical goals. In these cases, the arts "interventions" are commonly conducted or overseen by a therapist with special training in a given "modality", such as music, movement, visual art, poetry, or perhaps an "integrative creative arts" therapist. In other situations, professional artists are given basic training in dementia care and offer the programming themselves. There is also a third option – that artists provide training and model of arts programming to care staff who are able to continue the programming after the artists move on to another organization. This kind of approach, an "arts residency" of sorts, can ensure that we can fulfill what will be a tremendous need for such programming in dementia care as the number of people with dementia continues to grow.

Examples of arts programs

Over the last decade, there has been a proliferation of arts programming for people with dementia. I cannot provide an exhaustive list of those programs across the world, but rather share examples of this impressive breadth of programming. Here I address the most participatory models, which offer the greatest potential impact on well-being.

While these are discrete programs, they have the following qualities in common:

- They offer opportunities for improvisation and choice to people with dementia.
- They are beyond "right and wrong".
- They encourage play, exploration, and learning.
- They infuse value into the process and the products they produce.
- They view care partners and people with dementia as equal collaborators with expertise and as capable of learning and growth.

Clowning

The art of clowning is being taught to doctors and other clinical staff as a way to improve their relationships with patients. There are also professional groups of clowns that have residencies in care facilities to engage with residents and model/train care staff to embrace a sense of wonder and play. LaughterBosses and the "Elder Clown" program (humourfoundation.com.au/) in Australia, and the MiMakkus program in the Netherlands (mimakkus.nl) are just two of several examples.

Visual arts

Bringing the pleasure of creating visual art to people with dementia is to bring them choice (of materials), control (manipulating materials), and expression. Opening Minds Through Art at Miami University in Ohio (scrippsoma.org) is an excellent example of framing an arts program as an inter-generational learning opportunity. The I-Pad and other similar tablets are opening visual art-making to people with dementia who are living at home. Programs in New York (Self-Help, selfhelp.

net/virtual-senior-center) and the UK (Claire Ford, ipad-engage.blogspot.com/p/testimonials.html) enable people to "draw" and "paint" with the touch of a finger.

Film

Runaway Train, also based in Ohio, is an approach to writing and producing film scripts with people with dementia. Melissa Godoy, who made the documentary *Do Not Go Gently* on the power of the arts in aging, works with people with memory loss to create a screenplay and then to film the story itself.

Theater

Ladder to the Moon (laddertothemoon.co.uk/) uses culturally iconic stock characters to engage people with dementia in an immersive theater experience in which they can participate and shape. Theater Veder (theaterveder.nl) in the Netherlands uses a similar approach. The Penelope Project (thepenelopeproject.com) was a two-year collaboration with a professional theatre company (Sojourn Theatre) to explore Homer's *Odyssey* and devise and perform an original script for an outside, paying audience. To Whom I May Concern (towhomImayconcern.org) is an approach that invites people in early stages of memory loss to share their feelings through letters that are then performed for an audience.

Poetry and storytelling

TimeSlips (timeslips.org) is an improvisational form of storytelling that encourages people with dementia to exercise their imaginations. The Alzheimer's Poetry Project (alzheimerspoetry.com) draws on the familiar patterns of iconic poems and also invites people with dementia to create their own poetry.

Music

Songwriting Works (songwritingworks.org) invites people with dementia to write, perform, and record original music. The Unforgettables is a chorus of people with memory loss coordinated and evaluated by a team of researchers at New York University (aging.med.nyu.edu/research/chorus). In the UK, "Singing for the brain" has received considerable media attention (www.alzheimers.org. uk/singingforthebrain/).

Movement/dance

Mark Morris's Parkinson's (danceforparkinsons.org/) dance program has shown tremendous promise for helping people with Parkinson's limit their tremors. Kairos Alive! (MN) (kairosdance. org/) provides programming in storytelling and "chair" dancing, as well as training for staff to continue the programming. In the UK, there is a center of excellence in movement, dance, and dementia [http://www.creativedementia.org/project-centre/past-projects/example-project/88-centre-of-excellence-in-movement-dance-and-dementia].

Debates and controversies

Ethical imperative or empirical research evidence?

Anyone who has used creative engagement with people with memory loss can attest to its multi-fold powers. But to make the case for systemic adoption of arts-based methods requires that we have a significant body of data attesting to their effectiveness. This is particularly challenging because arts practices work on multiple levels (individuals, groups, care partners, systems) and are flexible to allow for individual preferences. As such, they are difficult to research in the traditional "gold standard" of randomized controlled trials (RCTs) where interventions need to be standardized and implemented in a uniform way for the whole group. Yet evidence-based policy initiatives tend to require RCT rather than accept single subject or other individualized research designs. Nor do the latter receive the same level of funding as RCT studies. Another challenge for arts programming is the duration of its impact. Dementia is a chronic condition that worsens over time. If an arts program yields a momentary improvement in quality of life, is that enough? Advocating for arts programming may be more a matter of ethics (in the frame of human rights and social justice) than an empirical research evidence-based prescription.

Sustainability of arts approaches

Even among the best arts programs for people with dementia, it is common to offer them as "one-offs", or as a drop-in program rather than one that builds skill and knowledge over time. While these "one-off" programs can indeed raise quality of life momentarily, these models miss an opportunity to build community, skill, and change on a deeper level. In my own experience, I found that staff members are reluctant to frame an arts program over a longer period of time as they might an arts program for children or young adults because they worry that the participants might pass away. With the Penelope Project, which took place over two years, we found that the duration of the project increased its meaning for participants and that the memory and contributions of those who passed away during it were woven into the community fabric and enabled people to grieve in a way they had previously been denied.

Lack of funding

Arts programming for people with dementia hovers between funding fields. Foundations that support health may decide that an arts program should be funded by an arts foundation, and the arts foundation might reject the proposal because they consider this applied use to be "less art and more medicine". Even artists battle the stereotype that non-artists cannot create "real art". We have a long way to go to taking art created by people with dementia seriously – as reflected in critical reviews and funding.

Conclusion

Arts have a unique role to play in excellence in dementia care. To have the most impact, they need to allow for individual choice and expression and to foster celebratory person-centered and relational care. They offer care practitioners and family members alternative routes to communication and celebration of life with people with dementia. In this way, people with dementia can feel connected and valued.

Further information

- National Center for Creative Aging: http://www.creativeaging.org
- The Society for the Arts in Dementia Care: http://www.cecd-society.org
- The Arts and Dementia Network: http://www.equalarts.org.uk

- Arts for Health: http://www.artsforhealth.org
- The Global Alliance for Arts & Health: http://www.thesah.org
- Arts and Health Australia: http://www.artsandhealth.org/
- The Creative Dementia Arts Network: http://www.creativedementia.org/

References

Boyle, P.A., Buchman, A.S., Barnes, L.L. and Bennett, D.A. (2010) Effect of a purpose in life on risk of incident Alzheimer disease and mild cognitive impairment in community-dwelling older persons, *Archives of General Psychiatry*, 67(3): 304–10.

Cohen, G., Perlstein, S., Chapline, J., Kelly, J., Firth, K. *et al.* (2006) The impact of professionally conducted cultural programs on the physical health, mental health, and social functioning of older adults, *The Gerontologist*, 46(6): 726–34.

De Medeiros, K. and Basting, A. (2013) 'Shall I compare thee to a dose of donepezil?': cultural arts interventions in dementia care research, *The Gerontologist* [DOI: 10.1093/geront/gnt055].

Fritsch, T., Kwak, J., Grant, S., Lang, J., Montgomery, R.R. *et al.* (2009) Impact of TimeSlips, a creative expression intervention program, on nursing home residents with dementia and their caregivers, *The Gerontologist*, 49(1): 117–27.

George, D.R., Yang, C., Stuckey, H.L. and Whitehead, M.M. (2012) Evaluating an arts-based intervention to improve medical student attitudes toward persons with dementia using the Dementia Attitudes Scale, *Journal of the American Geriatrics Society*, 60(8): 1583–5.

Killick, J. (2012) *Playfulness and Dementia: A Practice Guide.* London: Jessica Kingsley.

Langer, S.K. (1966) The cultural importance of the arts, *Journal of Aesthetic Education*, 1: 5–12.

Mello, R. (2012) *The Penelope Project, a Program Evaluation* [www.thepenelopeproject.com, accessed 28 May 2013].

Mental Health Foundation (2011) An Evidence Review of the Impact of Participatory Arts on Older People. 2011. London: Mental Health Foundation [http://www.baringfoundation.org.uk/EvidenceReview.pdf, accessed 28 May 2013].

National Endowment for the Arts (2013) *The Arts and Aging: Building the Science.* Washington, DC: National Endowment for the Arts [http://www.giarts.org/sites/default/files/Arts-and-Aging-Building-the-Science.pdf, accessed 28 May 2013].

Phillips, L.J., Reid-Arndt, S.A. and Pak, Y. (2010) Effects of a creative expression intervention on emotions, communication, and quality of life in persons with dementia, *Nursing Research*, 59(6): 417–25.

Rodriguez, J.J., Noristani, H.N., Olabarria, M., Fletcher, J., Somerville, T.D. *et al.* (2011) Voluntary running and environmental enrichment restores impaired hippocampal neurogenesis in a triple transgenic mouse model of Alzheimer's disease, *Current Alzheimer Research*, 8(7): 707–17.

Savundranayagam, M.Y., Dilley, L.J. and Basting, A. (2011) StoryCorps' memory loss initiative: enhancing personhood for storytellers with memory loss, *Dementia*, 10(3): 415–33.

van Dijk, A., van Weert, J.M. and Dröes, R. (2012) Does theatre improve the quality of life of people with dementia?, *International Psychogeriatrics*, 24(3): 367–81.

CHAPTER 11

Design matters in dementia care: the role of the physical environment in dementia care settings

Habib Chaudhury and Heather Cooke

66 It's how you use the space. They're very clever. You see, they tell people 'We're all going to the movies today!' then put chairs in rows, like the movies, and give them treats, then turn on the movie". It's really nice to get outside, to be able to access secure outside areas is great. It means people can experience something different, a different temperature, different things to look at, just different, not sitting inside the same building all the time. They can look at the garden. It's a nice garden. 99

—Carolyn Worth Melbourne, Australia

66 The nursing home is purpose built. It has wide corridors. It is light and airy. Well decorated. Well lit . . . On the EMI unit which is on the ground floor there is a doorway via a smaller sitting room into a secure garden. In the summer the residents often go in the garden by themselves. It's also used by the activities person sometimes for gardening activities. I thought this garden was an absolute boon. Residents in an EMI unit are usually quite physically fit and like to walk up and down. Therefore wide corridors and easy access to a garden is excellent. 99

—Brenda Smith Yorkshire, UK

Learning objectives

By the end of this chapter, you will:

- Understand the importance of the physical environment in enhancing quality of life for people with dementia
- Know about the conceptual issues and therapeutic goals that should inform the design of a dementia care environment
- Appreciate key findings of empirical studies on the effect of environmental design on behaviour and affect in people with dementia
- Be aware of how the physical environment can be modified to affect behavioural and emotional outcomes for people with dementia

Introduction

The physical environment is a critical component of a therapeutic setting for people with dementia. Over the last three decades, there has been a growing body of literature that has recognized and provided evidence on the effect of unsupportive physical environments that contribute to common challenging behaviours in people with dementia, such as spatial disorientation, anxiety, agitation, and social withdrawal. In contrast, a well-designed supportive physical environment has been shown to foster positive behaviours, such as reduced agitation, increased social contact, and less dependence in conducting activities of daily living. There is a fairly extensive body of research literature in the area of responsive physical environments for people with dementia that has arisen since the late 1980s (e.g. Calkins 1988; Cohen and Weisman 1991; Day *et al.* 2000; Brawley 2006). In the recent past, there has been a much needed increase in both fine-tuned design guidelines for design professionals and caregivers, and empirical studies examining the effectiveness of therapeutic physical environmental features supporting the quality of life for people with dementia in long-term care facilities (e.g. Zeisel *et al.* 2003; Brawley 2006; Calkins and Brush 2009; Fleming and Purandare 2010; van Hoof *et al.* 2010; Verbeek *et al.* 2010).

The purpose of this chapter is to review and synthesize the existing literature on the role of physical environment on the quality of life for people with dementia in long-term care settings. We begin with an overview of the theoretical issues that assist us in understanding the role of the physical environmental features in affecting, either positively or negatively, the behaviours, functioning, and affective responses of persons with dementia. An overview of the therapeutic goals of the physical environment in achieving behavioural outcomes will be presented. We then review the key environmental design features of the primary spaces of the long-term care facility, as evidenced in the extant empirical literature. Finally, we briefly highlight selected controversial issues and future research directions in this area. It is worth noting that although this chapter's focus is on the physical environment of long-term care facilities, a few of the discussed challenges and potential solutions are also relevant in home settings.

Key theories in design for dementia care

Three major theories in gerontology are briefly reviewed here along with a discussion of their relevance and implications for understanding the relationship between physical environment and psychosocial/behavioural outcomes for people with dementia. These theories are:

- individual competence and environmental press model (Lawton and Nahemow 1973)
- model of place (Weisman 1997; Calkins and Weisman 1999; Weisman *et al.* 2000)
- progressively lowered threshold model (Hall and Buckwalter 1987)

Individual competence and environmental press

Lawton and Nahemow's (1973) conceptualization of the interrelationship between individual competence and environmental demand is widely viewed as a landmark in advancing our understanding of person–environment interaction. Individual competence is defined as "a diverse collection of abilities residing within the individual, which differ among themselves and vary over time between minimum and maximum limits that are specific to the individual" (Lawton and Nahemow 1973: 659). Lawton (1982) expands on this concept by discussing five classes of competence:

- biological health
- sensory-perceptual capacity
- motor skills
- cognitive capacity
- ego strength

"Environmental press" is defined as "forces in the environment that together with an individual need evoke a response". These can be physical, social or interpersonal. In this model, individuals with lower competence are more vulnerable to environmental press, and are thus more likely to have maladaptive behaviour and affect. Similarly, individuals with higher competency have greater capacity and resilience to negotiate high environmental press. The key lessons from this model are as follows:

■ Behaviour and affect are natural outcomes of interactions between individual competencies and environmental factors.
■ Lowered physical and/or cognitive competence makes the individual more sensitive and susceptible to environmental features compared with those with higher competence.
■ The physical environment can be modified to compensate for the lowered individual competence to reach the desired behavioural and affective adaptation level.

This conceptual model is instrumental in our understanding of the behaviours and affective responses among people with dementia in long-term care facilities. Individual competence would vary for people with dementia, based on multiple factors including cognitive status, type of diagnosis, functioning abilities and challenges, personal preferences, and life history. Notable physical environmental press in a typical institutional long-term care facility would relate to multiple environmental features, such as long hallways with resident rooms along both sides, double occupancy resident rooms, large social spaces (e.g. dining area or lounge), prominent nursing station, consistent background noise, and lack of outdoor space. The social environmental press would likely be associated with large group size in dining and activities, unfamiliar people and activities, and communication challenges. Conceptually, the common behavioural and affective symptoms or expressions in persons with dementia, such as pacing, repetitive behaviours, inability to recognize once-familiar objects, anxiety, agitation, aggression, social withdrawal, and random vocalizing may be linked with the demands or stressors that originate from the combined social and physical environmental press.

From an intervention perspective, the negative environmental press resulting from a long hallway can be eliminated or greatly reduced by allowing direct visual access and close physical proximity between the resident's bedroom and the social spaces. In such an environment, the level of physical environmental press is lowered to compensate for the reduced spatial cognitive ability of the individual with dementia, which would increase the likelihood of a person finding their way.

Case example 11.1: Finding my way

Martha walks out of her bedroom, pausing for a moment at the door. She looks to the left and then to the right. She sees a long hallway with no immediate end in sight. The doors lining the hallway, which are painted the same colour as the walls, all look the same. "Where is everyone? ", she wonders. She feels thirsty and would love to have a cup of tea and a chat; however, there is no cue indicating which way she should go to get to the lounge or dining room. She sighs, frustrated – if only she could figure this place out. She turns around and walks back into her room.

The model of place

This model consists of four interacting subsystems and an emergent fifth element. The four subsystems are: people with dementia, social context, organizational context, and physical setting

(Weisman 1997; Weisman *et al.* 2000). The fifth element in this model is described as "therapeutic dimensions of the environment as experienced" (Weisman 1997: 326), which emerges out of the interactions among the four subsystems indicated earlier. The inclusion of social and organizational contexts is an important advance in understanding the complexity of multiple factors and their influencing role on the lived experience of persons with dementia. There are several organizational policy and practice factors that shape the organization's care philosophy, staff care practice, social interaction, and programmed activities. These in turn shape the quality of life for the persons with dementia living in the care home. The organizational and social factors include:

- organizational structure and hierarchy
- quality and commitment from leadership
- care vision
- funding level
- staff communication methods
- staff culture
- staff training on various aspects of dementia care (e.g. communication, interaction, "management" of challenging behaviours)
- everyday care practices

These factors interact with each other and with people with dementia and the physical setting to create and shape the therapeutic dimensions of the environment as experienced by people with dementia. This latter element is phenomenological in its orientation to the experiential quality of life for people with dementia. The therapeutic dimensions are based on therapeutic goals articulated by several researchers (e.g. Calkins 1988; Cohen and Weisman 1991; Moos and Lemke 1994). Arguably, this model comes closest in articulating the position of person-centred dementia care approaches (e.g. Kitwood 1997; Brooker 2007).

Progressively lowered threshold model

This model's premise is that each person has a stress threshold and this is lowered for persons with dementia (Hall and Buckwalter 1987; Smith *et al.* 2004), such that people with dementia have challenges in processing and making sense of the stressors. This in turn contributes to anxious and dysfunctional behaviours. This model also suggests that stressors come in various forms, including changes in routine, caregiver or environment. This model has a distinct applied orientation by recommending strategies for the caregivers to identify the triggers that produce stress responses with a view to modifying them to reduce or prevent the behaviours. For example, this model recommends reducing environmental stimuli to make them more easily processed by persons with dementia. These stimuli might include the television being continuously on, unending long spaces, and unnecessary noise. This model provides an important perspective on the processes by which environment influences behaviour.

One cautionary note is the potential to reduce environmental stimuli to the extent that it leads to sensory deprivation or an austere and clinical environment. This concern can be addressed by introducing positive stimulation appropriate for persons with dementia (e.g. smell of baked goods or foods that provide familiar memory cues).

These three theoretical models are helpful in understanding the key concepts in person–environment interaction in general and the particular challenges that people with dementia have in interacting with and navigating in the physical context of a care facility. The following section presents a synthesis of substantive physical environmental features and their effect on the functioning of people with dementia. Before getting into the literature synthesis, we recommend that you try the following exercise.

Exercise 11.1: Thinking about your physical environment in your everyday life

Create a three-column table.
In the left column, create a list of *your typical activities* on any given day, i.e. dressing, eating, and using the bathroom.

In the second column, record the *physical environmental features* with which you interact to accomplish this, e.g. wardrobe, kitchen cupboard, toilet.

In the last column, write down the *cognitive decisions* you consciously and sub-consciously make to do the activities.

This exercise will make you recognize the innumerable decisions we make in our everyday functioning in an autonomous manner. This will help you to understand how difficult and frustrating it might be for someone with impaired cognitive abilities. These make it difficult for them to make decisions to successfully interact with the environment, such as difficulty in choosing clothing to wear from the wardrobe, and forgetting where various cooking ingredients are kept in the kitchen cupboards. A mismatch between cognitive abilities and environmental features (i.e. resulting environmental press) would likely affect behaviour and performance.

Evidence-based design features for dementia care

This section provides an overview of the empirical research examining the therapeutic impact of key environmental design features, including unit size, residential design, sensory stimulation, and spaces (i.e. dining areas, resident rooms, outdoor areas, toilets and bathing areas), on individuals with dementia in long-term care settings.

Unit size

There is increasing recognition that large nursing home units (e.g. 30+ residents) do not meet the needs of residents with dementia. Larger unit sizes are associated with increased agitation and aggression, greater intellectual deterioration and emotional disturbance, and more frequent territorial conflicts and invasions of space (Annerstedt 1994; Morgan and Stewart 1998; Sloane et al. 1998). Reimer and colleagues (2004) followed 185 residents with dementia over a one-year period and found that those living in small, 10-bed bungalows exhibited less decline in activities of daily living, less negative affect, and more sustained interest in their environment than those in traditional, larger facilities. Similarly, in a two-year study by Kane et al. (2007), residents with and without dementia living in small-scale homes of 10 people (i.e. Green Houses™) experienced higher scores on a number of quality of life domains (privacy, dignity, autonomy, food enjoyment, meaningful activity, relationship, individuality), compared with residents of two traditional (i.e. 50- and 80-bed) nursing homes. Green House™ residents also reported significantly higher satisfaction and better emotional well-being.

Mixed results have been observed among residents of Dutch group-living units (i.e. small-scale homes of six to eight residents). While their overall quality of life, agitation levels, and behavioural problems do not differ from residents of larger, more traditional units (i.e. more than 20 beds), group-living residents have better social relationships, greater positive affect, feel more at home, and have higher quality of life scores for "having something to do" (te Boekhorst *et al.* 2009; Verbeek *et al.* 2010; de Rooij *et al.* 2012).

Relocation studies in Japan, Australia, and the USA reveal similar findings. Upon relocation to smaller units (i.e. 9- to 15-bed households or cottages), residents maintained their cognitive, intellectual, and motor functioning, and exhibited less behavioural impairment, increased engagement in activity, and an increase in non-verbal social behaviours (Suzuki *et al.* 2008; McFadden and Lunsman 2010; Smith *et al.* 2010).

Residential (homelike) character

Residential or homelike characteristics include furnishings (e.g. upholstered armchairs and sofas with different patterns and textures, coffee tables, bookcases), décor (e.g. wall coverings, pictures, paintings), and smaller-scale common areas (Cohen and Weisman 1991; Brawley 2006). The challenge with assessing the effect of residential character is that it is frequently accompanied by other physical and organizational features (e.g. smaller unit size, care philosophy, staffing patterns, management practices), which make it it difficult to determine the relative contribution of each. For example, the smaller-sized Dutch group-living units are noted for their resemblance to an archetypal home, featuring small-scale common areas, an open kitchen connected to the living room, and spaces decorated to specifically create a homelike feeling (Verbeek *et al.* 2010; de Rooij *et al.* 2012).

More homelike or enhanced residential environments (e.g. large windows, increased space for personal memorabilia and furniture in residents' rooms, open-plan lounge and dining areas, and paintings in the common areas/corridors) are associated with improved emotional and intellectual functioning, increased social interaction, autonomy, and community participation, less exit-seeking and lower levels of overall and verbal aggression and agitation (Annerstedt 1994; McAllister and Silverman 1999; Zeisel *et al.* 2003; Wilkes *et al.* 2005). An enhanced environmental ambience (e.g. one that is warm, embellished, welcoming, colourful, and novel) has also been shown to be associated with fewer pacing episodes, shorter pacing duration, and longer sitting duration (Yao and Algase 2006).

Residents of Dutch facilities with more group-living characteristics tend to be involved in significantly more overall and preferred activities, as well as more task-related and leisure activities and social interaction, than those in facilities with fewer group-living characteristics. Homelike environments not only offer more opportunities and an enhanced ambiance for residents to participate in everyday activities, but may also make it easier for staff to engage residents in such activities (Smit *et al.* 2012). This highlights an important point with regards to residential character – homelike design requires supportive caregiving practices to be effective (Day *et al.* 2000). Institutional or restrictive caregiving practices may undermine the therapeutic aspects of homelike features (e.g. locked doors to outdoor areas, restricted access to kitchenette unless accompanied by a staff member).

The variability of common spaces has also been observed to influence resident outcomes. Barnes (2002) found that residents in homes with a higher gradation of space (i.e. a range of private, semi-private, and public spaces) displayed higher levels of active behaviour and well-being than those in homes with a low gradation of space. Similarly, Zeisel and colleagues (2003) found that as the variability of common spaces increased (i.e. the extent to which interior décor, furniture, and natural light contributed to the uniqueness and mood of the spaces), social withdrawal decreased. In other words, greater socialization occurred in facilities with more diverse common spaces.

Sensory stimulation

For individuals with dementia, sensitivity to lighting and noise levels may be exacerbated by the hearing and visual deficits associated with ageing, thereby making it difficult for them to understand their surrounding environment (Day *et al.* 2000). Nursing home residents with dementia are typically exposed to considerably lower than recommended (i.e. <2000 lux) lighting levels as they spend most of their days in dim room light (Shochat *et al.* 2000; De Lepeleire *et al.* 2007). Recent research indicates that exposure to higher lighting levels has beneficial effects on sleep and behaviour. Exposure to morning bright light, via the use of a bright light box (ranging from 2500 to 10,000 lux), is associated with increased night-time sleep, improved circadian rhythm quality, increased daytime wakefulness, and decreased agitation and disruptive behaviour (Thorpe *et al.* 2000; Ancoli-Israel *et al.* 2003; Fetveit and Bjorvatn 2005). Similarly, residents exposed to all-day bright light have been found to experience significantly increased total sleep duration, as well as modest benefits in mood, cognition, and functional decline (Sloane *et al.* 2007; Riemersma-van der Lek *et al.* 2008). While the clinical significance of increased sleep duration is unclear, Sloane and colleagues (2007) point out that the sleep gains observed exceed those achieved by hypnotic drug use. Such findings have led researchers to suggest increasing ambient lighting levels in common areas where residents spend the majority of their days.

Although no sound level standards exist for nursing homes, recommended levels for hospital ward rooms range from 30 to 40 dB (i.e. level of a whisper and a quiet room), and for residential dwellings from 35 to 45 dB (i.e. level of a quiet room to a moderate rainfall) (World Health Organization 1999). However, several recent studies have found noise levels within nursing homes to exceed such recommendations; mean noise levels ranged from 52 to 57 dB in residents' rooms and from 59 to 60 dB in common areas (Bharathan *et al.* 2007; Joosse 2011). Peak noise levels have been found to range from 69 dB (i.e. level of busy traffic) to as high as 105–109 dB (i.e. level of a gas lawn mower, snow blower or chainsaw) (Joosse 2011; Garre-Olmo *et al.* 2012). Common sound sources included human background noise (e.g. staff conversations not involving residents), alarms, intercoms, ringing phones, loud televisions, and other equipment noise (e.g. ice/juice makers in adjacent kitchens). Such noise levels are associated with reduced social interaction, and increased agitation and wandering (Garre-Olmo *et al.* 2012; Joosse 2012).

Case example 11.2: Sensory overload

Anita sits at her table in a corner of the dining room with three other residents. Their table is close to the door to the kitchen, which opens and shuts with a bang each time a staff member enters or leaves the dining room. Two carers approach their table with the meal cart, talking to each other as they go. They pause briefly to dish out the food for Anita and her tablemates, continuing their conversation about their upcoming holidays as they do so. Anita studies the food in front of her but the lighting in the corner is so dim she finds it hard to recognize what is on her plate. A resident calls out from across the dining room. One of Anna's tablemates yells back, telling the resident to "shut up". Feeling increasingly anxious, Anna pushes her chair backwards, stands up, and looks around for the exit.

Dining spaces

Design guidelines emphasize the importance of creating small dining areas that evoke associations of home and regulate sensory stimulation to encourage eating (Cohen and Weisman 1991;

Brawley 2006). Interestingly, Swedish nursing homes base their unit or cluster size around the number of residents who can fit comfortably around a large dining room table (Regnier and Scott 2001). Smaller-sized, less institutional dining rooms have been found to result in fewer incidents of disruptive and agitated behaviours, more sustained conversations between residents and staff, and increased food and fluid intake (Schwarz et al. 2004; Reed et al. 2005; Desai et al. 2007) In a recent study, the introduction of three smaller dining rooms, each of which accommodated 25–30 residents and featured a variety of homelike features, including a fireplace, sideboard, bookshelves, plants, objects d'art, tablecloths, table centrepieces, and aromas of freshly baked bread and brewed coffee, significantly increased residents' caloric intake, which increased again (although not significantly) when combined with additional staff training (Perivolaris et al. 2006). Several studies have demonstrated that by enhancing lighting and maximizing the visual (i.e. colour) contrast between plates and table settings during meal times, residents with dementia eat more, display less agitation, and exhibit improved functional independence (Koss and Gilmore 1998; Brush et al. 2002). Focusing explicitly on the provision of high-contrast tableware, Dunne and colleagues (2004) substituted red plates, red cups, and red cutlery for white plates, white cups, and stainless steel cutlery, and observed a 25% increase in food intake and an 84% increase in fluid intake among individuals with severe dementia. High-contrast blue tableware was also effective, while low-contrast tableware (i.e. pastel red and blue) was not.

Exercise 11.2: Visit a long-term care facility to observe the physical environment

Locate a care home that has a specialist dementia care unit. Contact the manager to request a tour of the care unit. While you tour the facility, pay attention to and take notes on the following:

- How many residents live there?
- In what ways is there a homelike environment? Could it be made to be more homelike?
- What is the unit configuration or overall spatial layout of the unit like? How supportive is the layout for residents' mobility and comprehension of the environment?
- What is your impression of the level of sensory stimulation in the social spaces, i.e. dining and activity areas? Do you think the amount and quality of the stimulation is appropriate for persons with dementia?
- Did you observe any residents in the social spaces? What were they doing? Do you think the environment could be different to enhance the residents' experience?

Resident rooms

Personalized and private resident rooms are frequently advocated as key features of a dementia-friendly environment; however, research in this area is limited, and potentially confounded, by the fact that facilities with private bedrooms typically feature additional architectural and/or programmatic differences (e.g. Wilkes et al. 2005; Kane et al. 2007). Morgan and Stewart (1998) documented a number of positive effects of private rooms on resident behaviour following relocation to a new, lower-density special care unit. Residents experienced more privacy, improved night-time sleep, decreased agitation, reduced use of sedating medications, and reduced conflict with other residents. The latter finding is highlighted in focus group research, in which staff indicated spending anywhere from two to 25 hours per week managing roommate conflict (Calkins and Cassella 2007). Residents with dementia emphasize the importance of being able to create their own private area and personalize it with familiar and treasured items (Innes *et al.* 2011). Residents in facilities with more privacy have been found to show less anxiety and aggression, and have fewer psychotic problems (Zeisel *et al.* 2003).

Bathing and toilet rooms

In many care facilities, the design and layout of the bathing area is dictated by efficiency and utility, and sometimes this compromises resident comfort, dignity, and autonomy. Recommendations for improving the bathing environment typically focus on the provision of privacy, appropriate temperature control, lighting and noise levels, and a more homelike décor (Sloane *et al.* 1995; Brawley 2006).

Mechanical lifts (used to elevate and then lower residents into a water-filled tub), privacy intrusions (by care aides accessing supply carts stored in the bathing room), inappropriate water and air temperature (too hot and too cold), running water, loud noises, and mechanical bathtub devices have all been observed to be associated with resident confusion and agitation (Kovach and Meyer-Arnold 1996; Namazi and Johnson 1996). A recent study exploring the immediate antecedents of assaultive behaviour against care aides during bathing found such behaviour stemmed primarily from caregiver behaviour, although assaults were more likely when residents exhibited signs of temperature discomfort and multiple care aides were present (Somboontanont *et al.* 2004).

In terms of toilet rooms, design guidelines highlight the importance of making toilets readily accessible and identifiable so as to assist in maintaining independence in toileting (Day *et al.* 2000). Empirical evidence in this area is extremely limited – to date, only two studies (Namazi and Johnson 1991a, 1991b) have examined the impact of design interventions on toileting behaviour. The first quasi-experimental study compared the effectiveness of several types of signage – wall signs with the word "restroom", the word "toilet", the image of a toilet, or a combination of navigational arrows and the word "toilet" affixed to the floor (Namazi and Johnson 1991a). Of all the wall signs, the word "toilet" appeared the most meaningful; however, residents located and utilized the public toilets most frequently when the navigational arrows and word "toilet" were placed on the floor, due likely to the tendency of cognitively impaired individuals to walk with their heads down. In the second study, 14 residents were randomly assigned to one of two conditions to determine whether the visibility of ensuite toilets influenced toilet use. In the control condition, privacy curtains were secured to conceal, but not prohibit, access to the toilet, while in the intervention condition, the curtains remained open such that the toilet was highly visible from within the room. Frequency of toilet use increased dramatically in the open-curtain condition (Namazi and Johnson 1991b).

Case example 11.3: Bath time

Gladys is resting on her bed when there is a knock at her door. A carer walks into the room and announces that it's time for her bath. Gladys really doesn't feel like getting up, but the carer insists and so Gladys grudgingly gets out of bed. The carer leads her down the hallway and opens the door to a large tiled room. Gladys scans the room trying to figure out why the carer has brought her here. There is a large machine in the middle of the room, with a seat beside it. The yellow-tiled

(continued)

walls are bare. The carer goes over to the machine and turns a knob. The sound of rushing water fills the room. The carer seats Gladys next to the machine and begins to take off her clothes. Gladys tries to stop her – it's so cold in this room. All of a sudden the chair begins to rise, Gladys starts to panic – she looks around frantically but sees no escape. The chair swings to the left – Gladys looks down and sees water below her. The chair starts to descend and water slowly rises over her. Still panicked, she strikes out with her arm. The carer ignores her and starts to wash her. As the bath draws to an end, Gladys starts to shiver. The water has begun to drain around her and the small, scratchy towel the carer has draped around her shoulders isn't doing much to keep her warm. The chair begins to rise again. Gladys has had enough – "get me out of here", she thinks, as she lashes out at her carer in frustration.

Outdoor areas

Outdoor areas are increasingly recognized as a key design feature in residential care settings given the opportunities they provide for visual, olfactory, auditory, and tactile stimulation, exposure to sunlight, and normalized, meaningful activity and socialization (Cohen and Weisman 1991; Brawley 2006). To date, however, much of the literature on outdoor space is descriptive or preference-based.

Initial longitudinal research found that residents in facilities with garden areas experienced a significant decrease in the rate of violent incidents, while residents in facilities without garden areas experienced a significant increase in such incidents (Mooney and Nicell 1992). More recently, residents with dementia who spent increased time outdoors participating in activities exhibited improved sleep efficiency and sleep duration, and less verbal agitation than residents who participated in similar activities indoors (Calkins *et al.* 2007; Connell *et al.* 2007).

Detweiler and colleagues (2008, 2009) examined the influence of a wander garden on the behavioural outcomes of 34 male veterans with dementia. Twelve months following the garden opening, all participants experienced a decreased need for PRN medications, while participants in the high-use group (i.e. more than 22 visits) also experienced a significant decrease in anti-psychotic medication use, fewer scheduled psychiatric medications, and a greater reduction in the number of falls and fall severity than those in the low-use group (Detweiler *et al.* 2008, 2009). Further analyses revealed that while visiting the wander garden resulted in reduced agitation levels, there was a differential effect depending on residents' ambulatory status. For ambulatory residents, low, medium or high garden usage was accompanied by a decrease in agitation, yet for non-ambulatory residents, only those with a high number of garden visits experienced decreased agitation (Murphy *et al.* 2010). As such, staff support and commitment likely play a crucial role in the success of outdoor space.

Debates and controversies

There are several debates and controversies in theory, research, and methods in this area. The conceptual frameworks in environmental design for dementia need to meaningfully align with the growing recognition of the importance of person-centred care philosophy and practice. Also, on an applied level, it remains somewhat challenging as to how a purposefully designed environment could best meet diverse and varying individual needs and preferences of residents in a group care environment setting.

Feasibility challenges exist in physical environmental assessment of dementia care settings from individual residents' perspectives versus collective environmental assessment. Environmental features would likely have variable effects on persons with dementia depending on a host of individual level factors, such as type of dementia, stage of disease, cognitive status, and physical functioning. However, an environmental assessment tool or method that is not sensitive to the variability in person–environment interactions and resultant outcomes would only provide a global evaluation of the physical environment. On the other hand, an assessment focusing on individual-level interactions with environmental features might be inadequate to provide meaningful data for environmental modifications responsive to group needs. An approach combining both of these assessment methods would be most suitable: however, the feasibility of such an approach is yet to be determined.

Another subject of debate is related to the need for balancing the issues of ensuring safety and supporting personal autonomy. The need for safety and security often impacts design decisions that limit people's mobility and increase staff surveillance. On the other hand, choice and personal control are important aspects of design that are grounded on a person-centred care approach.

Implications for research

Issues and directions for theoretical and empirical research in this area of dementia care are numerous. A few noteworthy ones are identified here. First, a strong business case for stand-alone small group homes or households would benefit from research. Although there is much research evidence on the benefits of small unit sizes or households for enhanced quality of life for people with dementia, the operational cost issues and organizational challenges are not fully identified and they remain unclear. Second, a sophisticated understanding of the relationship between small care unit and staffing model would be useful. Without a clear understanding of the implications of household models on staffing structure, staff responsibilities, training, and so on, a homelike physical environment will fail to achieve its full potential. Third, we need more research focusing on the broader "quality of life" aspects (e.g. the physical environment's effect on positive engagement in an activity, planned or spontaneous), rather than research primarily focusing on environment and challenging behaviours or functional abilities. Fourth, empirical work in this area is plagued by small sample sizes and an absence of comparison groups. Future studies need to address these limitations in existing research. Finally, there is very little empirical research on the unique needs of ethnically diverse resident populations; this relates both to an ethnically mixed resident population in a single care facility and care facility design for particular ethnic groups.

Exercise 11.3: Alice Choi's heightened anxiety

Alice Choi is an immigrant Korean-Canadian woman. She is 86 years old, has Alzheimer's disease, and now lives in a large traditional long-term care facility in Vancouver, Canada. Over the course of any given day, her anxiety level goes up in the late afternoon and she speaks out wanting to "go home". Alice begins to pace and hover around the unit's exit and occasionally pushes furniture in the dining room.

- What might be some of the physical environmental factors affecting Alice's anxiety?
- What kinds of spaces in the facility environment might help her and/or staff to reduce her anxiety levels?
- What life-history issues might be worth exploring to understand her anxiety experience?

Conclusion

The physical environment of a long-term care facility has a salient role in enhancing the quality of life of people with dementia and the quality of care practices. It is important to recognize and appreciate the environment's influences on reducing behavioural and affective symptoms associated with cognitive losses and its potential as a therapeutic resource. As people with dementia have heightened sensitivity to environmental stressors and cues, it is vital that the designed environment is appropriate and responsive to their cognitive abilities and functioning. At the same time, we need to acknowledge that a good physical environment alone cannot create a therapeutic milieu. The potential of a therapeutic physical setting is meaningfully utilized only when there is a corresponding recognition of the importance of appropriately inspired organizational policies and care/relational practices.

Further information

The Environmental Design Research Association (EDRA) is an international, interdisciplinary organization founded by design professionals, social scientists, students, educators, and facility managers. The purpose of this organization is advancement and dissemination of environmental design research. There are resources on their web site on the topic of environment–behaviour research and practice for various settings.

The Society for the Advancement of Gerontological Advancement (SAGE) is a multidisciplinary and multi-sectoral organization that advocates improving the built environment for older adults. The resource links on their web site identify several key organizations and entities focused on physical environments in long-term care facilities.

The Environments for Aging Resource Directory is an initiative to showcase strategies and design best practices in planning and developing responsive environments for older adults. The annual conference on environments and ageing and digital publications are excellent resources on environmental design for older adults. More information is available on this initiative's web site.

References

Ancoli-Israel, S., Gehrman, P., Martin, J.L., Shochat, T., Marler, M. *et al.* (2003) Increased light exposure consolidates sleep and strengthens circadian rhythms in severe Alzheimer's disease patients, *Behavioral Sleep Medicine*, 1(1): 22–36.

Annerstedt, L. (1994) An attempt to determine the impact of group living care in comparison to traditional long-term care on demented elderly patients, *Aging: Clinical and Experimental Research*, 6(5): 372–80.

Barnes, S. (2002) The design of caring environments and the quality of life of older people, *Ageing and Society*, 22 (6): 775–89.

Bharathan, T., Glodan, D., Ramesh, A., Vardhini, B., Baccash, E. *et al.* (2007) What do patterns of noise in a teaching hospital and nursing home suggest?, *Noise and Health*, 9(35): 31–4.

Brawley, E.C. (2006) *Design Innovations for Aging and Alzheimer's: Creating Caring Environments*. New York: Wiley.

Brooker, D. (2007) *Person-centred Dementia Care: Making Services Better*. London: Jessica Kingsley.

Brush, J.A., Meehan, R.A. and Calkins, M.P. (2002) Using the environment to improve intake for people with dementia, *Alzheimer's Care Quarterly*, 3(4): 330–8.

Calkins, M. (1988) *Design for Dementia: Planning Environments for the Elderly and Confused.* Owings Mills, MD: National Health Publishing.

Calkins, M. and Brush, J. (2009) Evidence-based long-term care design, *Neurorehabilitation*, 25(3): 145–54.

Calkins, M. and Cassella, C. (2007) Exploring the cost and value of private versus shared bedrooms in nursing homes, *The Gerontologist*, 47(2): 169–83.

Calkins, M. and Weisman, G.D. (1999) Models for environmental assessment, in B. Schwarz and R. Brent (eds.) *Aging, Autonomy and Architecture: Advances in Assisted Living*. Baltimore, MD: Johns Hopkins University Press, pp. 130–42.

Calkins, M., Szmerekovsky, J. and Biddle, S. (2007) Effect of increased time spent outdoors on individuals with dementia residing in nursing homes, *Journal of Housing for the Elderly*, 21(3/4): 211–28.

Cohen, U. and Weisman, G.D. (1991) *Holding on to Home: Designing Environments for People with Dementia*. Baltimore, MD: Johns Hopkins University Press.

Connell, B.R., Sanford, J.A. and Lewis, D. (2007) Therapeutic effects of an outdoor activity program on nursing home residents with dementia, *Journal of Housing for the Elderly*, 21(3/4): 195–209.

Day, K., Carreon, D. and Stump, C. (2000) The therapeutic design of environments for people with dementia: a review of the empirical research, *The Gerontologist*, 40(4): 397–416.

De Lepeleire, J., Bouwen, A., De Coninck, L. and Buntinx, F. (2007) Insufficient lighting in nursing homes, *Journal of the American Medical Directors Association*, 8: 314–17.

de Rooij, A.M., Luijkx, K.G., Schaafsma, J., Declercq, A.G., Emmerink, P.J. *et al.* (2012) Quality of life of residents with dementia in traditional versus small-scale long-term care settings: a quasi-experimental study, *International Journal of Nursing Studies*, 49(8): 931–40.

Desai, J., Winter, A., Young, K.W. and Greenwood, C.E. (2007) Changes in type of foodservice and dining room environment preferentially benefit institutionalized seniors with low body mass indexes, *Journal of the American Dietetic Association*, 107(5): 808–14.

Detweiler, M.B., Murphy, P.F., Myers, L.C. and Kim, K.Y. (2008) Does a wander garden influence inappropriate behaviors in dementia residents?, *American Journal of Alzheimer's Disease and Other Dementias*, 23(1): 31–45.

Detweiler, M.B., Murphy, P.F., Kim, K.Y., Myers, L.C. and Ashai, A. (2009) Scheduled medications and falls in dementia patients utilizing a wander garden, *American Journal of Alzheimer's Disease and Other Dementias*, 24(4): 322–32.

Dunne, T.E., Neargarder, S.A., Cipolloni, P.B. and Cronin-Golomb, A. (2004) Visual contrast enhances food and liquid intake in advanced Alzheimer's disease, *Clinical Nutrition*, 23: 533–8.

Fetveit, A. and Bjorvatn, B. (2005) Bright-light treatment reduces actigraphic-measured daytime sleep in nursing home patients with dementia: a pilot study, *American Journal of Geriatric Psychiatry*, 13(5): 420–3.

Fleming, R. and Purandare, N. (2010) Long-term care for people with dementia: environmental design guidelines, *International Psychogeriatrics*, 22(7): 1084–96.

Garre-Olmo, J., López-Pousa, S., Turon-Estrada, A., Juvinyà, D., Ballester, D. *et al.* (2012) Environmental determinants of quality of life in nursing home residents with severe dementia, *Journal of the American Geriatrics Society*, 60(7): 1230–6.

Hall, G. and Buckwalter, K. (1987) Progressively lowered stress threshold: a conceptual model for care of adults with Alzheimer's disease, *Archives of Psychiatric Nursing*, 1: 399–406.

Innes, A., Kelly, F. and Dincarslan, O. (2011) Care home design for people with dementia: what do people with dementia and their family carers value?, *Aging and Mental Health*, 15(5): 548–56.

Joosse, L.L. (2011) Sound levels in nursing homes, *Journal of Gerontological Nursing*, 37(8): 30–5.

Joosse, L.L. (2012) Do sound levels and space contribute to agitation in nursing home residents with dementia?, *Research in Gerontological Nursing*, 5(3): 174–84.

Kane, R., Lum, T., Cutler, L., Degenholtz, H. and Yu, T. (2007) Resident outcomes in small-house nursing homes: a longitudinal evaluation of the initial Green House program, *Journal of the American Geriatrics Society*, 55: 832–9.

Kitwood, T. (1997) *Dementia Reconsidered: The Person Comes First*. Buckingham: Open University Press.

Koss, E. and Gilmore, G. (1998) Environmental interventions and functional ability of AD patients, in B. Vellas, J. Filten and G. Frisoni (eds.) *Research and Practice in Alzheimer's Disease*. New York: Springer, pp. 185–93.

Kovach, C.R. and Meyer-Arnold, E.A. (1996) Coping with conflicting agendas: the bathing experience of cognitively impaired older adults, *Scholarly Inquiry for Nursing Practice: An International Journal*, 10(1): 23–36.

Lawton, M.P. (1982) Competence, environmental press, and the adaptation of older people, in M.P. Lawton, P. Windley and T. Byerts (eds.) *Aging and the Environment: Theoretical Approaches*. New York: Springer.

Lawton, M.P. and Nahemow, L. (1973) Ecology and the aging process, in C. Eisdorfer and M.P. Lawton (eds.) *The Psychology of Adult Development and Aging*. Washington, DC: American Psychological Association, pp. 619–74.

McAllister, C.L. and Silverman, M.A. (1999) Community formation and community roles among persons with Alzheimer's disease: a comparative study of experiences in a residential Alzheimer's facility and a traditional nursing home, *Qualitative Health Research*, 9(1): 65–85.

McFadden, S.H. and Lunsman, M. (2010) Continuity in the midst of change: behaviors of residents relocated from a nursing home environment to small households, *American Journal of Alzheimer's Disease and Other Dementias*, 25 (1): 51–7.

Mooney, P. and Nicell, P.L. (1992) The importance of exterior environment for Alzheimer residents: effective care and risk management, *Healthcare Management Forum*, 5(2): 23–9.

Moos, R. and Lemke, S. (1994) *Group Residences for Older Adults: Physical Features, Policies, and Social Climate*. New York: Oxford University Press.

Morgan, D.G. and Stewart, N.J. (1998) Multiple occupancy versus private rooms on dementia care units, *Environment and Behavior*, 30(4): 487–503.

Murphy, P., Miyazaki, Y., Detweiler, M. and Kim, K. (2010) Longitudinal analysis of differential effects on agitation of a therapeutic wander garden for dementia patients based on ambulation ability, *Dementia*, 9(3): 355–73.

Namazi, K. and Johnson, B. (1991a) Physical environmental cues to reduce the problems of incontinence in Alzheimer's disease units, *American Journal of Alzheimer's Care and Related Disorders and Research*, 6: 22–8.

Namazi, K. and Johnson, B. (1991b) Environmental effects on incontinence problems in Alzheimer's disease patients, *American Journal of Alzheimer's Care and Related Disorders and Research*, 6: 16–21.

Namazi, K.H. and Johnson, B.D. (1996) Issues related to behavior and the physical environment: bathing cognitively-impaired patients, *Geriatric Nursing*, 17(5): 234–9.

Perivolaris, A., LeClerc, C.M., Wilkinson, K. and Buchanan, S. (2006) An enhanced dining program for persons with dementia, *Alzheimer's Care Quarterly*, 7(4): 258–67.

Reed, P.S., Zimmerman, S., Sloane, P.D., Williams, C.S. and Boustani, M. (2005) Characteristics associated with low food and fluid intake in long-term care residents with dementia, *The Gerontologist*, 45(1): 74–80.

Regnier, V. and Scott, A.C. (2001) Creating a therapeutic environment: lessons from Northern European models, in S. Zimmerman, P.D. Sloane and M.G. Ory (eds.) *Assisted Living: Needs, Practices and Policies in Residential Care for the Elderly*. Baltimore, MD: Johns Hopkins University Press, pp. 53–77.

Reimer, M.A., Slaughter, S., Donaldson, C., Currie, G. and Eliasziw, M. (2004) Special care facility compared with traditional environments for dementia care: a longitudinal study of quality of life, *Journal of the American Geriatrics Society*, 52(7): 1085–92.

Riemersma-van der Lek, R.F., Swaab, D., Twisk, J., Hol, E., Hoogendijk, W. *et al.* (2008) Effect of bright light and melatonin on cognitive and non-cognitive function in elderly residents of group care facilities: a randomized controlled trial, *Journal of the American Medical Association*, 299(22): 2642–55.

Shochat, T., Martin, J., Marler, M. and Ancoli-Israel, S. (2000) Illumination levels in nursing home patients: effects on sleep and activity rhythms, *Journal of Sleep Research*, 9: 373–9.

Schwarz, B., Chaudhury, H. and Tofle, R. (2004) Effect of design interventions on a dementia care setting, *American Journal of Alzheimer's Disease and Other Dementias*, 19(3): 172–6.

Sloane, P.D., Honn, V.J., Dwyer, S.A., Wieselquist, J., Cain, C. *et al.* (1995) Bathing the Alzheimer's patient in long-term care: results and recommendations from three studies, *American Journal of Alzheimer's Disease*, 10(4): 3–11.

Sloane, P.D., Mitchell, C.M., Preisser, J.S., Phillips, C., Commander, C. *et al.* (1998) Environmental correlates of resident agitation in Alzheimer's disease special care units, *Journal of the American Geriatrics Society*, 46(7): 862–89.

Sloane, P.D., Williams, C.S., Mitchell, C.M., Preisser, J.S., Wood, W. *et al.* (2007) High-intensity environmental light in dementia: effect on sleep and activity, *Journal of the American Geriatrics Society*, 55(10): 1524–33.

Smit, D., de Lange, J., Willemse, B. and Pot, A. (2012) The relationship between small-scale care and activity involvement of residents with dementia, *International Psychogeriatrics*, 24(5): 722–32.

Smith, M., Gerdner, L., Hall, G. and Buckwalter, K.C. (2004) History, development, and future for the Progressively Lowered Threshold Model: a conceptual model for dementia care, *Journal of the American Geriatrics Society*, 52: 1755–60.

Smith, R., Mathews, R. and Gresham, M. (2010) Pre- and post-occupancy evaluation of new dementia care cottages, *American Journal of Alzheimer's Disease and Other Dementias*, 25(3): 265–75.

Somboontanont, W., Sloane, P.D., Floyd, F.J., Holditch-Davis, D., Hogue, C.C. *et al.* (2004) Assaultive behaviour in Alzheimer's disease: identifying immediate antecedents during bathing, *Journal of Gerontological Nursing*, 30(9): 22–9.

Suzuki, M., Kanamori, M., Yasuda, M. and Oshiro, H. (2008) One-year follow-up study of elderly group-home residents with dementia, *American Journal of Alzheimer's Disease and Other Dementias*, 23(4): 334–43.

te Boekhorst, S., Depla, M., de Lange, J., Pot, A. and Eefsting, J. (2009) The effects of group living homes on older people with dementia: a comparison with traditional nursing home care, *International Journal of Geriatric Psychiatry*, 24(9): 970–8.

Thorpe, L., Middleton, J., Russell, G. and Stewart, N. (2000) Bright light therapy for demented nursing home patients with behavioral disturbance, *American Journal of Alzheimer's Disease and Other Dementias*, 15: 18–26.

van Hoof, J., Kort, H.S.M., van Waarde, H. and Blom, M.M. (2010) Environmental interventions and the design of homes for older adults with dementia: an overview, *American Journal of Alzheimer's Disease and Other Dementias*, 25(3): 202–32.

Verbeek, H., Zwakhalen, S., van Rossum, E., Ambergen, T., Kempen, G. *et al.* (2010) Dementia care redesigned: effects of small-scale living facilities on residents, their family caregivers, and staff, *Journal of the American Medical Directors Association*, 11(9): 662–70.

Weisman, G.D. (1997) Environments for older persons with cognitive impairments, in G.T. Moore and R.W. Marans (eds.) *Advances in Environment, Behavior and Design*. New York: Plenum, pp. 315–46.

Weisman, G.D., Chaudhury, H. and Diaz Moore, K. (2000) Theory and practice of place: toward an integrative model, in R. Rubinstein, M. Moss and M. Kleban (eds.) *The Many Dimensions of Aging: Essays in Honor of M. Powell Lawton*. New York: Springer, pp. 3–21.

Wilkes, L., Fleming, A., Wilkes, B.L., Cioffi, J. and Miere, J. (2005) Environmental approach to reducing agitation in older persons with dementia in a nursing home, *Australasian Journal on Ageing*, 24(3): 141–5.

World Health Organization (WHO) (1999) Guidelines for Community Noise. Geneva: WHO [http://www.who.int/docstore/peh/noise/guidelines2.html, accessed 12 March 2003].

Yao, L. and Algase, D. (2006) Environmental ambiance as a new window on wandering, *Western Journal of Nursing Research*, 28(1): 89–104.

Zeisel, J., Silverstein, N.M., Hyde, J., Levkoff, S., Lawton, M.P. *et al.* (2003) Environmental correlates to behavioral health outcomes in Alzheimer's special care units, *The Gerontologist*, 43(5): 697–711.

Best practice dementia care for the person

Understanding and enhancing the relationship between people with dementia and their family carers

Carol J. Whitlatch

> 66 Having a loving and caring wife, who encourages me to 'push the boundaries' of what I am able to do helps enormously, even if she has to listen to me asking the same question that I asked half an hour before. 99
>
> —Doug Jenks London, UK

Learning objectives

By the end of this chapter, you will be able to:

- Describe evidence that confirms the ability of persons with dementia to be actively engaged in psychosocial interventions and research
- Appreciate the "partnership", mutuality, and reciprocity involved in the giving and receiving of care and support
- Utilize strategies for improving communication between care partners and developing a mutually agreed upon plan of care

Introduction

Families provide the majority of care and support to the millions of people with dementia worldwide (see Chapter 1). Family members assist with instrumental and personal care tasks such as finances, housework, transportation, bathing, feeding, dressing, and toileting. This chapter looks at the experience of dementia for both the person and carer, how interactions, communication, and relationship quality of people with dementia and their carers are affected by changes in memory during the earliest stages of dementia, and the experience of recognizing and accepting symptoms of dementia. Interventions that can improve communication between people with dementia and their care partners and help them develop a plan of care are described.

> **"Family"** is defined most inclusively and broadly to include persons related by blood, marriage, adoption, fostering, and choice.

The reciprocity of family care: the giving and receiving of support

Family members often share in provision of support for their relatives with dementia. Yet, there is typically one family member with primary responsibility for the care. There is an unwritten but widely followed "hierarchy" of who will become this primary carer (Cantor 1979). As noted in Chapter 14, if the person with dementia has a partner, then that partner will most likely provide the majority of care over time. If the person has no partner or the partner is unable to assist (the partner may be too ill or physically unable to help), then adult children are next in line to provide support, most frequently an adult daughter. Adult sons are also care providers, although their wives are often more involved in hands-on and emotional support (Noelker and Whitlatch 2005). In addition, grandchildren, nephews, nieces, close friends, and neighbours provide support to the millions of adults with dementia.

The care partnership in dementia

It is critical to understand that care provision within families is not one-sided. Persons with dementia continue to be very involved in social and physical activities, careers, community service, family gatherings, self-care, and other activities well into the disease process. They continue to "give back" and remain significant contributors to their families and communities. Indeed, the terms "carer," "caregiver", and "care recipient" connote a uni-directional relationship with one person only giving and the other only receiving support. Increasingly, the more inclusive and accurate term "care partner" is used, which reflects the mutuality and reciprocity that both members of the "care dyad" experience. "Care partner" evokes the experience of partnership characteristic of living with dementia and other chronic conditions. Although reciprocity will diminish with increasing dependency, there are strategies to ensure that the spirit of partnership is maintained through the later stages of dementia. Before we describe these strategies, we move to a discussion of how care partners (both the person with dementia and their carer) come to understand and accept the disease that will have a lasting impact on their lives.

Stages leading to acceptance that "something is not right"

As described in Chapter 22, families face a tremendous uncertainty as they begin to recognize the changes in memory that are beyond "normal ageing". This recognition varies by person, family, situation, illness severity, and culture.

Pre-diagnosis: first recognizing symptoms of memory loss

For each person with dementia, a unique process unfolds as the person:

1 first recognizes symptoms of memory loss or dementia
2 discloses this recognition to others, and
3 obtains a formal diagnosis

Very little empirical evidence exists on recognizing early symptoms of dementia. There is, however, a growing body of anecdotal evidence that indicates that many people who receive a diagnosis of dementia describe feeling that "years ago I knew something was wrong". Persons in this earliest pre-diagnosis phase are often keenly aware of very subtle changes in memory and attention – changes that often go unnoticed by the care partner or others. Many people begin to establish compensatory routines to help organize their lives so that less information needs to be remembered and processed. The belief that this is "normal ageing" gives some people a sense that the changes they are experiencing are "to be expected and lived with".

> I tried to keep everything in its place. Keys on the hook, grocery lists on the refrigerator, appointments on the calendar.
>
> —75-year-old mother with dementia

Similarly, care partners describe many different reactions to their loved one's cognitive changes. Some care partners do not notice the subtle lapses in memory or organization, while others may be keenly aware that "something is not quite right". Moreover, many family members do not self-identify as a "carer": "I'm his wife, he's my husband. We take care of each other." Practitioners need to be sensitive to the language they use when working with families.

> Mom had developed elaborate routines that helped her shop for groceries, pay bills, and do laundry.
>
> —Daughter whose mother with early-stage dementia lives alone

As described in Chapter 22, differences across cultures affect how families view symptoms and when symptoms are recognized. Often there is an attempt to normalize symptoms with the belief that normal ageing is the cause. People with dementia and their families may seek assistance later in the disease progression, potentially missing important opportunities for intervention and support.

Diagnosis: a time for understanding the cause of changes in memory and cognition

What do care partners experience as they approach the time of diagnosis? Must changes in memory or behaviour reach a specific level of decline before diagnosis is sought? Is there a crisis or serious event ("Dad was found driving the wrong way on the motorway") that acts as the "last straw" or final catalyst leading to the need for medical oversight? Little is known about what predicts the timing of diagnosis. Again, our limited knowledge draws upon anecdotal evidence from the field and from research interviews.

> I don't really want to know. I'm in denial.
>
> —Husband whose wife has vascular dementia

Some people with dementia want to know the cause of their memory changes, hoping that the decline can be halted or reversed through medication, diet, or targeted intervention. The case example of Mr. Juarez illustrates this approach and worldview.

> ## Case example 12.1: Mr. Juarez
>
> Mr. Juarez has noticed a change in his memory dating back two years. He describes his first experiences as trouble remembering words. During that first year, Mr. J attributed his changes in memory to increasing stress at his job and dissatisfaction in his marriage. After he retired, he expected his memory problems to end, but they only worsened, as did his marital difficulties. Mr. J. sought diagnosis with the hope that there would be a cure for his worsening memory. A neurologist tells Mr. J that he has experienced mini strokes and that better adherence to his high blood pressure medications could prevent further decline. The neurologist tells Mr. and Mrs. J that his memory loss is a symptom of these mini strokes and suggests that his memory problems may be contributing to their marital troubles as well. Mr. J. follows the neurologist's advice about medication adherence, exercise, and diet, and the couple seeks counselling with a practitioner knowledgeable about dementia and memory loss. For Mr. and Mrs. Juarez, diagnosis is the first step towards preventing further decline.

Unlike Mr. Juarez, who wanted to know the cause of his memory loss, other individuals prefer to ignore changes and blame "normal ageing"; they may believe that nothing can be done to reverse or prevent further decline. When working with families who are at this early stage of recognition, it is important to meet them at their level of understanding and acceptance. Ideally, each care partner has the same view and understanding of the situation: "We both understand she has dementia and we both want help." More common, however, is a mismatch between care partners: one care partner has accepted the diagnosis and is ready to move forward, whereas the other person denies anything is wrong. Patient and persistent discussions with the care partners combined with education about the disease will help them come to a more common understanding.

> **❝** I was so relieved when I was told I had dementia. Finally, I had a reason for my bad memory. It's not that I wasn't trying hard enough to remember . . . I really just COULDN'T remember. It wasn't my fault. **❞**
>
> —80-year-old husband with Alzheimer's disease

Our work with families suggests that differences in reactions to or interest in obtaining a diagnosis is based on socioeconomic status and perceived access to diagnostic procedures. For families facing multiple stressors associated with day-to-day living (e.g. affordable housing, permanent employment, lack of access to health care), obtaining a diagnosis and follow-up support may not be a priority. If symptoms become too disruptive to the family, the advice of a medical provider may be sought. Education about dementia and memory loss and encouragement to seek diagnosis and appropriate assistance may be the most effective strategies for supporting at-risk families.

Issues specific to young-onset families

In addition to the millions of older adults with dementia, there is a smaller yet growing number of middle-aged adults who are experiencing symptoms of dementia (see Chapters 1 and 7). The National Alzheimer's Association (USA) estimated that in 2013 there were approximately

200,000 persons under the age of 65 living with Alzheimer's disease (Alzheimer's Association 2006, 2013). It is likely that many of these persons may not even know they have Alzheimer's because it is so often under-diagnosed (Alzheimer's Association 2013). A dementia diagnosis before the age of 65 is considered "early" or "young" onset dementia (Alzheimer's Association 2012).

For adults in their forties, fifties, and early sixties, a diagnosis of dementia is considered an "off-time" and unexpected event. Many people with young-onset dementia have children living at home, are involved in careers, and reliant on work-provided health care for themselves and their families. These individuals and their families face unique stressors throughout the course of their illness.

❝I want to know more about what to expect.❞

—Mother with early memory loss (daughter carer)

Off-time event

Adults diagnosed with dementia in their forties and fifties often report that they had to change their retirement plans, that their children (some very young) helped them with a variety of personal care needs, and that their careers abruptly ended. These and other "off-time events" are unique to the young-onset experience and can be a significant source of distress for both care partners.

Misdiagnosis

Until recently, many health care providers were unaware of young-onset dementia. Many families we have interviewed report that their lifelong physician was unable to determine the cause of their loved one's memory and behaviour change; diagnosis did not occur until a specialist (e.g. neurologist, geriatrician) was brought in. Luckily, education about young-onset dementia has improved diagnostic accuracy so that few families face the uncertainty of no diagnosis or misdiagnosis.

Juggling multiple roles

Many people with young-onset dementia report a significant amount of stress from their attempts to maintain multiple roles. People with young-onset dementia who have children continue to be very involved as parents. Young-onset individuals report being at the height of their careers with little thought of retirement. Relationships with family and friends can be stressful for the young-onset individual.

Lack of appropriate services

Currently, there are very few services or programmes specifically designed to meet the needs of young-onset families. Many younger onset families feel out of place in support groups or other programmes where the majority of participants are much older and facing very different care and life challenges. Some services available to people with dementia and their families are not available to young-onset families because of age restrictions; many programmes do not serve people under the age of 60. Sadly, young-onset families report feeling isolated, unsupported, and, as a result, unprepared to meet the challenges they will face.

> ### Case example 12.1: Mr. Ross
>
> Mr. Ross is in his early forties and lives with his 43-year-old wife and two young children. He recently received a diagnosis of fronto-temporal dementia (FTD) after speaking with a handful of medical doctors, only one of whom recognized his symptoms as "young-onset" or "early-onset" FTD. He is a machinist who works second shift and is required to operate large and heavy equipment. Mr. Ross is a life-long diabetic who manages his glucose testing and monitoring on his own. The family lives in a rural area and Mr. Ross operates large farm equipment. He owns guns, which are kept unloaded and locked in a secure area of the basement. Mrs. Ross works full time so that Mr. Ross is alone much of the day and is home when their children get off the school bus. He still drives and is very self-aware of his memory symptoms.

Exercise 12.1: Helping the Ross family

You are a social service provider working with the Ross family to help them plan for current and future care needs. What issues are unique to this young-onset family compared with the issues facing a retired couple who receive a diagnosis when they are in their eighties?

- You should make time to have an open and frank discussion about the family's expectations for the future. This diagnosis is an "off time and unexpected event" and while they may be experiencing emotions similar to older couples, the Ross family may be experiencing emotions more intensely (e.g. extreme sadness, grief, resentment, fear for their children, anxiety about losing Mr. Ross's income, health care coverage).
- Education about fronto-temporal dementia is critical, including information about symptoms and progression.
- Issues of safety are very important to this family: operating large machinery and farm equipment, guns, and diabetes self-management could be problematic as Mr. Ross's memory symptoms worsen.

Maximizing personhood in early dementia

Early diagnosis brings with it critical opportunities for targeted interventions (pharmacological and psychosocial) with potential to address the cognitive and social needs of the person and his or her family carer. Yet, few interventions are designed to meet the needs of both care partners. Interventions that target the carer are typically designed to ameliorate stress and improve outcomes for carers of persons in the more moderate to later stages of dementia. Intervention strategies include education about how to manage difficult behaviours (e.g. agitation, wandering), support provided by family, friends, and formal providers, and enhancing healthy behaviours (see Chapter 14).

A small but growing number of interventions are meeting the needs of persons with early-stage dementia. Many of these interventions are designed as support groups for both the person with early-stage dementia and their family carer (Zarit *et al*. 2004; Logsdon *et al*. 2010; D. Coon and C.J. Whitlatch, unpublished). Some groups are designed so that the carers and persons with dementia meet together. Another design offers separate groups for persons and carers. Other strategies offer a mixed approach: first everyone meets together, then participants separate into different peer groups, and then everyone comes together at the end. The feasibility, acceptability, and efficacy of these various group approaches are encouraging, although large comparative effectiveness trials have not yet established whether one strategy is more effective. Overall, the programmes that include the person with dementia offer the greatest opportunity for maximizing personhood.

Understanding care values and preferences for care in early-stage dementia

The person's perspective

A common misperception of many well-meaning service providers and family members is that people with dementia are unable to answer questions, and thus should be limited in their involvement in their own decision-making. A growing literature reflects an alternative view, indicating that persons with mild to moderate cognitive loss are able to respond accurately and consistently to questions about health, preferences, instrumental activities of daily living or functional problems (Lai and Karlawish 2007; Clark *et al.* 2008; Lai *et al.* 2008). For more impaired persons, it is possible to measure four decision-making abilities that are highly related to executive functioning – understanding, appreciation, reasoning, and expressing a choice (Lai *et al.* 2008). This assessment can help the person and carer to understand more clearly if there are areas of strength, weakness, and changing circumstances that could make living independently safe or unsafe. Interventions that enhance or preserve decision-making capacity can help empower people with dementia to voice their preferences (Whitlatch and Feinberg 2003).

Care values of persons with early-stage dementia

One strategy to help mitigate conflict around decisions and enhance planning for current and future care is to engage people with dementia and their carers together in a discussion around values for care. A structured assessment or informal discussion can help clarify the person's values for care and illuminate the carer's accurate and inaccurate perceptions about the person's values. The 34-item Care Values Scale (formerly Values and Preferences Scale [VPS]; Whitlatch *et al.* 2005; Whitlatch 2010) has been developed to help facilitate a structured dialogue around the care dyad's values for care. Five subscales focus on values for care: (1) not being a burden on family, (2) being independent, (3) activities with family and friends, (4) keeping safe, and (5) having a say in who helps out.

Box 12.1: Care Values Scale (shortened version)

For the person with dementia:
   "How important is it for you to . . ."

For the carer:
   "How important is it for your relative to . . ."

Not important	Somewhat important	Important	Very important
0	1	2	3

Burden

- Avoid being a physical burden

(continued)

- Avoid being an emotional burden
- Avoid being a financial burden
- Not make your carer put his/her life on hold to provide care

Safety and quality of care

- Be safe from crime
- Have a say in who helps out
- Have reliable help

Activities with others

- Do things with other people
- Be part of family celebration
- Be with family and friends

Independence

- Do things for yourself
- Come and go as you please
- Feel useful
- Have something to do

After collecting information about care values, a trained clinician engages the dyad in a discussion about their perceptions, pointing to similarities and differences in responses. There are no right or wrong answers: the goal is for the dyad to gain a better understanding of the person's values for care. Does Mr. Gardiner value independence over not being a burden? Is his daughter surprised by this? Are other family members surprised? Again, the goal is to understand each person's perceptions and reactions and to use the information to inform current and future decision-making that reflects the family's collective understanding.

Our longitudinal research indicates that people with dementia remain consistent in their values for care (Reamy *et al.* 2013). Thus, the values for care that people with dementia feel are important to them at the early stages of memory loss, remain important throughout the more moderate stages as well. The implications of these findings are critical to families, practitioners, and most importantly, people with dementia. If a person's values for care are elicited early in the disease, the family can be assured that these values will remain consistent over time. Communication about care values has the potential to decrease the family stress that stems from not knowing the person's values for care.

> 66 We made good progress in getting issues on the table. In discussing care values, I was very surprised that his perception of safety was far different from mine. I know I need to listen more to him. 99

—Wife whose husband has mild cognitive impairment

Care preferences of persons with dementia

An additional source of stress for the carer and conflict within families stems from the burdensome number and intensity of care tasks requiring increasing attention as dementia symptoms worsen. These "care tasks" range from housework, yard work, shopping, and getting to appointments, to more personal tasks such as eating, bathing, dressing, toileting, and help at night. Family conflict arises when there are disagreements about who should help with these tasks, when help should be introduced, and how often support is required. To prevent carer stress and family conflict, we recommend engaging the dyad (and larger family as appropriate) in discussions about the person's preferences for who will "help out". The 19-item Preferences for Care Tasks scale (Whitlatch 2010) is designed to assess the person's preferences for who will provide help and the carer's perceptions of their relative's preferences. Exercise 12.2 provides examples of questions from the Preferences for Care Tasks scale and strategies for engaging families in discussions around these preferences.

Exercise 12.2: Preferences for Care Tasks scale

For the person with dementia:
"Who would you prefer help you with these tasks if there comes a time when you need help or support?"

For the carer:
"Who do you think your relative would prefer to help him/her with these tasks if there comes a time when she/he needs help or support?"

	Carer	Family and friends	Paid providers
Cooking meals			
Dressing			
Eating			
Toileting			
Shopping			
Bathing			
Housework			
Help at night			
Getting to appointments			

Circles diagram

1 For the person with dementia: within each empty circle, write the task that the person with dementia assigned to each person/group.
2 For the carer: using a second set of empty Circles diagrams, within each circle, write the task that the carer thought the person with dementia would assign to each person/group.
3 Typically, the "care partner" circle is overloaded with tasks, which offers an alarming, but impressive visual of potential carer burden (see Figure 12.1).

Create more balanced Circles diagram

Take a few minutes to try to move some tasks out of the "care partner" circle and into another circle, thus creating a more balanced visual. This is a step towards creating a plan of care that balances (a) the best interests of both care partners, and (2) the provision of care across multiple sources of potential support (see Figure 12.2).

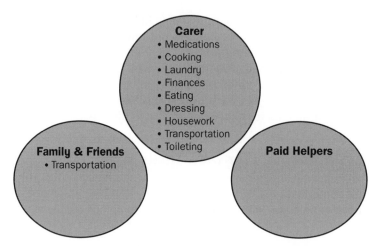

Figure 12.1: Circles diagrams for care tasks: example of an initial SHARE plan

Similar to care values, people with dementia maintain consistency over time concerning who they would prefer help them with various care tasks. Not surprisingly, the carer remains the person of choice for the majority of tasks.

Do carers know their relative's values for care and preferences for care tasks?

The carer's perspective: care values

Do carers know what their loved one values most for their own care in the future? Growing evidence indicates that carers have a general idea about their loved one's care values, but carers typically underestimate how important certain values are to the person.

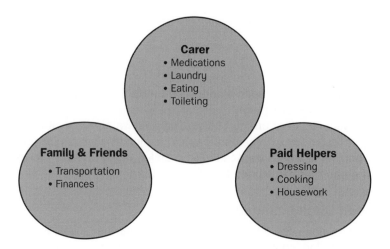

Figure 12.2: Circles diagrams for care tasks: a more balanced SHARE plan

There can be significant challenge for families who are unaware of their loved one's values for care. Research by Reamy and colleagues (2011) suggests that carers consistently underestimate their relative's involvement in decision-making. These discrepancies in perceptions about decision-making seem to be related to discrepancies in the importance placed on care values. In other words, for dyads where the person with dementia is more involved in decision-making, the dyad's view of the person's care values are more consistent and congruent. To avoid conflict, it may be in the family's best interests to engage in discussions about decision-making and care values as early in the disease progression as possible.

To illustrate, a daughter caring for her father believes he values "not being a burden on family". However, she is unaware of how strongly he values not being a burden over all other values. Consider the potential stress that could be eliminated from her care responsibilities if she were to understand that her father, above all other values, did not want her to be burdened by his care. We have seen many carers in our intervention studies experience great relief when they hear their relative say, "I am very concerned with your [the carer's] well-being" or gives the carer "permission" to take steps to decrease burden (e.g. ask for and bring in help, take time away from caring). Facilitating a conversation between the carer and the person with dementia about the person's values for care and mutual best interests has the potential to relieve anxiety and distress for both care partners. Moreover, because people with dementia are consistent in their values for care over time, these discussions could have a lasting positive impact on both care partners.

The carer's perspective: preferences for care tasks

In contrast to a general underestimation of the importance of their relative's values for care, family carers are very accurate in their understanding of who their relative would prefer to provide assistance. In our interviews with families, we learned that, typically, both the carer and person with dementia believe that the person would prefer that the carer assume most if not all care responsibilities. To illustrate, a wife caring for her husband is very aware that her husband would prefer for her to help him with all care tasks. She likely agrees with his preferences, noting: "I know better than anyone what he wants and how he wants it." However, this shared and often agreed upon understanding of who is preferred to provide support may be very burdensome to the carer.

SHARE: Support, Health, Activities, Resources, and Education

One of the only interventions to engage both care partners in discussions about care values and preferences is the SHARE programme: Support, Health, Activities, Resources, and Education. This seven-session in-home intervention targets care partners in the early stages of dementia and is designed to engage care partners in structured discussions about their plans for care currently and in the future. This dyadic evidence-based intervention utilizes unique visual and hands-on instructional strategies that help carers to understand their relative's care values and preferences. The Care Values Scale (see Box 12.1) and the Preferences for Care Tasks scale (see Exercise 12.2) are examples of innovative techniques used in the SHARE programme. SHARE counsellors use these tools to help families come to a shared understanding of the person's values for care and preferences for who they prefer to assist them with a variety of care tasks. Subsequent discussions draw on these values and preferences as a strategy to encourage the care dyad to maintain healthy activities and supportive relationships, and to reach out for assistance if the provision of care becomes unmanageable.

> ### Case example 12.3: Kelly
>
> Kelly was frustrated with her father with dementia who could no longer get his clothes out and dress himself after breakfast. She would tell him: "After you put your breakfast dishes away, go upstairs, pick out a long sleeved shirt and pants, and get dressed." Her dad became agitated when he could not follow her multiple commands or when she became frustrated. Kelly learned from her SHARE counsellor that people with dementia can remember only one step at a time and that she should try to keep her directions "short and simple". This technique is called "KISS": Keep It Short and Simple. Kelly completely changed how she spoke to her father: "Dad, let's get you dressed." "Let's go upstairs." After getting upstairs: "Let's go in your room." After going into his room: "Here are some clothes for you." He notices his pants. "Let's get these pants on you." And so on. Kelly's new approach and communication strategies lessened her frustration, helped her father maintain his ability to dress himself with prompts, and significantly decreased his agitation. Education about dementia and help using more appropriate communication techniques dramatically helped this family.

Upon completion of the seven SHARE sessions, care partners have developed a "SHARE plan". This plan draws upon the dyad's values and preferences for care and provides a blueprint for who will provide support so that the carer is not overburdened with the provision of care. In addition to the exercises around care values and preferences, a few SHARE programme techniques are described in the following sections.

Education about dementia and techniques to enhance communication and decision-making

It is critical to communication and decision-making that both care partners understand the symptoms and progression of dementia. SHARE provides care partners with information about dementia and teaches them to use communication strategies that enhance optimal functioning, improve communication strategies, and help to decrease stress for both care partners.

The SHARE plan

Families involved in the SHARE programme work towards developing a plan of care that suits both care partners' preferences. This "SHARE plan" builds from discussions and exercises about care values, preferences for who will help with care tasks, how to balance the best interests of the person and the carer, and how to maintain healthy activities even under stress. We have described these strategies and provided examples of how to engage a dyad in these exercises. The goal is for the dyad to leave the SHARE programme with a list of potential helpers (i.e. family, friends, and service providers), their contact information, and the types of assistance each person can provide. The dyad signs their SHARE plan thus acknowledging their intent to refer to it in the future.

> What a help to me to verbalize and put in writing the kind of help I will need. I am very grateful for this session and the program.
>
> —Wife whose husband has dementia

The interface between professionals and the care dyad: an extended care "triadic" partnership

As described in Chapter 22, partnerships between people with dementia, their carers, and health care professionals have great potential for improving outcomes for both the person and carer. The positive outcomes from this "triadic" relationship (Nolan *et al.* 2002) centre around a positive influence on decision-making within families and enhancing the relationship between the person and carer (Clissett 2007, as noted by Davies and Nolan 2008). Interactions with social service providers are also common among families, although even less literature exists about the quality and usefulness of these interactions. Although many people with dementia and their carers report positive interactions with social service and health care providers, there are also many families who describe their interactions with them as unsatisfying and inadequate. As noted by one person with dementia: "The doctor never spoke to me. He spoke to my (carer). It was as if I didn't exist." In addition, families note that the physician provided very little information about dementia and even less information about supportive services. This anecdotal evidence reflects both positive and negative reactions to interactions. Clearly, there is a need for further empirical research that explores these triadic relationships.

Debates and controversies

Although our experience in working with families is growing, many debates and controversies remain. One controversy concerns *genetic testing* and whether this should be required of people with a family history of dementia. We know that many people do not want to be diagnosed and that mandatory testing could be very stressful for these individuals and their families. Similarly, we know very little about the experiences of *young-onset families*. Precious research dollars have been reallocated to investigate how best to support these families and their unique needs. Knowing more about these families would position us to design interventions that meet their unique needs.

Additional controversy centres on the utility of developing *interventions and public policies that include both care partners*. One barrier to the development of programmes for both care partners is the limited public funding mechanisms targeting dyads. It is much more common for policies to support programmes for either the person with dementia or the carer, but rarely both. Until public policies become more inclusive and allow for programmes to work with both care partners, it is likely we will see neither an increase in the number of dyads served nor improvements in outcomes for these at-risk families.

Conclusion

This chapter has described evidence documenting the ability of people with dementia to answer questions about values for care and preferences for care tasks. We have noted that carers are not always accurate in their perceptions of their loved one's values for care. On the other hand, carers are very accurate in their understanding of who their loved one would prefer to provide assistance if their loved one was unable to assist him or herself. Typically, both carer and person with dementia believe that the person would prefer that the carer assume most if not all care responsibilities. This unbalanced plan for care has the potential to cause significant stress for the carer. Coming to a more balanced and realistic plan of care can be achieved if both care partners engage in discussions about care values and preferences. As a result, distress and other negative outcomes can be lessened for both the person with dementia and the family carer.

Further information

In the USA, the Alzheimer's Association works to provides support and assistance to persons and families affected by Alzheimer's disease and other dementias. The mission of the Association is to "eliminate Alzheimer's disease through the advancement of research; to provide and enhance care and support for all affected; and to reduce the risk of dementia through the promotion of brain health" [http://www.alz.org].

In the UK, Uniting Carers is an involvement network of family carers of people with dementia. The aim of the network is to give carers the opportunity to raise awareness and increase people's understanding of dementia. Over 1000 members throughout the country have now joined the network – people who want to use their experience of caring for someone with dementia to make a difference [https://www.dementiauk.org/what-we-do/uniting-carers/].

The Caregiving Resource Center of the American Association of Retired Persons (AARP) provides online support, education, and linkages to local support for caregivers of persons with a variety of chronic physical and cognitive conditions [http://www.aarp.org/home-family/caregiving/?intcmp=HP-LN-sec2-pos1].

The Cares Trust has published a report about the caring journey in the UK undertaken by carers of people with dementia and the challenges they face, from initial concerns to experiences at the end of life and afterwards [http://www.carers.org/sites/default/files/dementia_executive_summary_english_only_final_use_this_one.pdf].

The National Center on Caregiving of the Family Caregiver Alliance provides online support, education, and results of research studies related to caregiving for adults with chronic disabling health conditions. The Family Caregiver Alliance is one of 11 Caregiver Resource Centers in California that provide programmes and support to families statewide. The FCA is located at 785 Market Street, Suite 750, San Francisco, CA 94103; call 800.445.8106 [http://caregiver.org].

The National Alliance for Caregiving is a national resource for caregivers of persons of all ages and physical and cognitive conditions. The NAC is located at 4720 Montgomery Lane, 2nd floor, Bethesda, MD 20814-3425; call 301.718.8444 [http://ww.caregiving.org].

References

Alzheimer's Association (2006) *Early-onset Dementia: A National Challenge, A Future Crisis*. Washington, DC: Alzheimer's Association.
Alzheimer's Association (2012) 2012 Alzheimer's disease facts and figures, *Alzheimer's and Dementia*, 8(2): 131–68.
Alzheimer's Association (2013) 2013 Alzheimer's disease facts and figures, *Alzheimer's and Dementia*, 9(2): 208–45.

Cantor, M.H. (1979) The informal support system of New York's inner city elderly: is ethnicity a factor?, in D. Gelfand and A. Kutzik (eds.) *Ethnicity and Aging: Theory, Research, and Policy*. New York: Springer, pp. 67–73.

Clark, P.A., Tucke, S.S. and Whitlatch, C.J. (2008) Consistency of information from persons with dementia: an analysis of differences by question type, *Dementia*, 7(3): 341–58.

Clissett, P. (2007) A constructivist investigation into relationships between community dwelling older people and their carers. Unpublished PhD thesis, University of Sheffield.

Davies, S. and Nolan, M. (2008) Attending to relationships in dementia care, in M. Downs and B. Bowers (eds.) *Excellence in Dementia Care: Research into Practice*. Maidenhead: Open University Press.

Lai, J.M. and Karlawish, J. (2007) Assessing the capacity to make everyday decisions: a guide for clinicians and an agenda for future research, *American Journal of Geriatric Psychiatry*, 15: 101–11.

Lai, J.M., Gill, T.M., Cooney, L.M., Hawkins, K.A. and Karlawish, J. (2008) Everyday decision-making ability in older adults with cognitive impairments, *American Journal of Geriatric Psychiatry*, 16(8): 693–6.

Logsdon, R.G., Pike, K.C., McCurry, S.M., Hunter, P., Maher, J. *et al*. (2010) Early-stage memory loss support groups: outcomes from a randomized controlled clinical trial, *Journals of Gerontology B: Psychological and Social Sciences*, 65(6): 691–7.

Noelker, L.S. and Whitlatch, C.J. (2005) Informal caregiving, in C.J. Evashwick (ed.) *The Continuum of Long-term Care* (3rd edn.). Stamford, CT: Delmar.

Nolan, M., Ryan, T., Enderby, P. and Reid, D. (2002) Towards a more inclusive vision of dementia care practice and research, *Dementia*, 1(2): 193–211.

Reamy, A.M., Kim, K., Zarit, S.H. and Whitlatch, C.J. (2011) Understanding discrepancy in perceptions of values: individuals with mild to moderate dementia and their family caregivers, *The Gerontologist*, 51(4): 473–83.

Reamy, A., Kim, K., Zarit, S.H. and Whitlatch, C. (2013) Values and preferences of individuals with dementia: perceptions of family caregivers over time, *The Gerontologist*, 53: 293–302.

Whitlatch, C.J. (2010) Assessing the personal preferences of persons with dementia, in P. Lichtenberg (ed.) *Handbook of Assessment in Clinical Gerontology* (2nd edn.). San Diego, CA: Elsevier, pp. 557–80.

Whitlatch, C.J. and Feinberg, L.F. (2003) Planning for the future together in culturally diverse families: making everyday care decisions, *Alzheimer's Care Quarterly*, 4(1): 50–61.

Whitlatch, C.J., Feinberg, L.F. and Tucke, S.T. (2005) Measuring the values and preferences for everyday care of persons with cognitive impairment and their family caregivers, *The Gerontologist*, 45(3): 370–80.

Zarit, S.H., Femia, E.E., Watson, J., Rice-Oeschger, L. and Kakos, B. (2004) Memory Club: a group intervention for people with early-stage dementia and their care partners, *The Gerontologist*, 44(2): 262–9.

CHAPTER 13

Supporting families coping with dementia: flexibility and change

Steven H. Zarit and Judy M. Zarit

66 Well meaning people would make unwelcome comments that my family should come first, meaning my husband and children. If my mother wasn't part of my family then whose was she? 99

—Sue Tucker Yorkshire, UK

66 And it's always this problem that what you don't need is a whole list of email addresses. You don't need even a list of Alzheimer's Cafés in your area, because you don't even know that you need an Alzheimer's Café. Does that make sense? Because Peter's early, both age and early in the disease process, it didn't occur to me to go to an Alzheimer's Café, because they were for demented old people. And therefore, that's what I'm saying, the personal contact who would've said, 'Look, there's this really nice café that goes on once a week, a mile down the road from you, why don't you come in and see what goes on?' would've been fantastic. 99

—Tricia Dunlop Greater Manchester, UK

66 I was lucky, I joined lots of services. I was directed to the Social Services here in (name of town). They ran a service for family carers and provided us with advice - with input from CPNs, GPs, the hospital pharmacist etc. As carers we made close friendships with each other, but when we had completed all the educational aspects of the service we were asked to leave, as they didn't want us to mix with carers who had just joined the service and were not at the late stages of dementia with their relative. This was a difficult period for us all – we felt abandoned by the service; but luckily we had become close friends with each other and we started our own carer group and met at the local pub! Having a two-tier service would have been beneficial and I think that this should be part of a care pathway. 99

—Vivienne Cooper Yorkshire, UK

Learning objectives

By the end of this chapter, you will be able to:

- Distinguish between primary and secondary stressors in caring
- Discuss how carers' views affect their experience of caring
- Describe the satisfactions and rewards of caring
- Outline the steps carers can take to improve quality of life for themselves and their relatives with dementia

Introduction

As our population ages, more people develop disabilities that require assistance (see Chapter 1) and more family members are called upon to lend a hand. Families provide most of the care received by older people, with paid help and institutional care playing a surprisingly small role, often mainly near the end of life (Spillman and Black 2005). This commitment of families to their older relatives has remained strong, despite all the changes that have taken place during the past half a century in family roles and relationships. Family carers provide this help, however, often at considerable risk to their own health and well-being. Studies have consistently found that providing care to a disabled elder is associated with increased rates of depression and other mental health symptoms (Aneshensel et al. 1995; Schulz et al. 1995). The health of carers can also suffer, either directly due to the stressors associated with care, or because carers do not take the time to attend to their own health needs (Schulz and Beach 1999).

In this chapter, we look at the adjustments and adaptations that occur within families caring for someone with dementia. We draw upon the research on caregiving, as well as our clinical experience and discussions with carers over the past 30 years. We consider both the main carer as well as other family members who provide a portion of the help. We examine the stressors and challenges carers experience, as well as the satisfactions and rewards of caring for a relative with dementia.

Caregiving stressors and their impact

Much of the focus of research on caring has been on stressors and their consequences. Examination of stressors has been guided by a "stress and coping" framework (Lazarus and Folkman 1984; Pearlin et al. 1990). From this perspective, stressful events lead to a mobilization of psychological and social resources for managing or coping with these events and their consequences. In the case of caregiving, stressors are not one-off events but are ongoing. How much impact particular stressors will have on carers' lives is influenced by:

- the meanings that people give to events
- their beliefs about their ability to manage the events
- the skills and resources they have

From our clinical experience we know that for some carers even mild perturbations can overwhelm their poor coping resources, while other people can take on an exhausting routine without much difficulty. Of course, symptoms of dementia worsen over time, which can diminish the carer's coping resources. As discussed in Chapter 14, when people are unable to contain the effects of stressors, they will experience anxiety, depression or other psychological distress. Chronic stress also affects the body's hormonal and immune systems, and these changes can lead to an increased vulnerability to disease (Vitaliano et al. 2003).

Caregiving stressors can be divided into two main types: primary stressors or those events and challenges directly related to their relative's illness; and secondary stressors, the ways in which primary stressors may interfere with the carer's other roles, involvements, and activities (Pearlin et al. 1990; Aneshensel et al. 1995).

Primary caregiving stressors

Primary stressors fall into three categories:

- changes in the person's cognition and abilities
- behavioural and emotional changes
- changes in the relationship between the carer and person with dementia, including a sense of loss

Cognition and day-to-day abilities

Changes in cognition and abilities include being able to look after oneself and to initiate and engage in activities. We have observed that initially families typically respond to memory lapses with commonsense approaches that worked in the past, such as giving reminders or encouraging the person to remember on his or her own, but these strategies have limited utility for people experiencing dementia-related progressive memory loss. For example, people with dementia may ask where their mother is, even though their mother may have died 20 or 30 years earlier. They may be concerned that their purse or wallet was stolen. In response, families often contradict the person with dementia, saying: "I've already told you your mother died 20 years ago" or "No one stole your wallet, it's under your bed." While attempting to resolve their relative's concern, carers frequently ignite an argument instead.

Instead of trying to reason with or reorient the person with dementia, we encourage carers to take a two-step approach (Zarit and Zarit 2007):

- think about why their relative would behave in this way
- think about what their relative might be feeling

For example, we encourage carers to consider why their relative would ask to see their mother. For one thing, the request suggests that the person's cognitive impairment is severe enough that he does not remember that his mother is dead. Presenting the fact that she is dead can sometimes produce a grief reaction. We suggest that it is better to focus on the underlying feeling – what emotions might underlie the request to see one's mother? The person may be seeking comfort and reassurance. A carer can respond by providing comfort, rather than directly challenging the request, for example, stating: "Let's sit down and have a cup of tea and talk about your mother." In other words, carers need to learn not to argue over the facts of a situation, but instead to identify and respond to the feelings that are embedded in these communications, and to provide comfort or reassurance, when needed (see Chapter 12).

As memory problems and other cognitive difficulties worsen, people with dementia gradually require assistance with a variety of daily tasks, as well as supervision to make sure that they do not get into difficulty, for example, by getting lost. Another complex area to negotiate is driving (Breen et al. 2007). Providing help with personal care can be problematic for some carers. Persons with dementia may resist help, insisting they can look after themselves, or in other ways be uncooperative. In late-stage dementia, care may become physically challenging for carers, as persons with dementia may need help with transfers from bed to chair, and chair to standing.

An often overlooked problem is that people with dementia become increasingly unable to initiate or sustain meaningful activities on their own (Perrin and May 1999). The lack of activity, combined with taking frequent naps during the day, can lead to a variety of other problems, including restlessness and not sleeping at night.

Behavioural and emotional changes

Behaviour and emotional disturbances are typically experienced as the most stressful events by carers (Aneshensel et al. 1995). These problems, which constitute the second area of primary stressors, are called the behavioural and psychological symptoms of dementia (BPSD) (Finkel *et al.* 1996; see Chapter 11). These symptoms can include depressive symptoms, agitation and restlessness, angry or aggressive actions, and hallucinations and delusions. They also include problems discussed above, such as resisting help and problems sleeping at night.

Carers can feel helpless in the face of behavioural problems, a reaction that is reinforced by physicians who too often have limited knowledge of the strategies that are helpful. Medications, though sometimes useful, can have significant adverse effects (Ballard and Cream 2005). As an alternative or to complement medications, carers can learn to use a simple behavioural management approach called "problem-solving" (Zarit and Zarit 2007). Carers learn to look for antecedent events, that is, triggers that lead to problem behaviour, and for consequences or how people respond to problems that can inadvertently reinforce problem behaviour. This approach has been empirically validated with various behavioural and sleep problems (Teri *et al.* 1997; McCurry *et al.* 2005).

Case example 13.1: A person with dementia becoming restless

A person with dementia might become restless after a long period of inactivity (the antecedent), and the restlessness would be reinforced by the attention that the carer gives to the person. In this case, carers could prevent restlessness by addressing the antecedent (i.e. inactivity) by engaging the person with dementia in meaningful activities. The carer could also direct attention (i.e. reinforcement) to the person with dementia at times when he or she is engaging in socially appropriate behaviour, in other words, reinforce adaptive rather than problem behaviour.

Relationship with carer

With improved diagnostic processes, early diagnosis of dementia is now common, which makes it possible to engage both the carer and the person with dementia in conversations about the illness and its implications (Clare 2002; Clare *et al.* 2002; Whitlatch *et al.* 2006; Reamy *et al.* 2011). These conversations can help the dyad to learn more about what lies ahead, and to begin making plans for the future. Carers also have the opportunity to hear about the preferences of the person with dementia. In turn, people with dementia who still have an awareness of their problem can talk about how they would like to be cared for without becoming overwhelmed or depressed. They may be able to help carers develop realistic plans by indicating that the carer does not have to provide all the help him or herself (Whitlatch *et al.* 2006). See Chapter 12.

Living with dementia can change the relationship between the person with dementia and his or her carer. As discussed in Chapter 21, carers may grieve or experience a sense of loss as their relative loses cognitive and functional abilities. Some carers may also lose the tangible benefits they received from the relationship. For a spouse, the relationship probably provided companionship, affection, and intimacy, as well as some division of labour around household tasks. Adult children may feel a loss of the support they received from a parent, including advice, assistance, and affection.

The carer's reactions to these changes depend partly on his or her past relationship with the person with dementia. When that relationship has been positive, the carer may feel a greater sense of loss, but also have a strong commitment to providing the needed care. A relationship that has been more conflicted often leaves carers feeling ambivalent. They may have a sense of obligation, but may also resent or be angry over being put in this position. Wives who become carers sometimes feel that they have been cheated out of the benefits of retirement, such as opportunities to travel, and instead they must reassume the roles of homemaker and carer that they have played their whole lives. Children who are carers may similarly struggle with the ambivalence they feel towards a parent. Long-standing dysfunctional relationships in the family will be carried forward into caregiving and complicate the process of giving care and receiving help from others.

Another important source of stress is that the contributions that the person with dementia made to the family system are lost. This loss can have a considerable impact, for example, when the person with dementia previously functioned as kin-keeper, bringing everyone else in the family together.

From our experience, carers need opportunities to address their feelings of grief, loss, and ambivalence (see Chapter 21). Carers who are grieving the loss of the person or their relationship with that person cannot do the planning needed or learn the skills that will help them manage other stressors effectively. They must first be able to get beyond their grief and reconceptualize their relationship with the person with dementia as one in which they have to take the initiative. Carers who do well are those who see themselves as maintaining continuity of the relationship through the help they are giving. Their role is an extension of the love and obligation they feel for the person with dementia, and they accept that these feelings cannot be reciprocated. Helping carers reach this understanding, of course, is not accomplished by pointing it out to them, but through open and non-judgemental discussions about the meaning the relationship holds for them and their goals in providing care.

In a similar fashion, carers who have ambivalent and conflicted feelings about providing care can benefit from opportunities to talk with a supportive person, such as a counsellor. These conversations can help carers realize that they have a choice in the matter. They may decide to continue to provide care, or they can set limits on the amount of help they are willing to provide. Helping carers restructure their commitment to a level that they are willing to make can reduce their ambivalence.

Exercise 13.1: Rating the stressfulness of care demands

For each category of primary stressors, i.e.

- changes in the person's cognition and abilities
- behavioural and emotional changes
- changes in the relationship between carer and person with dementia

do the following:

- Identify one or two problems that would be relatively easy for you to manage, and one or two problems that you would find very difficult or stressful to manage.
- For each problem, write down what makes it stressful or easy for you to manage.
- Review the reasons why you found some problems easy to manage and some problems stressful. What coping strategies could you use for managing the problems you found stressful?

Secondary stressors: changes in the carer's life

Secondary stressors include:

- the impact of caring on the carer's usual activities, including work and leisure
- conflict or strain in family relationships and friendships
- economic strains

The impact of caring on the carer's usual activities, including work and leisure

The increasing demands of caring can disrupt and absorb a carer's other roles and activities, leaving little time for anything except providing care. Leisure and social activities are often the first to go. Carers may give up these activities because the person with dementia can no longer participate, or because of embarrassing or socially inappropriate behaviour. Friends and relatives may feel uncomfortable around the person with dementia and decrease contact.

Not surprisingly, carers with more stress in their daily lives are less likely to engage in positive health behaviours (Son et al. 2007). They may no longer exercise regularly, may not eat a healthy diet, may increase smoking or alcohol use, or may not go to the doctor when they have a health problem.

Many carers continue to work outside the home. For them, daily routines are a continuing challenge, juggling multiple responsibilities and hoping that the care arrangements that they have made for their relative will continue to be adequate. For some carers, however, working is associated with positive experience (Aneshensel et al. 1995; Zarit et al. 2013). Going to work gives carers time away from the person with dementia, as well as leading to positive experiences and the feeling that they can accomplish something.

The carers that we have known who successfully managed the challenges they faced maintained significant activities apart from the person with dementia. One man who was caring for his wife worked for many years as a volunteer at a local radio station. The enjoyment and recognition he received from this weekly show helped carry him through the rest of the week.

Conflict or strain in family relationships and friendships

Tensions among siblings or between parents and their children add considerable stress to the primary carer (Aneshensel et al. 1995) and, in the end, erode the family's ability to provide care. Families may argue over whether care is needed, how it should be provided, and if people are contributing their fair share. Resentment can even develop over which one of them is helping, as shown in case examples 13.2 and 13.3.

Case example 13.2: Lesley

Lesley was the younger of the two children in her family. Her brother was an international businessman, who travelled extensively and was rarely at home. Their mother had doted upon him when he was a child. Their father had died in his early sixties. When their mother began to show signs of dementia, Lesley sought help from the local public agency that provides help to older people. Her mother's financial resources were modest, and she qualified for some public help. Her brother, whose main contact with his mother was over the telephone, questioned the need for help, since she sounded fine to him when they talked. As the dementia progressed, there were repetitions of the following scenario. The brother would fly into town, spend time in the family home with their mother, and then declare that she was "just fine" and that she did not need help. Of course, he was not listening carefully to the emptiness of her responses to him, nor did he challenge her memory at all. Instead, he talked about himself, and she smilingly listened to him, which was a pattern in their relationship all along.

Another family we have worked with had a similar pattern of sibling tensions.

Case example 13.3: Ruth

Ruth, the eldest of three children, took on the care of her mother. She had two siblings, a sister who lived in another part of the country, and a much younger brother who lived nearby. Ruth carefully researched her mother's problems and accompanied her to medical appointments. When the neurologist explained that her mother had dementia and would eventually need caretakers, Ruth initiated a family consultation with an elder law specialist, with all three children and her mother present. As her mother continued to deteriorate, the various provisions that had been agreed upon with the attorney were invoked, but at each step the two younger children opposed them. Ruth's brother did not see the need to pay for help in the home. He visited his mother frequently, but he minimized her problems until she was so far into her dementia that she could not live alone at all. The out-of-town sister was actually a nurse but she, too, minimized her mother's problems. After their mother ended up in a personal care home for dementia patients, she would swoop in, criticize the care, make the staff defensive and agitated, then leave for another several months. After several years of this pattern of interactions, the relationships among the three children were severely strained.

Exercise 13.2: Expectations about caring in your family

This exercise is designed to help you understand the expectations in your family about caring. You can do the exercise if you are already in a caring relationship or in a hypothetical way if you are not.

1. Identify a person in your family currently receiving care, or an older relative who might need care in the future.
2. Identify the people in that individual's immediate family. These could include a spouse, children (including sons-in-law and daughters-in-law), grandchildren, and anyone else who has a close relationship to the older person.
3. For each person, including yourself, write down the strengths and limitations of that person as a primary carer.
4. Who is, or who would probably become, the primary carer for this person? Why would that person be selected?
5. Review the strengths of everyone in the family network, and highlight those strengths that would be helpful to the primary carer.

At this point, you have a plan for drawing on the available resources within the family network. This plan can help the main carer share the demands and responsibilities. Families often have long-standing points of conflict or tension, but it is possible to focus on what each person can contribute, rather than on limitations.

Although families can be a source of strain, the assistance they provide may make the situation bearable for many carers (Aneshensel *et al*. 1995). Besides kin, carers may receive help from friends, neighbours, and other informal helpers. Assistance may be tangible, such as staying with the person with dementia, or it may involve emotional support, for example, having an understanding person to talk with in person or on the phone.

Support, however, is not always forthcoming. As noted, there can be conflict in the family over what help is needed and who should provide it. Some family and friends offer only advice and criticism. Often, friends and family wait to be asked to assist, or do not realize that the carer needs help. And finally, some carers have difficulty asking for the help that they need, or think that help should be forthcoming without their having to ask. All of these scenarios have the same result – the carer ends up up providing most of the help, and feeling isolated and unsupported by family and friends.

The example in case example 13.4 describes problems that can develop around giving and receiving assistance.

Case example 13.4: Marie

Marie had a mild vascular dementia when she and Phil moved back to her home town to be near her sister, Connie. As Marie's dementia progressed, Phil tried the medications that the neurologist prescribed for her memory problems, but Connie was very critical of this decision. She had worked in a doctor's office and she did not "believe" in taking medication. She also thought that Phil was just using the medication to keep Marie docile. Tension developed between Connie and Phil, which was very upsetting to Marie.

Phil did a heroic job of keeping Marie independent in her activities of daily living (ADL), encouraging her and never accepting "I can't do it" as an answer. Consequently, she surprised even her doctors with how much she continued to do for herself. But Phil had great difficulty accepting the fact the Marie could not control her symptoms. He thought that she should try harder to remember and that if she had a more positive attitude, she would be able to do more. Even as her memory deteriorated, Phil held onto a belief that she could remember if he reminded her enough times, or if she would just rehearse things more. He would get frustrated and impatient and raise his voice at her, which in turn would cause her to cry.

The solution came from an outside source. One of the carers that Phil hired to help with Marie's physical care was a retired nurse who developed a true fondness for her patients. She spent enough time with Marie, Phil, and Connie to observe all of the dynamics, and then took it upon herself to teach Marie to be assertive with both of them. She taught Marie that when Phil started to raise his voice, she should put her index finger to her lips and say, "Shhh", and that was the signal to him that he was too loud and he was upsetting her. Similarly, Marie learned to tell Connie that while she appreciated her concern, she was going to let her doctors decide which medications she should take. And with enough reminders, Marie was able to do just that.

As another source of misunderstandings and conflict over care and support, we pioneered the use of family meetings (Zarit and Zarit 1982, 2007; Zarit et al. 1985). The family meeting brings together everyone involved or who could potentially be involved in care. Goals are to address the current care needs of the person with dementia and answer everyone's questions about care. A counsellor leads the family meeting, answering questions about dementia and helping carers discuss what help could be of assistance. The counsellor also avoids focusing on old conflicts and instead directs the conversation to what can be done to help both the person with dementia and his or her carer. Solutions emerge from the family, who will come up with a plan for helping, once they have a better understanding of the carer's needs.

Economic strain

Finally, caregiving may place considerable economic strain on the family. The carer or, in some instances, the person with dementia, may leave the workforce, decreasing the income available. Medical and care-related expenses may place an increasing burden on the family budget. Tensions can flare up when the carer expects children or siblings to pay a portion of the cost for care, but they are unwilling. If the person with dementia has financial assets, children may argue about the proper ways of using the money. Some children see their parents' estate as their rightful inheritance, and resent using assets to pay for care. If one or more of the children has financial pressures of their own and may have been dependent on the parent for assistance, they may continue to try to divert money for their own needs.

Case example 13.5: Lesley (Continued)

Lesley did not have a large income herself, but assumed much of the financial burden of paying for home helpers in order to keep her mother in the family home as long as possible. Her brother had a much higher income, but contributed very little. Lesley did not resent spending the money, and did not really see any other choice. In some ways, she found compensation in how her mother responded to the care she gave. As her mother's dementia progressed and her brother visited less and less frequently, Lesley began receiving the attention she had always craved from her mother. Her mother enjoyed spending time with her and no longer compared her unfavourably to her brother.

Caring for a relative at the end of life

Perhaps the most challenging situation for families is the decisions they must make at the end of their relative's life (see Chapter 20). The emotional burden is especially great when the dying person has dementia or other cognitive impairment. In that case, unless that person has written an advance directive or communicated his or her preferences, the family must guess about what their relative would have wanted. Before we examine the issues that families face, conduct Exercise 13.3 in which you examine your own preferences and values.

Exercise 13.3: Planning your end-of-life directive

For this exercise, plan your own advance directive for end-of-life care, addressing each of the following points:

1. What would you want to emphasize, prolonging life at any cost or maintaining your comfort?
2. If your condition were terminal, would you want to use any of these medical devices?

- feeding tube
- intravenous hydration
- respirator

3. What regimen of pain medication would you prefer: maximum dosage even though it might impair cognition, or minimal dosage to preserve awareness, but not fully control your pain?

4. Would you want heroic efforts to be made on your behalf, such as a surgical procedure, even though it would prolong life only a short while longer?

Although some people with dementia die during the early and middle stages of the disease, others live to a point where illness has caused massive impairment. Patients gradually lose their ability to communicate verbally so that little or no conversation is possible, and they often have trouble recognizing familiar people. They also become increasingly frail, and may end up spending most or all of their time in bed. They are prone to infections, injury, and aspirating food.

Late-stage care poses four main challenges to the family:

- grappling with the definition of quality of life for the person with dementia
- deciding how to respond to the various medical crises that will arise
- deciding on the location for late-stage care
- finding closure

Quality of life for the person with dementia

With limited verbal communication, pleasure and discomfort often have to be discerned from non-verbal signs (see Chapter 27). Care at this stage should emphasize keeping the person comfortable and, to the extent possible, free from pain and other sources of discomfort. People at this stage of their life value contact with the people with whom they have been close, such as a spouse or child, even though it may not always be apparent that they recognize those people.

Deciding how to respond to the various medical crises that arise

In an optimal situation, the person with dementia would have previously prepared a living will and discussed it with the main carer long before the onset of the disease. When the patient's wishes about end-of-life decisions are well known, the choices for the family are simpler, although not without potential hazards. One dilemma for the family is in understanding the implications of the choices they are asked to make when there is a medical problem. A physician may present an intervention such as the use of an intravenous tube for hydration as addressing an immediate problem, yet it may be difficult to stop the procedure once it has been started. Thus, the person who did not want life prolonged artificially may now be headed down that pathway. In a way, the family need to decide something that physicians cannot tell them, that is, when the time has come to let go, so that they do not authorize further treatment. This decision becomes much harder when the person with dementia has not left a living will, or any other clear directives. The other dilemma is that whether or not there is a living will, some family members may dispute the decisions that the main carer makes. Often, the child or other relative who is pushing to prolong life at any cost hangs on to the belief that a cure will be found that restores the person to health. This type of conflict is very distressing for the primary carer.

Choosing the location for care for relatives with dementia at the end of their life

Some carers keep their relative at home through the whole course of the disease. They have observed that care gets easier in some ways when the person with dementia is no longer mobile. With some help in the home, they find they are able to provide highly personal care at the end of life. Institutions also provide care for people at the end of life. As with the traditional hospice, the emphasis is on comfort, not intervention. The staff in a good care facility will also be comfortable with letting a medical crisis run its natural course if that has been the preference of the person with dementia, instead of rushing the person to the emergency room or insisting on invasive treatment.

Finding closure

Carers have been involved for years by the time the end comes. They can take pride in the many ways they made the person's life better, and reminisce about the good times they spent together before the illness.

Satisfactions and rewards of caring

We have emphasized the challenges associated with care of people with dementia, but many carers report positive experiences or find their activities to be meaningful and satisfying. We have seen carers provide help at home for as long as 20 years, which is well past the time when most people would have given up. Our discussions with these carers suggest that they are not acting out of guilt, but rather they have made considerable sacrifice because of a genuine commitment to and affection for the person for whom they are caring.

Positive emotions in caring may be an important buffer against stress and lead to personal growth (Levesque *et al.* 1995; Robertson *et al.* 2007). Carers who experience positive emotions in the face of stressors are more likely to build resources and identify possible solutions to address the problems they are facing (Folkman 1997; Fredrickson and Joiner 2002). In case example 13.5, when Lesley talks about what gives her satisfaction in her life, that her mother is happy is always the first thing she mentions. Her mother no longer knows her name, but always gives her a big smile and is happy to see her.

Debates and controversies

What should the obligation of families and government be to help older people with dementia? The increase in the older population throughout Europe, North America, and parts of Asia raises a fundamental question of whether and to what extent government can afford to provide supportive services to families and, in turn, to what extent families will be expected to provide care for their older relatives. Should families be expected to help, either financially or by providing direct assistance? Should family help be a legal obligation? Or should families be guaranteed a certain level of support from government-funded programmes when they provide help to an older relative? Economic and demographic pressures suggest that these questions may be re-examined, even in countries that previously made a commitment to provide extensive services to their older population. In Sweden, for example, economic factors led to cutbacks in services to older people, which have shifted some types of assistance back to the family (Sundström *et al.* 2002). Should families be obliged that way to give care, or should help be completely voluntary?

How should we weigh the welfare of the carer with that of the person with dementia? As documented in this and other chapters in the book, there is extensive evidence that the interests of the carer and the person with dementia diverge. Carers' health and well-being often improves if they turn the care over to an institution, while the older person will usually function better at home (Aneshensel *et al.* 1995). Should public policy and the efforts of clinicians favour one person over the other? If a carer makes the commitment to provide help, whatever the cost, should that person be supported, or should clinicians encourage giving up the carer role?

Conclusion

The role of families is critical in the care of persons with dementia. Not only do people with dementia need assistance with daily tasks, but because of their cognitive impairment they also require that someone look out for their best interests, whether in everyday decisions, medical care or financial management. We know that dementia care can be very stressful, leading to harmful effects on health and well-being. From our understanding of the family carer's experience, we can make some observations that can guide the development of programmes and services to help carers as well as the person with dementia. First, caregiving stress is multidimensional. There is no single measure of stress or burden that can tell us what we need to know about a particular family. Rather, whether for planning services or conducting research, we need to consider the multiple stressors associated with care. Second, carers are characterized by a great deal of individual variability. There is no one pattern of stressors or adaptation, and no normative patterns. Carers should not be encouraged to act or feel in a certain way because of our expectations that a particular type of adaptation is better. Rather, our goal should be to facilitate carers to find their own goals and make their own decisions. And third, towards that end, we can provide valuable information and tools for stress management that can help carers reach their goals more effectively, and thereby allow them to provide assistance for as long as they want without undue harm to themselves.

Further information

Carers UK is an organization of carers fighting for society and government to recognize the true value of carers' contribution to society, so that carers get the practical, financial, and emotional support they need. Their web site has information about policy and campaigns [http://www.carersuk.org/].

The Family Caregiver Alliance is a pioneer in the development of programmes and services for carers of people with dementia and other brain disorders. Their web site contains extensive information on a wide range of topics [https://www.caregiver.org/caregiver/jsp/home.jsp].

The National Alliance for Caregiving is a coalition of organizations in the USA that focuses on issues of family caregiving. Their web site includes useful survey data that document the extent of family involvement in caregiving, as well as resources for family carers [http://www.caregiving.org/].

References

Aneshensel, C.S., Pearlin, L.I., Mullan, J.T., Zarit, S.H. and Whitlatch, C.J. (1995) *Profiles in Caregiving: The Unexpected Career.* New York: Academic Press.

Ballard, C. and Cream, J. (2005) Drugs used to relieve behavioral symptoms in people with dementia or an unacceptable chemical cost?, *International Psychogeriatrics*, 17(1): 12–22.

Breen, D.A., Breen, D.P., Moore, J.W., Breen, P.A. and O'Neill, D. (2007) Driving and dementia: a clinical review, *British Medical Journal*, 334: 1365–9.

Clare, L. (2002) We'll fight it as long as we can: coping with the onset of Alzheimer's disease, *Aging and Mental Health*, 6(2): 139–48.

Clare, L., Wilson, B.A., Carter, G. and Hodges, J.R. (2002) Relearning face–name associations in early Alzheimer's disease, *Neuropsychology*, 16(4): 538–47.

Finkel, S.I., Costa de Silva, J., Cohen, G., Miller, S. and Sartorius, N. (1996) Behavioural and psychological signs and symptoms of dementia: a consensus statement on current knowledge and implications for research and treatment, *International Psychogeriatrics*, 8 (Suppl. 3): 497–500.

Folkman, S. (1997) Positive psychological states and coping with severe stress, *Social Science and Medicine*, 45(8), 1207–21.

Fredrickson, B.L. and Joiner, T. (2002) Positive emotions trigger upward spirals toward emotional well-being, *Psychological Sciences*, 13(2): 172–5.

Lazarus, R.S. and Folkman, S. (1984) *Stress, Appraisal, and Coping*. New York: Springer.

Levesque, L., Cossette, S. and Laurin, L. (1995) A multidimensional examination of the psychological and social well-being of caregivers of a demented relative, *Research on Aging*, 17(3): 332–60.

McCurry, S.M., Gibbons, L.E., Logsdon, R.G., Vitiello, M.V. and Teri, L. (2005) Nighttime insomnia treatment and education for Alzheimer's disease: a randomized controlled trial, *Journal of the American Geriatrics Society*, 53(5): 793–802.

Pearlin, L.I., Mullan, J.T., Semple, S.J. and Skaff, M.M. (1990) Caregiving and the stress process: an overview of concepts and their measures, *The Gerontologist*, 30(5): 583–94.

Perrin, T. and May, H. (1999) *Well-being and Dementia: An Occupational Approach for Therapists and Carers*. Edinburgh: Churchill Livingstone.

Reamy, A.M., Kim, K., Zarit, S.H. and Whitlatch, C.J. (2011) Understanding discrepancy in perceptions of values: individuals with mild to moderate dementia and their family caregivers, *The Gerontologist*, 51: 473–82.

Robertson, S.M., Zarit, S.H., Duncan, L.G., Rovine, M. and Femia, E.E. (2007) Family caregivers' patterns of positive and negative affect, *Family Relations*, 56: 12–23.

Schulz, R. and Beach, S.R. (1999) Caregiving as a risk factor for mortality: the caregiver health effects study, *Journal of the American Medical Association*, 282(3): 2215–19.

Schulz, R., O'Brien, A.T., Bookwala, T. and Fleissner, K. (1995) Psychiatric and physical morbidity effects of dementia caregiving: prevalence, correlates, and causes, *The Gerontologist*, 35(6): 771–91.

Son, J., Erno, A., Shea, D.G., Femia, E.E., Zarit, S.H. *et al.* (2007) The caregiver stress process and health outcomes, *Aging and Health*, 19(6): 871–87.

Spillman, B.C. and Black, K.J. (2005) *Staying the Course: Trends in Family Caregiving*. Washington, DC: AARP Public Policy Institute.

Sundström, G., Johansson, L. and Hassing, L. (2002) The shifting balance of care in Sweden, *The Gerontologist*, 42(3): 350–5.

Teri, L., Logsdon, R.G., Uomoto, J. and McCurry, S.M. (1997) Behavioral treatment of depression in dementia patients: a controlled clinical trial, *Journals of Gerontology B: Psychological Sciences and Social Sciences*, 52(4): 159–66.

Vitaliano, P.P., Zhang, J. and Scanlan, J.M. (2003) Is caregiving hazardous to one's physical health? A meta-analysis, *Psychological Bulletin*, 129(6): 946–72.

Whitlatch, C.J., Judge, K., Zarit, S.H. and Femia, E.E. (2006) A dyadic intervention for family caregivers and care receivers in early stage dementia, *The Gerontologist*, 46: 688–94.

Zarit, S.H. and Zarit, J.M. (1982) Families under stress: interventions for caregivers of senile dementia patients, *Psychotherapy: Theory, Research and Practice*, 19(4): 461–71.

Zarit, S.H. and Zarit, J.M. (2007) *Mental Disorders in Older Adults*, 2nd edn. New York: Guilford Press.

Zarit, S.H., Orr, N.K. and Zarit, J.M. (1985) *The Hidden Victims of Alzheimer's Disease: Families Under Stress*. New York: New York University Press.

Zarit, S.H., Kim, K., Femia, E.E., Almeida, D.M. and Klein, L.C. (2013) The effects of adult day services on family caregivers' daily stress, affect and health: outcomes from the Daily Stress and Health (DaSH) Study, *The Gerontologist* [DOI: 10.1093/geront/gnt045].

CHAPTER 14

Supporting cognitive abilities

Jan Oyebode and Linda Clare

66 I have a diary. I've always had a diary. I have a daily diary. What I've done through the day. I can look at what happened yesterday and then pull that back. It brings the day back. Otherwise I can't remember and I don't know what I've done today. So I read the diary and then Oh yes, that's right, and that was lovely. Otherwise it's just empty. 99

—Sheila Varo Yorkshire, UK

66 It's embarrassing and just humiliating. If you were on your own, you would just sink. 99

—Jenny Reid Melbourne, Australia

66 I have to learn how to do things that I used to be able to do without thinking! 99

—Tony Oates Yorkshire, UK

Learning objectives

By the end of this chapter, you will:

- Be aware of factors that affect the choice of strategies for supporting cognitive functioning
- Know about the major domains of cognitive functioning and how impairment in each might affect a person's day-to-day functioning
- Be aware of the three major types of cognitive intervention – cognitive stimulation, cognitive training and cognitive rehabilitation, and the level of evidence for their effectiveness
- Be able to plan cognitive stimulation sessions to suit people from a variety of backgrounds
- Know about the steps involved in developing a cognitive rehabilitation intervention
- Know about the different strategies (internal and external, compensatory and restorative) that can be used to enhance memory functioning

Introduction

Managing life with increasing cognitive impairment is at the centre of adapting to living with dementia. Damage to cognitive functions often starts with memory impairment, and progressively widens to other cognitive functions and worsens. As a consequence, over time a person with dementia will experience increasing problems in many aspects of everyday functioning, thus impairing independence and making social functioning difficult. Loss of memory means that the person's sense of identity and sense of self are threatened. The person may have limited awareness and understanding of their situation. Some of the internal resources the person might formerly have used to cope are depleted by the dementia. Given this, it is evident that, as time goes by, those with dementia will require increasing assistance and support with aspects of life that depend on cognitive functioning.

This chapter considers how service providers can support the person with dementia, and those close to him or her, in managing increasing intellectual impairment. The goal is to enable individuals with dementia to function to their maximum capacity, giving them more efficient and effective ways of using their remaining cognitive capacity, eroding any excess disability that has arisen through lack of opportunity or loss of confidence, and enabling effective use of external environmental support.

Several ways exist of intervening to address intellectual functioning. We outline here the drugs that aim to enhance cognitive functioning as well as the three main direct psychosocial approaches of cognitive rehabilitation, cognitive stimulation, and cognitive training. Each of these approaches is supported at least to some extent by research evidence. Interventions may involve working directly with the person with dementia and their family or, when the person is living in supported housing or a care home, intervention may be through staff.

This chapter is not focused solely on cognitive interventions. To achieve a positive outcome, any intervention needs to consider the wider context, as well as the person's cognitive capacity. This chapter therefore situates work on cognitive functioning within a holistic framework, enabling interventions that directly target cognitive problems to be understood as part of wider person-centred and relationship-centred care.

Contextual factors affecting choice of strategies for supporting intellectual functioning

The degree of awareness, the person's coping style, and the availability of social support affect whether work to address difficulties can be carried out directly with the individual or whether it would be more effective to work with or through others. Each of these factors is briefly considered below.

Awareness

Awareness refers to the accuracy with which people judge aspects of their own situation and level of functioning, including their cognitive functioning and any associated difficulties. Where there is a specific issue causing concern that might become the focus of an intervention, the professional needs to explore the person's awareness of that area in particular. People with dementia vary in the degree of awareness of their memory functioning from being fully aware to having limited awareness (Clare 2004a).

Case example 14.1: Mrs. Patel and Mr. Squires

Mrs. Patel goes to her GP concerned about her tendency to be increasingly forgetful and provides examples of forgetting appointments. She demonstrates a high level of awareness. Mrs. Patel might welcome the opportunity to develop strategies for addressing these difficulties. This contrasts markedly with Mr. Squires, who repeatedly loses items and accuses his wife of hiding them. In the latter case, it is his wife who goes to the doctor to express her concern. This situation suggests a possible lack of awareness that would make it more difficult to work directly with Mr. Squires.

To explain the person's level of awareness, we need to take a bio-psycho-social approach (Clare 2004b) (see Chapter 8). When a person lacks awareness, this may result from his or her social context, personal reactions or cognitive impairment *per se*. Consideration of biological, psychological, and social factors may provide ideas for how to raise awareness.

Case example 14.2: Mrs. Brown and Mr. Williams

Mrs. Brown is making constant errors but her husband Mr. Brown constantly covers up for her. This protection adds to her lack of awareness about the errors she is making. It may be possible to discuss with Mr. Brown the costs and benefits of providing more honest feedback to his wife. Mr. Williams, on the other hand, has recently become increasingly forgetful but refuses to discuss the subject when his daughter brings it up, denying that he ever forgets things. His apparent lack of awareness may actually be denial, caused by embarrassment. Providing a chance to talk about how he is managing with a professional, without his daughter present, may be a way of helping him save face.

Coping

People with dementia have been described as using ways of coping that fall on a continuum from *self-maintaining* to *self-adjusting* (Clare 2002). Clare reported that those with a self-maintaining position aimed to continue to live life in their usual way without necessarily absorbing the notion of having dementia into their identity, whereas those with self-adjusting ways of coping were more willing to accommodate dementia into their identity. A person with a more self-adjusting style might be more willing to take part in open discussion of their difficulties, whereas a person with a self-maintaining style might be more defensive, though possibly still willing to put effort into employing memory aids or trying memory strategies if this could help them maintain their usual way of life and avoid the risk of exposing their difficulties to others.

Social context

A final contextual factor to consider is the person's social network (see Chapter 8). Care and intervention are provided through relationships, whether with relatives (see Chapters 13 and 21) or with paid carers (see Allan and Killick). The knowledge, resources, and feelings of these carers need to be considered. In designing interventions, it is necessary to pay attention to how much energy and time it is feasible for them to commit. Collaboratively designed interventions will have a better chance of success than those formulated by expert professionals alone.

If an intervention needs to rely on others, then their understanding of the situation and their ways of coping will be important.

Case example 14.3: Mr. Baytree

Mr. Baytree has memory loss that leads him to keep asking the same questions. His wife, Mrs. Baytree, feels that he is asking the same thing repeatedly not because of cognitive impairment but to annoy her. Mrs. Baytree could be given further information about the impact of memory loss that would help her to understand and have patience with Mr. Baytree. Such work would need to be undertaken before she could be enlisted to help in finding ways of addressing the asking of repeated questions.

In this section of the chapter, we have outlined why the person's awareness, coping, and social context are important to consider when thinking about how to support cognitive functioning in someone with dementia. It is suggested that at this point you use the information from this section to consider the position of Mrs. Margery Gubbins, who is described in Exercise 14.1.

Exercise 14.1: Identifying contextual influences

Mrs. Margery Gubbins is a 76-year-old woman who lives at home with her husband, Roy. He has noticed that Margery has recently had difficulty with some everyday tasks. She seems to buy washing-up liquid every time she goes shopping so that they now have six unused bottles in their kitchen cupboard. He got quite cross about this but she said it would be useful if there was a shortage. More recently, he found a bottle hidden in their medicine cabinet. She seems to keep starting shopping lists but doesn't finish them or forgets to take them with her. She recently came home without her shopping and it turned out that she had forgotten to take her purse. She said it was Roy's fault for taking it out of her handbag. Their grown-up son recently bought them a new washing machine but Margery cannot seem to learn to use it. She says all these modern appliances have complicated instructions. Roy does not want his son to think he has bought something too hard for Margery to use, and so has not told him she is having problems with it. He thinks his son means well, but he would rather he came over and took them out from time to time rather than keep buying them things. Apart from these issues, Roy has noticed that Margery is not being as sociable as usual and seems to look for excuses not to go to the club where they would usually meet their friends. He has been trying to persuade her to go for a check-up at the doctor's as he thinks this is a developing problem, but Margery says it is only to be expected that someone her age will occasionally forget things and in any case, nothing could be done to improve her memory even if it is faulty.

Consider the above information and complete the following:

- List three things that may indicate that Margery has some awareness of her memory problems.
- List four ways of coping that Margery is using. Would you say these are predominantly self-maintaining or self-adjusting?
- List three sources of actual or potential social support for Margery.

The nature of cognitive impairments in dementia

This section provides a brief overview of ways of understanding cognitive functioning in dementia.

Domains of cognitive functioning

Cognitive functioning can be divided into several domains, each of which contributes to effective cognitive functioning. The different cognitive functions vary in their importance in relation to different activities. The major domains are shown and defined in Table 14.1.

Which domain to focus on when considering cognitive interventions

In Alzheimer's disease, the most common form of dementia, memory is usually the first function to be affected. People with Alzheimer's disease have difficulty developing new long-term memories.

Domain	Abilities subsumed	Everyday impact if impaired
Executive functions	Initiation of ideas and actions	Apathy
	Switching of ideas and actions	Perseveration
	Planning and monitoring of ideas and actions	Impulsive behaviour or actions not addressed in a logical sequence
Attention and concentration	Focusing on and sustaining attention to pertinent aspects of the environment	Distractibility
	Dividing attention as necessary between tasks	Concentrating on one task to exclusion of another, e.g. attending to doorbell and forgetting tap running in kitchen
Memory	Encoding new material	No new memories formed
	Storing memories	Recent events forgotten
	Recalling memories as necessary	Inability to recall events or names as needed
Language	Understanding what is said (i.e. receptive language)	Misunderstanding of conversations or instructions
	Being able to use words to express oneself (i.e. expressive language)	Lack of ability to express self verbally to others.
	Understanding written language	"Challenging behaviour" may occur as a form of communication
	Writing	Fails to understand labels, instructions, etc.
		Fails to fill out forms, write cards, etc.
Visuospatial skills	Being able to identify objects	Misidentifies objects, e.g. unable to recognize a plate or a toilet seat
	Being able to recognize faces	Unable to find objects
	Being able to perceive orientation and positioning of objects in three-dimensional space	Lack of recognition of people
		Lack of recognition of things
Psychomotor skills	Being able to manipulate objects singly or in relation to each other	Problems with activities such as dressing, brushing teeth, using a knife and fork
	Being able to fit parts together to make a whole	
	Being able to string together a series of actions	
Social and emotional intelligence	Understanding social cues	Engages in socially unacceptable and uncharacteristic behaviour, causing offence or embarrassment to others
	Being able to put oneself in another's position	
	Having empathy for others	

Table 14.1 Major domains of cognitive functioning and the impact of impairment on everyday life

This is partly due to a difficulty in encoding, or laying down, new memories (Morris 2008). Interventions targeting coping with memory difficulties, and especially encoding, therefore have particular importance in early dementia. Addressing them can have a major beneficial impact on the person's day-to-day life. In addition, attention, concentration, executive function, and word-finding may also be affected in the early stages, so these may also be early targets.

The pattern and progression of changes across domains varies between types of dementia (see Chapter 1), and this demands careful assessment and a focus on other areas for those with different diagnoses. Social cognition, for example, may be affected early in fronto-temporal dementia and so may be a particular focus where this is the diagnosis.

As cognitive impairment spreads to affect a greater range of cognitive domains, new problems are likely to emerge and therefore the appropriate focus of intervention may change. In moderate dementia, in the face of difficulty with tasks and activities, the person with dementia may withdraw and develop "excess disability" – that is, disability that is greater than that warranted by the cognitive impairment alone. The focus may then be on providing an appropriately stimulating and enriching environment and maintaining practical skills and engagement in conversation (see Chapters 2 and 17). As dementia progresses, it also becomes more likely that cognitive impairment, being more widespread and severe, will lead to emotional reactions and behaviours that can be distressing for the person and others close to them. For example, when people with dementia do not recognize their surroundings or are unable to engage with their environment, they may seek to leave where they are for somewhere that is more familiar. Finding ways to prevent this distress may also be an appropriate focus of cognitive interventions.

Identifying the cognitive domains that are impaired can help to explain why a particular problem has arisen and can therefore also suggest possible ways of intervening. Similarly, identifying relatively preserved cognitive domains can suggest resources that can be harnessed to find ways around difficulties. Both require knowledge of the person.

Case example 14.4: Mary

Mary is increasingly experiencing episodes of incontinence. Her disorientation for time may mean she forgets that she needs to visit the toilet, whereas spatial disorientation may mean she cannot find her way there. Visuospatial impairment may cause difficulties identifying the toilet and psychomotor problems (in this case as "apraxia") may impair manipulating her clothing. A timely prompt, a clearer sign on the toilet door, and a cognitive rehabilitation programme using rehearsal (see below) and simple adjustments to clothing may all help to avoid episodes of incontinence.

Interventions to support cognitive functioning

This section defines the main interventions that have been used to support cognitive functioning in people with dementia. It reviews evidence for their effectiveness and looks at ways of applying them in dementia care.

Anti-dementia drugs

Three drugs (donepezil, rivastigmine, and galantamine) have been shown, over a 6-month period, to produce small improvements in overall cognitive functioning, activities of daily living, and behaviour

Type	Definition	Aims
Cognitive training	Structured exercises that focus on practice of defined cognitive functions such as memory, visuospatial reasoning or problem-solving	To give sufficient practice to ensure that skills in particular cognitive domains are maintained or improved
Cognitive stimulation	Group activities centred on presentation and rehearsal of cognitive material in a social context	To reduce excess disability, rebuild self-esteem, and enhance general social and cognitive functioning
Cognitive rehabilitation	Bespoke goal-oriented intervention, based on knowledge of cognition and behaviour, which is applied directly in the real-life setting to address a particular difficulty	To improve quality of life and well-being through optimizing cognitive functioning in relation to everyday problems, and prevent or reduce excess disability

Table 14.2 Types of intervention to support cognitive functioning in people with dementia

in people with mild to moderate Alzheimer's disease, with some evidence that improvements are similar in individuals with severe dementia (see Birks 2006). They are collectively known as cholinesterase inhibitors (ChEIs) because they inhibit (i.e. delay) the breakdown of one of the brain chemicals (acetylcholine). This particular chemical is lost during Alzheimer's disease and the drugs enable the small amount that the brain still produces to work more effectively by enabling it to remain in the brain for longer.

It is important to note that ChEIs cannot be prescribed for many people with Down syndrome and dementia as they cannot be used with people who have heart or breathing problems, which are common in Down syndrome, and also it is not clear that they are of benefit to those in this population (Mohan *et al.* 2009).

A fourth drug, memantine, has been found to provide benefits in cognitive functioning and functional activities in people with moderate to severe Alzheimer's (NICE 2011). This works by a different mechanism associated with the reduction of glutamate (a brain chemical that causes brain damage).

In addition to drug treatments, there are a range of psychosocial interventions available to support people with dementia and their families (Olazaran *et al.* 2010), and some of these target cognitive functioning. These cognition-focused interventions can be divided into three main types: cognitive training, cognitive stimulation, and cognitive rehabilitation (Clare and Woods 2003/2007; Clare 2008). Each is described in Table 14.2, followed by a description of current research evidence for effectiveness.

Cognitive training

Cognitive training is based on the assumption that exercising cognitive functions in a particular cognitive domain will strengthen performance, either slowing deterioration or leading to a degree of improvement. An appropriate domain can be selected according to the needs of the person with dementia. The training may be offered through a number of modalities, such as pencil and paper exercises, computerized programs or analogues of everyday tasks, and through a number of settings, including one-to-one interaction with relatives or staff and in group settings.

Variability in the way cognitive training has been used makes its effectiveness hard to review. However, Clare (2008) provides a thorough discussion of studies evaluating individual and group cognitive training. The level of training that has been tested is fairly intense with typical studies involving 30–60 minute sessions delivered three to seven times per week by staff or relatives. Some studies have reported significant improvements in the areas specifically targeted; however, these benefits do not seem to generalize to wider aspects of daily life. Bahar-Fuchs and colleagues (2013) conducted a systematic review of RCTs of cognitive training and found 11 relevant studies in the field, adding three to their earlier reviews (Clare and Woods 2003/2007). The studies were evaluated as being of low to moderate quality rather than being of high quality, and no differences were found in outcomes for those in the cognitive training conditions versus those in the control conditions, who did not receive cognitive training. On this basis, we cannot say whether cognitive training has a positive impact for people with dementia.

Cognitive stimulation

In tune with the aim of general enhancement of cognitive and social functioning, cognitive stimulation encompasses reality orientation, which focuses predominantly on current time; reminiscence therapy, which focuses on past memories; activities that provoke thought, such as puzzles and word games; and activities that necessitate planning and activity, such as collage or baking. Reality orientation and reminiscence therapy are described in more detail below.

Reality orientation operates through the presentation of information about orientation for time, person, and place (Holden and Woods 1995). The assumption is that enabling someone to feel more orientated will increase well-being by providing anchors to the current environment and setting. The information is generally presented in a group setting and through various modalities. For example, participants may say the name of the day aloud, using prompting or cued recall if necessary, they may read and write it, and it may also be presented on a noticeboard in the general environment. Reality orientation has traditionally included other elements of orientation to the environment such as consideration of the weather, the season, and topical associations with it, such as daffodils in springtime, and the news. Where orientation information can be tangibly provided, members are encouraged to use all their senses, for example feeling, smelling, and tasting an apple as well as looking at it. In the USA, the early studies of reality orientation were conducted in a classroom to encourage pride in learning. In the UK, they were conducted in an informal setting, with a cup of tea provided, to encourage a relaxed atmosphere and social interaction. These differences indicate the need to adapt therapies in a culturally sensitive way that will encourage motivation and participation.

In contrast to reality orientation, reminiscence therapy focuses on past memories (see Chapter 15). Topics might relate to particular periods of life, life events or daily activities. So, for example, discussion might focus on playground games, or rituals of courting the opposite sex. Materials such as photographs, recordings or objects can often prompt memories. An old skipping rope with wooden handles might provoke richer memories than an abstract conversation.

A systematic review of 15 randomized controlled trials (RCTs) of cognitive stimulation (Woods *et al.* 2012) found significant benefits for individuals with mild to moderate dementia in cognition and memory, which lasted at follow-up of 1-3 months. Where people with dementia were consulted, they reported improved quality of life as a result of taking part, and staff reported improvements in communication and social interaction. One study trained relatives to provide cognitive stimulation, but the results were inconclusive.

Overall, the research findings suggest that it is worth providing sessions for individuals with mild to moderate dementia, initially more intensively but later continuing on a weekly basis.

Exercise 14.2: Cognitive stimulation

Outline a schedule for a cognitive stimulation session for each of the following groups:

- a group of Irish elders meeting in the spring
- a group of retired men in a rural area meeting in the summer
- a group of African Caribbean women meeting in the autumn
- a group of women over 65 years of differing backgrounds meeting in the winter

Each schedule should include:

- a symbol for group identity that can be drawn on the reality orientation board
- a non-cognitive warm-up exercise that will encourage group participation, and be acceptable to group members
- a reminiscence activity that will be enjoyable and relevant to the group as well as being cognitively stimulating, with a list of possible props to bring back memories
- an appropriate seasonal activity that will encourage multi-sensory stimulation

Cognitive rehabilitation

Although the term "rehabilitation" implies recovery of function, the main focus of cognitive rehabilitation in progressive conditions such as dementia is on optimizing remaining cognitive functioning, finding ways around difficulties, reducing their impact or helping someone to live more comfortably with their limitations. Cognitive rehabilitation does not aim to improve cognitive functioning in the sense of improving scores on cognitive tests, although such improvement might occur in some cases; instead, this approach aims to help people manage the impact of dementia on their everyday lives, and to reduce disability by identifying specific difficulties that have a cognitive basis and applying strategies derived from knowledge of cognition and behaviour to address these difficulties. The focus is on understanding and intervening in relation to *specific* aspects of everyday functioning (usually referred to as "goals") that are important to the person and those close to them. Given that the approach is centred on the person's unique needs, it fits well with the principles of person-centred dementia care.

In a review of 43 studies, Hopper *et al.* (2013) assessed the evidence for the effectiveness of cognitive rehabilitation. They concluded that evidence was gradually accumulating to show good outcomes from cognitive rehabilitation for people with mild to moderate dementia but that further development and testing of methods is needed. There have been no large-scale RCTs of cognitive rehabilitation, and most evidence is from smaller-scale studies and reports. A pilot RCT (Clare *et al.* 2013) compared participants who each received eight sessions of cognitive rehabilitation with control groups receiving the equivalent number of sessions of relaxation therapy or no treatment. The cognitive rehabilitation focused on individually relevant goals that were negotiated with each participant. Clare and colleagues found that compared with the control groups, those who took part in cognitive rehabilitation reported better performance on their selected goals. In addition, people with cognitive rehabilitation did better on measures of attention and memory, quality of

1	Determine whether the person is able or willing to indicate something that she or he would like to be different.
2	Identify the area to focus on – for example, memory problems, family relationships, participation in activities.
3	Identify the specific issue to focus on – for example, remembering the names of people met during an activity.
4	Establish the baseline level of performance.
5	Identify the goal in clear behavioural terms.
6	Identify the level of performance that will indicate that the goal has been wholly or (partially) achieved.
7	Plan the intervention to address the goal, using appropriate methods and techniques.
8	Implement the intervention.
9	Monitor progress and adjust the intervention as necessary.
10	Evaluate the outcome of the intervention and decide on any further steps that may be needed.

Source: Based on Clare (2008)

Table 14.3 Steps in cognitive rehabilitation

life and mood, than people in the other two groups. The carers of those who took part in cognitive rehabilitation also reported improved quality of life. This is therefore a promising intervention to help support people with dementia.

Examples of the principal techniques and their application are given below. There are a number of steps involved from setting appropriate feasible goals, through to assessment of outcome (see Table 14.3).

The first step is to work with the person with dementia and other key individuals to decide on a meaningful, potentially achievable goal. Goals selected by people with dementia and their families in our teams have included being able to take the correct number of tablets at the correct time, being able to use the remote control for the television, and being able to heat up meals using a microwave oven.

Where the person has more severe dementia and cannot provide consent, it is important to consult others and explicitly consider whether the proposed goal is in the person's best interest. For example, a goal to find ways of stopping Mrs. Jamieson from shouting might make for a more peaceful environment for staff and fellow residents but might deprive her of her only means of gaining social contact. In this case, it would be important to have a modified goal such as "to find a means for Mrs. Jamieson to gain social contact without shouting".

Once a clear and focused goal has been agreed upon, the professional needs to decide what sort of strategies or techniques may enable this to be achieved. These may be internal or external to the person with dementia. *Internal strategies*, often called "restorative" strategies, involve helping the person with dementia to optimize use of their own cognitive resources. *External strategies*, often called "compensatory" strategies, involve manipulation of the environment or the use of memory and cognitive aids.

Internal learning strategies that can be used to promote effective encoding into episodic memory and retrieval include (Clare 2008; Hopper *et al.* 2013):

- reducing the number of errors made during learning
- encouraging deep rather than superficial processing of the information
- practising remembering or re-learning facts, such as names, by rehearsing the answer a number of times at intervals (e.g. 10 seconds apart) – known as "spaced retrieval"

- encouraging encoding based on "doing" rather than "talking"
- encouraging encoding based on using several sorts of memory processes rather than one (e.g. visual, verbal and action memory; recognition and recall)

A focus on the external environment includes supporting memory and cognitive functioning through:

- the use of external memory aids and modern technologies
- life-history books and memory wallets
- the creative use of physical design

Use of external memory aids

External memory aids can be used to prompt appropriate action, convey information that otherwise would not be remembered, or trigger episodic memories that might be hard to access otherwise. Typical actions that may require prompting include taking tablets, preparing food, and remembering an appointment. Typical prompts might include diaries, notebooks, signs, buzzers or phone calls. The prompt needs to be *timely*, *specific*, and *accurate*.

Case example 14.5: Dennis

The buzzer that Dennis uses to remind him to take his tablets needs to go off at the moment the tablets need to be taken (timely); he needs to realize the buzzer is reminding him to take his tablets (specific); and it needs to be reset to buzz again when he needs to take the next dose (accurate).

Enlisting the help of others to ensure aids are up-to-date and timely makes their use more efficient. Where possible, it is best to adapt aids the person already uses. For example, if a person uses a board to list their shopping requirements in their kitchen, then its use might be expanded to include important appointments.

When new aids are introduced, a person is likely to need practice, using the internal strategies described above, to learn to use them.

Case example 14.6: A woman with dementia

A woman with dementia asked her husband repeatedly about the date, causing friction in their relationship. An intervention was introduced using prompts to look at a calendar rather than ask her husband. This simple aid, combined with practice in its use, led to a reduction in questioning and a reduction in tension in the relationship.

Source: Clare *et al.* (2000)

Modern technology has great potential to provide effective memory aids. Studies have looked at a range of devices that can support independent living, including: the use of electronic, computer-based devices that can give specific reminders (Baruch *et al.* 2004); devices to support sequences of activities (Orpwood *et al.* 2007); and devices to decrease risk due to forgetting, such as cooker and tap monitors (Orpwood *et al.* 2004). This is an area that will develop markedly in the future.

Life-history books and memory wallets

As you will see in Chapter 15, external reminders of past events can be helpful in reinforcing biographical memory. Life-story books, into which a person can paste reminders such as photos and postcards alongside diary-type entries, may be particularly helpful at a particular transition such as when a person moves from home into residential care. They also enable staff to have a feeling for the character and life of the person who is in their care. On a less grand scale, memory wallets containing pictures and photographs of personally relevant events and people can easily be carried in a handbag or pocket and can enhance memories and interactions between a person with dementia and others (Bourgeois 1992).

Physical design

Physical aspects of buildings can be used to support cognitive functioning, helping to reduce cognitive errors and to promote independence and orientation. Features that can be taken into account range from basic design through to décor, furnishings, and lighting. Although a detailed report on this area is outside the scope of this chapter, a good review is provided by Day *et al.* (2000).

In practice, a combination of internal strategies and external aids often works best.

Case example 14.7: A woman in a residential home

A woman living in a residential home became upset at not having her belongings and accused staff of taking them. A relative and staff worked with her to establish a list of some of her favourite things, indicating who she had given each to. She signed this list and it was made into an attractive poster for the wall of her room (an external aid). An intervention was used to teach her to go and look at the poster when she became concerned about the whereabouts of her possessions (encoding based on doing rather than talking). This was done by asking her: "What do you do when you worry about where your things have gone?" If she was unable to answer, she was given cues until she went to the poster (reducing the number of errors during learning). After regular practice, this response became well established, leading to the point where the worry in itself led the woman to go and look at the poster in order to know where her belongings were and feel settled again.

Source: Bird (2001)

Exercise 14.3: Designing a cognitive rehabilitation intervention

At the time of Exercise 14.1, Margery was having problems with her memory but was reluctant to openly acknowledge this or seek medical advice. Since that time, Margery has had a memory clinic assessment, which concluded that she has dementia. She has become a little more willing to accept that she has difficulties and is pleased to hear there may be some assistance available.

You meet Margery and her husband Roy to discuss areas that are stressful and find out where they might appreciate help. They say they wish she could still go shopping without buying the same item several times on successive trips, or forgetting to take her purse.

- Develop a plan for steps 2–7 of a cognitive rehabilitation programme (see Table 14.3 for steps) to address these issues.

Debates and controversies

Some might argue that focusing on improving and supporting cognitive functioning in people with dementia is putting effort into the wrong place. Progressive cognitive impairment is, after all, an inevitable consequence of having dementia. Trying to hold it back takes a lot of effort and is only likely to yield modest gains. It might be seen as more constructive to put our energies into supporting emotional functioning and adaptation so as to ensure that those with dementia "live well" with the condition.

However, we would argue that finding ways of enabling people with dementia to manage with the cognitive impairments that are core to the condition, can make a significant contribution to day-to-day functioning and hence self-esteem and well-being. Small gains in everyday functioning may make a great difference to people's lives as long as the effort is carefully targeted towards personally tailored, meaningful goals. We hope this chapter has convinced you that cognition-focused intervention and rehabilitation have a key place in excellent dementia care.

Conclusion

By drawing on research and practice in this chapter, we have attempted to demonstrate the place of drug therapy, cognitive training, cognitive stimulation, and cognitive rehabilitation in holistic person-centred care for people with dementia.

Cognitive stimulation involves engagement in a range of group activities and discussions aimed at generally enhancing cognitive and social functioning. Cognitive training involves systematic practice of standardized tasks focused on particular cognitive domains. Cognitive rehabilitation comprises the personally tailored application of strategies derived from knowledge of cognition and behaviour to address specific difficulties. There is a growing body of evidence to suggest that all these approaches have a positive impact.

Possibilities for cognitive interventions are influenced by a person's awareness, ways of coping, and social supports. A holistic assessment is therefore needed to inform any intervention. Furthermore, people vary in their cognitive strengths and weaknesses and a comprehensive assessment of cognitive functioning will therefore help to identify which preserved abilities to build on and which impaired functions to address or circumvent.

Further information

Clare, L. (2008) *Neuropsychological Rehabilitation and People with Dementia,* Hove: Psychology Press. This book provides a readable overview of the field.

http://www.cstdementia.com/: A web site about cognitive stimulation that is linked with the work of Dr. Aimee Spector, Professor Bob Woods, and Professor Martin Orrell, and includes links to manuals and information about training.

References

Bahar-Fuchs, A., Clare, L. and Woods, B. (2013) Cognitive training and cognitive rehabilitation for mild to moderate Alzheimer's disease and vascular dementia, *Cochrane Database of Systematic Reviews*, 6: CD003260.

Baruch, J., Downs, M., Baldwin, C. and Bruce, E. (2004) A case study in the use of technology to reassure and support a person with dementia, *Dementia*, 3: 372–7.

Bird, M. (2001) Behavioural difficulties and cued recall of adaptive behaviour in dementia: experimental and clinical evidence, *Neuropsychological Rehabilitation*, 11: 357–75.

Birks, J. (2006) Cholinesterase inhibitors for Alzheimer's disease, *Cochrane Database of Systematic Reviews*, 1: CD005593 [http://www.mrw.interscience.wiley.com/cochrane/clsysrev/articles/CD005593, accessed 9 August 2007].

Bourgeois, M. (1992) Evaluating memory wallets in conversations with persons with dementia, *Journal of Speech and Hearing Research*, 35: 1344–57.

Clare, L. (2002) We'll fight it as long as we can: coping with the onset of Alzheimer's disease, *Aging and Mental Health*, 6: 139–48.

Clare, L. (2004a) Awareness in early-stage Alzheimer's disease: a review of methods and evidence, *British Journal of Clinical Psychology*, 43: 77–96.

Clare, L. (2004b) The construction of awareness in early-stage Alzheimer's disease: a review of concepts and models, *British Journal of Clinical Psychology*, 43: 155–75.

Clare, L. (2008) *Neuropsychological Rehabilitation and People with Dementia*. Hove: Psychology Press.

Clare, L. and Woods, B. (2003/2007) Cognitive rehabilitation and cognitive training for early-stage Alzheimer's disease and vascular dementia, *Cochrane Database of Systematic Reviews*, 4: CD003260.

Clare, L., Wilson, B.A., Carter, G., Breen, K., Gosses, A. *et al.* (2000) Intervening with everyday memory problems in dementia of Alzheimer type: an errorless learning approach, *Journal of Clinical and Experimental Neuropsychology*, 22: 132–46.

Clare, L., Linden, D., Woods, R.T., Whitaker, R., Evans, S. *et al.* (2013) Goal-oriented cognitive rehabilitation for people with early stage Alzheimer's disease: a single-blind randomised controlled trial of efficacy, *American Journal of Geriatric Psychiatry*, 18: 928–39.

Day, K., Carreon, D. and Stump, C. (2000) The therapeutic design of environments for people with dementia: a review of the empirical research, *The Gerontologist*, 40: 417–21.

Holden, U. and Woods, R.T. (1995) *Positive Approaches in Dementia Care* (3rd edn.). Edinburgh: Churchill Livingstone.

Hopper, T., Bourgeois, M., Pimental, J., Qualis, C., Hickey, E. *et al.* (2013) An evidence-based systematic review on cognitive interventions for individuals with dementia, *American Journal of Speech-Language Pathology*, 22: 126–45.

Mohan, M., Carpenter, P.K. and Bennett, C. (2009) Donepezil for dementia in people with Down syndrome, *Cochrane Database of Systematic Reviews*, 1: CD007178.

Morris, R.G. (2008) The neuropsychology of dementia: Alzheimer's disease and other neurodegenerative disorders, in R.T. Woods and L. Clare (eds.) *Handbook of the Clinical Psychology of Ageing* (2nd edn.). Chichester: Wiley, pp. 161–84.

National Institute for Clinical Excellence (NICE) (2011) Donepezil, galantamine, rivastigmine and memantine for the treatment of Alzheimer's disease, *Technology Appraisal TA 217*.

Olazaran, J., Reisberg, B., Clare, L., Cruz, I., Peña-Casanova, J. *et al.* (2010) Non-pharmacological therapies in Alzheimer's disease: a systematic review of efficacy, *Dementia and Geriatric Cognitive Disorders*, 30: 161–78.

Orpwood, R., Bjørneby, S., Hagen, I., Mäki, O., Faulkner, R. *et al.* (2004) User involvement in dementia product development, *Dementia*, 3: 263–79.

Orpwood, R., Sixsmith, A., Torrington, J., Chadd, J., Gibson, G. *et al.* (2007) Designing technology to support quality of life in people with dementia, *Technology and Disability*, 19: 103–12.

Woods, B., Aguirre, E., Spector, A.E. and Orrell, M. (2012) Cognitive stimulation to improve cognitive functioning in people with dementia, *Cochrane Database of Systematic Reviews*, 2: CD005562.

CHAPTER 15

Working with life history

Errollyn Bruce and Pam Schweitzer

The importance of a cup of tea: ❝My parents loved their tea – the kettle and teapot were always on the go and if they weren't actually drinking tea their cups were lined up ready for the next 'mash'. On Mum going in to a nursing home I wondered what would happen about this very important ritual. The first thing that struck me was the crockery – cheap, heavy white cups and mugs that Mum could hardly lift, and many of them were chipped. Tea was supposed to be served at 3 o'clock every afternoon as I found out when I complained about Mum not having had a drink. I think everyone thought that it was someone else's job and not that important.❞

—Anne Warburton Yorkshire, UK

❝While Mum was well enough I used to take her to Sunday evensong at the local church. This church has an excellent choir. Mum had been a church goer all her life. She therefore still knew all the responses from memory and all the hymns from memory. She also greatly enjoyed the other music sung by the choir and the organ music. She came away absolutely uplifted. This was the power of music and reminiscence. She found the repetition of the order of service she had known for so long as comforting.❞

—Brenda Smith Yorkshire, UK

❝In the office in the unit of the care home was a big sign saying what to do in the event of a bomb alert, they also had a reminiscence room completely done out to be like a room from the thirties/forties. It even had tape on the windows in the event of bomb blast and was full of old artifacts. Initially I thought the room was interesting and tried to coax my mum in but she became very distressed saying 'come on we have to get out of here there's a bomb'. I didn't understand. It was only afterwards when I saw the sign in the office that I realised how my mother was interpreting the situation. I believe in reminiscence work as a therapy but never recommend putting people into time-warps by having a full room done out to one specific era. Mum had lived in Hull, which was heavily bombed during the war.❞

—Sue Tucker Yorkshire, UK

Learning objectives

By the end of this chapter, you will:

- Understand the key role of life history in providing person-centred care
- Be familiar with ways to work with life history in dementia care
- Understand the essentials of good practice in life-history work

Introduction

Life history is now firmly established as central to achieving excellence in person-centred care for people with dementia. It is now considered essential to know where people have come from and what they have lived through in order to understand who they are now and provide high-quality care. We now know that past experiences, especially if emotionally significant, influence how people perceive events in the present, and how they respond to them (Kitwood 1997; Cheston and Bender 2000; Bell and Troxel 2001). Knowledge of life history can provide caregivers with valuable clues about the meaning of words and actions that might at first sight appear meaningless or baffling.

As Sabat explains in Chapter 8, neurological impairment is not the only factor that explains why a person with dementia does what they do. Kitwood (1993) suggested five factors that influence behaviour, illustrating this with the equation:

$$SD = P + B + H + NI + SP$$

where SD = clinical presentation of dementia, P = personality, B = biography or life history, H = health, NI = neurological impairment, and SP = social psychology.

Kitwood (1997) stressed that life history helps us to understand people's experience of dementia, their needs, and their behaviour. Bell and Troxel (2001) argue that life history is as central to person-centred care as medical history is to medical care. Both recent experiences and those from the long past can be significant. While the effects of distressing parts of a person's life history can be very striking, it is clear that positive memories of the past can also shape the way that people experience the present.

The significance of life history is underlined if we see emotional care as a central element in dementia care, as it is widely recognized that an understanding of life history is important when working with emotional distress (Cheston and Bender 2000). Dementia is a very frightening condition, sometimes described as ongoing trauma (Miesen 2004). It puts people into an altered world (Perrin and May 2000), and the strangeness of the experience tends to activate the alarm system (Miesen 1992; Cheston and Bender 2000). The typical losses of late life mean that many people are coping with their dementia while destabilized by a series of unwelcome life changes (Kitwood 1997).

Profound insecurity, anxiety, depression, and above all, loss, are features of the emotional experience of dementia (Cheston and Bender 2000; see also Chapter 21). Loss of identity is a significant hazard. Loss of autobiographical memory weakens the narratives that contribute to identity (Cheston and Bender 2000), and appears to leave some people with dementia with a vague and shadowy sense of self (Bruce et al. 2002). Emotional care is needed to enable people to achieve tolerable levels of security, stability, and confidence. This can be delivered in a more sensitive, appropriate, and personalized way when the carer has, and reveals, a knowledge of the person's past.

Exercise 15.1: Exploring our own life stories

Find a friend to work with. (1) Ask your friend to tell you about a grandparent (or another older person who was a significant figure in their childhood) while you listen. (2) Swap roles, so you talk and your friend listens. Allow about three minutes each way for this. (3) Reflect back what you heard about your friend's grandparent while she or he listens. (4) Listen while your friend tells you what she or he heard about your grandparent. Then discuss how it felt.

Questions for reflection: As tellers – How did it feel to tell someone about your grandparent? Were you surprised by how much you could remember? How did it feel to hear the listener telling your

Reminiscence work	Reminiscence work ranges from making positive responses to spontaneous reminiscence to using a wide range of methods to trigger memories of the past. It can be a done as a one-to-one activity or with groups. Its main emphasis is working with memories to stimulate conversation and communication in the present. Creative reminiscence uses drama, dance, music, and visual arts to stimulate recall and celebrate stories and may sometimes involve working towards a group or individual end-product, e.g. collage, mural, memory box, book, film, quilt, exhibition, performance
Life-story work	Typically, life story places an emphasis on recording a person's life story. This can be done by collecting information from family, friends, and general sources, but Gibson (2004) believes that wherever possible people with dementia should be involved and have a say in the selection and arrangement of material. Like reminiscence, life-story work can involve working with groups as well as individuals
Oral history	Oral history work involves collecting personal accounts of past times and past events, usually with a view to including them in a book, report or archive. Typically, oral historians are selective, including the most interesting material from reliable informants. However, some of the work done by oral historians has been very similar to life-story and reminiscence work
Life review	Life review is a planned one-to-one structured intervention (Haight and Haight 2007) that can lead to a personal history record. The worker needs counselling skills and the ability to act as a therapeutic listener (Gibson 2004)

Table 15.1 Ways of working with life history

story? How well did your listener capture the emotional tone of your story? As listeners – How did it feel to listen to your friend's account? How well did you remember the details of their story? Were you able to pick up on the emotional aspects? Was she or he happy with your version of the story?

Ways of working with life history

Practitioners are often committed to a particular type of life-history work, but in practice the different ways of working overlap and are intertwined (Bornat 2001), and there are a range of different interventions within each category (Table 15.1). The overlap between life story and reminiscence is most marked, but we have also come across projects presented as oral history and life review, which could equally well be described as life-story work and reminiscence. Thus, while each of these ways of working has its own emphasis, they draw upon similar methods and approaches. Reminiscence, in the sense of talking and thinking about the past, is a central element in them all. For these reasons – and because most of our own work in this area has been reminiscence work – reminiscence is the main focus in the chapter.

The value of working with life history in dementia care

The evidence base

As we have seen, the terms used to describe different ways of working are not used consistently, and there are many different interventions with a variety of different aims and objectives. These interventions are complex, and are at their best when tailored to individual needs. This presents a challenge for research methods designed to investigate standard treatments that are expected to affect everyone in much the same way. Diversity in aims and approaches is reflected in diverse research methods (Moos and Bjorn 2006). Discussing life-story work undertaken with a view to having an impact on care, McKeown *et al.* (2005) conclude that it has potential benefits, but high-quality research is scarce. Discussing reminiscence, Woods (2002) suggests the need to use different outcome measures depending upon the aims and type of work done. He points out that we should not expect reminiscence to result in cognitive and behavioural improvement – more realistic aims might be to stimulate communication, foster identity, enhance mood and well-being, promote individualized care, and improve autobiographical memory. Woods and colleagues' (2009) recent systematic review of reminiscence suggests that while there are promising indications of effectiveness, there remains an urgent need for more and better designed studies so that more robust conclusions can be drawn.

Moos and Bjorn (2006) note a trend towards more rigorous quantitative studies but suggest that this is premature, since we still have a great deal to learn about how best to make use of life histories in the delivery of sensitive, individualized, and effective support and care to people with dementia.

Evidence from practice and qualitative studies suggests that working with life history can be very valuable to care workers, family members, and people with dementia themselves (Bender *et al.* 1999). However, some older people are reluctant to talk about the past, and many people have aspects of their lives they do not want to talk about (Gibson 2004). A recent randomized controlled trial evaluating joint reminiscence with people with dementia and their carers found no significant differences between intervention and control groups on the outcome measures used (Woods *et al.* 2012). Yet there was positive feedback from people involved in the reminiscence groups. Indeed, their main complaint was that these sessions had to end. In our view, this result says more about the difficulties of evaluating complex psychosocial interventions, and the limitations of classic randomized controlled trials for this purpose, than the value of reminiscence-based interventions. However, it is a reminder that we need to be cautious about making grandiose claims for what can be achieved.

Box 15.1: A current research project

A research project called "Life story work with people with dementia: an evaluation" is being conducted at the University of York by Kate Gridley and her colleagues. The objectives of the research are to:

- develop a theoretical model of life-story work
- establish core elements of good practice in using the life-story work approach
- benchmark the current use of life-story work in dementia services in England against good practice
- scope the potential effects and costs of using life-story work
- explore the feasibility of formal evaluation of life-story work
- disseminate findings

The research includes:

- a systematic literature review on life-story work with people with dementia
- focus groups with people with early-stage dementia, carers, and professionals
- a survey of care providers and informal carers
- two small-scale feasibility studies to examine outcomes and costs of using life-story work
- disseminate findings using a short film, designed and produced with the help of people with dementia and their carers

For further information, see http://php.york.ac.uk/inst/spru/research/summs/life.php

The functions of reminiscence

As most life-history work involves reminiscence (i.e. thinking and talking about the past), discussions of the functions of reminiscence (Bender *et al.* 1999; Webster 2002; Coleman 2004; Gibson 2004) can shed light on the value of life-history work. Reminiscence was once thought to be an unhealthy diversion from the present, but over the past 40 years there has been growing recognition that it can be positive and constructive. People of all ages enjoy reminiscing, but it has been suggested that it can have a number of important functions for older people. These may be different for different people and vary over time (Gibson 2004). It has been suggested that reminiscence can be of value to people with dementia when it helps them to:

- maintain a sense of coherence and continuity
- retain autobiographical memory
- retain a strong and positive sense of self
- re-experience the "feel" of happier times in life
- communicate with others
- be sociable and build relationships
- engage in intimacy
- remember how past adversities were dealt with and use this experience with present difficulties
- engage in life review and preparation for death
- pass on family history and cultural heritage
- participate in enjoyable, stimulating, and creative activities
- remember, share, and use retained skills
- find an outlet for creativity

Research on reminiscence has tended to focus on outcomes for clients but we also need to look at the impact of life-history work on carers to fully appreciate its value (Gibson 2004). In a study by Pietrukowicz and Johnson (1991), care workers reported warmer feelings and better understanding of the people with dementia they cared for when they had knowledge of life histories. Warmth and understanding are clearly important for good relationships (Bender *et al.* 1999).

Family carers may also find that re-visiting the past improves their current relationship with the person they care for. For example, they may find that recalling happier times can help them to set current difficulties into the context of the relationship as a whole, and give meaning to their caring role (Schweitzer and Bruce 2008). Knowledge of life stories, whether gained from reminiscence work or elsewhere, has the potential to alter how people are perceived and understood by their carers, and thereby to influence relationships. However, any effects are most likely to be subtle; we should not expect a small reminiscence project to have a dramatic impact on relationships that have lasted a lifetime.

Ways in which life history is valuable in person-centred practice

Life history is central to person-centred care because it helps with:

- understanding the meaning behind what people say
- understanding the messages in behaviour
- providing individualized care
- reinforcing a person's identity
- facilitating interaction
- facilitating relationships between people with dementia
- providing ideas for occupation, engagement, and activity

Understanding the meaning behind what people say

To keep communication going, carers need to believe that there is meaning in what people with dementia say, and be prepared to make efforts to find meaning (see Chapter 17). Life history can often provide clues to meaning in metaphor, stories, and speech that seems confused or irrelevant to the present (Barnet 2000; Killick and Allan 2001; Cheston et al. 2004).

Case example 15.1: Sam

As a young man, Sam was in the RAF. At his day centre, he repeatedly told a story about his time in the Far East. While there, he went on many missions in small planes to tiny airstrips deep in the Malaysian jungle. Navigational aids were primitive, and the planes had small fuel tanks. As they approached their destination, he remembered the mounting anxiety in the plane as pilot and crew scanned the seemingly unending spread of trees looking for signs of an airstrip. On one trip, they only had enough fuel for a few more minutes in the air when someone gave a shout and the pilot turned the plane to investigate. Sam described the enormous feeling of relief as the airstrip came into view and the plane was able to land. After each mission, he thanked "the fates" for his safe return.

The significance of this story to Sam's experiences in the present came to light during a focus group set up to explore people's experiences of their day centre. After making some hesitant and confused comments about finding the day centre toilet, and his fears of being shown up, he gave us a fluent and coherent account of his RAF experiences. Putting two and two together, we suggested that finding the day centre toilet might feel similar to searching for airstrips in the jungle, and he gave a chuckle of recognition. It seemed that he would leave the lounge and go into the corridor when he needed to use the toilet, but once in the corridor he wasn't sure where it was. As he went looking for it, he became increasingly anxious, fearing that he would wet himself if he didn't find it soon. When he found the toilet he had an enormous feeling of relief, and afterwards felt thankful to have avoided humiliation.

The hazards in the two situations – crashing in the depths of the jungle, having an incontinence accident – are very different, but the emotional experience follows the same pattern.

Understanding the messages in behaviour

Understanding the language of behaviour requires us to work out the message or need conveyed by a person's actions (see Chapter 16). To do this we need an empathic understanding of the person's present experience, something that is often only possible if we have some knowledge about their past.

Case example 15.2: Celia

When Celia Conway moved in to Mossycroft House after the death of her sister she settled in remarkably well, and staff found her cooperative, apart from two particular moments in the day. As soon as she had finished breakfast she wanted to go outside. If the doors to the garden were locked she became agitated and incoherent, banging on the doors and trying to open windows.

(continued)

During the day she showed little interest in going outside, but when the light began to fade in the evening she wanted to go outside again, becoming angry if anyone tried to prevent her. It was often inconvenient for staff to help Celia into her coat at these times, and some felt that it was wrong to give in to her "tantrums", but most thought it better to let her go out. Once outside, Celia always took the same route around the garden before coming back inside. When a niece from Australia came to visit she was able to explain Celia's behaviour. Celia had moved into her sister's house after her husband died, and her sister had a dog. Her sister asked her to take the dog out for its early morning and late evening runs, and although not fond of dogs, she took her responsibility very seriously. Despite her deteriorating memory, she continued to take the dog out twice a day. When the dog died, she carried on going out at these times.

The links between current behaviour and the past are not always obvious, and it can sometimes take a considerable amount of detective work to find a plausible explanation.

Providing individualized care

Life history can often provide ideas about important details that can be used to make care personal rather than impersonal. In this context, recent life history may be as relevant as the deep past. For example, changes in routine have been identified as life events that have a clear impact on people with dementia (Orrell and Bebbington 1995). Allowing people to stick to habitual routines (e.g. getting up time, a sherry before lunch) is a relatively simple way to provide individualized care. In the case of Celia, finding out about her old habits helped staff to accept her need to go outside at inconvenient times.

Reinforcing a person's identity

Oyebode and Clare (Chapter 14) remind us that memories of the past contribute to identity in the present. When dementia undermines autobiographical memory and disrupts the narratives that are important to identity, reminders of life history can be helpful. As Sabat (Chapter 8) points out, recall is more severely impaired in people with dementia than recognition. People often retain the ability to recognize their own story when they can only recall fragments, or have difficulty communicating what they remember. If stories are collected and recorded well, carers can tell people their own stories (Naess 1998), which may help them maintain a stronger sense of self as dementia becomes more severe. However, Kitwood (1998: 106) stresses the "great moral responsibility" of telling someone's story for them. Whereas it can be affirming and comforting to hear one's story told by someone who has understood it well, it can be confusing, irritating or insulting if misunderstood or told incorrectly. It is therefore very important to "check back" with the person during the telling of their experience, which also helps the person to retain a sense of ownership of their story.

Tangible reminders of past times can be valuable in reinforcing identity. They include carefully chosen photographs, objects, work tools, souvenirs, school reports, prizes, everyday objects, songs (sung live or recorded by favourite stars of the past), local newspaper items from the past, and even familiar packaging from a previous era. Items like these can be used to make reminiscence products, such as life-story books, collages, display boards, memory boxes, memory wallets, and the life books made in structured life review (Haight and Haight 2007). These products need to be attractive and recognizable records capturing important elements in people's lives.

Reminiscence products can be a stimulus for communication and further reminiscence. They can be particularly helpful when identity is threatened by disorientating changes, such as hospitalization, bereavement or when moving into long-term care. By providing a reminder of the story so far, these records can help people construct narratives that put difficult changes in context. They also provide staff with useful information and a valuable starting point for conversation, enabling them to support the person's identity in a new environment. In the absence of an existing record, it is helpful if families compile an annotated photo album or use a life-story template such as the Alzheimer's Society's "this is me" book.

Case example 15.3: Erroll

Erroll lived a very active life but in his eighties became increasingly frustrated by dementia and general frailty. After falling into the sea early one January morning, he had to give up his favourite activity – going out alone in his boat at dawn. By this time his memories of his past life had become hazy, but as he had been a lifelong writer and journalist, he had diaries and copies of his books and articles, and he was persuaded to write his memoirs. He worked on this for many months and eventually produced a manuscript. He was extremely put out when he could not find a publisher, but reluctantly settled for self-publication. The arrival of the books brought a lift in spirits and a new activity – packing them up and sending them to friends and family. As time went on, he always had a copy of his book at his side, and took great pleasure in reading it. When he had strokes, it went with him to hospital, and was a stimulus for conversation with visitors and staff. When he was found with his wheelchair teetering at the top of a flight of stairs, staff commented wryly that it was only to be expected from a man with a life of adventure. When visitors came he would gesture towards the book and comment, with an expression of mild surprise, "I've been reading this, and I must say, I have had a very interesting life."

Taking time to do reminiscence work with people with dementia can convey powerful messages to support a positive identity. Examples of these messages are "We value you as person", "We are interested in you as an individual", "We respect you and your experience" (Woods 1998: 143–4). Tangible products of reminiscence can help to reiterate these messages over a longer period of time.

Facilitating interaction

For many people, the loss of enjoyable conversation is a consequence of the biological and psychosocial changes associated with dementia. They may be psychologically isolated though surrounded by others. Knowing about people's lives makes it easier to communicate with them, and to find suitable memory triggers (e.g. pictures, objects, music) to stimulate interaction, whether based on verbal or non-verbal exchange. As well as being a convenient stimulus for interaction for staff and visitors, having objects that trigger memories to handle in the care environment can encourage conversation between users. The tangible reminders mentioned above can be particularly helpful in stimulating interaction, especially if they provide an attractive and accessible record of life stories (e.g. Bourgeois 1992). Computer-based systems using reminiscence to enhance communication are an interesting innovation (e.g. Alm *et al.* 2007).

Facilitating relationships between people with dementia

Shared experience is the basis of friendship. The experience of needing care is one that few people welcome, and is often not, on its own, a good basis for friendship among users of care services. Knowledge of life histories can help us to identify common ground between clients, and use this to foster relationships (Schweitzer and Bruce 2008). Bell and Troxel (2001) suggest introducing clients to each other repeatedly (saying, for example, "Bill, this is Fred, he was a truck driver too, you know"), while Bender *et al.* (1999) stress the value of reminiscence groups both for discovering common ground and for kindling interest in differences. Good use of life histories can help transform the experience of receiving care from feeling disconnected and misplaced among strangers, to finding some comfort from a sense of belonging and making meaningful connections with others.

Case example 15.4: Ethel

Ethel O'Neill, mother of nine, worked hard in a biscuit factory all her life, and had a robustly positive attitude to living in a care home, saying she was delighted to have others doing all the cooking and cleaning. Margaret Conway was in the room next door. She had been a doctor's receptionist, married a doctor, and was sad to be childless. Although well settled in the home, she was anxious, easily upset, and grieving for her husband and brothers who were all dead. She often said "these are not my people" and that she wanted to move out to live with her cousins. Ethel thought Maggie was fussy, stuck up – "a tuppenny snob" – and they often rubbed each other up the wrong way. However, in an impromptu reminiscence session that took place when three of Ethel's daughters came to visit, it emerged that their fathers had sung in the same church choir, and that Ethel's daughters had been Brownies in a pack where Maggie was a helper. This connection helped to soften their feelings of animosity.

Providing ideas for occupation, engagement, and activity

A person's life story can provide clues about the kind of occupation or activity that might suit them. Information has to be used thoughtfully, and ideas tested to see if they are appropriate. Tastes can change, and past passions may lose their appeal, but there can be some surprising threads of continuity. The skill often lies in seeing a way to evoke the "feel" of an activity enjoyed in the past, without engendering any anxiety about performance.

Case example 15.5: Betty

Betty was once a skilled dressmaker but no longer enjoyed sewing. It frustrated her, and was a distressing reminder of the skills she had lost. However, she still loved to handle fabrics, and enjoyed folding laundry. When given a basket of fabric samples, she enjoyed sorting through them and deciding what each could be used for. She enjoyed hearing and saying the names of the different fabrics and what they were used for.

Well-run reminiscence activities appeal to many people. For example, Brooker and Duce (2000) observed higher levels of well-being during a group reminiscence activity than during other group activities.

Exercise 15.2: Making use of what we know

Return to each of the vignettes in this section, and for each person with dementia:

- consider how carers could make best use of life-history information given in order to provide person-centred care
- comment on what more they might need to find out about the person's life to develop their work further

Good practice when working with life history in dementia care

Valuing people

Good practice in life-history work is achieved by combining person-centred principles with creative, communication-centred approaches to reminiscence. Whether we are gathering and recording information about life stories, running reminiscence sessions or responding to spontaneous reminiscence, it is important to value people and their stories, be sensitive to their emotional needs, and careful to avoid malignant social psychology (Brooker 2007). This is not always easy – for example, it is very tempting to exchange looks that say "there she goes again" when stories are repeated many times. However, a more compassionate response is to strive to understand why a particular story is repeated, and to find out whether there is a connection – possibly at an emotional level – with the story told and a person's experiences in the present.

Attitudes and skills

The attitudes and skills needed for reminiscence work are listed in Table 15.2. These are applicable to other ways of working with life history in dementia care. They are not tied to a particular background or training (Gibson 1998). They are closely related to the principles of person-centred care as described by Brooker (2007) – valuing people regardless of cognitive ability, approaching them as unique individuals, understanding the world from their perspective, and creating a social environment that supports their psychological needs.

- Respecting and valuing people as unique individuals
- Having a genuine interest in the past and in people's life stories
- Being willing to listen to both painful and happy memories
- Not being frightened by strong emotions
- Paying good attention with active listening and a sense of being genuinely available to people
- Empathizing – sharing another's world without losing hold of your own
- Relating sensitively – not being a bull in a china shop or over-interpreting
- Being able to reflect critically on your own work

Source: Based on Gibson (1998: 18)

Table 15.2 Attitudes and skills for reminiscence work in dementia care

Skills and techniques are not everything. Believing that meaningful communication with people with dementia is possible, and having both the desire to communicate and the patience to keep trying are possibly the most important qualifications for reminiscence work (Gibson 1998).

Good practice in reminiscence work

There are different approaches to reminiscence work. Oyebode and Clare (see Chapter 14) characterize "reminiscence therapy" as cognitive stimulation, and this may be appropriate in the case of "recall and tell" approaches to reminiscence that are predominantly reliant on verbal communication, and delivered without particular attention to person-centred practice. However, the creative, communication-based approach is better suited to meet the needs of people with dementia (Schweitzer and Bruce 2008) and shares many of the characteristics of cognitive rehabilitation.

The principles of good practice we set out here follow from combining a creative communication-based approach to reminiscence with a person-centred approach to dementia (Table 15.3). They need to be applied appropriately, given the context and the needs of particular individuals.

Good practice in creative communication-based reminiscence work requires us to be alert to ways to support each person, and careful to avoid anything that might undermine them. For example, we need to find ways around the fear of failure, and to play to the strengths of the people with whom we are working. If questioning seems to make a person's mind go blank, we

---

- Establishing rapport – e.g. making people feel that you are pleased to see them, and are happy to spend time in their company

- Being attentive to basic needs – e.g. check that people are comfortable and able to hear and see; reassure people if they are agitated or anxious, and do not expect them to concentrate on reminiscence if they are preoccupied by worries or distress

- Showing interest – e.g. being attentive, showing no signs of boredom or needing to be elsewhere

- Sensitivity – e.g. being receptive to the feelings people express, responding supportively; respecting people's interests and preferences

- Being non-judgemental – e.g. showing that you respect people's views and experiences, even if you disagree or feel shocked by what they are telling you

- Using cooperative conversational strategies – e.g. making sure that people with dementia take their turns in the conversation, leaving long pauses for them to come in; checking out your understanding by saying something like, "Have I got this right – you were saying that ... ?"

- Having the ability to create an easy atmosphere – e.g. sharing the funny side of things, showing delight in what people are able to remember, appreciating the efforts they are making to participate

- Respecting the right to tell the story as they choose – e.g. recognizing that there may be an emotional truth in a story, even though "the facts" are not accurate; avoiding showing people up by correcting mistakes or indicating that you don't believe what they are saying

- Approaching reminiscence with enthusiasm – e.g. modelling the activities by briefly relating an experience of your own, but not taking too much time over this

- Being prepared to let your hair down, thus licensing others to do the same (Schweitzer and Bruce 2008)

- Being person-centred – e.g. avoiding personal detractions, and making use of personal enhancers

Source: Brooker (2007)

Table 15.3 Good practice in reminiscence work

need to avoid direct questions. If verbal communication has become difficult, we need to support it (for example, by allowing time for people to collect and express their thoughts) and explore other, non-verbal channels of communication (for example, asking people to show us, rather than tell us, how things were). We need to give people the best chance of receiving an idea and responding to it by stimulating all the senses (sight, hearing, touch, taste, smell, and the body's sense of its own movements).

Group activities

When doing reminiscence work with a group, leaders need group skills. All members of the group need to feel secure and that their contributions are valued. Everyone needs to be given the opportunity to present something to the whole group, but no-one should feel under pressure to do so if they do not want to. People can gain a great deal by watching and listening to others' contributions and their incapacity or reluctance to join in should not be seen as a failure or met with disappointment. Group leaders need to build a sense of belonging, for example, by pointing out common ground and connections between people in the group. Leaders can "amplify" people's contributions by repeating their story to the whole group, showing their appreciation of each individual, and making connections with stories told by others in the group.

There need to be plenty of people available to listen to people with dementia, one-to-one wherever possible, because they often need to speak immediately to avoid forgetting what they want to say. If you are working alone, it is generally better to work with groups of three or four people (Heathcote 2007). In larger groups, it is a good idea to have a balance between small and large group activities, and there needs to be a leader or volunteer to work with each of the small groups (Schweitzer and Bruce 2008). Planning needs to take account of things such as deafness, and how long participants are able to concentrate when other people are speaking. There can be a great deal of humour and fun in reminiscence groups, but leaders should also be able to handle serious stories, and any feelings of anger or distress that arise from them (Gibson 1998; Bruce *et al.* 1999).

Spontaneous reminiscence and conversation

Recalling and talking about the past without being prompted by a question or a planned reminiscence activity is known as spontaneous reminiscence. Most carers are familiar with spontaneous reminiscence because many people with dementia enjoy talking about the past, describing how things used to be long ago or commenting on differences between then and now. Some have a story, or stories, which they tell repeatedly. Others may talk as though they are living in the past, for example, saying that they need to go out to fetch the children – who are now adults – from school.

Spontaneous reminiscence provides a springboard for conversation and understanding a person in the present, and best practice involves making the most of these opportunities. However, there are a number of reasons why family and paid carers do not encourage spontaneous reminiscence and the challenge for best practice is finding ways around these barriers.

Family carers often feel that chatting about the past is irrelevant when what they are missing and needing is talk about the present. However, some family members discover the power of the past to keep conversation going in the present, and are able to "hold" a person's memories for them. In Box 15.2, an interview with the son of a man with dementia illustrates this phenomenon of "holding" a person's memories.

> ### Box 15.2: An interview
>
> So I could get him to talk about these things from years and years and years ago and I can remember these things too . . . And he liked that, so we always therefore managed to have quite a healthy little conversation going . . . we had to talk about things he knew . . . his old work colleagues and some of those fund of stories which came out of all that . . . it's like pressing buttons . . . immediately he'd be smiling and laughing and he'd remember . . . And after a while he'd forget what the stories were but I could tell him them and then he'd remember . . .

Not all family carers find this easy to do. For example, in Box 15.2, the wife of the man with dementia felt much less able to use the past as a way to connect with her husband than her son did. Deeply upset by her husband's decline, and resentful that he would chat to others, but not to her, she was unable to settle for conversation that did not meet her needs. The communication gap between them was widened by her stress, her deafness, and her tendency to scold when he made mistakes. Family carers who are feeling overwhelmed by dementia and finding it hard to adjust their expectations need a lot of support and understanding. Given this, they may then be able to appreciate the importance of the past for those they are caring for, and change a little. Joint reminiscence sessions (Bruce *et al.* 1999) or other interventions that work with people with dementia and carers together may be helpful here.

Finding repeated stories boring, and feeling that "living in the past" puts a person beyond their reach can be barriers for both family carers and paid staff. They may feel better about these things if they understand that listening to the person and responding positively may be helping that person cope with very difficult present-day experiences. Remembering your own life story can be an important way to maintain identity, and repetition is a good way to remember. Believing that your mother is not far away is a reassuring thought when faced by a strange and threatening situation (Bruce 1999). These are examples of taking the perspective of a person with dementia – an important principle in both person-centred practice and reminiscence work.

For care workers, the culture of care can be a barrier. Findings from studies in long-term care settings suggest that people with dementia have very little conversation with care workers. Conversations tend to be brief and superficial; there is surprisingly little interaction during personal care (Hallberg *et al.* 1990; Ward *et al.* 2005; Cohen-Mansfield *et al.* 2007). However, in settings where communication and relationships are seen as a priority, there is evidence to suggest that staff can act very differently. There are reports of staff responding warmly to what people say, and using their knowledge of their clients' lives to facilitate further conversation (Vittoria 1998; Bell and Troxel 2001).

Ongoing support as well as education and training may be needed by both family and paid carers to facilitate best practice in this area. Carers need to know how to make the most of spontaneous reminiscence as an opportunity for conversation and communication, but to act on this knowledge they need to be in a supportive context.

Exercise 15.3: Learning from experience

Reminiscence was the scheduled activity on the day I visited Chestnut Grove Care Home. Staff had been very busy due to a resident having a fall, and being taken to hospital in an ambulance, so the activity started later than planned. The activity worker brought a box of reminiscence objects into the lounge and quickly helped a few people to move their chairs to make a group of nine people. The three other people in the room were not asked if they wanted to join in. Despite the moves, the chairs were not well placed and some people could not see or hear each other very well. A care worker joined the group and the activity was run like a quiz game – residents who named an object correctly were praised. Those who didn't were asked to pass it on. Hilda held a pack of penny blue for quite a while, looking at it intently. She was asked to pass it on to the next person, and when she eventually spoke, no-one noticed. Lizzie was given the thimble and said quietly, "A silver thimble. Mother had one. She made all our dresses – we had lovely clothes." The activity worker said, "That's a lovely memory, Lizzie", and repeated what she had said so everyone could hear. Several other people chipped in with memories triggered by Lizzie's story. Sally began to cry when she was holding the darning mushroom. The care worker glanced at me and said, "Sally cries a lot, don't you Sally?" Sally continued to cry quietly. She was given no further attention. When she smelt the carbolic soap, Hetty began to talk fondly about her grandmother's dog. When she paused the care worker said, "You loved that dog didn't you Hetty, but we're not talking about animals today, we're talking about laundry and mending." Fred could not hear what was going on, and pointed out that it was raining outside. The activity ended abruptly without explanation when there was some shouting in the corridor and both workers went out to investigate.

- What went well in the above example?
- What areas of practice could be improved?

Debates and controversies

Family members and practitioners often express concern that working with life history may be harmful if it causes traumatic memories from the past to resurface. Many psychologists argue that recalling and speaking about unresolved distress is unlikely to lead to lasting harm, and may be necessary for resolution. However, the prospect of dealing with strong emotions can be alarming. In this debate, it is important to consider what problems the recall of painful memories is likely to cause both for clients and for their caregivers – and how they can be handled in each case.

A very different area of debate concerns the place of psychosocial interventions (such as reminiscence work and life review) in dementia care. There is increasing evidence to support the view that psychosocial interventions compare well with current drug treatments in maintaining quality of life for people with dementia and their carers. They are free from adverse side-effects, and not necessarily more expensive than drugs. Thus it can be argued psychosocial interventions should be available on the same basis as medication, given that the available drugs are unsuitable for many people and, where tolerated, may be less effective than psychosocial interventions. The opposing view is that while psychosocial interventions may be valuable as an adjunct to medication, they should take second place. More effective drug treatment will eventually become available and will be the best way to intervene in the long run. A question for this debate is whether the expectation that more effective medication will be found in the future is good reason to limit the interventions offered to those who are living before this comes about.

Conclusion

While it is not easy to quantify and measure the benefits of life-history work, ignoring the life stories of people with dementia is short-sighted and arguably irresponsible. Taking account of life history is essential for person-centred practice. The key question for practitioners is not whether to work with life history, but how best to do this work.

Further information

Age Exchange was established in 1983 to improve quality of life by valuing people's reminiscences [http://age-exchange.org.uk/about_us/index.html].

The European Reminiscence Network aims to promote best practice in reminiscence work and to share experience across national frontiers [http://www.europeanreminiscencenetwork.org/].

Facilitated life-story writing is a research project at the Sheridan Elder Research Center at McMaster University, Hamilton, Ontario, which aims to promote quality of life through the sharing of personal life stories.

The Life Story Network (LSN) is an organization that works with a range of partners, and individuals, to promote the value of using life stories to improve the quality of life and well-being of people and communities, particularly those marginalized or made vulnerable through ill health or disability. The work of the LSN will considerably enhance the quality of care, and support, delivered to individuals and communities, through embedding a human rights-based approach [http://www.lifestorynetwork.org.uk/].

The Sporting Memories Network promotes and develops the use of sporting memories to improve well-being of people through conversation and reminiscence [http://www.sportingmemoriesnetwork.com/].

References

Alm, N., Dye, R., Gowans, G., Campbell, J., Astell, A. *et al.* (2007) A communication support system for older people with dementia, *Computer*, 40(5): 35–41.

Barnet, E. (2000) *Including the Person with Dementia in Designing and Delivering Care: 'I Need to be Me!'* London: Jessica Kingsley.

Bell, V. and Troxel, D. (2001) *The Best Friends Staff: Building a Culture of Care in Alzheimer's Programs*. Baltimore, MD: Health Professions Press.

Bender, M., Bauckham, P. and Norris, A. (1999) *The Therapeutic Purposes of Reminiscence*. London: Sage.

Bornat, J. (2001) Reminiscence and oral history: parallel universes or shared endeavour?, *Ageing and Society*, 21(2): 219–41.

Bourgeois, M. (1992) Evaluating memory wallets in conversations with persons with dementia, *Journal of Speech and Hearing Research*, 35: 1344–57.

Brooker, D. (2007) *Person-centred Dementia Care: Making Services Better*. London: Jessica Kingsley.

Brooker, D.J.R. and Duce, L. (2000) Well-being and activity in dementia: a comparison of group reminiscence therapy, structured and goal-directed group activity and unstructured time, *Aging and Mental Health*, 4: 356–60.

Bruce, E. (1999) Holding onto the story: older people, narrative and dementia, in G. Roberts and J. Holmes (eds.) *Healing Stories: Narrative in Psychiatry and Psychotherapy*. Oxford: Oxford University Press, pp. 181–205.

Bruce, E., Hodgson, S. and Schweitzer, P. (1999) *Reminiscing with People with Dementia: A Handbook for Carers*. London: Age Exchange.

Bruce, E., Tibbs, M.A. and Surr, C. (2002) *A Special Kind of Care: Improving Well-being in People Living with Dementia*. Bradford: Bradford Dementia Group, University of Bradford [http://www.brad.ac.uk/acad/health/dementia/research/methodist.php, accessed 12 April 2008].

Cheston, R. and Bender, M. (2000) *Understanding Dementia: The Man with the Worried Eyes*. London: Jessica Kingsley.

Cheston, R., Jones, K. and Gilliard, J. (2004) 'Falling into a hole': narrative and emotional change in a psychotherapy group for people with dementia, *Dementia,* 3(1): 95–103.

Cohen-Mansfield, J., Creedon, M.A., Malone, T., Parpura-Gill, A., Dakheel-Ali, M. *et al.* (2007) Dressing of cognitively impaired nursing home residents: description and analysis, *The Gerontologist*, 46: 89–96.

Coleman, P.G. (2004) Uses of reminiscence: functions and benefits, *Aging and Mental Health*, 9(4): 291–4.

Gibson, F. (1998) *Reminiscence and Recall: A Guide to Good Practice* (2nd edn.). London: Age Concern.

Gibson, F. (2004) *The Past in the Present: Using Reminiscence in Health and Social Care*. Baltimore, MD: Health Professions Press.

Haight, B.K. and Haight, B.S. (2007) *The Handbook of Structured Life Review*. Baltimore, MD: Health Professions Press.

Hallberg, I.R., Norberg, A. and Eriksson, S. (1990) A comparison between the care of vocally disruptive patients and that of other residents at psychogeriatric wards, *Journal of Advanced Nursing*, 15: 267–75.

Heathcote, J. (2007) *Memories are Made of This: Reminiscence Activities for Person-centred Care*. London: Alzheimer's Society.

Killick, J. and Allan, S. (2001) *Communication and the Care of People with Dementia*. Buckingham: Open University Press.

Kitwood, T. (1993/2007) Person and process in dementia, in C. Baldwin and A. Capstick (eds.) *Tom Kitwood on Dementia: A Reader and Critical Commentary*. Maidenhead: Open University Press.

Kitwood, T. (1997) *Dementia Reconsidered*. Buckingham: Open University Press.

Kitwood, T. (1998) Life history and its vestiges: reminiscence work with people with dementia, in P. Schweitzer (ed.) *Reminiscence in Dementia Care*. London: Age Exchange.

McKeown, J., Clarke, A. and Repper, J. (2005) Life story work in health and social care: systematic literature review, *Journal of Advanced Nursing*, 55(2): 237–47.

Miesen, B.M.L. (1992) Attachment theory and dementia, in G.M.M. Jones and B.M.L. Miesen (eds.) *Care-giving in Dementia: Research and Applications*, Vol. 1. London: Routledge, pp. 38–56.

Miesen, B.M.L. (2004) The psychology of dementia care: awareness and intangible loss, in G.M.M. Jones and B.M.L. Miesen (eds.) *Care-giving in dementia: Research and Applications*, Vol. 4. London: Routledge, pp. 183–213.

Moos, I. and Bjorn, A. (2006) Use of the life story in the institutional care of people with dementia: review of intervention studies, *Ageing and Society*, 26: 431–54.

Naess, L. (1998) Reminiscence work with people with dementia, in P. Schweitzer (ed.) *Reminiscence in Dementia Care*. London: Age Exchange.

Orrell, M. and Bebbington, P. (1995) Life events and senile dementia: admissions, deterioration and social environment change, *Psychological Medicine*, 25(2): 373–86.

Perrin, T. and May, H. (2000) *Well-being in Dementia: An Approach for Therapists and Carers*. Edinburgh: Churchill Livingstone.

Pietrukowicz, M.E. and Johnson, M.M.S. (1991) Using life histories to individualise nursing home staff attitudes towards residents, *The Gerontologist*, 31: 105–6.

Schweitzer, P. and Bruce, E. (2008) *Remembering Yesterday, Caring Today – Reminiscence in Dementia Care: A Guide to Good Practice*. London: Jessica Kingsley.

Vittoria, A.K. (1998) Preserving selves: identity work and dementia, *Research on Aging*, 20(1): 91–136.

Ward, R., Vass, A.A., Aggarwal, N., Garfield, C. and Cybyk, B. (2005) What is dementia care? 1. Dementia is communication, *Journal of Dementia Care*, 13(6): 16–19.

Webster, J.D. (2002) Reminiscence functions in adulthood: age, race and family dynamics correlates, in J.D. Webster and B.K. Haight (eds.) *Critical Advances in Reminiscence Work: From Theory to Applications*. New York: Springer.

Woods, R.T. (1998) Reminiscence as communication, in P. Schweitzer (ed.) *Reminiscence in Dementia Care.* London: Age Exchange.

Woods, R.T. (2002) Non-pharmacological techniques, in N. Qizilbash, L. Schneider, H. Chui, P. Tariot, H. Brodaty *et al.* (eds.) *Evidence-based Dementia Practice.* Oxford: Blackwell Science.

Woods, R.T., Bruce, E., Edwards, R.T., Hounsome, B., Keady, J. *et al.* (2009) Reminiscence groups for people with dementia and their family carers: pragmatic eight-centre randomised trial of joint reminiscence and maintenance versus usual treatment: a protocol, *Trials*, 10: 64 [http://www.trialsjournal.com/content/10/1/64, accessed 25 May 2014].

Woods, R.T., Bruce, E., Edwards, R.T., Elvish, R., Hoare, Z. *et al.* (2012) REMCARE: reminiscence groups for people with dementia and their family caregivers – effectiveness and cost-effectiveness pragmatic multicentre randomised trial, *Health Technology Assessment*, 16 (48) [http://www.hta.ac.uk/fullmono/mon1648.pdf, accessed 25 May 2014].

CHAPTER 16

Understanding behaviour

Jiska Cohen-Mansfield

"It was so uncharacteristic. Totally uncharacteristic aggression from this lovely, gentle man. He was just so frustrated."

—Frances Annal Melbourne, Australia

Learning objectives

By the end of this chapter, you will be able to:

- Recognize that behaviour is a form of communication
- Recognize that behaviour is often used to address unmet need
- Identify a range of psychosocial approaches that can address needs
- Appreciate the importance of knowing the individual person and their circumstance when seeking to understand the language of behaviour

Introduction

How we make sense of a person's behaviour, its cause, and its purpose is one of the most controversial issues in dementia care. This is an important area in dementia care because how we interpret a person's behaviour will influence how we respond. For example, if we consider a person's behaviour to result directly from brain dysfunction via disinhibition or via direct neurological activation of certain behaviours, such as screaming, we are more likely to propose drugs as a solution. Such a perspective has led to an over-reliance on anti-psychotic medication (see, for example, Child *et al.* 2012). If, on the other hand, we adopt a more bio-psycho-social approach to understanding dementia, we are more likely to seek explanations in the interaction between the person and their environment. As we have seen in Chapter 8, a bio-psycho-social approach argues that a person's behaviour is the result of interplay between neurobiology and the psychological and social environment. This chapter challenges the notion that behaviour is the direct result of neuropathology and argues instead that much behaviour is an attempt to address unmet needs – whether physical, psychological or social. According to this model, behaviour is a complex phenomenon affected by an interaction of cognitive impairment, physical health, mental health, past habits and personality, and environmental factors.

The chapter describes how a person with dementia experiences a decreased ability to meet their own needs. At the same time, people with dementia often find themselves in living or care situations that are either in direct opposition to, or in other ways fail to meet, their needs. Thus people with dementia rely on behaviour to fulfil and/or to communicate those needs. When this fails, they experience frustration and act in ways that others find challenging. The chapter presents a range of psychosocial interventions that can be employed to address the physical and psychosocial needs of people with dementia and argues for increased advocacy to support their research and use. Throughout the chapter, evidence will be drawn from research with people with dementia in a range of care settings.

Needs and dementia

Maslow (1968) argued that humans are motivated by a group of hierarchically organized innate needs. The lowest layer involves mostly physiological needs (hunger, sleep, etc.), whereas the next layers include safety, belongingness and love, esteem, and other higher-order needs. Once the lower need is satisfied, a person focuses on satisfying the higher needs. Results of observational studies of persons with severe cognitive impairment demonstrate that people with dementia, in common with all people, have higher-order needs, such as those for social contact and sensory stimulation. While change has occurred in the person's ability to recognize, express, and resolve these needs independently, and the environment often proves inadequate to address the needs, this does not mean the person no longer has such needs (see Table 16.1). People with dementia express needs in common with all human beings (Cohen-Mansfield and Werner 1995), and as such these can be summarized under the hierarchy described by Maslow (1987).

Similar to Maslow's hierarchy of needs, Kitwood (1997) proposed a cluster of overlapping needs that, in his view, fall within one all-encompassing need, the need for love. These include the needs for comfort, attachment, inclusion, occupation, and identity. By comfort he meant the need for tenderness and soothing of psychological pain; by attachment, the need for bonds with others; by inclusion, the need to be part of the group, part of the people club; by occupation, the need to be "involved in the process of life"; and by identity, the need to "know who one is" (Kitwood 1997: 83). He contended that many of these psychological needs are unmet in care environments. For Kitwood (1997), the key task of person-centred care is to meet these needs.

In our empirical research, we have identified a range of physical, psychological, and social needs. Physical needs include those related to pain, ill health, and physical discomfort, including uncomfortable environmental conditions. Psychological and social needs include the need for

Human needs	Cognitive impairment	Unfavourable environment
Physiological – pain, health, physical discomfort	Unable to communicate needs	Environment does not comprehend the needs
Safety – uncomfortable environmental conditions	Unaware of needs of self	Environment does not provide for the needs
Love and belonging – need for social contacts	Unable to communicate the needs effectively	
Esteem – type of stimulation	Unable to use prior coping mechanisms	
Self-actualization – level of stimulation	Unable to obtain the means for meeting the need	

Source: Based on Cohen-Mansfield (2000)

Table 16.1 Unmet needs: the effect of an interaction between human needs, cognitive impairment, and an unfavourable environment

social contacts and stimulation and those related to emotional discomfort (evident in affective states: depression, anxiety, frustration).

What makes the discussion of needs and dementia unique is that the dementia process results in a decreased ability to meet one's needs because of a decreased ability to communicate the needs, and a decreased ability to provide for oneself. As a result, there is an imbalance in the interaction between lifelong habits and personality, current physical and mental states, and less than optimal environmental conditions. As such, most unmet needs arise because of the interaction between dementia-related impairments in communication and a reduced ability to utilize the environment appropriately to fulfil the needs together with a social and physical environment that neither meets nor facilitates the meeting of these needs.

Understanding behaviour as an expression of unmet need

Exercise 16.1: Imagining unmet need

Think of the last time you felt hungry.

- What led you to know that you were hungry? What did you do in response?
- Were you able to meet your needs? What might you have done if you were unable to meet your needs?
- How did your hunger affect your thinking? How did your hunger affect your behaviour?

Think of the last time you felt the need to talk to someone about something.

- What happened in this circumstance? Were you able to meet your needs?
- How did your need to talk to someone affect your thinking? How did it affect your behaviour?

There is a developing evidence base in support of the argument that behaviour is an expression of unmet needs (Cohen-Mansfield and Werner 1995; Algase et al. 1996; Cohen-Mansfield and Deutsch 1996; Miranda-Castillo et al. 2010; Beck et al. 2011). Thought of in this way, behaviour is a complex phenomenon affected by an interaction of cognitive impairment, physical health, mental health, past habits and personality, and environmental factors. Behaviour can be seen as an attempt to address unmet needs in one of several ways:

- The behaviour can aim to directly meet the need, e.g. when pacing may provide stimulation to alleviate the unmet needs for engagement, occupation, and stimulation.
- The behaviour may aim to communicate the need, e.g. repetitious vocalizations that aim to draw attention to an unmet need.
- The behaviour may represent the outcome of having an unmet need, e.g. screaming as a result of frustration or pain.

From our research, we have concluded that the main needs people with dementia seek to address through their behaviour include:

- unaddressed physical pain or discomfort
- lack of social contacts and loneliness
- boredom, inactivity, and sensory deprivation
- depression, which may be the result of lack of positive experiences or lack of control

Behaviour as an expression of physical pain and discomfort

Physical pain and ill health factors are associated with a range of verbal and vocal behaviours (Cohen-Mansfield et al. 1990). Hurley et al. (1992) reported an increase in vocalizations among patients experiencing fevers. The behaviour may be a direct manifestation of discomfort, a natural response to pain, and may be exacerbated in persons who are unable to communicate and, therefore, express their suffering through screaming. Alternatively, the vocally disruptive behaviour may be an attempt to communicate the discomfort under circumstances in which a cognitively impaired individual is no longer able to communicate more directly. While the relationship between health and physically aggressive behaviour is less clear, a positive association between aggressive behaviour and urinary tract infections has been reported (Ryden et al. 1991).

In contrast, people who engage in physically non-aggressive behaviour (e.g. pacing) have been reported to have fewer medical diagnoses than other nursing home residents, and have better appetites (Cohen-Mansfield et al. 1990). However, some people who pace suffer from akathaesia, an inner sense of restlessness, due to neurodegenerative disease or as an extrapyramidal reaction to anti-psychotic or other drugs (Mutch 1992).

Sleep disturbance and fatigue are another aspect of health that has been linked to behaviour (Cohen-Mansfield and Marx 1990; Cohen-Mansfield et al. 1995). The impairment of circadian rhythms that is characteristic of Alzheimer's disease (e.g. Bliwise 1993) may also be related to behaviour. In particular, an increase in active behaviour in older individuals with dementia that occurs in the evening hours, beginning at a time near sunset, has been termed "sundowning" (Bliwise 1994). It should be noted, however, that such behaviour is not related to the sunset or to the time of sunset. Many people experience restless behaviour more often in morning hours, while others manifest those at relatively uniform levels throughout the day (Cohen-Mansfield 2007).

Behaviour as an expression of uncomfortable environmental conditions

In an observational study of the nursing home environment, most behaviours that staff found difficult tended to increase when it was cold at night, and requests for attention increased when it was hot during the day (Cohen-Mansfield and Werner 1995). These findings suggest that discomfort may cause some behaviours.

Behaviour as an expression of need for social contact

Verbal/vocal behaviours, as well as some physically non-aggressive behaviours other than pacing and wandering, tended to increase in frequency when nursing home residents were alone, and to decrease when they were with others. Similarly, such behaviours decreased when staffing levels increased (Cohen-Mansfield and Werner 1995). These findings suggest that loneliness or the need for social contact may be at the root of verbal or vocal behaviours that distress others. This idea is supported by an intervention study (Cohen-Mansfield and Werner 1997) in which social interaction was more beneficial in decreasing verbal and vocal problem behaviours than the mere provision of pleasant stimuli, such as music.

Behaviour as an expression of need for stimulation

In the past, problem behaviours have been attributed to over-stimulation or too much stimulation, which cannot be processed because of the dementia. An observational study of a nursing home (Cohen-Mansfield et al. 1992a) did not support this hypothesis. In fact, observations from this study found that the nursing home was a relatively monotonous place. Routine is the rule and activities and stimulation are infrequent (Cohen-Mansfield *et al.* 1992b). People often have nothing to do in long-term care settings. Most behaviours that others found difficult to manage increased when the older person was inactive, and decreased when structured activities were offered (Cohen-Mansfield and Werner 1995).

It has thus been suggested that problem behaviours result from under-stimulation and sensory deprivation. According to this view, the person with dementia has a reduced ability to obtain stimulation and process it. In addition, many of those living with dementia also have vision and hearing impairments which further decrease their ability to process stimuli. Finally, many of the nursing homes in which persons with dementia reside offer few activities or other positive stimuli. All of these factors result in insufficient stimulation, which, at times, reaches a state of sensory deprivation with the person responding through either self-stimulation or behaviours that manifest discontent because of this unmet need for stimulation. Studies on social deprivation in younger populations have shown that sensory deprivation can result in hallucinations and perceptual distortions, which may in turn lead to behaviours that others find difficult. Even without hallucinations or perceptual changes, the sensory deprivation may evoke feelings of fear, loneliness, and boredom, all resulting in the manifestation of problem behaviours. Several studies have shown that providing sensory stimulation to nursing home residents decreases behavioural disturbances in general, and vocally disruptive behaviours in particular (Birchmore and Clague 1983; Zachow 1984; Mayers and Griffin 1990). Similarly, the systematic provision of stimuli with which nursing home residents could engage themselves resulted in the prevention of behavioural disturbances (Cohen-Mansfield *et al.* 2010).

Behaviour in response to delusions and hallucinations

Delusions and hallucinations provide inappropriate internal stimuli, which may result in behaviour that others find difficult to understand. The relationship between behaviours and delusions or hallucinations has been documented repeatedly (Deutsch *et al.* 1991; Steiger *et al.* 1991; Lachs *et al.* 1992; Cohen-Mansfield *et al.* 1998). It is possible that, like other behaviours, those that are considered to be delusions and hallucinations also result from the interaction of the limited capabilities of the person with dementia and psycho-social and environmental situations that do not support the person (Cohen-Mansfield *et al.* 2011).

Exercise 16.2: Needs-related behaviour

Think of the last time you saw someone with dementia behaving in a way you did not understand and which you found distressing. What was the person doing?

Thinking of this same person, do you think their needs for comfort, attachment, inclusion, occupation, and identity were being met at the time? Which needs may not have been met? How might they have been?

Psychosocial interventions for meeting needs

Psychosocial interventions for meeting needs include those that address the need for social contact, engagement, and relief from discomfort (see Table 16.2). Many interventions address

Need

General treatment approach	Social contacts			Engagement				Discomfort		
		Simulated significant others	Non-human	Provide		Accommodate behaviour		Pain/ discomfort	Sleep	Discomfort during ADL
	Real human			Active	Passive	Decrease risk	Make more acceptable			
Interventions	One-on-one social interaction	Simulated presence therapy	Pets	Walking	Provide hearing aids and glasses to help process ongoing simulation	Environmental design, e.g. tape on floor, covering doors and exits, relocating areas	Activity apron	Pain medication	Light therapy	Environmental redesign of bathing process (e.g. bird pictures and sounds in baths, offering food)
	Small group interaction	Family videotapes	Dolls	Exercise	Sensory stimulation		Provide materials to handle	Re-positioning	Melatonin	Music during bath
	Activity programmes	Music					Environmental design	Remove restrictions	Increase exercise and decrease awakening at night	Use of sponge bath rather than shower or bath
	Flower arranging	Aroma therapy					Changing the visual, auditory, and olfactory stimuli on corridors			Change location of meal
	Massage	Massage								

Source: Based on Cohen-Mansfield (2000)

Table 16.2 Psychosocial interventions to address needs

more than one of these, such as meaningful social contact alleviating both loneliness and boredom. A variety of psychosocial interventions have been described in the literature and summarized in reviews (Allen-Burge *et al.* 1999; Opie *et al.* 1999; Kasl-Godley and Gatz 2000; Cohen-Mansfield 2001, 2003, 2004; Grasel *et al.* 2003; Snowden *et al.* 2003; Bates *et al.* 2004; Siders *et al.* 2004).

Psychosocial approaches to the care of persons with dementia differ from pharmacological treatment in that they consider the interaction between the person, caregiver, environment, and system of care. Such interventions generally provide more person-centred, individualized, and personalized care, addressing their needs and considering their preferences.

Providing social support and contact

At the most basic level, providing social support and contact involves talking to persons with dementia, even if the caregiver conducts the majority of the conversation. One-on-one interaction is a potent intervention that can be provided by relatives, paid caregivers or volunteers. There are two major difficulties in providing positive social contact for persons with dementia: (1) these individuals may prefer socializing with loved ones rather than formal caregivers, and (2) providing one-on-one interaction with staff members can become costly. Two successful interventions that have addressed both of these issues are video-tapes of family members addressing their relative with dementia (Cohen-Mansfield and Werner 1997; Werner *et al.* 2000), and simulated presence therapy (Camberg *et al.* 1999; Woods and Ashley 1995) in which a family member audio-tapes his or her side of a telephone conversation, which is then played for the older person. Interventions addressing cost issues include training staff members to view all interactions with individuals in their care as opportunities for social contact (including during activities of daily living) and interaction videos for persons with dementia. These commercially produced video-tapes often incorporate memories from the past and viewers are invited to sing along to familiar music. Pet therapy is another option (Churchill *et al.* 1999), and may include visits with dogs, cats, fish or even plush stuffed animals or robotic pets (Libin and Cohen-Mansfield 2004). In addition to interaction with the animal, pet therapy provides a topic for interaction with other people. Dolls have also been used to simulate companions/babies, and massage may be an effective mechanism for social contact with persons with advanced dementia who lack verbal language.

Research indicates that verbally disruptive behaviours often relate to social isolation, and that these behaviours decrease with the provision of appropriate ongoing social contact. In a study of verbally disruptive behaviours in the nursing home, both one-on-one social interaction and watching a video-tape of a relative talking to the older person decreased verbal and vocal disruptive behaviours among residents who had manifested these behaviours at very high frequencies, compared with a no-intervention condition (Cohen-Mansfield and Werner 1997). One-on-one interaction was more effective, though also more costly. There were also noticeable individual differences in response, with some persons benefiting more from one type of intervention. This suggests that additional factors, such as the person's prior relationship with relatives, must be taken into account when customizing the specific programme for each individual.

The ability of an individual with dementia to communicate verbally declines as the condition becomes more advanced (see Chapter 12). As a result, communication skills on the part of the carer are crucial for maintaining quality of life and for understanding the perspective of the person with dementia. Caregivers must be educated in communication techniques, learning to observe, listen, speak, ask questions, and offer alternatives in ways that will maximize the individual's ability to receive and transmit information. Communication training for caregivers of persons with dementia focuses on environmental aspects of communication (e.g. approaching slowly, communicating at eye level), content, phrasing, and interpreting non-verbal or confused verbal communication. Phrasing sentences in a short and clear way (Small *et al.* 2003), on a level compatible with the person's understanding (Hart and Wells 1997), and asking questions in a simple, "yes/no" format is considered helpful. Others have advised using broad opening sentences, treating the person with dementia as an equal, sharing experiences and feelings, and finding topics that are meaningful (Tappen *et al.* 1997). Finally, caregivers must be aware that even when individuals with dementia do not speak in coherent sentences, their individual words may be meaningful, and their messages may be embedded in those words (see Chapter 12). It is most essential that one does not ignore, discount or negate the verbalizations of persons with dementia, but rather view these as insights into their perspectives and to use them to improve their situations whenever possible (Ripich 1994; Ripich *et al.* 1995; Small and Gutman 2002).

Providing relief from discomfort – medical and nursing care

To address discomfort, pain, hearing and vision impairments, positioning problems, difficulties adjusting to activities of daily living (ADLs), and unmet ADL-related needs, interventions such as pain management, light therapy to improve sleep, reduction of discomfort through improved seating or positioning, and removal of physical restraints have been related to improvements in behaviour. Once needs have been identified, the interventions often call for straightforward medical or nursing interventions, while others require more complex approaches, such as assessing pain.

Many articles have described the difficulties involved in assessing pain in this population (Cohen-Mansfield and Lipson 2002), and recent findings suggest strategies for dealing with these complexities (Feldt 2000; Huffman and Kunik 2000; Cohen-Mansfield and Lipson 2008). One small study found that pain medication reduced difficult behaviours and allowed discontinuation of psychotropic medication (Douzjian *et al.* 1998). In a study of the implementation of a systematic pain protocol with persons with dementia and agitation, Husebo *et al.* (2011) showed that pain treatment resulted in a significant reduction in agitated behaviours.

Owing to the difficulties of pain assessment, statements about not feeling well, or about being in pain, and unusual movements need to be examined. Looking at the person carefully for several minutes while sitting and during transfer may be beneficial for detecting signs of pain. Similarly, a change from the person's usual behaviour may be a sign of physical pain (Cohen-Mansfield *et al.* 1989). Caregivers' ratings for the assessment of pain together with a pain relief protocol may be especially useful for detection and treatment of pain in persons with dementia (Cohen-Mansfield and Lipson 2008).

Physical discomfort is very common in the nursing home and can include thirst, needing to go to the bathroom, and an uncomfortable sitting position. The reasons for such needs may be complex, such as insufficient staff to take persons to the bathroom, frequent urges to go to the bathroom, or the fear that the resident may choke if given regular liquids. Nevertheless, such issues need to be addressed.

One specific type of physical discomfort is the use of physical restraints, which have been shown to result in increased levels of agitation (Werner *et al.* 1989). The removal of physical restraints may eliminate those behaviours (Werner *et al.* 1994; Yeh *et al.* 2001).

A number of methods have been used to improve sleep and thereby decrease agitation, including bright light therapy (Okawa *et al.* 1991; Mishima *et al.* 1994), melatonin, which has been tried (Cohen-Mansfield *et al.* 2000a) but not found to be effective (Serfaty *et al.* 2002; Gehrman *et al.* 2009), increased exercise (Zisselman *et al.* 1996), and a decrease in night-time interruptions (Alessi *et al.* 1999).

Improvement in eating or drinking, resulting from the use of enhanced light during meals, has been linked with a decrease in inappropriate behaviours (Koss and Gilmore 1998), as has the use of hearing aids (Leverett 1991; Palmer *et al.* 1999).

Changes in the methods and environment of providing activities of daily living have also been associated with a reduction in inappropriate behaviours. For example, tape-recordings and pictures of birds, flowing water and small animals in baths, as well as offering food during bathing have been associated with a decrease of such behaviours during bathing (Whall *et al.* 1997). Person-centred showering and towel baths resulted in decreased agitation compared with usual bathing routines (Sloane *et al.* 2004). Similarly, changing the location of meals from central dining to dining on the unit was effective in reducing patient-to-patient assaults on an Alzheimer's and related dementias unit (Negley and Manley 1990).

Providing engaging activities

Engaging persons with dementia can be accomplished by providing them with stimulation (passive engagement), providing activities (active engagement), and facilitating self-stimulation by accommodating inappropriate behaviours (see Table 16.2). Engaging persons may also involve the reduction of sensory barriers, as in the case of providing hearing aids. Providing stimulation includes the use of music, which should be tailored to the person's preferences (Gerdner 2000), and other sensory stimulation such as aromatherapy or touch therapy (Snyder *et al.* 1995). Music interventions take many forms, including listening to recorded music, playing musical games, dancing or moving to music, playing musical instruments (Sung *et al.* 2012), and singing. (Prior to initiating music therapy, hearing must be tested, and an amplifier, headphone or hearing aid may be necessary.) One example of sensory stimulation is the "Snoezelen" programme, which was developed in Holland and includes a variety of relaxing stimuli (Baillon *et al.* 2004).

More active engagement is usually offered in the form of structured activities, including group and individual activities. One such intervention, known as "simple pleasures", includes a range of activities such as tetherball (Buettner 1999). Activity interventions may involve manipulation (e.g. ball throwing), nurturing (e.g. watering a plant), sorting, cooking, sewing or sensory interventions as described above, such as music or tactile stimulation with a fabric book. Montessori-based activities are a set of activities based on Maria Montessori's principles (Camp *et al.* 2002), such as task breakdown, immediate feedback, and use of everyday, real-world materials. Alternatively, the content of activities may be based on information regarding "pleasant activities" – that is, activities that were or are reinforcing to the individual (Teri and Logsdon 1991) – or on information about the individual's role-identity in the past or in the present (Cohen-Mansfield *et al.* 2000b, 2006a, 2006b; Parpura-Gill and Cohen-Mansfield 2006). Activities can involve exercise (Zisselman *et al.* 1996), or they may incorporate an adaptation of activities of daily living, such as setting the table or cooking (Marsden *et al.* 2001). Cognitive tasks are activities that stimulate cognitive and memory skills. Group examples include "question asking readings", in which a group reads a script accompanied by questions typed on cards that encourage participants to discuss related topics. Another group memory task is memory bingo, a game in which participants match beginnings and endings of popular sayings, which can also stimulate group discussion (Camp *et al.* 1996). Individual cognitive tasks include sorting cards or objects by category.

Interventions for accommodating pacing or wandering behaviour include outdoor walks (Cohen-Mansfield and Werner 1998a) and the use of wandering areas. Outdoor walks may take place in the company of a caregiver, in which case they also involve a social component, or they may occur in secure outdoor wandering areas (Namazi and Johnson 1992; Cohen-Mansfield and

Werner 1999). Accommodating pacing and wandering often involves protection of others' privacy from trespassing while wandering. To prevent trespassing into another person's room or through emergency exit doors, doors and doorknobs can be camouflaged with cloth panels or murals, thereby disguising the doors. Additionally, providing alternative doors, which can be controlled by the person with dementia and permit movement into another secured area, can be useful in preventing people from getting into other people's rooms (Namazi *et al.* 1989).

Inappropriate handling or the constant manipulation of objects can be accommodated by providing appropriate materials, such as books and pamphlets for handling (Cohen-Mansfield and Werner 1998a), and activity aprons (aprons that have buttons, zippers, and other articles sewn on) providing appropriate and safe items for persons to handle. Similarly, rocking chairs and gliding swings have been used to accommodate restless behaviour and provide more acceptable stimulation.

Some verbally disruptive behaviour may serve self-stimulatory functions and may be associated with inactivity and boredom. Such behaviour is likely to be reduced when structured activities are offered. In the study described above (Cohen-Mansfield and Werner 1997), music chosen on the basis of the older person's past preferences significantly reduced verbally disruptive behaviours compared with a no-treatment condition, although it was less effective than interventions aimed at social contact. The importance of individualizing an intervention was highlighted by Gerdner (2000), who showed that music matched to the person's past preferences was more effective than merely providing soothing music.

When the person's need calls for an activity, the specific type of activity offered needs to be matched to the person's level of cognitive functioning, sensory and physical abilities and deficits, as well as sense of identity and preferences (Parpura-Gill and Cohen-Mansfield 2006).

The specific choice of activity for the intervention would be determined by evaluating the older person on the following dimensions:

■ current *sense of identity*, which usually includes some retained aspects of previously held identities, such as work role, family relationship, or preference for a certain type of leisure activity
■ current *sensory abilities*, which include visual, auditory, smell, and touch modalities. Mechanisms for augmentation of sensory abilities should be explored, including simple ones, such as better-fitting eyeglasses, an auditory amplifier, and better-fitting hearing aids
■ current *motor abilities*, including ability to walk, to wheel oneself, as well as dexterity
■ an enhanced understanding of current *needs*, including social contact of any kind, longing for family, for daytime activity, for stimulation, for physical exercise, or for a specific meaningful activity, such as helping or working
■ an understanding of the person's past and present *habits and preferences* for daily life activities and the manner and environment in which they take place (Cohen-Mansfield and Jensen 2005a, 2005b, 2007a, 2007b)

The interaction of these factors will define the intervention that is most appropriate for the individual. A hypothetical-planning grid for matching activities to the needs of individuals is presented in Table 16.3. Examples of the range of possible activities to use as stimulation can be found in Zgola (1987), Teri and Logsdon (1991), Bowlby (1993), Russen-Rondinone and DesRoberts (1996), and Hellen (1999).

The actual utilization of psychosocial interventions in dementia falls far short of its potential. A number of systemic issues are responsible for this gap. Funding is lacking both for the practice of these interventions and for the acquisition of knowledge about them through systematic

	Needs/activity domains				
	Social contact	Family contact/home environment	Stimulation	Physical exercise/self-stimulation	Meaningful activity/increased sense of identity
Seeing	Home movies (H) Mirror (L) Video-tape of someone talking to the person (E)	Video-tape of family (E) Picture album of family (E) Increase family visits (E)	Show old movies (H) Place near a window with view to street or other activity (L) Display moving objects, such as bubbles and strands (L) Flower arranging, sorting shapes and colours, colouring (L)	Dancing (E)	Sheltered workshop (H)
Hearing	One-on-one social interaction (H) Group activities (H) Audio-tape of someone talking to person (L)	Telephone calls with family (H) Audio-tape of family member (L) Simulated presence therapy (L)	Books or tape (H) Trivia (H) Card games (H) Tapes of music the person used to like (E)	Moving to music (E)	Listening to religious services or music (E)
Moving	Arrange social visits (tea) (H) Go to religious services (H)		Rocking chair (E)	Walk in sheltered area (E) Going outside (E)	Assembling materials (H) Cooking (H) Simulating work environment (H)
Touching	Use of soft dolls (L) Massage therapy (E)	Use of object from home (E)	Massage therapy (E) Jacuzzi (E)	Handling different materials (L) Activity apron (L)	Caring for or petting a dog or a cat (E)

H = Activities appropriate for higher cognitively functioning residents. L = Activities appropriate for lower cognitively functioning residents.
E = Activities appropriate for both groups of residents.

Table 16.3 Choosing activities to suit needs and abilities

research. In the USA, the commonly used alternative intervention of psychoactive medication is reimbursed, and the underlying structure for its delivery, such as physicians, medicine aids, pharmacy, monitoring, and quality control systems, are largely in place. However, the provision of psychosocial interventions is generally not reimbursed, and a system for providing them is often absent. No-one in the care system is currently responsible for assessing, observing, and analysing behaviour in order to determine its underlying cause and its impact on individuals' lives. The ability of paid carers to provide psychosocial interventions is further limited by lack of staff knowledge, insufficient staffing levels, and stressful experiences within and outside the care situation (see Chapter 23).

Individualizing care for people with dementia: treatment routes for exploring agitation (TREA)

Exercise 16.3: Individualizing care

Think of a time when you felt very sad. It is possible that several people tried to comfort you. You may have accepted some people's support while pushing others away.

- What might explain your willingness to accept help from one person while rejecting it from another?
- Might it have anything to do with how well understood you felt?
- Might it be related to the way you were approached? In what way?

Addressing people's behavioural communication requires us to adopt a cyclical approach. This starts with assessment of the behaviour – describing the behaviour in detail and the circumstances in which it occurs. We then go on to hypothesize the cause of the behaviour – the need that is striving to be met. Finally, we propose an intervention, implement that intervention, and then undertake a reassessment some time later.

Once we have explored the possible causes for the person's behaviour – understanding what the person is communicating through their behaviour – we then identify an intervention to match. The intervention may target a change in the environment, the behaviour of a staff member, the system of care, or the person with dementia. After the intervention is implemented, another evaluation is performed to determine whether the approach was helpful or whether it should be changed. A change may require a different intervention entirely, or may focus on a specific aspect of the intervention, such as timing, dosage or presentation style.

The aim of our care should be about improved quality of life and pleasure. To achieve this goal, we aim to either fulfil the person's need or to accommodate the behaviour that fulfils the need for the person. Therefore, the target of the intervention may be to reduce behaviour, or it may be to make it acceptable to the persons around. The job of care for people with dementia requires empathy, caring, and love for the person. This type of care has to be present throughout the different care activities. For example, one-to-one dressing is an opportunity for human contact, an opportunity for intimacy.

On the basis of our research, we have proposed Treatment Routes for Exploring Agitation (TREA) as an approach for individualizing treatment plans in response to behaviours that others find distressing, or that seem to indicate that the older person may be distressed. Such a plan involves three stages:

1. Hypothesize which need underlies the behaviour.
2. Characterize the way in which the behaviour results from the need: does the behaviour attempt to accommodate the need? Does it express discomfort? Does it attempt to communicate the need?
3. Provide an intervention that either provides for the unmet need or, alternatively, when the behaviour itself is alleviating the need, provide a method in which the behaviour can be accommodated.

When an intervention to provide for the unmet need is required, it needs to be matched to the person's sensory, mental, and physical abilities, as well as to the person's habits and preferences. The goal of the plan is to improve the quality of life for the patient and to reduce the burden on caregivers.

The assumptions and principles underlying TREA

- A methodology for detecting the needs of the person with dementia is essential for proper caregiving.
- The first step in developing a specific treatment plan for a specific person is to attempt to understand the cause of the behaviour or the need it signals.
- Psychosocial approaches to behaviour should precede pharmacological approaches.
- Psychosocial approaches to behaviour need to be individualized.

Maximizing function and well-being requires a focus on the person–environment fit – both lifelong and current attributes must be considered in the development of methods to optimally address needs. Therefore, in developing a treatment plan, the remaining abilities, strengths, memories, and needs should be utilized, as well as recognition of impairments, especially those in sensory perception and mobility. Unique characteristics of the individual such as past work, hobbies, important relationships, and sense of identity need to be explored to best match current activities to the person.

Key elements of the TREA approach

Individualization of treatment as opposed to care for a group

In general, persons with dementia are usually treated alike. In a typical nursing home, wake-up time and dining times are frequently guided by state regulations and by staffing issues more than by individual habits. Medication for dementia is guided more by market forces and by prescription habits than by individual differences. Group activities do not necessarily fit the participants' abilities and interests.

The detective rather than resigned approach

- Rather than assuming that the person suffering from dementia has lost all sense of self, our treatment of them should be a constant search for their personhood within the dementia.
- There should be a commitment to understanding the person with dementia through communication with that individual and with appropriate informants.
- Formal caregivers' knowledge of their patients' past daily habits and identities are extremely limited (Cohen-Mansfield et al. 2000b) and need to be augmented by reports from other sources, most often family members (see Chapter 10). Communication with the older person

also needs to be enhanced, so that the communicator listens to the underlying message rather than to the exact message conveyed.

Focus on prevention, accommodation, and flexibility as essential elements of intervention

- Prevention refers to structuring the environment in a manner that prevents the development of unmet needs. Examples include better control of temperature, facilitating activities, monitoring pain, and providing stimulation and social contact.
- Accommodation involves ensuring that the design of the environment permits the person to express themselves through behaviours, in a manner that fulfils the needs of the older person without imposing an undue burden on caregivers. Even when the need is unclear, if the behaviour is not harmful, it is frequently best to accommodate it. Thus, simply accommodating the person's wish, even without understanding it, is frequently an appropriate route.
- Flexibility refers to the willingness and ability of caregivers to adjust elements of the older person's daily routine and environment to meet the resident's needs and/or wishes. This pertains to flexibility to accommodate biological needs (e.g. toileting times, feeding times) and psychosocial needs (e.g. social contacts, meaningful activities) that are tailored to the person's lifelong habits, identity, current physical disabilities (e.g. incontinence), and remaining abilities. Flexibility in meal times, type of food (e.g. finger food vs. regular cooked food), sleep times, and type of bathing (bath vs. sponge bath) can all reduce the amount of conflict and ensuing disruptive behaviour by modifying the activities of daily living to accommodate the individual's needs, habits, moods, and tolerance.

Case example 16.1: Mr. Baker – accommodation and flexibility

Mr. Baker had a long-standing love of being out of doors. Staff members often found him at the glass door pushing hard against it trying to get outside. Care staff asked the nurse if the door could be left unlocked. This was agreed and allowed Mr. Baker to walk in the sheltered garden. Walking around in the garden did not place him at risk or place a great burden on the caregiver (Namazi and Johnson 1992; Cohen-Mansfield and Werner 1998b). Over time, staff and family members developed the sheltered garden further by populating the glasshouse and adapting the outdoor area to allow yearlong use.

Case example 16.2: An older woman

An older woman was screaming next to the locked dining room door, obviously wanting to get in. It was not clear why she wanted to get in, as the room held no objects of interest or entertainment. Staff opened the door for her and she went in and sat quietly at one of the tables. It appeared she had wanted to get away from the busy sitting room.

The TREA approach, shown to be efficacious in several studies (Cohen-Mansfield *et al.* 2007, 2012), utilizes a decision tree algorithm by which one arrives at the most likely cause of an agitated behaviour via assessment of the type of behaviour manifested, conditions surrounding the behaviour, and information about the individual's past preferences and needs. Once a cause has been hypothesized, a corresponding treatment is attempted. This effort is evaluated for effectiveness. If effective, the treatment is continued; if ineffective, or only partially effective, the next most likely cause is found and the corresponding treatment provided. The decision tree itself is a series of questions, beginning with the type of agitated behaviour (i.e. physically non-aggressive, physically aggressive, or verbally disruptive behaviours). Within each category, the decision tree guides the caregiver through the steps to be explored in order to ascertain the need most likely contributing to the manifested behaviour. Studies using other algorithms based on the unmet needs model also found them useful in decreasing agitated behaviors (Bédard *et al.* 2011; Kovach *et al.* 2012; Mowrey *et al.* 2013).

Debates and controversies

There is little consensus in either the literature or clinical practice about the definition of problem behaviours and theoretical frameworks used to understand and treat the problem behaviours of persons with dementia. Even the terminology used has been controversial. Some argue that terms such as problem behaviours, disruptive behaviours, challenging behaviours, disturbing behaviours, behavioural problems, and agitation are pejorative, as they suggest the behaviour is intrinsically problematic rather than an indication of an environment that is failing to address people's needs.

Implications for research

Greater monetary resources must be allocated for research to develop the knowledge necessary for optimizing psychosocial care and for understanding dementia in diverse populations. There is an urgent need to improve our ability to answer basic questions: which interventions are efficacious for which individuals? Which aspects of an intervention are necessary for it to be efficacious? What are the active ingredients, or principles at work, in different interventions? Which personal characteristics (gender, culture, prior stress) should be considered in matching an intervention with an individual? What is the impact of the person delivering the intervention and the manner in which it is delivered? Only once these basic questions are answered can the issues of effectiveness and costs be properly addressed.

To increase the use of psychosocial interventions in dementia care, there is a need for public education and advocacy concerning the importance of such interventions and their support. Psychosocial interventions generally provide more personalized care for persons with dementia, addressing their needs, and thereby promoting quality of life.

Conclusion

There are several prerequisites to good psychosocial care of persons with dementia. To provide psychosocial interventions, the system of care must promote an atmosphere and practice of caring that goes beyond what is currently found in most care settings. A practice style that includes good communication skills, compassion and empathy by caregivers, as well as a high level of flexibility of direct care staff and the larger organization are needed, and are often lacking. To allow for alternative interventions, the system of care must promote autonomy and respect for the person with dementia and maximize flexibility in all procedures.

Further information

The Alzheimer's Association is involved in direct support, research, and advocacy for individuals living with and affected by Alzheimer's and related dementias in the USA. Their web site includes tips on how to deal with problem behaviours and also directs caregivers to their 24-hour helpline, local support groups and message board for further support [http://www.alz.org].

The National Dementia Behaviour Advisory Service (NDBAS) within Alzheimer's Australia provides advice on managing behaviours of concern to those who care for a person with dementia. This confidential assistance is available 24 hours a day to respite care staff, health professionals, and carers [http://www.nican.com.au/service/national-dementia-behaviour-advisory-service].

The Alzheimer Society Canada provides information on support, resources, education, and public awareness for caregivers dealing with problem behaviours of people with Alzheimer's as well as links to local support resources [http://www.alzheimer.ca].

The Alzheimer's Society in the UK provides tips for dealing with problem behaviours. See, for example, their information sheets on aggression and also on anti-psychotic medication. They also provide a helpline and email support during business hours for those living in the UK [http://www.alzheimers.org.uk].

The Right Prescription: A Call to Action is a call to action on the use of anti-psychotic drugs for people with dementia [http://www.alzheimers.org.uk/site/scripts/news_article.php?newsID=984].

References

Alessi, C.A., Yoon, E.J., Schnelle, J.F., Al-Samarrai, N.R. and Cruise P.A. (1999) A randomized trial of a combined physical activity and environmental intervention in nursing home residents: do sleep and agitation improve?, *Journal of the American Geriatrics Society*, 47(7): 784–91.

Algase, D., Beck, C., Kolanowski, A., Whall, A., Berent, S. *et al*. (1996) Need-driven dementia-compromised behavior: an alternative view of disruptive behavior, *American Journal of Alzheimer's Disease*, 11: 10–19.

Allen-Burge, R., Stevens, A.B. and Burgio, L.D. (1999) Effective behavioral interventions for decreasing dementia-related challenging behavior in nursing homes, *International Journal of Geriatric Psychiatry*, 14(3): 213–28.

Baillon, S., Van Diepen, E., Prettyman, R., Redman, J., Rooke, N. *et al*. (2004) A comparison of the effects of Snoezelen and reminiscence therapy on the agitated behaviour of patients with dementia, *International Journal of Geriatric Psychiatry*, 19: 1047–52.

Bates, J., Boote, J. and Beverley, C. (2004) Psychosocial interventions for people with a milder dementing illness: a systematic review, *Journal of Advanced Nursing*, 45(6): 644–58.

Beck, C., Richards, K., Lambert, C., Doan, R., Landes, R. *et al*. (2011) Factors associated with problematic vocalization in nursing home residents with dementia, *The Gerontologist*, 51(3): 389–405.

Bédard, A., Landreville, P., Voyer, P., Verreault, R. and Vézina, J. (2011) Reducing verbal agitation in people with dementia: evaluation of an intervention based on the satisfaction of basic needs, *Aging and Mental Health*, 15(7): 855–65.

Birchmore, T. and Clague, S. (1983) A behavioural approach to reduce shouting, *Nursing Times*, 79: 37–9.

Bliwise, D.L. (1993) Sleep in normal aging and dementia, *Sleep*, 16(1): 40–81.

Bliwise, D.L. (1994) What is sundowning?, *Journal of the American Geriatrics Society*, 42(9): 1009–11.

Bowlby, C. (1993) *Therapeutic Activities with Persons Disabled by Alzheimer's Disease and Related Disorders*. Gaithersberg, MD: Aspen.

Buettner, L.L. (1999) Simple pleasures: a multilevel sensorimotor intervention for nursing home residents with dementia, *American Journal of Alzheimer's Disease and Other Dementias*, 14(1): 41–52.

Camberg, L., Woods, P., Ooi, W.L. Hurley, A., Volicer, L. *et al.* (1999) Evaluation of simulated presence: a personalized approach to enhance well-being in persons with Alzheimer's disease [see comments], *Journal of the American Geriatrics Society*, 47: 446–52.

Camp, C.J., Foss, J.W., O'Hanlon, A.M. and Stevens, A.B. (1996) Memory interventions for persons with dementia, *Applied Cognitive Psychology*, 10: 193–210.

Camp, C., Cohen-Mansfield, J. and Capezuti, E. (2002) Nonpharmacological interventions for dementia: enhancing and maintaining mental health in long-term care residents, *Psychiatric Services*, 53(11): 1397–1404.

Child, A., Clarke, A., Fox, C. and Maidment, I. (2012) A pharmacy led program to review anti-psychotic prescribing for people with dementia, *BMC Psychiatry*, 12(1): 155.

Churchill, M., Safaoui, J., McCabe, B. and Baun, M. (1999) Using a therapy dog to alleviate the agitation and desocialization of people with Alzheimer's disease, *Journal of Psychosocial Nursing and Mental Health Services*, 37(4): 16–24.

Cohen-Mansfield, J. (2000) Nonpharmacological management of behavioural problems in persons with dementia: the TREA model, *Alzheimer's Care Quarterly*, 1(4): 22–34.

Cohen-Mansfield, J. (2001) Nonpharmacologic interventions for inappropriate behaviors in dementia: a review, summary, and critique, *American Journal of Geriatric Psychiatry*, 9(4): 361–81.

Cohen-Mansfield, J. (2003) Nonpharmacologic interventions for psychotic symptoms in dementia, *Journal of Geriatric Psychiatry and Neurology*, 16(4): 219–24.

Cohen-Mansfield, J. (2004) Cognitive and behavioral interventions for persons with dementia, in C.D. Spielberger (ed.) *Encyclopedia of Applied Psychology*. Oxford: Elsevier.

Cohen-Mansfield, J. (2007) Temporal patterns of agitation in dementia, *Journal of the American Geriatrics Society*, 15(5): 395–405.

Cohen-Mansfield, J. and Deutsch, L. (1996) Agitation: subtypes and their mechanisms, *Seminars in Clinical Neuropsychiatry*, 1(4): 325–39.

Cohen-Mansfield, J. and Jensen, B. (2005a) Sleep-related habits and preferences in older adults: a pilot study of their range and self rated importance, *Behavioral Sleep Medicine*, 3(4): 209–26.

Cohen-Mansfield, J. and Jensen, B. (2005b) The preference and importance of bathing, toileting, and mouth care in older persons, *Gerontology*, 51(6): 375–85.

Cohen-Mansfield, J. and Jensen, B. (2007a) Self-maintenance habits and preferences in elderly (SHAPE): reliability of reports of self-care preferences in older persons, *Aging: Clinical and Experimental Research*, 9(1): 61–8.

Cohen-Mansfield, J. and Jensen, B. (2007b) Dressing and grooming preferences of community-dwelling older adults, *Journal of Gerontological Nursing*, 33(2): 31–9.

Cohen-Mansfield, J. and Lipson, S. (2002) Pain in cognitively impaired nursing home residents: how well are physicians diagnosing it?, *Journal of the American Geriatrics Society*, 50(6): 1039–44.

Cohen-Mansfield, J. and Lipson, S. (2008) The utility of pain assessment for analgesic use in persons with dementia, *Pain*, 134(1/2): 16–23.

Cohen–Mansfield, J. and Marx, M.S. (1990) The relationship between sleep disturbances and agitation in a nursing home, *Journal of Aging and Health*, 2(1): 153–65. [Also abstracted in *Abstracts in Social Gerontology*, 33(1): 114.]

Cohen-Mansfield, J. and Werner, P. (1995) Environmental influences on agitation: an integrative summary of an observational study, *American Journal of Alzheimer's Care and Related Disorders and Research*, 10(1): 32–7.

Cohen-Mansfield, J. and Werner, P. (1997) Management of verbally disruptive behaviors in nursing home residents, *Journals of Gerontology: Biological Sciences and Medical Sciences*, 52A(6): 369–77.

Cohen-Mansfield, J. and Werner, P. (1998a) The effects of an enhanced environment on nursing home residents who pace, *The Gerontologist*, 38(2): 199–208.

Cohen-Mansfield, J. and Werner, P. (1998b) Visits to an outdoor garden: impact on behavior and mood of nursing home residents who pace, in B. Vellas, J. Fitten and G. Frisoni (eds.) *Research and Practice in Alzheimer's Disease*. Paris: Serdi, pp. 419–36.

Cohen-Mansfield, J. and Werner, P. (1999) Outdoor wandering parks for persons with dementia: a survey of characteristics and use, *Alzheimer's Disease and Associated Disorders*, 13: 109–17.

Cohen-Mansfield, J., Marx, M.S. and Rosenthal, A.S. (1989) A description of agitation in a nursing home, *Journals of Gerontology: Biological Sciences and Medical Sciences*, 44A(3): M77–M84.

Cohen-Mansfield, J., Billig, N., Lipson, S., Rosenthal, A. and Pawlson, L. (1990) Medical correlates of agitation in nursing home residents, *Gerontology*, 36(3): 150–8.

Cohen-Mansfield, J., Marx, M.S. and Werner, P. (1992a) Observational data on time use and behavior problems in the nursing home, *Journal of Applied Gerontology*, 11(1): 111–21.

Cohen-Mansfield, J., Marx, M.S. and Werner, P. (1992b) Agitation in elderly persons: an integrative report of findings in a nursing home, *International Psychogeriatrics*, 4(Suppl. 2): 221–41.

Cohen-Mansfield, J., Werner, P. and Freedman, L. (1995) Sleep and agitation in agitated nursing home residents: an observational study, *Sleep*, 18(8): 674–80.

Cohen-Mansfield, J., Taylor, L. and Werner, P. (1998) Delusions and hallucinations in an adult day care population, *American Journal of Geriatric Psychiatry*, 6(2): 104–21.

Cohen-Mansfield, J., Garfinkel, D. and Lipson, S. (2000a) Melatonin for treatment of sundowning in elderly persons with dementia: a preliminary study, *Archives of Gerontology and Geriatrics*, 31: 65–76.

Cohen-Mansfield, J., Golander, H. and Arnheim, G. (2000b) Self-identity in older persons suffering from dementia: preliminary results, *Social Science and Medicine*, 51: 381–94.

Cohen-Mansfield, J., Parpura-Gill, A. and Golander, H. (2006a) Utilization of self identity roles for designing interventions for persons with dementia, *Journals of Gerontology: Psychological Sciences*, 61B(4): 202–12.

Cohen-Mansfield, J., Parpura-Gill, A. and Golander, H. (2006b) Salience of self-identity roles in persons with dementia: differences in perceptions among patients themselves, family members and caregivers, *Social Science and Medicine*, 62(3): 745–57.

Cohen-Mansfield, J., Libin, A. and Marx, M. (2007) Non-pharmacological treatment of agitation: a controlled trial of systematic individualized intervention, *Journals of Gerontology: Biological Sciences and Medical Sciences*, 62A(8): 908–16.

Cohen-Mansfield, J., Marx, M., Regier, N.G., Dakheel-Ali, M., Thein, K. *et al.* (2010) Can agitated behavior of nursing home residents with dementia be prevented with the use of standardized stimuli?, *Journal of the American Geriatrics Society*, 58(8): 1459–64.

Cohen-Mansfield, J., Golander, H., Ben-Israel, J. and Garfinkel, D. (2011) The meanings of delusions in dementia: a preliminary study, *Psychiatry Research*, 189(1): 97–104.

Cohen-Mansfield, J., Thein, K., Marx, M.S., Dakheel-Ali, M. and Freedman, L. (2012) Efficacy of nonpharmacologic interventions for agitation in advanced dementia: a randomized, placebo-controlled trial, *Journal of Clinical Psychiatry*, 73(9): 1255–61.

Deutsch, L.H., Bylsma, F.W., Rovner, B.W., Steele, C. and Folstein, M.F. (1991) Psychosis and physical aggression in probable Alzheimer's disease, *American Journal of Psychiatry*, 148(9): 1159–63.

Douzjian, M., Wilson, C., Shultz, M., Berger, J., Tampino, J. *et al.* (1998) A program to use pain control medication to reduce psychotropic drug use in residents with difficult behavior, *Annals of Long Term Care*, 6(5): 174–9.

Feldt, K.S. (2000) Improving assessment and treatment of pain in cognitively impaired nursing home residents, *Annals of Long Term Care*, 8(9): 36–42.

Gehrman, P.R., Connor, D.J., Martin, J.L., Shochat, T., Corey-Bloom, J. *et al.* (2009) Melatonin fails to improve sleep or agitation in a double-blind randomized placebo-controlled trial of institutionalized patients with Alzheimer's disease, *American Journal of Geriatric Psychiatry*, 17(2): 166.

Gerdner, L.A. (2000) Effects of individualized versus classical "relaxation" music on the frequency of agitation in elderly persons with Alzheimer's disease and related disorders, *International Psychogeriatrics*, 12(1): 49–65.

Grasel, E., Wiltfang, J. and Kornhuber, J. (2003) Non-drug therapies for dementia: an overview of the current situation with regard to proof of effectiveness, *Dementia and Geriatric Cognitive Disorders*, 15(3): 115–25.

Hart, B. and Wells, D. (1997) The effects of language used by caregivers on agitation in residents with dementia, *Clinical Nurse Specialist*, 11(1): 20–3.

Hellen, C. (1999) *Alzheimer's Disease: Activity Focused Care*. Woburn, MA: Butterworth-Heinemann.

Huffman, J.C. and Kunik, M.E. (2000) Assessment and understanding of pain in patients with dementia, *The Gerontologist*, 40(5): 574–81.

Hurley, A.C., Volicer, B.J., Hanrahan, P.A., Houde, S. and Volicer, L. (1992) Assessment of discomfort in advanced Alzheimer patients, *Research in Nursing and Health*, 15: 369–77.

Husebo, B.S., Ballard, C., Sandvik, R., Nilsen, O.B. and Aarsland, D. (2011) Efficacy of treating pain to reduce behavioural disturbances in residents of nursing homes with dementia: cluster randomised clinical trial, *British Medical Journal*, 343: d4065.

Kasl-Godley, J. and Gatz, M. (2000) Psychosocial interventions for individuals with dementia: an integration of theory, therapy, and a clinical understanding of dementia, *Clinical Psychology Review*, 20(6): 755–82.

Kitwood, T. (1997) *Dementia Reconsidered: The Person Comes First.* Buckingham: Open University Press.

Koss, E. and Gilmore, G.C. (1998) Environmental interventions and functional ability of AD patients, in B. Vellas, J. Fitten and G. Frisoni (eds.) *Research and Practice in Alzheimer's Disease.* Paris: Serdi, pp. 185–92.

Kovach, C., Simpson, M., Joose, L., Lorgan, B., Noonan, P. *et al.* (2012) Comparison of the effectiveness of two protocols for treating nursing home residents with advanced dementia, *Research in Gerontological Nursing*, 5(4): 251–63.

Lachs, M.S., Becker, M., Siegal, A., Miller, R. and Tinetti, M. (1992) Delusions and behavioral disturbances in cognitively impaired elderly persons, *Journal of the American Geriatrics Society*, 40(8): 768–73.

Leverett, M. (1991) Approaches to problem behaviors in dementia, *Physical and Occupational Therapy in Geriatrics*, 9(3/4): 93–105.

Libin, A. and Cohen-Mansfield, J. (2004) Therapeutic robocat for nursing home residents with dementia: preliminary inquiry, *American Journal of Alzheimer's Disease and Other Dementias*, 19: 111–16.

Marsden, J.P., Meehan, R.A. and Calkins, M.P. (2001) Therapeutic kitchens for residents with dementia, *American Journal of Alzheimer's Disease and Other Dementias*, 16: 303–11.

Maslow, A.H. (1968) *Toward a Psychology of Being.* New York: D. Van Nostrand.

Maslow, A.H. (1987) *Motivation and Personality* (3rd edn.). New York: Harper & Row.

Mayers, K. and Griffin, M. (1990) The Play Project: use of stimulus objects with demented patients, *Journal of Gerontological Nursing*, 16(1): 32–7.

Miranda-Castillo, C., Bob, W., Kumari, G., Sabu, O., Charles, O. *et al.* (2010) Unmet needs, quality of life and support networks of people with dementia living at home, *Health and Quality of Life Outcomes*, 8: 132–45.

Mishima, K., Okawa, M., Hishikawa, Y., Hozumi, S., Hori, H. *et al.* (1994) Morning bright light therapy for sleep and behavioral disorders in elderly patients with dementia, *Acta Psychiatrica Scandinavica*, 89(1): 1–7.

Mowrey, C., Parikh, P.J., Bharwani, G. and Bharwani, M. (2013) Application of behavior-based ergonomics therapies to improve quality of life and reduce medication usage for Alzheimer's/dementia residents, *American Journal of Alzheimer's Disease and Other Dementias*, 28(1): 35–41.

Mutch, W.J. (1992) Parkinsonism and other movement disorders, in J.C. Brocklehurst, R.C. Tallis and H.M. Fillit (eds.) *Book of Geriatric Medicine and Gerontology.* Edinburgh: Churchill Livingstone, p. 423.

Namazi, K.H. and Johnson, B.D. (1992) Pertinent autonomy for residents with dementias: modification of the physical environment to enhance independence, *American Journal of Alzheimer's Care and Related Disorders and Research*, 7(1): 16–21.

Namazi, K.H., Rosner, T.T. and Calkins, M.P. (1989) Visual barriers to prevent ambulatory Alzheimer's patients from exiting through an emergency door, *The Gerontologist*, 29(5): 699–702.

Negley, E.N. and Manley, J.T. (1990) Environmental interventions in assaultive behavior, *Journal of Gerontological Nursing*, 16: 29–33.

Okawa, M., Mishima, K., Hishikawa, Y., Hozumi, S., Hori, H. *et al.* (1991) Circadian rhythm disorders in sleep – waking and body temperature in elderly patients with dementia and their treatment, *Sleep*, 14(6): 478–85.

Opie, J., Rosewarne, R. and O'Connor, D. (1999) The efficacy of psychosocial approaches to behaviour disorders in dementia: a systematic literature review, *Australia and New Zealand Journal of Psychiatry*, 33: 789–99.

Palmer, C.V., Adams, S.W., Bourgeois, M., Durrant, J. and Rossi, M. (1999) Reduction in caregiver-identified problem behavior in patients with Alzheimer disease post hearing-aid fitting, *Journal of Speech, Language and Hearing Research*, 42: 312–28.

Parpura-Gill, A. and Cohen-Mansfield, J. (2006) Utilization of self-identity roles in individualized activities designed to enhance well-being in persons with dementia, in L. Hyer and R.C. Intrieri (eds.) *Geropsychological Interventions in Long-Term Care.* New York: Springer, pp. 157–84.

Ripich, D.N. (1994) Functional communication with AD patients: a caregiver training program, *Alzheimer's Disease and Associated Disorders*, 8(3): 95–109.

Ripich, D.N., Wykle, M. and Niles, S. (1995) Alzheimer's disease caregivers: the focused program. A communication skills training program helps nursing assistants to give better care to patients with disease, *Geriatric Nursing*, 16(1): 15–19.

Russen-Rondinone, T. and DesRoberts, A.M. (1996) Success through individual recreation: working with the low-functioning resident with dementia or Alzheimer's disease, *American Journal of Alzheimer's Disease and Other Dementias*, 11(1): 32–5.

Ryden, M., Bossenmaier, M. and McLachlan, C. (1991) Aggressive behavior in cognitively impaired nursing home residents, *Research in Nursing and Health*, 4: 87–95.

Serfaty, M., Kennell-Webb, S., Warner, J., Blizard, R. and Raven, P. (2002) Double blind randomised placebo controlled trial of low dose melatonin for sleep disorders in dementia, *International Journal of Geriatric Psychiatry*, 17(12): 1120–7.

Siders, C., Nelson, A., Brown, L.M., Joseph, I., Algase, D. *et al.* (2004) Evidence for implementing nonpharmacological interventions for wandering, *Rehabilitative Nursing*, 29(6): 195–206.

Sloane, P.D., Hoeffer, B., Mitchell, C.M., McKenzie, D.A., Barrick, A.L. *et al.* (2004) Effect of person-centered showering and the towel bath on bathing-associated aggression, agitation, and discomfort in nursing home residents with dementia: a randomized, controlled trial, *Journal of the American Geriatrics Society*, 52: 1795–804.

Small, J.A. and Gutman, G. (2002) Recommended and reported use of communication strategies in Alzheimer caregiving, *Alzheimer's Disease and Associated Disorders*, 16: 270–8.

Small, J.A., Gutman, G., Makela, S. and Hillhouse, B. (2003) Effectiveness of communication strategies used by caregivers of persons with Alzheimer's disease during activities of daily living, *Journal of Speech, Language and Hearing Research*, 46: 353–67.

Snowden, M., Sato, K. and Roy-Byrne, P. (2003) Assessment and treatment of nursing home residents with depression or behavioral symptoms associated with dementia: a review of the literature, *Journal of the American Geriatrics Society*, 51: 1305–17.

Snyder, M., Egan, E.C. and Burns, K.R. (1995) Interventions for decreasing agitation behaviors in persons with dementia, *Journal of Gerontological Nursing*, 21(7): 34–40.

Steiger, M., Quin, N., Toone, B. and Marsden, C. (1991) Off-period screaming accompanying motor fluctuations in Parkinson's disease, *Movement Disorders*, 6: 89–90.

Sung, H.C., Lee, W.L., Li, T.L. and Watson, R. (2012) A group music intervention using percussion instruments with familiar music to reduce anxiety and agitation of institutionalized older adults with dementia, *International Journal of Geriatric Psychiatry*, 27(6): 621–7.

Tappen, R.M., Williams-Burgess, C., Edelstein, J., Touhy, T. and Fishman, S. (1997) Communicating with individuals with Alzheimer's disease: examination of recommended strategies, *Archives of Psychiatric Nursing*, 11 (5): 249–56.

Teri, L. and Logsdon, R.G. (1991) Identifying pleasant activities for Alzheimer's disease patients: the Pleasant Events Schedule–AD, *The Gerontologist*, 31(1): 124–7.

Werner, P., Cohen-Mansfield, J., Braun, J. and Marx, M.S. (1989) Physical restraints and agitation in nursing home residents, *Journal of the American Geriatrics Society*, 37(12): 1122–6.

Werner, P., Cohen-Mansfield, J., Koroknay, V. and Braun, J. (1994) Reducing restraints: impact on staff attitudes, *Journal of Gerontological Nursing*, 20(12): 19–24.

Werner, P., Cohen-Mansfield, J., Fischer, J. and Segal, G. (2000) Characterization of family-generated videotapes for the management of verbally disruptive behaviors, *Journal of Applied Gerontology*, 19(1): 42–57.

Whall, A., Black, M., Groh, C., Yankou, D., Kupferschmid, B. *et al.* (1997) The effect of natural environments upon agitation and aggression in late stage dementia patients, *American Journal of Alzheimer's Disease and Other Dementias*, 12(5): 216–20.

Woods, P. and Ashley, J. (1995) Simulated presence therapy: using selected memories to manage problem behaviors in Alzheimer's disease patients, *Geriatric Nursing*, 16(1): 9–14.

Yeh, S.H., Lin, L.W., Wang, S.Y., Wu, S.Z., Lin, J.H. *et al.* (2001) The outcomes of restraint reduction programme in nursing homes, Abstract [article in Chinese], *Hu Li Yan Jiu*, 9(2): 183–93.

Zachow, K.M. (1984) Helen, can you hear me?, *Journal of Gerontological Nursing*, 18(8): 18–22.

Zgola, J.M.L. (1987) *Doing Things: A Guide to Programming Activities for Persons with Alzheimer's Disease and Related Disorders*. Baltimore, MD: Johns Hopkins University Press.

Zisselman, M.H., Rovner, B.W., Shmuely, Y. and Ferrie, P. (1996) A pet therapy intervention with geriatric psychiatry inpatients, *American Journal of Occupational Therapy*, 50(1): 47–51.

CHAPTER 17

Communication and relationships: an inclusive social world

Kate Allan and John Killick

> ❝It makes you feel silly. You lose confidence. You don't want to start something different. Just stay home and hide. But my husband won't let me. He nudges me on. I'm quite lucky.❞
>
> —Jenny Reid Melbourne, Australia

> ❝I remember one time visiting my father in the EMI nursing home where he had been living for a year or so. It was tea time and sandwiches and cake were on the menu. The staff carers had been remarking about how my dad, never a greedy man, was always quick to come to the tea trolley. One of the nurses lightheartedly thrust a sandwich at him. At this stage of his disease he had lost the power of speech but he had lost neither his intelligence nor his sensitivity. He correctly read her body-language and was, quite rightly, hurt and upset, but did not have the wherewithal to challenge her. He cried – she had unintentionally humiliated him. It was obvious then that, although mostly hidden from view by his disease, the essence of my proud and gentlemanly father remained on the inside.❞
>
> —Fiona Hardy Yorkshire, UK

> ❝One of the big problems I faced when my relative's dementia was in the middle stage was the way members of the family and some of her friends, became frightened to communicate with her – this was reflected in many different ways. In social settings she was often disregarded and not included in the conversation – also people failed to say goodbye to her when they were leaving. I did try to overcome this with very close members of the family by telling them that she was more aware than they realized but I didn't feel it was appropriate to tell everybody. But I know she often felt isolated and lonely even in company.
>
> During the last year of her life, she said, 'What would I have done without you?' This remark came as a complete surprise to me, as she hadn't spoken any full sentences for at least six months prior to this comment. But, it illustrates that she was aware of her situation.❞
>
> —Vivienne Cooper Yorkshire, UK

Learning objectives

By the end of this chapter, you will:

- Understand the significance of communication in the lives of people with dementia, and those who support them
- Have an appreciation of both the possibilities and challenges in terms of achieving genuine communication with people who have dementia in various contexts
- Have considered a range of value-laden issues that are raised in the exploration of this subject
- Learn about a particular strand of communication work that shows real promise in relating to people with advanced dementia and expanding our nature of dementia as a condition

Introduction

As social animals, we conduct our lives in the context of relationships that rely on communication. Communicating with others – friends, relatives, colleagues, neighbours, and fellow citizens – allows us to achieve the things we need to do to survive and flourish in all sorts of ways: physically, emotionally, in terms of activity and occupation, and at a spiritual level. Each of our individual relationships is unique and differs along a multitude of dimensions, including how the relationship formed, its purpose or core activities, its level of intimacy, and style of communication involved. Our changing networks of relationships reflect the stage we are at in life and what is important to us.

Human communication is highly diverse. The use of language has been identified as one of the defining characteristics of the human species. Linguistic communication can take a variety of forms – spoken, written, and signed. Alongside and interacting with language, we rely on many aspects of non-verbal communication, including facial expression, gesture, eye contact, and touch. Art forms such as drama, painting, photography, dance, film, and literature offer further channels that cross the boundary between language and non-verbal communication.

Communication plays a central role in our concept of identity, both as individuals and as members of groups. The particular ways in which each of us communicates form a large part of how others come to recognize us as unique individuals. However, the fact of our personal uniqueness exists within a wider social context that engenders another dimension of identity, that of a person's culture.

As well as being very much a day-to-day, practical reality, human interaction is underpinned by many complex and value-laden issues, including:

- what counts as a valid relationship
- what is regarded as meaningful communication
- what happens to relationships when there are differences in power between people

Work with people with dementia has a way of highlighting many of these issues, as we shall see in what follows.

We begin by describing why communication is so fundamental to work with people with dementia. We then go on to chart the progress which brought about agreement that people continue to communicate no matter how cognitively disabled they are. Following this, we describe the current state of knowledge in the field, opening with a description of the changes typically associated with dementia which impact on communication and relationships, and highlight the role of psychological and social factors in such changes. This is followed by a discussion of the issues raised within families, recognizing that most people with dementia are supported by family members, before going on to examine communication and relationships between care staff and people with dementia. Arguments for the usefulness of the concept of relationship-centred care in making explicit the centrality of relationship to good dementia care are discussed. Finally, we focus on a significant area in the field: communication with people with advanced dementia.

Dementia, communication, and relationships

Twenty years ago, it was generally believed that the development of dementia gradually destroyed the capacity of an individual to communicate and have meaningful relationships with others (Kitwood 1997). As discussed in Chapter 8, during this period there has been a move away from a purely medical understanding of dementia to recognition of the psychological and social factors that influence its development. Another significant change during the last two decades has been the recognition that persons with dementia are still, first and foremost, persons, and with this comes the realization that just as communication plays a central role in all of our lives, the same applies to people with dementia.

The subject of communication can be seen as pertinent to work with people with dementia for a number of reasons:

1. In relation to personhood, Tom Kitwood (1997) asserts that all of us are only persons by virtue of being in relationship with others, meaning that communication is crucial to the reality of personhood. Whenever we stop attempting to communicate with those around us, we are withdrawing our regard for them as persons. And since we rely on others for the maintenance of our own personhood, we also damage ourselves by doing so.

2. There is no doubt that one of the major changes we see in persons with dementia is in the sphere of communication. More detailed discussion of the specific ways in which communication is commonly affected in dementia follows later.

3. A third reason why communication is a key issue to consider in understanding the needs of people with dementia arises out of the fact that although we have seen much progress in the past 20 years or so, we are still at an early stage of understanding the nature of dementia as a condition. Progress in this area must rely on genuine communication with those who have experience of living with dementia and those who support them.

4. It is difficult to imagine any form of care or support which does not involve communication, and therefore quality care and effective support are dependent on achieving genuine communication. A large part of the rest of this chapter is concerned in various ways with this subject.

5. Our final reason for stressing communication in the understanding of dementia draws on a more values-orientated perspective. The attempt to achieve genuine communication with persons who are experiencing such profound changes in their lives and relationships forces us to confront what are essentially moral issues about why and how we value persons. The bioethicist Stephen Post has drawn our attention to the "hypercognitive" nature of much of western culture, in which "clarity of mind and economic productivity determine the value of a human life" (Post 1995: 3). Within such a culture, our natural bias is to disregard or devalue the kinds of relationships and communication (with adults at least) that seem to lie outside the domain of full cognitive competence. Contact with people with dementia can invite us to value different aspects of being human, and to engage with others in different ways, for example at a physical, emotional or spiritual level.

In addressing some of these issues, we will look not only at problems but also provide examples of situations in which the creativity and resourcefulness of those involved have resulted in new ways forward being found, and unhelpful assumptions being challenged.

Richard Taylor, a man with a diagnosis of dementia, issues the challenge of involving people with dementia in our explorations in the following words:

> ❝Why not spend a bit more time and effort talking with people who have the disease? Studying our needs? Coming up with ideas to make our lives both safer and more fulfilling (and not necessarily in that order)? Why not spend less time with nude mice and more time with early-stage, early-onset folks?❞

—Taylor (2007: 67)

Changes in communication

We begin with a brief description of the changes in communication commonly seen in persons with dementia. The term "aphasia" is a general one used to refer to a range of difficulties with language, including those observed in dementia. Typical features include difficulties with word-finding, which may result in the person "talking around" the word that is causing difficulty, confusion with pronouns such as "he" and "she", and reduced fluency overall. Difficulties with the comprehension of language can unfold alongside problems with expression. This is how one woman with dementia described this experience:

> " You See?
>
> I'll tell you something about myself:
>
> when I'm having a conversation
>
> with someone like yourself
>
> whenever I say "I see"
>
> I do not see,
>
> because when I see
>
> I don't say that but make
>
> a sensible observation,
>
> but when I don't quite follow
>
> I say "I see".
>
> That's the conclusion I've come to anyhow. "
>
> —Killick (2008: 48)

More advanced dementia is frequently characterized by features such as reduction in language use, difficulties producing sounds, repetitions of words and phrases, and the person becoming "stuck" on certain sounds. Whereas it is broadly true that individuals with dementia demonstrate a progressive picture as regards difficulties with language, research shows that considerable variability exists in patterns of change even between individuals diagnosed with the same form of dementia, and between different forms of the condition (Bryan and Maxim 2006).

It is important to note that the kinds of changes we see in the way individuals with dementia communicate cannot be assumed to arise directly from damage to the brain. Psychological factors such as loss of confidence, anxiety, and depression can all have a profound effect on this capacity. Furthermore, a major aspect of Kitwood's (1997) contribution to the reconceptualization of dementia was his illumination of the impact of a range of interpersonal processes that he termed "malignant social psychology". An example of this is "objectification", which refers to the act of treating the person as if an inanimate object. Another example is "outpacing", when others consistently act or communicate at a pace that is too fast for the person with dementia.

Case example 17.1

A friend of Kate's was involved in research investigating people's experiences of ageing. She remembers one participant talking about how she dislikes being the person everyone else is overtaking when out walking. Since then, when in similar circumstances Kate's friend always makes a point of trying to make contact with the older person, even if it is just a brief nod or smile, "excuse me" or other words of acknowledgement. While the reality of being overtaken on the pavement hasn't changed, the act of communication seems to help. Through saying "I know you are a person", perhaps some of the power differential is neutralized.

Such processes, while not consciously intended to be damaging, have the effect of undermining the person's opportunities to communicate with others in a meaningful way and therefore to have their personhood enacted. Les, a man with dementia, expressed his feelings about this issue in strong terms:

> Once you've got Alzheimer's, you're branded. That was terrible. It still is terrible. I can't come to grips with that at all. It is so frustrating. Because I have Alzheimer's, what I say is irrelevant: nobody will listen.

—in Crisp (1995: 52)

Whatever the underlying cause, changes in how people communicate often bring real distress to all parties, and can have a considerable impact on relationships. However, although such changes have traditionally been framed as evidence of an irreversible process of loss, the last decade or so has seen the emergence of alternative perspectives that question this kind of hopelessness.

Much less attention has been given to the changes in the use of non-verbal forms of communication in persons with dementia, although Kitwood (1993) argued that persons with dementia have a heightened capacity for communicating in non-verbal ways. However, a study by Gill Hubbard and colleagues (2002) has made an important contribution to the subject. Researchers spent time in a day centre identifying the incidence of non-verbal communication, both as an adjunct to speech and as a form of communication in its own right. They observed instances of people with dementia using non-verbal means to initiate interactions, to describe their own difficulties, and to signal needs such as visiting the toilet. Non-verbal humour was apparent, as was evidence that participants with dementia were active in interpreting others' non-verbal communication. The authors concluded that: "recognizing and working with nonverbal communication may be one of the ways in which caregivers can contribute towards the preservation of self-identity and personae, and thus contribute towards improving quality of life and care" (Hubbard et al. 2002: 164). An example of how non-verbal expression can be used actively and creatively by an individual with dementia in order to influence the quality of communication is provided by Wilson et al. (2007). They report how one man with significant dementia used laughter in the course of a one-to-one interaction with a researcher to establish that the researcher was listening attentively to him. This strategy enabled him to share his insights about life, as well comment humorously on features of the immediate situation, and sustain a collaborative and enjoyable quality of communication.

Case example 17.2

People with dementia can be really playful. John was interacting one day with someone who did not use verbal language. He sensed she wanted to look at him but would not do so while he was looking at her. So John looked away and gave her the opportunity, which, out of the corner of his eye, he saw that she took. After a while he signalled that he was shortly going to look back at her in order to give her time to withdraw her gaze. After the third or fourth exchange he did something different: he took her by surprise by looking back at her quickly and caught her scrutinizing him. They both burst out laughing.

The subject of non-verbal communication, and the strengths of people with dementia in this regard, needs much more exploration and development work.

The role of communication in understanding dementia

Exercise 17.1: Using humour

Cary Smith Henderson, a man with dementia, said: "Laughing is absolutely wonderful. A sense of humour is probably the most important valuable thing you can have when you have Alzheimer's" (Henderson and Andrews 1998: 14).

■ What roles do you think humour could play in helping people to live with dementia?
■ Think of an example of the successful use of humour in a situation with someone with dementia.

We now move to considering the developments that have occurred in the dementia field following the positive impact of Kitwood's (1997) argument for a relationship-based concept of personhood, and attention to the social and psychological aspects of dementia. This has triggered a flourishing of many new and exciting ways of working, and many of these are concerned directly or indirectly with the subjects of communication and relationships. There is a considerable wealth of findings from research, practice experience, and accounts from people with dementia themselves, and their relatives and friends, to demonstrate that genuine communication is possible and vital to the well-being of all involved. This section of the chapter will present an overview of this learning.

Malcolm Goldsmith's book *Hearing the Voice of People with Dementia* (1996) represents a landmark in terms of thinking about communication. Based mainly on the views of those working in the field, Goldsmith's conclusion is unequivocal:

> ❝It is possible to be involved in meaningful communication with the majority of people with dementia *but* we must be able to enter into their world, understand their sense of place and time, recognize the problems of distraction and realize that there are many ways in which people express themselves and *it is our responsibility* to learn how to recognize these. ❞

> —Goldsmith (1996: 165; emphases in original)

Among many key messages of this work, including the importance of slowing the pace of communication, understanding the effect of the environment on interaction, and the communicative function of so-called "challenging behaviour", Goldsmith stresses the need to recognize the distinctiveness of the person's own subjective experience of dementia. We need to continue to find ways of learning more about the inner world of the person with dementia, and to understand the implications of this dimension for how we think about dementia as a condition and offer support to those who live with it.

One very positive development of this need has come about through people with dementia themselves speaking out about their experiences, needs, and views. This activity has taken a variety of forms, including the publication of writing of various sorts. An example that is highly relevant to the subject of this chapter is an article written by James McKillop, who has a diagnosis of vascular dementia, giving practical advice for enhancing communication (McKillop 2011). We now have videos featuring people with dementia talking about their perspectives; people with dementia are voting members of organizations such as the Alzheimer's Society; they speak at conferences and other events; and they get involved in research projects and advisory groups. In 2002, the Scottish Dementia Working Group was launched, the first organization run by people with the condition whose aim was to campaign for changes in attitudes and improvement in services. (Details of this and other organizations are provided at the end of the chapter.) This emergence of people with dementia themselves as a force for social change represents a significant step forward in addressing the problem of their long-standing exclusion.

Communication in family contexts

In setting out to explore this subject, we are usefully reminded of the complexity of the terrain by Cary Smith Henderson, a man with early onset dementia who kept a journal about his experiences. He wrote:

> 66One of the things about this is – it's in the family and the family has not only me and my wife, but we have our children and the children have their spouses. In other words, this whole thing about Alzheimer's is not just about two people; it's about a whole mess of people. Not only our families but our extended families and their friends. It gets very very involved.

—Henderson and Andrews (1998: 65)

As Cary Smith Henderson so eloquently describes, the development of a condition such as dementia in one of its members is bound to affect the whole family. And, as we all know, families are complex! In addition to practical day-to-day routines and arrangements, financial matters, and how decisions are made, there are all the intricate and involved emotional dimensions of relationships. Some of these relate to issues of power and deeply held values and beliefs. Most family relationships have a long history, and of course issues that go back many years usually have an ongoing influence on the quality of our relationships with relatives. These multifaceted and personal issues are fundamental to our sense of who we are and how we fit into our social worlds. As each family is unique in its strengths and vulnerabilities, the effect of dementia in one party will be unique. However, the changes that accompany dementia will represent a profound challenge to how most families function, and as relatives provide most of the care required by people with dementia, the likelihood of difficulties arising is high.

There is now a considerable body of work exploring ways for those who have known the person prior to the onset of their dementia to adjust their styles of communicating in order to support the continuation of relationships. An important contribution is that of Steven Sabat. His book, *The Experience of Alzheimer's Disease: Life Through a Tangled Veil* (2001), largely consists of painstaking analyses of a series of interactions with a small number of individuals, and he describes some of the characteristics of successful conversations. He draws attention to the importance of turn-taking, of not interrupting and thus breaking the pattern, speaking clearly and slowly, and allowing the other person time to collect their thoughts. He has formulated the concept of "indirect repair", which he defines as follows:

> ❝Inquiring about the intention of the speaker, through the use of questions marked not by interrogatives but by intonation patterns, to the use of rephrasing what you think the speaker said and checking to see if you understood his or her meaning correctly.❞

—Sabat (2001: 38–9)

By using such subtle "cooperative strategies", one can help conversation to flow smoothly without outpacing the other person or otherwise over-exposing their difficulties.

Using her knowledge and skills as a communication scientist and drawing on her experience of supporting her mother who had dementia, Jane Crisp (2000) has written about ways of "keeping in touch" with a person with dementia. This includes advice about strategies for making sense of apparently confused speech, and also responding in empathic and creative ways to the stories the person with dementia tells rather than dismissing a narrative as confused or simply untrue. There is also very good advice about understanding how non-verbal aspects of communication contribute to the whole picture.

While progress has been made in this area, we are some way from developing the kinds of policies and practices that properly support the large number of people who provide care within a family context for people with dementia. However, despite the difficulties, we have begun to see the emergence of a kind of writing that demonstrates a balanced approach to both the possibility of gain and development, as well as the reality of loss. A notable example comes from a book written by Sunny Vogler called *Dementia: The Loss . . . The Love . . . The Laughter* (2003). The author had a very difficult relationship with her mother during her early life that was characterized by turmoil and estrangement. Having taken the decision to care for her mother when she developed dementia, she writes:

> ❝Mother was different, and discovering who she was each day was a delight. The bitterness she had lived with was draining from her mind – and in its place was a new pleasant outlook that seemed to surprise and please us both. More than once she gave me a loving look and simply whispered 'Thank you'. These were the rewards I had missed in my childhood and were so welcome now.❞

— Vogler (2003: 37)

Exercise 17.2: Dealing with a dilemma

You visit a service where you meet a number of people with dementia for the first time. One person seems especially drawn to you, and on engaging in conversation, it becomes clear that the person is convinced that you are a much-missed relative, and is delighted that you have at last come to visit them.

- How would you handle this situation?
- What does this tell you about your values?

Communication and relationships with care staff

While most care for people with dementia is provided within the family, many experience care in an institutional setting. Here, we consider two research projects that have closely examined the nature of communication and relationships in care homes. First, however, it is important to remind ourselves that Kitwood's understanding of personhood emphasizes that one can only be truly a person if we are recognized as such by others, and that this applies as much to staff as it does to the person with dementia. It follows, then, that the personhood of care staff is put at risk when communication is absent. This is demonstrated in the following quotation from a member of staff in a Swedish care setting:

> 66 When you cannot get into contact with the patient you feel insufficient, without hope, dissatisfied or burnt out. Care seems meaningless. You lose your commitment. 99

—Ekman *et al*. (1991: 168)

The first study discussed here was carried out by Richard Ward and colleagues and used video-recording, observation, and interviews to examine patterns of communication within various sorts of services over a period of three years. The findings reported in Ward *et al*. (2008) concentrate on care homes, and they do not make comfortable reading. Analysis revealed that residents with dementia spend only an average of 10% of their day engaged in interaction with others. Of this, 75% takes place between residents and with visitors. It was apparent that some residents who were able sought to maximize their experiences of contact with others by positioning themselves strategically within the care setting, and certain residents were observed helping each other to overcome obstacles to communication arising out of mobility issues, memory loss, and the sequelae of stroke. These findings make it clear that opportunities for interaction with others were important to residents in the care homes.

Focusing in on the small amount of communication between residents and staff (averaging approximately 2.5% of residents' days), Ward and colleagues revealed a number of concerning patterns. Among these were that episodes of direct interaction usually (in about 77% of instances) occurred only at times when a care task was being carried out. The majority of such contacts were extremely short, and non-verbal means of interacting with the resident in order to execute a task predominated, meaning that encounters were conducted in silence. Where verbal communication was used, this was generally in response to the resident failing to cooperate with the carer's intentions. Interactions involving speech overwhelmingly conformed to a remarkably standardized and deeply impoverished format that neither took account of the communicative capacity of the resident, nor invited any input from them. The researchers labelled this kind talk "carespeak". It took the form of a series of instructions directed to the resident, or a commentary on the care task being performed, punctuated by brief expressions of approval, all of which proceeded at a pace set by the member of staff. Such a pattern raises the question of whether, in order to have some verbal communication, however unsatisfying, a resident may intentionally obstruct the process of care tasks.

A particular strength of this study arises out of the very extensive use of video-recording, allowing the researchers to discern patterns in how residents communicate with others in non-verbal terms. They provide an account of how one man, Michael, expressed his mood and influenced how much contact he had with care staff despite the fact of having extremely limited means of communication. Through careful analysis of recordings made over time and in different situations, it became clear that the speed of Michael's body movements (including folding and unfolding his arms and legs) corresponded to his events, which affected his emotional state, and he used body posture (specifically sliding down in his chair) to attract the attention of staff, who, while helping him to sit in a more upright position, would address some words to him and engage in physical contact by holding his hand. Despite this evidence of meaningful expression, Michael was regarded as being unable to communicate.

Ward and colleagues' description of infrequent, brief, and impoverished acts of communication in the course of care provision makes for disheartening reading, but these findings are not surprising in the context of what the study revealed about attitudes towards communication. The general belief expressed by those in both junior and senior roles, and those involved in the regulation and inspection of services, was that people with dementia generally were simply unable to communicate due to their dementia. We can see here that the many examples of malignant social psychology – outpacing, objectification, infantilization – that dominated contact between staff and residents follow directly from this more fundamental belief. Why would a member of staff put time and effort into attempting to make genuine contact with a person with dementia if they believe it simply isn't possible?

Other findings showed that the chances of real communication occurring in the contexts studied could not be attributed solely to the attitudes and behaviour of individuals: they were further diminished by the physical layout of the environment, the ways in which tasks were organized and carried out, and the emphasis on how residents look as an indicator of quality care. The picture is of a whole range of interrelated barriers to those living in the homes being recognized as persons and offered opportunities to connect authentically with others. The combined effect of these barriers "effectively excludes people with dementia from any form of participation in or influence over the support they receive" (Ward et al. 2008: 645). While the primary impact of this state of affairs was borne by the residents, we have to wonder how such a situation affected the self-image, morale, and health of the staff too. And yet, despite all this, encounters characterized by warmth, sensitivity, and creativity between carers and those with significant disabilities were observed, and the authors emphasize that valuable lessons could be learned by studying such exceptions to the norm.

We now consider the findings of another study that investigated the use of one of the earliest approaches to communicating with persons with dementia, which was developed by Naomi Feil (2002) and is known as "Validation". Validation stresses the importance of recognizing and engaging with the individual's emotional world and subjective experience in the moment, and responding by means of verbal and non-verbal interaction. In a year-long study in Sweden (Söderlund et al. 2012), training was provided to help nursing staff in a care home develop both the necessary guiding values or "approach" and specific empathic and communicative skills consistent with what was termed the "Validation Method". The authors emphasize that in striving to communicate more meaningfully the technical aspects of what is done differently cannot be applied in isolation from a values-based approach.

The participating staff underwent extensive theoretical and practical instruction, and applied what they were learning in the course of their daily work. Evaluation was carried out through interviews with participating staff, and this process included reflection on video-recordings of encounters with individuals with dementia.

Feil found that as the Validation Method was applied, nursing staff noticed significant changes in how individuals with dementia seemed to feel, in how they interacted with staff and other residents, and in more general aspects of their day-to-day conduct, for example in improved initiative, self-care, and participation in activities. When situations arose involving conflict or expression of aggression, these were less intense.

Among the significant themes to emerge from analysis of the interviews was that while learning and using the approach was demanding, it was associated with the development of a more trusting "atmosphere" between the persons with dementia and the nursing staff, with residents being more open to interaction and appearing to enjoy it more. The staff talked about having a greater sense of enjoyment and confidence in their work, and felt that use of the Validation Method helped them to develop professionally and to feel "stronger, happier, less stressed and more secure". This study provides an illustration of how engaging in genuine communication affirms and strengthens the personhood of both the individual with dementia and those in supporting roles.

While this study provides an encouraging and inspiring example of what is possible when communication is accorded its rightful place, the former demonstrates that we clearly have a long way to go in putting what we know into action.

From person-centred to relationship-centred care

The impetus for much of the progress in this field has come from the emergence of the concept of person-centred care. The robustness and practical implications of this concept continue to be a focus of discussion and debate (Brooker 2006), and partly as a response to the problems of implementing such a model and a recognition that people exist within a network of relationships, the concept of "relationship-centred care" has developed (Nolan et al. 2004).

In this vein, Trevor Adams and Paula Gardiner (2005) explored different patterns of communication within dementia care triads, which typically comprised the person with the condition, a relative, and a professional. They describe "enabling dementia communication", which:

> [o]ccurs when informal carers or health and social care professionals either help the person with dementia express their thoughts, feelings and wishes or represent the person with dementia as someone who is able to make decisions about their own care.

—Adams and Gardiner (2005: 190)

Such communication arises through efforts to remove unwanted stimuli, get in the right position physically, promote equal participation, and be sensitive to non-verbal cues. "Disabling" communication is characterized by practices such as interrupting, speaking on behalf of the person, using language that is too technical or complex, and talking out of earshot.

John Keady and Mike Nolan (2003) carried out a study exploring how couples, who were still at an early stage of coming to terms with the condition, coped with the challenge. They interviewed both family members and persons with dementia. As a result of this, they identified four kinds of relationship. Three of these are variants on both partners working as single units, but one describes the partners working together to make the best of the situation.

Ingrid Hellström and colleagues describe an example of what could be considered the latter type of relationship (Hellström et al. 2005). They present a case study of a couple, Mr. and Mrs. Svensson, who are in their eighties and live in Sweden. Mrs. Svensson developed dementia within four years of them getting married. This study provides indications of what are successful approaches to communication, as well as an example of how dementia is not always a burden that has a damaging effect on relationships. They describe how "whilst surprised by the diagnosis, for both partners this turn of events provided yet further meaning as to why they married late in life". The researchers identified ways in which Mr. Svensson included his wife in communication, and "demonstrated both remarkable sensitivity to her needs and great ingenuity in providing assistance that actively reinforced, rather than undermined, his wife's sense of agency" (Hellström et al. 2005: 19).

Nolan *et al.* (2004) admit that the concept of relationship-centred care needs further clarification and development. Certainly, while the model can be considered to correspond more closely to the reality of most people's lives, it does not seem likely that implementing such care on a widespread basis will prove any less of a challenge than that of delivering so-called person-centred care.

Communication with people with advanced dementia

This is the strand of development work we have chosen to feature in this chapter. Considerable progress has been made in exploring communication and relationships in the earlier years of dementia, but making meaningful contact with those with much more profound disabilities and those close to death has been comparatively neglected.

> ### Case example 17.3: Peggy
>
> John and Kate both worked on a project exploring the capacity for communication with people with advanced dementia. On the fourth occasion John met Peggy, it took her 25 minutes to become fully aware of his presence. A powerful encounter then ensued when Peggy seized his hands in hers and rubbed them, manipulating them vigorously, and digging her nails into them. This went on for about 17 minutes, before she released his hands and turned away, seemingly having been able to express something deeply felt and painful. This encounter demonstrated the importance of remaining available to an individual even when what they express is unclear or uncomfortable.

Within the last few years in the UK, and partly as a result of the growing recognition of the need for people with dementia to have access to palliative care services, there are signs that the challenges of communicating with people whose disabilities are profound are receiving attention.

In 2004, an article by Rosemary Clarke was published which described her experience of using an approach for communicating with people in coma (Mindell 1997) with her mother, who at the time had advanced dementia. The approach involves close observation of movement, posture, and position, and a wide range of other non-verbal signals and feeding back observations to the person, together with attempting to match breathing, and use the voice and touch in time with breathing rhythm. Clarke comments:

> 66 My experience has been, at times, sublime, and I believe for her empowering . . . [It has] been infinitely precious and enriching for me, and I commend this approach to others who would like to both give and gain deep satisfaction in their contact with those with dementia who are largely beyond words. 99

—Clarke (2004: 23)

Research on the capacity of persons with advanced dementia to engage in communication has been undertaken by Maggie Ellis and Arlene Astell, who used a modified form of Intensive Interaction (II), a communication approach developed for use with people with profound learning disabilities (Caldwell 2005), which they call Adaptive Interaction (AI). In common with II and coma work, AI involves using imitation or mirroring of the vocalizations and non-verbal actions of the person in order to establish interaction. In one study (Astell and Ellis 2006), they found that Jessie, a woman with advanced dementia living in a care home, retained the capacity and desire to interact, as evidenced by her use of turn-taking, eye contact, and gestures such as nodding. Part of the study included observing Jessie's responses to the use of "still face", when a communication partner stops responding and appears impassive. Her use of vocalization, decreased eye contact, and body movements demonstrated that she was aware of the violation of the normal give and take of interaction and had a desire to resume contact. Ellis and Astell (2011) report the use of AI with a variety of individuals with dementia revealed a hitherto hidden range of communicative capacity, and a small-scale training programme with members of staff was found to be successful and indicated that it is possible to enable those supporting people with advanced dementia to learn how to engage in meaningful and satisfying ways with them.

While such work should encourage and inspire us, it also has deeply challenging implications about the neglect of the human needs for contact of so many people and the seemingly ever-expanding scope of the work which faces those in a caring role. And discovering that people who can seem unreachable remain able to respond to others demands that we question assumptions about the nature of dementia itself.

Exercise 17.3: Exploring silence

- Think of some reasons why periods of silence during interactions with a person with dementia might be helpful.
- Try having conversations with family, friends, and persons with dementia where silence is a more prominent feature than usual.
- Reflect on how these experiences felt, and any effects silence had on other aspects of communication.

Debates and controversies

We have already referred to how work with very advanced dementia raises ethical issues. This situation embodies the most extreme example of a power differential that has to be handled with great care. For example, how might we know if a person welcomes our attention or wishes to be left alone? How should we interpret very minimal or ambiguous signals that may or may not constitute an act of communication? In a world where resources are limited, how much time and energy should be devoted to attempts to connect with a person who may or may not appear to respond? And with increased emphasis on evidence-based care, how should we value outcomes that are transient and difficult to record, such as the squeeze of one's hand or simply having a strong sense of the person being engaged and present?

A lively debate has developed about whether it is ever justified to lie to a person with dementia. Research suggests that it is common practice among care staff, such as when, for example, confronted by a person asking where their long-dead spouse is, they are told that their wife has gone out and will be back later. For some, such an approach may be the most "therapeutic" one if others, such as attempting to meet their needs or distracting them, have failed. Another view sees such situations as more symbolic in nature and in need of nuanced interpretation. Yet again there are those who see anything other than a straightforward approach as disrespectful to the person.

The whole issue of deception has been thrown into relief by the SPECAL approach, promulgated by the psychologist Oliver James in his book *Contented Dementia* (2008). Here the primary object is to keep the person with dementia safe from any uncomfortable issues or questions in a kind of protective bubble.

Conclusion

This chapter has argued that communication is essential to being a person and to our relationships with others. While it is usual to see changes in ways of communicating in the person with dementia, the need to maintain contact with others, and do so in a range of ways, remains and is crucial to well-being. Those in a supporting role are equally reliant on authentic communication if they are not to experience a sense of alienation and perhaps burnout.

Work in this field has looked at ways of enhancing communication in both professional care and family contexts, and we have seen the emergence of people with dementia themselves speaking out about their experiences and needs. Despite the development of greater understanding of what is needed and what works, however, research indicates that communication still does not have its rightful central place in how care is organized and provided.

We end with a quotation from Faith Gibson, which is an answer to her own question: can we risk person-centred communication?

> 66 We must employ whatever power we have in the world of dementia care for this purpose. We must use our present knowledge, our skills and feelings, to communicate. We are morally obliged to continue working in extending our limited understanding, developing our embryonic skills, and taming our deep anxieties. 99

—Gibson (1999: 24)

Further information

The Scottish Dementia Working Group provides extensive resources for people with dementia, caregivers and friends of people with dementia, and professionals engaged in providing care. There is basic information on dementia, symptoms, treatments, legal and financial issues, as well as conferences and formal training programmes on a range of issues. Each section includes advice for people newly diagnosed with dementia, including guidance on "what next". The site also includes a charter of rights and an outline of important policy issues related to dementia [http://www.alzscot.org/campaigning/scottish_dementia_working_group].

The Dementia Engagement and Empowerment Project (DEEP) aims to explore, support, promote, and celebrate groups and projects led by or actively involving people with dementia across the UK that are influencing services and policies affecting the lives of people with dementia [http://www.mentalhealth.org.uk/our-work/research/dementia-engagement-and-empowerment-project/].

The Dementia Advocacy and Support Network is an international group of people with dementia. Founded in 2000, this organization provides a forum for exchanging information, advocating for services, and promoting respect for people with dementia [http://www.dasninternational.org/].

Memory Bridge is devoted to connecting people with dementia to their communities and to promoting companionship for people with dementia. Memory Bridge also provides educational programmes for the public, specifically focusing on understanding what is not erased by dementia – the memory that endures. They also foster opportunities for people to learn from the voices of people with dementia, and what these voices have to "teach us about our own humanity" [www.memorybridge.org].

Innovations in Dementia Care is a consultancy group of dementia care experts, partnering with organizations and communities for the purpose of supporting people with dementia to maintain control over their lives. Innovations in Dementia Care employs people with dementia as advisors on projects [http://www.innovationsindementia.org.uk/who.htm].

Alzheimer's from the Inside Out is the web site of Richard Taylor, a man with a PhD in psychology who was diagnosed with dementia 10 years ago. The web site provides an "insider's" view of living with dementia while also providing information and training opportunities [http://www.richardtaylorphd.com].

Dementia Positive is a web site that gathers work from many people and places that celebrates the creativity, strengths, and insights of people living with dementia. It includes examples of creative arts that people with dementia participate in, books and films that celebrate continued enjoyment in life for people with dementia, and organizations that have developed creative programmes for people with dementia [www.dementiapositive.co.uk].

The Social Care Institute for Excellence: Research Briefing 3: Aiding communication with people with dementia [http://www.scie.org.uk/publications/briefings/briefing03/].

The Social Care Institute for Excellence: Dementia Gateway: Living with dementia – Communicating well [http://www.scie.org.uk/publications/dementia/living-with-dementia/communication/].

References

Adams, T. and Gardiner, P. (2005) Communication and interaction within dementia care triads: developing a theory for relationship-centred care, *Dementia*, 4(2): 185–205.

Astell, A.J. and Ellis, M.P. (2006) The social function of imitation in severe dementia, *Infant and Child Development*, 15(3): 311–19.

Brooker, D. (2006) *Person-centred Dementia Care: Making Services Better*. London: Jessica Kingsley.

Bryan, K. and Maxim, J. (2006) *Communication Disability in the Dementias*. London: Whurr.

Caldwell, P. (2005) *Finding You Finding Me: Using Intensive Interaction to Get in Touch with People whose Severe Learning Disabilities are Combined with Autistic Spectrum Disorder*. London: Jessica Kingsley.

Clarke, R. (2004) Precious experiences beyond words, *Journal of Dementia Care*, 12(3): 22–3.

Crisp, J. (1995) Dementia and communication, in S. Garratt and E. Hamilton-Smith (eds.) *Rethinking Dementia: An Australian Approach*. Melbourne: Ausmed Publications.

Crisp, J. (2000) *Keeping in Touch with Someone who has Alzheimer's*. Melbourne: Ausmed Publications.

Ekman, S.L., Norberg, A., Vitanen, M. and Winblad, B. (1991) Care of demented patients with severe communication problems, *Scandinavian Journal of Caring Sciences*, 5(3): 163–70.

Ellis, M. and Astell, A. (2011) Adaptive interaction: a new approach to communication, *Journal of Dementia Care*, 19(3): 24–6.

Feil, N. (2002) *The Validation Breakthrough*. Baltimore, MD: Health Professions Press.

Gibson, F. (1999) Can we risk person-centred communication?, *Journal of Dementia Care*, 7(5): 20–4.

Goldsmith, M. (1996) *Hearing the Voice of People with Dementia: Opportunities and Obstacles*. London: Jessica Kingsley.

Hellström, I., Nolan, M. and Lundh, U. (2005) "We do things together": a case study of "couplehood" in dementia, *Dementia*, 4(1): 7–22.

Henderson, C.S. and Andrews, N. (1998) *Partial View: An Alzheimer's Journal*. Dallas, TX: Southern Methodist University Press.

Hubbard, G., Cook, A., Tester, S. and Downs, M. (2002) Beyond words: older people with dementia using and interpreting non-verbal behaviour, *Journal of Aging Studies*, 16(2): 155–67.

James, O. (2008) *Contented Dementia: 24-hour Wrapped Around Care for Lifelong Well-being*. London: Vermilion.

Keady, J. and Nolan, M. (2003) The dynamics of dementia: working together separately, or working alone?, in M. Nolan, U. Lundh, G. Grant and J. Keady (eds.) *Partnerships in Family Care: Understanding the Caregiving Career*. Buckingham: Open University Press.

Killick, J. (2008) *Dementia Diary: Poems & Prose*. London: Hawker Publications.

Kitwood, T. (1993) Towards a theory of dementia care: the interpersonal process, *Ageing and Society*, 13(1): 51–67.

Kitwood, T. (1997) *Dementia Reconsidered: The Person Comes First*. Buckingham: Open University Press.

McKillop, J. (2011) Top tips for good communication, *Journal of Dementia Care*, 19(2): 14–15.

Mindell, A. (1997) *Coma, a Healing Journey: A Guide for Families, Friends and Carers*. Portland, OR: Lao Tse Press.

Nolan, M.R., Davies, S., Brown, J., Keady, J. and Nolan, J. (2004) Beyond "person-centred care": a new vision for gerontological nursing, *International Journal of Older People Nursing*, 13(3a): 45–53.

Post, S.G. (1995) *The Moral Challenge of Alzheimer's Disease*. Baltimore, MD: Johns Hopkins University Press.

Sabat, S.R. (2001) *The Experience of Alzheimer's Disease: Life Through a Tangled Veil*. Oxford: Blackwell.

Söderlund, M., Norberg, A. and Hanselbo, G. (2012) Implementation of the validation method: nurses' description of caring relationships with residents with dementia disease, *Dementia*, 11(5): 569–87.

Taylor, R. (2007) *Alzheimer's from the Inside Out*. Baltimore, MD: Health Professions Press.

Vogler, S. (2003) *Dementia: The Loss . . . The Love . . . The Laughter*. Bloomington, IN: 1st Books.

Ward, R., Vass, A.A., Aggarwal, N., Garfield, C. and Cybyk, B. (2008) A different story: exploring patterns of communication in residential dementia care, *Ageing and Society*, 28: 629–51.

Wilson, B.T., Muller, N. and Damico, J.S. (2007) The use of conversational laughter by an individual with dementia, *Clinical Linguistics and Phonetics*, 21(11/12): 1001–6.

CHAPTER 18

Supporting health and physical well-being

John Young and Amy Illsley

66 My relative had recurring UTI infections and these were missed by the care-staff and they did not pick up the signs up until a later stage in the infection. If I was away I knew that my relative's health would suffer. I could tell by my relative's body language when she was developing an infection. Regular tests for a patient with urinary tract infections would be beneficial for patients at risk of infection. 99

—Vivienne Cooper Yorkshire, UK

66 You said they were valuable so we put them away"– (Nurse at an inpatient dementia assessment unit when I asked where my father's hearing aids were), "I'm not sure they make much difference anyway" – (another nurse at the same unit discussing what had happened.) 99

—Anne Warburton Yorkshire, UK

Learning objectives

By the end of this chapter, you will:

- Understand actions needed to promote health and well-being for people with early dementia
- Understand how delirium and falls might be prevented in people with moderate dementia
- Understand swallowing difficulties common in more advanced dementia
- Understand the range of interventions helpful in maintaining health and physical well-being during the "career" of people living with dementia

Introduction

Evidence-based best practices for health promotion and disease prevention that constitute routine care for people in later life are equally applicable to people with dementia. Indeed, people with dementia may accrue increased benefits due to their additional vulnerability to common forms of ill health that can arise in later life. Unfortunately, people with dementia are often excluded from routine best clinical practice due to pervading professional stigmatism, ignorance, and misunderstandings (Iliffe and Manthorpe 2002). We present the arguments for a considered, proactive style of clinical care. Such an approach ensures that people with dementia achieve optimum health and physical well-being.

We first look at health promotion for people in the early stages of dementia, focusing on diet, prevention of vascular disease, exercise promotion, and flu prevention. We then look at the definition, prevention, and treatment of delirium, and falls. Finally, we discuss strategies for ameliorating the swallowing impairment that affects people at the end of their journey with dementia.

The beginning of the journey

Case example 18.1: Marjorie, recently diagnosed with dementia

Marjorie is a 75-year-old lady who has always lived in the same area. Since retiring as a teacher, she has written a weekly column in her local newspaper. Her husband died five years ago and, after a period of bereavement, she re-formed her social life to include twice weekly luncheons with her daughter who lives nearby. Marjorie has had good health and rather dismisses her mini-stroke two years ago and high blood pressure that was diagnosed at that time. Recently, her memory has deteriorated and, on her daughter's insistence, she has attended the local memory clinic where a diagnosis of early mixed-type dementia has been established and explained to Marjorie and her daughter. Marjorie's daughter wants to know what should be done to keep her mother independent and living at home for as long as possible.

■ What might you suggest?

We know that co-existing medical conditions in people with dementia are common and that they are at increased risk of developing new physical conditions. A study of 671 patients with Alzheimer's disease reported that 61% had three or more co-morbid conditions and that medical co-morbidity increased with advancing dementia (Doraiswamy *et al*. 2002). Another study found that patients with dementia presenting to primary care have, on average, 2.4 chronic conditions and receive 5.1 medications (Schubert *et al*. 2006). To promote health and physical well-being, the following areas could be highlighted for Marjorie:

■ diet
■ prevention of heart attacks and strokes
■ promoting activity
■ flu prevention

Diet

The World Health Organization has a nutritional goal to increase fruit and vegetable intake to at least 400g per day in order to reduce the burden of long-term conditions (WHO 2005). For example, in the UK the national dietary scheme is called the "5 A DAY" programme. It involves promotion of a simple message: "to eat at least five portions (400g) of a variety of fruit and vegetables each day" (Department of Health 2003) (see Box 18.1).

Box 18.1: The 5 A DAY Programme: key messages

■ Eat a least five portions of a variety of fruit and vegetables each day.
■ Fresh, frozen, chilled, canned, and dried fruit and vegetables and 100% juice all count.
■ 1 portion is 80 g of fruit or vegetables, for example: 1 medium apple **or** 1 medium banana **or** 3 tablespoonfuls of cooked vegetables **or** 1 cereal bowl of mixed salad **or** 1 glass (150 ml) or 100% orange juice.

(*continued*)

> ■ The fruit and vegetables contained in convenience foods – such as ready meals, pasta sauces, soups, and puddings – can contribute towards 5 A DAY. But convenience foods can also be high in added salt, sugar or fat – which should only be eaten in moderation – so it's important always to check the nutrition information on food labels.
>
> *Source*: Department of Health (2003)

Increasing the consumption of fruit and vegetables is associated with reduced risk for cancer, coronary heart disease, and stroke, while also delaying cataract development and improving bowel function. Although the effects of diet on dementia progression are unclear (see Chapter 1), increasing the intake of fruit and vegetables is equally valuable for people with or without early dementia. Studies involving over 250,000 participants demonstrated a 26% risk reduction in stroke associated with eating more than five portions of fruit and vegetables per day compared with less than three (He *et al.* 2006), particularly important for preventing the further cognitive decline resulting from stroke. It is ethically unjust to limit access to dietary advice on the basis of co-existing dementia.

Prevention of heart attacks and strokes

Vascular disease, primarily coronary heart disease and stroke, is the leading cause of death in most regions of the world. As discussed in Chapter 1, epidemiological evidence has demonstrated a link between hypertension (high blood pressure) and dementia – both future dementia and accelerated progress of existing dementia. Given Marjorie's history of hypertension and mini-strokes, she is at high risk of future vascular disease and she would benefit from vascular disease prevention measures.

What steps should be taken?

First, an assessment of vascular risk should be performed. In addition to ageing, several lifestyle factors (smoking, poor diet, low activity) and clinical factors (hypertension, diabetes, obesity, high cholesterol) predispose to vascular disease. Estimating Marjorie's vascular risk will involve questioning and testing to detect these factors, for example, urine dip testing to detect possible kidney damage from hypertension. Blood glucose should be checked to test for diabetes. Measurement of total blood cholesterol and high-density lipoprotein should be done. Several blood pressure recordings and 24-hour ambulatory blood pressure monitoring, where appropriate, should be undertaken to assess for hypertension (NICE 2011).

Should Marjorie's hypertension be treated, and if so, what benefits might she get?

Treating hypertension

High blood pressure increases the chance of strokes, heart attacks, heart failure, kidney failure, and poor circulation in the legs. In a major review involving over one million people, increased blood pressure was conclusively linked to vascular disease risk (Lewington *et al.* 2002). This has been confirmed in many subsequent studies – reducing blood pressure saves lives and improves quality of life by preventing heart disease and strokes. Recent research has clearly demonstrated *reduced* cognitive decline in people with both dementia and hypertension receiving treatment to lower blood pressure. It is therefore clear that people like Marjorie should be offered treatment for their hypertension.

Treatment of hypertension consists of lifestyle advice and drug therapy. Lifestyle advice for adults aged over 65 includes:

- a healthy diet
- regular exercise for 150 minutes per week and muscle strengthening activities on two or more days each week
- avoidance of excess alcohol (men: less than three–four units of alcohol per day; women: less than two–three units units of alcohol per day)
- reduction of dietary salt
- support to quit smoking

In most people, this advice will need to be supplemented by long-term medication with blood pressure lowering drugs. In the UK, NICE guidelines on diagnosis and management of dementia recommend that vascular risk factors should be identified and treated in the secondary prevention of dementia (NICE 2006a). Risk of vascular disease can be minimized by reducing blood cholesterol to reduce the chance of blocked arteries (British Cardiac Society *et al*. 2005).

Promoting activity

Exercise and activity are associated with health benefits at any age, including people with dementia. It is never too late to commence regular exercise, which can prevent or delay the onset of several diseases, including osteoporosis, diabetes, hypertension, heart disease, stroke, and possibly some cancers. Regular exercise can also improve sleep, prevent falls and fractures, and there are social benefits with amelioration of loneliness and depression.

The potential benefits of exercise have been investigated and confirmed in people with dementia. A systematic review (30 randomized controlled trials; 2020 participants) summarized the evidence and demonstrated that exercise increases fitness, physical function, cognitive function, and positive behaviour in people with dementia (Heyn *et al*. 2004). People with dementia should be encouraged to maintain, or if possible increase, their levels of activity, as it represents an important protective factor for cognitive decline.

In a review of the exercise literature in relation to older people, McMurdo (2000) concluded: "Most of the health benefits (of exercise) can be gained by performing regular moderate intensity physical activity", such as "walking, dancing, bowling or gardening". These activities should be well within the grasp of the majority of older people, including those with early dementia. Even frail older people in care homes (many of whom will have had dementia) can have their physical functioning stabilized and possibly even improved with tasks such as chair exercises (Crocker *et al*. 2013).

Flu prevention

Influenza is a highly infectious disease that occurs every year, usually in winter. It spreads rapidly, from person to person, mainly by airborne respiratory droplets, particularly in highly populated environments such as care homes. Most people with flu feel severely unwell with aches and pains, high fever, sore throat, and runny nose. A few develop complications: viral pneumonia, secondary bacterial pneumonia, or exacerbations of chronic medical conditions such as heart failure and bronchitis, more common in older people, with poor background health.

Flu infections can be reduced in people with dementia and their carers by an annual flu vaccination each autumn. This provides 70–80% protection against infection lasting about one year. For example, UK Government policy is to offer flu vaccination to the "at risk" groups in society (Department of Health 2007). This includes people over 65 years, people who have chronic diseases such as heart disease, renal disease or diabetes, and those who live in a residential care home. People with dementia are not a specified group but will be largely subsumed in the "all people over 65 years" category and those who live in a long-care facility. Flu vaccination is also recommended for those who are the main carer for an older person (Department of Health 2007).

The middle of the journey

Case example 18.2: Marjorie (continued) – experiencing delirium and dementia

Marjorie is now 81 years old. Her daughter phones to say that she is worried, explaining that her mother has been coping satisfactorily at home but two days ago became incontinent of urine (unusual for her) and more confused and that the home care team found her rather sleepy. She seems reluctant to get out of bed and doesn't seem interested in eating or drinking but appears uncomfortable, frequently rubbing her tummy. Sometimes her speech is slurred and it's hard to make out what she is trying to say.

■ What might be causing these changes in Marjorie?
■ What advice might you give?

Delirium

Marjorie has delirium (also called acute or toxic confusion) and needs urgent medical attention. Delirium is common in people who have a dementia, between 22% and 89% in hospitalized and community populations aged over 65 years with the condition (Fick et al. 2002). Delirium is characterized by fluctuating inattention and confusion, linked to one or more triggering factors. Marjorie's presentation of new-onset urinary incontinence suggests the triggering factor may be a urinary infection. Delirium is serious with mortality rates of 25–33%, functional decline, and symptoms that may persist for up to 12 months (Young and Inouye 2007). One large prospective cohort study found that delirium significantly accelerates irreversible cognitive decline in patients with Alzheimer's (Fong et al. 2009).

Detecting delirium

As is discussed in Chapter 22, delirium is poorly detected, being missed in about half of cases in hospital, and therefore poorly managed, resulting in sub-optimum outcomes. NICE recommends screening at hospital admission with the aim of preventing delirium in people identified to be at risk using a targeted, multi-component intervention that addresses modifiable risk factors. (NICE 2010). They advise that at-risk patients are screened using a validated tool such as the Confusion Assessment Method (CAM) (see Box 18.2).

Box 18.2: The Confusion Assessment Method (CAM)	
	SCORE
1. Is there a history of recent-onset confusion that has fluctuated? And	0 or 1
2. Attention impairment (count backwards from 20) And either	0 or 1
3. Disorganized thinking or incoherent speech? Or	0 or 1
4. Is the patient sleepy or lethargic?	0 or 1
If a score of 3 or more, consider delirium.	

Causes of delirium: risk factors and precipitants

Delirium is a complex clinical syndrome that rarely has a single cause. A useful approach is to consider delirium as an interaction between underlying risk factors and precipitants (or triggering events). Recognition of the risk factors for delirium opens up the important issue of delirium prevention, and timely identification of delirium precipitants leads to early treatment, before the delirium syndrome has become fully established (Young and Inouye 2007).

Box 18.3: Risk factors for delirium	
Old age	Deafness
Physical frailty	Polypharmacy (multiple medications being taken at the one time)
Severe illness	Surgery (especially fractured neck of femur)
Dementia	Alcohol excess
Infection	Renal impairment
Dehydration	Pain
Visual impairment	

For Marjorie, age and dementia are obvious risk factors. There are also clinical clues for pain (rubbing her tummy), constipation (abdominal discomfort, restlessness, reduced mobility, and reluctance to eat), and dehydration (reluctance to drink). Tackling her constipation and dehydration at this early stage could minimize the impact of the delirium.

Precipitants of delirium

Precipitants are factors that can be identified as the event that triggered the delirium.

Box 18.4: Common precipitants for delirium

■ lower respiratory tract infection
■ urinary infection/urinary retention
■ faecal impaction/constipation
■ electrolyte disturbance (dehydration, renal failure, high or low sodium levels)
■ drugs (especially those affecting blood pressure or sedatives)
■ alcohol withdrawal
■ severe pain
■ neurological (stroke, epilepsy)

Note: Many patients have more than one cause.

Precipitants alone do not cause delirium but interact with the underlying individual predisposition. Thus, a major insult, such as a serious infection, is required to trigger delirium in a previously fit person, but only a minor change (e.g. a change in medication) can result in delirium in a person at high risk such as someone like Marjorie with dementia.

Preventing delirium

Perhaps the most important aspect of delirium is that there is good evidence it can be prevented in about one-third of cases (Young and Inouye 2007). As we have seen, many risk factors have been identified and many can be modified. In the UK, for example, NICE suggest a team trained in management of delirium should address dehydration, constipation, hearing and visual disturbance, hypoxia, infection, immobility, pain, nutrition, sleep disturbance, environment, and multiple medications (NICE 2010). The latter is particularly important, as inappropriate medications may be the sole precipitant of delirium in 12–39% of cases (Young and Inouye 2007). To prevent episodes of delirium for Marjorie, the following steps should be taken.

Medication review

People with dementia are likely to be taking several medications for a range of conditions. This is called "polypharmacy". Taking more than six drugs is associated with major risk of delirium development, and more than four medications is a risk factor for falls. Marjorie might have been advised to take hypertension medication to reduce her risk of stroke. However, we know that in the middle part of the dementia journey blood pressure can fall due to dementia-related weight loss and changes in cardiovascular reflexes. Thus a treatment that was once highly appropriate may become potentially harmful. Key risk factors for medication-related adverse events have been identified as inappropriate prescribing, old age, adherence issues, drug interaction, co-morbidity, and polypharmacy (Gomez-Pavon et al. 2010). Although dementia is not an independent risk factor for adverse drug reactions, the above risk factors are more prevalent in patients with dementia.

Polypharmacy in the UK was recognized in the National Service Framework for Older People with a recommendation for six-monthly medication reviews (Department of Health 2001). It is important that people with moderate dementia obtain regular drug reviews from their general practitioner, to review each medication and to discuss if it is still necessary.

Patients with dementia are sometimes prescribed anti-psychotic medication to manage challenging behaviour (HSCIC 2012). These medications cause a significant increase in adverse cardiovascular events and death. Living Well with Dementia: A National Dementia Strategy (Department of Health 2009) has a target of reducing prescriptions of these medications by two-thirds.

Prevention of dehydration

Dehydration can develop insidiously in people with moderate dementia and will be an important risk factor for delirium for Marjorie. The causes are usually several: dementia-associated loss of thirst sensation, drinks placed out of reach, diuretic medication, and loss of body fluids through diarrhoea or vomiting. Early recognition of dehydration is difficult but a slow spring-back of the skin on the forehead after gently pinching it can be a useful indication. Dehydration can be confirmed through a blood sample.

Prevention of constipation

Prevention of constipation is important for people with dementia because it is a common problem and a risk factor for delirium: about one-third of older people suffer from constipation (Petticrew *et al.* 1997).

There are many causes of constipation, including serious disease such as colon cancer (alarm symptoms are rectal bleeding, alternating diarrhoea and constipation, weight loss, anaemia). For Marjorie, the most likely reasons will be medications, a diet low in fibre, dehydration, and lack of activity. A dementia-specific factor is impaired attention to the call-to-stool sensation. Constipation can progress to faecal impaction where the large bowel becomes loaded with hard faeces that irritate the colon lining, causing a mucus-rich form of diarrhoea: a trap for the unwary – diarrhoea that is due to severe constipation.

Prevention involves withdrawal of constipating drugs (commonly codeine preparations, tricyclic anti-depressants, and some hypertension medications), the promotion of mobility, and increasing fluids and dietary fibre.

Prevention of malnutrition

The adverse health consequences of obesity have absorbed the attention of the media. But the main risk to people with dementia is under-eating and weight loss. "Thousands . . . are annually starved in the midst of plenty from want of attention to the ways which make it possible for them to take food." So wrote Florence Nightingale in 1859 – it is sad that her observation is still applicable in the twenty-first century. The cause of under-eating is multi-factorial. For Marjorie, her cognitive impairment and living alone will be two important risk factors but there may well be others, as listed in Box 18.5.

Box 18.5: Common risk factors for malnutrition in older people

Isolation/living alone	Poor dentition/sore mouth
Poverty	Gastrointestinal diseases
Disability/chronic disease	Loss of manual dexterity
Lack of easy access to shops	Cold house
Depression/loss of interest in food	Bereavement
Impaired taste, vision, smell, hearing	Cognitive impairment

Marjorie may be one of the 40% of older people with malnutrition when admitted to hospital. A quality standard from NICE requires all care services to take responsibility for identification of people at risk of malnutrition using a validated screening tool and provide nutrition support where appropriate. Inpatients are required to be screened weekly, those in a care home monthly, and outpatients on their first attendance. Screening should assess body mass index (BMI), percentage unintentional weight loss, and the time over which nutrient intake has been unintentionally reduced alongside the likelihood of future impaired nutritional intake (NICE 2006b, 2012). Nutritional support should then be considered for people identified as at risk of malnutrition, or who are malnourished, typically with a BMI of less than 18.5 (see Box 18.6).

Box 18.6: Identifying people with malnutrition

Calculation of body mass index (BMI):

$$BMI = weight/(height)^2$$

where weight is measured in kilograms and height in matres.

BMI < 18.5 is indicative of under-nutrition

People at risk of malnutrition:

a) Have eaten little or nothing for five days
b) Unable to take in food properly
c) Have conditions causing increase nutritional needs

People who are malnourished:

a) BMI < 18.5
b) Unintentional weight loss of more than 10% over three to six months
c) BMI < 20 and unintentional weight loss of more than 5% over three to six months

---

If Marjorie has a BMI of less than 18.5, further enquiry is necessary to identify causes and remedies. These may include ill-fitting dentures, loss of interest in food (ensure depression is not overlooked), forgetfulness about meals, difficulty planning meals, or difficulty cooking meals. Providing meals at home or increasing the social opportunities for meals may be required. Marjorie is more likely to eat foods she is familiar with, she may require longer meals times with gentle encouragement, and finger foods can be enjoyable and increase intake (Biernacki and Barratt 2001).

Case example 18.3: Marjorie (continued) – falls at home

Marjorie has been finding it increasingly difficult to get up from her chair and often needs help. She has started walking in the house more slowly and places her hands on items of furniture for balance as she walks. She is found in the morning lying on the floor by the home care staff. Marjorie is upset and cannot recall what exactly happened but it seems she fell while going to the toilet during the night.

■   What would you suggest?

Reducing the risk of falls

Falls are a common occurrence in people like Marjorie who have dementia and are aged over 75 years, as age and cognitive impairment are both important risk factors for falls. The risk of falls associated with dementia is partly caused by impaired balance reactions due to slower brain processing as a consequence of the dementia, partly because dementia is associated with impairment of cardiovascular reflexes that help maintain blood pressure when standing, and partly due to risk factors common to many older people (e.g. multiple drugs, environmental hazards, poor eyesight, inappropriate footwear, painful feet). Marjorie might be expected to have an annual falls incidence of around 60% (twice that of people without dementia), and to have an increased risk of a head injury or a major injury such as a fracture (Tinetti et al. 1988). Head injury is a particular concern to people with dementia because observational studies have repeatedly identified head injury as associated with a steep change in cognitive decline. Preventing falls in people with dementia is therefore an important aspect of their care.

NICE produced guidance on the prevention of falls. The recommendation is for people like Marjorie who have a high risk of falls to be assessed by "healthcare professionals with appropriate skills and experience, normally in the setting of the specialist falls service" (NICE 2004). The assessment is designed to identify the risk factors for falls and to construct an individual treatment plan to address them. These multi-factorial prevention interventions have been successful in preventing falls in at-risk individuals, including people with cognitive impairment (Tinetti et al. 1994; Close et al. 1999).

Assessment of the home environment is also essential, including: attention to loose mats and carpets; provision of non-slip bathmats and rails in showers, around baths and toilets, and to stairs and steps; removal of trailing electric cords; and improved lighting, especially in critical areas such as stairwells. Equally important is to check footwear. There have been several "sloppy slipper" campaigns to replace inadequate slippers and reduce the risk of falls. Home modifications, provided after assessment by an experienced occupational therapist, have been associated with a reduction in falls (Cumming et al. 1999).

Promoting continence

Problems with urinary or bowel continence are common in people with dementia, and are commonly under-reported. Sensitive questioning about continence should therefore be part of usual care. Incontinence develops because of abnormalities in the pelvic, bowel or bladder wall muscles, or their nerve supply. People with dementia are particularly prone to "overflow" faecal incontinence (sometimes called faecal impaction), and so-called "functional" urinary incontinence. These conditions are related to, or exacerbated by, poor mobility, impaired manual dexterity or poor cognitive awareness of a full bladder or bowel. Easy access to toilets that are private, comfortable, and can be used safely and have clear signage (especially toilet facilities away from the home), and regular exercise are essential to maintain continence. Other simple measures to maintain urinary continence include caffeine reduction, advice on modifying fluid intake (an increase for people with low intake, and a decrease for people with high intake), and weight loss for people who are overweight. Faecal impaction can be avoided by ensuring good hydration and adjusting the diet (increased or reduced dietary fibre depending on individual assessment) to promote ideal stool consistency and predictable bowel emptying. Encouraging bowel emptying after a meal is also important.

Towards the end of the journey

Case example 18.4: Marjorie (continued) – difficulty swallowing

Marjorie is now 85 years old, still living at home but has become much more dependent such that she spends much of the day lying in bed with only brief periods sitting in a chair. Her daughter visits several times each day but Marjorie doesn't always recognize her. She now needs assistance to eat her food and the home care staff are worried because there have been some choking episodes.

■ What would you advise?

Impairment of swallowing

Marjorie now has advanced dementia and is developing a further problem – impaired swallowing. This is a common, probably inevitable, feature in people with more advanced dementia (Ratnaike 2002).

Difficulty swallowing liquids or solids is referred to as *dysphagia*. Swallowing is complex and involves a highly coordinated sequence of muscle contractions that move mouth contents safely over the upper airway and into the oesophagus. Initiation and control is by a swallowing centre located in one cerebral hemisphere. This centre can become damaged by the neuropathology of dementia (or by a stroke). A further issue is that the muscles involved with swallowing are subject to the generalized weakness that affects all muscles in people who adopt a chair-fast lifestyle. This weakness is progressive and a critical stage is reached when there is just sufficient swallowing function for usual health but with a loss of functional reserve such that a stressor event (commonly an infection) unmasks the loss of reserve and manifests as acute dysphagia. The principal complications of dysphagia are aspiration pneumonia, malnutrition, and dehydration, all of which are unpleasant and distressing and have a high mortality.

Timely identification of dysphagia is important, as it can prevent aspiration pneumonia and provide a window of opportunity to consider selected feeding techniques described below. Early features include a moist sounding voice or moist cough (due to liquid pooling in the pouches around the back of the throat), or coughing immediately after sipping a drink (implies abnormal penetration of fluid into the larynx). If any of these features is present, it is imperative that drinks and food are withheld and an urgent specialist swallowing assessment requested – usually from a speech and language therapist. Often compensatory measures will be recommended, such as careful head and body positioning, attention to consistency of food, smaller meals, a double swallow if cooperation is possible, frequent checking of mouth contents to ensure no accumulation is occurring, and watching for fatigue. Meals should be flexible and timed with periods of greatest wakefulness. Marjorie's concentration will be impaired and it is important that disturbances and distractions are minimized. "Feeders", cups with spouts, popular in elderly care settings, must be banned. They create a fast jet of liquid liable to overwhelm the deficient swallow mechanism landing the fluid at the back of the mouth and straight into the airway. When in doubt, use a thickening agent. Thickened fluids are much less likely to penetrate into the larynx.

If dysphagia is more severe and persistent, tube feeding may be considered. Nasogastric tubes with liquid feeds can be useful in the short term if swallowing deteriorates during an acute illness.

This can buy time for a few days while the swallowing hopefully improves. However, nasogastric tubes are poorly tolerated and are often quickly removed by the patient, particularly in people like Marjorie with advanced dementia who have difficulty retaining the information about the purpose of the tube.

Persistent dysphagia prompts consideration for a percutaneous endoscopic gastrostomy (PEG) feeding tube system. Here, a feeding tube is located in the stomach via the overlying skin under local anaesthetic using an upper gastrointestinal endoscope procedure. The procedure is usually well tolerated by people with dementia so that the immediate complication rate (haemorrhage, infection, and perforation) is very low. The main issue, however, is not the technical aspects of the procedure, but in determining whether it is the right course of action, and considering the long-term complications. A Cochrane review looked at the evidence for tube feeding in advanced dementia. They found no conclusive evidence that tube feeding prolongs survival, improves quality of life, improves nutrition or reduces the risk of pressure sores, but may actually increase the risk of aspiration pneumonia and even death (Sampson *et al.* 2009). The overriding ethical principle is to consider how the supported feeding will affect quality of life and to what extent the life of the person is meaningful. In the UK, a pragmatic approach is usually adopted such that when the dementia has severely affected awareness to an extent that, for example, the person no longer appears able to appreciate the presence and contact of people close to them, then prolonged PEG feeding has little to offer (see Chapter 25).

Debates and controversies

Primary care is pivotal to the delivery of good quality assessment and care for people with dementia. What the systems of care should look like to optimize this process is poorly evidence based. For example, the role and precise content of dementia registers, regular reviews, and care plans remains poorly defined. Many people with dementia will have other long-term conditions. How this co-morbidity should be managed, the inter-relationships of different conditions, and how to prioritize care components for different conditions is unclear. Another area of controversy surrounds the balance between primary/community and secondary care for people with dementia who become unwell. Can more people with dementia who become unwell be assessed and treated safely in their own homes? Related to this is the extent to which falls and delirium might be prevented for people with dementia living at home or in residential care. It would be eminently sensible to achieve this but we have little evidence of what to do and how to do it. Finally, with respect to people with advanced dementia, it is unclear whether we should struggle to maintain sufficient food intake, or if this apparently humane approach simply prolongs the period of decline and its associated poor quality of life. Associated with this is how to provide better dementia-specific end-of-life care training for primary care teams.

Conclusion

There is a range of interventions to promote and sustain optimal health and physical well-being for people with various stages of dementia. We have an established evidence base of their effectiveness. As dementia progresses, different priorities emerge. This implies that regular reviews are needed if health care crises are to be minimized and physical well-being promoted.

The aim should be to identify early indications of changing health to ensure there is the best opportunity to implement a process of proactive management. Involving family members is key to the success of this process.

There is much that can and should be done to promote and sustain optimal health and physical well-being for people with dementia. We can think of prevention and intervention as focusing on various points along on a person's journey with dementia. For people with mild dementia, as for all people, it is important to provide advice about health promotion including exercise, diet, and flu prevention, and to ensure they are assessed for vascular disease prevention. An increasing risk of delirium becomes a major issue for people with moderate dementia and this can be reduced by regular drug reviews and prevention of malnutrition, dehydration, and constipation. Also, the risk of falls and injury becomes an important threat to health. A falls risk assessment is needed to reduce this risk. In advanced dementia, a deterioration of swallowing is an important and distressing issue and some simple preventative measures can be helpful.

Further information

- Age Concern (2006) *Hungry to be Heard: The Scandal of Malnourished Older People in Hospital.* London: Age Concern [http://www.scie.org.uk/publications/guides/guide15/files/hungrytobeheard.pdf].

- National Institute for Health and Clinical Excellence (NICE) (2006) *Dementia: Supporting People with Dementia and their Carers in Health and Social Care.* Clinical Guideline No. 42. London: NICE [http://guidance.nice.org.uk/cg42/?c=91523].

- National Institute for Health and Clinical Excellence (NICE) (2010) Delirium: Diagnosis, Prevention and Management. Clinical Guideline No. 103. London: NICE [http://guidance.nice.org.uk/CG103/Guidance/pdf/English].

References

Biernacki, C. and Barratt, J. (2001) Improving the nutritional status of people with dementia, *British Journal of Nursing*, 10: 1104–14.

British Cardiac Society, British Hypertension Society, Diabetes UK, HEART UK, Primary Care Cardiovascular Society, The Stroke Association (2005) JBS 2: Joint British Societies' guidelines on prevention of cardiovascular disease in clinical practice, *Heart*, 91 (Suppl. V) [http://heart.bmj.com/cgi/content/extract/91/suppl_5/v1, accessed 29 April 2014].

Close, J., Ellis, M., Hooper, R., Glucksman, E., Jackson, S. *et al.* (1999) Prevention of falls in the elderly trial: the PROFET study, *The Lancet*, 353: 93–7.

Crocker, T., Young, J., Forster, A., Brown, L., Greenwood, D. *et al.* (2013) The effect of physical rehabilitation on activities of daily living in older residents of long-term care facilities: systematic review with meta-analysis, *Age and Ageing*, 42(6): 682–8.

Cumming, R.G., Thomas, M., Szongi, G., Salkeld, G., O'Neil, E. *et al.* (1999) Home visits by an occupational therapist for assessment and modification of environmental hazards; a randomised trial of falls prevention, *Journal of the American Geriatrics Society*, 47: 1397–1402.

Department of Health (2001) *National Service Framework for Older People.* London: Department of Health [https://www.gov.uk/government/uploads/system/uploads/attachment_data/file/198033/National_Service_Framework_for_Older_People.pdf, accessed 29 April 2014].

Department of Health (2003) *Booklet 2 – A Local 5 a Day Initiative: A Handbook for Delivery.* London: Department of Health.

Department of Health (2007) *Flu Prevention*. London: Department of Health.

Department of Health (2009) *Living Well with Dementia: A National Dementia Strategy*. London: Department of Health [https://www.gov.uk/government/uploads/system/uploads/attachment_data/file/168220/dh_094051.pdf, accessed 29 April 2014].

Doraiswamy, P.M., Leon, J., Cummings, J.L., Marin, D. and Neumann, P.J. (2002) Prevalence and impact of medical comorbidity in Alzheimer's disease, *Journals of Gerontology: Biological Sciences and Medical Sciences*, 57(3): M173–M177.

Fick, D.M., Agostinim, J.V. and Inouye, S.K. (2002) Delirium superimposed on dementia: a systematic review, *Journal of the American Geriatrics Society*, 50: 1723–32.

Fong, T.G., Jones, R.N., Shi, P., Marcantonio, E.R., Yap, L. *et al*. (2009) Delirium accelerates cognitive decline in Alzheimer disease, *Neurology*, 72(18): 1570–5.

Gomez-Pavon, J., Gonzalez Garcia, P., Frances Roman, I., Vidan Astiz, M., Gutierrex Rodriguez, J. *et al*. (2010). Recommendations for the prevention of adverse drug reactions in older adults with dementia, *Revista Española de Geriatría y Gerontología*, 45: 89–96.

He, F.J., Nowson, C.A. and MacGregor, G.A. (2006) Fruit and vegetable consumption and stroke: meta-analysis of cohort studies, *The Lancet*, 367: 320–6.

Health and Social Care Information Centre (HSCIC) (2012) *National Dementia and Antipychotic Prescribing Audit 2012: Key Findings on the Prescription of Antipsychotics for People with Dementia in England – Report for the Audit Period 2006 to 2011*. Leeds: HSCIC [www.ic.nhs.uk/dementiaaudit, accessed 29 April 2014].

Heyn, P., Abreu, B.C. and Ottenbacher, K.J. (2004) The effects of exercise training on elderly persons with cognitive impairment and dementia: a meta-analysis, *Archives of Physical Medicine and Rehabilitation*, 85:1694–1704.

Iliffe, S. and Manthorpe, J. (2002) Dementia in the community: challenges for primary care development, *Reviews in Clinical Gerontology*, 12: 243–52.

Lewington, S., Clarke, R., Qizilbash, N., Peto, R. and Collins, R. (2002) Age specific relevance of usual blood pressure to vascular mortality: a meta-analysis of individual data for one million adults in 61 prospective studies, *The Lancet*, 360: 1903–13.

McMurdo, M.E.T. (2000) A healthy old age: realistic or futile goal?, *British Medical Journal*, 321: 1149–51.

National Institute for Health and Clinical Excellence (NICE) (2004) *Falls: The Assessment and Prevention of Falls in Older People*. Clinical Guidance No. 21. London: NICE [http://guidance.nice.org.uk/CG21/guidance/pdf/English, accessed 29 April 2014].

National Institute for Health and Clinical Excellence (NICE) (2006a) *Dementia: Supporting People with Dementia and their Carers in Health and Social Care*. Clinical Guideline No. 42. London: NICE [http://guidance.nice.org.uk/CG42, accessed 29 April 2014].

National Institute for Health and Clinical Excellence (NICE) (2006b) *Nutrition Support in Adults: Oral Nutrition Support, Enteral Tube Feeding and Parenteral Nutrition*. Clinical Guideline No. 32. London: NICE [http://guidance.nice.org.uk/CG32/?c=91500, accessed 29 April 2014].

National Institute for Health and Clinical Excellence (NICE) (2010) *Delirium: Diagnosis, Prevention and Management*. Clinical Guideline No. 103. London: NICE [http://guidance.nice.org.uk/CG103/Guidance/pdf/English, accessed 29 April 2014].

National Institute for Health and Clinical Excellence (NICE) (2011) *Hypertension: Clinical Management of Primary Hypertension in Adults*. Clinical Guideline No. 127. London: NICE [http://publications.nice.org.uk/hypertension-cg127, accessed 29 April 2014].

National Institute for Health and Clinical Excellence (NICE) (2012) *QS24 Quality Standard for Nutrition Support in Adults*. London: NICE [http://publications.nice.org.uk/quality-standard-for-nutrition-support-in-adults-qs24, accessed 29 April 2014].

Petticrew, M., Watt, I. and Sheldon, T. (1997) Systematic review of the effectiveness of laxatives in the elderly, *Health Technology Assessment*, 1(13): 1–53.

Ratnaike, R.N. (2002) Dysphagia: implications for older people, *Reviews in Clinical Gerontology*, 12: 283–94.

Sampson, E.L., Candy, B. and Jones, L. (2009) Enteral tube feeding for older people with advanced dementia, *Cochrane Database of Systematic Reviews*, 2: CD007209 [http://onlinelibrary.wiley.com/doi/10.1002/14651858.CD007209.pub2/full, accessed 29 April 2014].

Schubert, C.C., Boustani, M., Callahan, C.M., Perkins, A.J., Carney, C.P. *et al*. (2006) Comorbidity profile of dementia patients in primary care: are they sicker?, *Journal of the American Geriatrics Society*, 54: 104–9.

Tinetti, M.F., Speechley, M. and Ginter, S.F. (1988) Risk factors for falls among elderly persons living in the community, *New England Journal of Medicine*, 319: 1701–7.

Tinetti, M.F., Baker, D., McAvay, G., Claus, E.B., Garrett, P. *et al.* (1994) A multifactorial intervention to reduce falls risk among elderly people living in the community, *New England Journal of Medicine*, 331: 821–7.

World Health Organization (WHO) (2005) *Fruit and Vegetables for Health: Report of a Joint FAO/WHO Workshop* [http://www.who.int/dietphysicalactivity/publications/fruit_vegetables_report.pdf, accessed 29 April 2014].

Young, J. and Inouye, S.K. (2007) Clinical review: delirium in older people, *British Medical Journal*, 334: 842–6.

Chapter contents

CHAPTER 19

Diagnosis and post-diagnosis support

Richard H. Fortinsky

> ❝Here's the medication now go away. It was three years down the line from diagnosis and I saw nobody. Diagnosing people early is good, you know, but if you're gonna diagnose people earlier you need to give them supports. It needs to be there before you give somebody a diagnosis. I was just given the diagnosis and medications. I was still working at the time. There was nothing. Like you know if you're a diabetic they don't just give you the insulin and say come back when your legs drop off.❞
>
> —Sheila Varo Yorkshire, UK

> ❝My mother was more than sad and embarrassed by her condition. She was in denial and tried to hide her failing memory. She was scared and confused. When she was diagnosed the consultant explained that she had a disease called Alzheimer's disease but she did not take it in. She had a friend who had AD who had to go into a care home.❞
>
> —Brenda Smith Yorkshire, UK

> ❝Every individual with dementia is different, every carer is different, everyone's journey is different. Therefore every service needs to be flexible. I'd really like to emphasise the need for flexibility, because as I said everyone is different. And in an ideal world what would've helped us is to be contacted a few weeks after the diagnosis by a named person at that point, even if I'd've said 'It's alright, we're fine', they could've then given me a name, a contact number, a few leaflets, and maybe kept in touch with me, so that I would have known where to turn to, instead of leaving it for a year and then bursting into tears and go 'No one's given me any information'.❞
>
> —Tricia Dunlop, Greater Manchester, UK

> ❝Sometimes with surprise, sometimes with worry, sometimes in horror, sometimes just feeling silly that something has changed and you just cannot do what you have always been able to do....but if someone opens the door, invites you in and tries to help then you are damn sight better off than you were without any help. In other words 'I' becomes part of 'us' and 'we'.❞
>
> —Tony Oates Yorkshire, UK

Learning objectives

By the end of this chapter, you will be able to:

- Discuss the importance and application of the principle of uncertainty from the first symptoms of dementia through diagnosis to the use of early support services
- Explain how people with dementia and their family carers view dementia-related symptoms and decide to seek information and help

- Explain implications of results from clinical trials intended to improve diagnosis and early support in the primary care setting for people with dementia and their families
- Explain recent evidence-based research findings and public policy initiatives on early support services and non-pharmacological interventions offered in community settings for people with dementia and their families

Introduction

In the twenty-first century, dementia has become a global health issue owing largely to the ageing of populations in all developed countries and many developing countries throughout the world. Symptoms characteristic of dementia, regardless of the cause, include (NICE-SCIE 2006; Alzheimer's Society 2007; Alzheimer's Association 2013):

- progressive loss of memory that disrupts daily life
- challenges in planning or solving problems
- increasingly impaired judgement, decision-making, and verbal communication
- mood changes
- withdrawal from work or social activities
- increased inability to conduct activities of living, ranging from driving to grocery shopping to personal care

Because the trajectory and accumulation of these symptoms vary widely among individuals in terms of time intervals and intensity, there is a tremendous amount of uncertainty among people affected by these symptoms and their family members regarding when to seek help from health care professionals to determine a diagnosis and answer questions they have about prognosis and treatment options. Once a diagnosis of Alzheimer's disease or other dementia is made, people with dementia and their families face questions about what support services are available in the community to help them plan for the future and manage symptoms as they worsen. For most families living with the daily challenges of dementia, the goal is to enable the person with dementia to live in the comfort of her or his home with as much dignity as possible, as long as support services in the local community can be identified and marshalled to help enable them to achieve this goal (see Chapters 13 and 21).

This chapter focuses on the phase of the dementia journey beginning with the initial recognition of symptoms, proceeding through the acquisition of a diagnosis, and ending when the person diagnosed with dementia is still living at home but with symptoms progressed to the point where they and their family carers receive some degree of health and social care assistance. For purposes of this chapter, then, "early support" refers to health and social care services in the statutory (public) and voluntary (private) sectors provided during the time that a person with dementia resides in a domestic home setting and any involved family carers are actively engaged in helping the person remain at home. As we will see, some early support services specifically target people in earlier stages of dementia and their families, while others offer service to people in any stage of dementia and their families.

The chapter is divided into four interrelated sections: time before the diagnosis, making the diagnosis, disclosing the diagnosis, and early support after the diagnosis. Each section highlights that uncertainty remains a key problem throughout the dementia journey among persons with dementia, family carers, and health and social care practitioners.

Before the diagnosis

The time between symptom development and diagnosis is characterized by increasing uncertainty for most people with dementia and their families. A large-scale survey of more than 600 family carers from six European countries found that the average length of time between symptom recognition and a diagnosis of symptoms was 20 months, with an average range from 10 months in Germany to 32 months in the UK (Bond *et al.* 2005). Research on the pre-diagnosis phase of the dementia journey, between memory symptom recognition and diagnosis by a health care practitioner, remains quite limited. Although there is growing research about the self-described experience of living with dementia, we are just beginning to understand the ways in which persons with dementia symptoms feel about and respond to their symptoms before a diagnosis is made. The challenge in this type of research is locating and interviewing persons living with dementia during the period between recognition of symptoms and receiving a diagnosis from a physician or memory clinic practitioner.

The earliest study to capture this pre-diagnosis window was conducted in England. The study included 48 people attending a memory clinic for assessment of their symptoms who were later diagnosed with Alzheimer's disease and/or vascular dementia as a result of this clinic assessment (Moniz-Cook *et al.* 2006). Separate interviews were conducted with these participants (age range 66–87 years) and with their accompanying family members. Study participants were exclusively British Caucasians residing in urban or suburban settings at the time of the study. Results from this study illustrated the principle of uncertainty at this pre-diagnosis stage of the dementia journey from the perspective of persons with dementia symptoms. Uncertainty arose primarily from not knowing whether the course of their symptoms would mirror those experienced previously by loved ones who had been affected by dementia. Findings also revealed uncertainty among persons with dementia and their family members in the form of a lack of awareness about support that might enable the person with dementia to live at home as long as possible.

A review of literature from several countries on the broader topic of living with dementia from the perspective of the person with dementia suggests that the uncertainty uncovered by this English study permeates the entire dementia journey (de Boer *et al.* 2007). Themes emerging from this literature review indicate that individuals who experience memory loss and associated symptoms respond with complex coping strategies ranging from the emotion-oriented (e.g. denial, avoidance of symptoms) to the problem-oriented (e.g. compensation for cognitive loss, finding other ways to be useful). Although little was found in this literature review regarding how these disparate reactions lead to seeking a diagnosis, an important lesson at the time of a diagnosis-oriented encounter is that health and social care professionals should be sensitive to and inquire about how the person has already reacted to their dementia-related symptoms (see Chapter 20).

There is a growing literature about how family members become aware and react to dementia symptoms prior to diagnosis. Although most published studies are based on small sample sizes, insights can be gained from this literature about the views of ethnically diverse family carers. Wilson (1989) developed an elegant model of co-resident family carer experiences based on retrospective reports, including three stages before diagnosis (see Box 19.1).

Box 19.1: Wilson's three stages before diagnosis

- Stage 1: Carers noticed behaviours that were out of the ordinary
- Stage 2: Carers became concerned when these behaviours began to accumulate and when the person with dementia could no longer rationalize, normalize or discount the behaviours

> ■ Stage 3: Carers realized that they needed to find an explanation. Often a sentinel event actually triggered the move to seek a diagnosis, such as a driving-related incident

Wilson's work and subsequent research by Keady and Nolan (2003) helped clarify that family members most often internalize their roles as "carers" only after seeking and receiving a diagnosis from a physician or other health care professional.

Research conducted with family members in the USA revealed that they often waited for a considerable time after first noticing symptoms before seeking a diagnosis (Boise *et al.* 1999; Wackerbarth *et al.* 2002). Reasons for this wait included those echoed in the study by Wilson (1989):

■ attributing memory lapses and other symptoms to normal ageing and not having proper information to distinguish symptoms as problematic
■ perceived barriers:
  ■ lack of confirmation of a problem by a physician
  ■ the cost of diagnostic services
  ■ lack of access to medical specialists

Diversity and the pre-diagnosis experience

Studies in the USA have also tapped ethnic diversity in searching for how family carers interpret dementia symptoms before seeking a diagnosis. Mahoney and colleagues (2005) conducted retrospective interviews in either focus group or personal interview format with small samples of African American, Chinese, and Latino family carers. The Latino group included individuals from six different countries of origin, including Puerto Rico and five Central or South American countries, providing clear evidence of the wide cultural heritage represented by Latinos in the USA (Gallagher-Thompson *et al.* 2003; Weineck *et al.* 2004). Across the three groups, initial impressions of their relatives' memory loss were attributed to normal ageing, although cultural explanations for this attribution varied:

■ African Americans: "old timer's disease"
■ Chinese: "hu tu", signifying forgetfulness in old age, as well as bad "feng shui" or negative environmental energies
■ Latinos: "el loco" or "craziness"

All family carer groups reported normalizing their response to early symptoms but tactics varied:

■ African Americans: the ethic of strong respect for elders supported quiet tolerance of symptoms while marshalling extended family support
■ Chinese: normalization was couched in terms of keeping mental health problems hidden to avoid community awareness and social stigmatization
■ Latinos: normalization was prompted mainly by not wishing to upset the person with symptoms

Triggering events to seek help outside the family were common across all three groups, leading to advice from community confidantes and subsequently medical sources to establish a diagnosis. Chinese carers mentioned the most hostility upon seeking informal advice due to the stigma attached to dementia in that community (Mahoney *et al.* 2005).

These results strongly suggest that remarkable cross-cultural similarities are found in the reactions of carers to symptoms in the pre-diagnosis phase of the dementia journey. Cultural differences tended to emerge, however, in the wider social world of these families as they sought information and support when symptoms persisted. Another study of carers from diverse ethnic backgrounds, including African Americans, Chinese, Latinos, and European Americans (whites) found subtle group differences in reasons that symptoms were attributed to old age rather than to a disease process, but more striking differences were seen in how cultural meanings were reinforced through immediate family members' interactions with other family and community members (Dilworth-Anderson and Gibson 2002). This study and another study comparing white American carers with African Americans, Asian Americans, and Latinos (Hinton *et al.* 2005) also found that whites were more likely to attribute biomedical – or disease – explanations to symptoms, while carers from other ethnic groups subscribed more often to folk or mixed folk/biomedical explanations. For additional literature on ethnic and cultural diversity in the context of dementia, see Chapter 3.

Case example 19.1: Mrs. Anderson

Mrs. Anderson, 70 years old, has been married for 46 years to her husband. She has been employed at the same insurance company for almost 25 years, but lately she has complained to her husband about how difficult her job has become and she has begun missing routine deadlines at the office. Recently, she forgot to organize a monthly dinner party at their home, which they have hosted for more than 10 years with the same three married couples in their neighbourhood. Mr. Anderson has confided in his pastor about his growing concerns about his wife's memory lapses. Mrs. Anderson is embarrassed and defensive when her husband mentions his concerns, but she has mentioned to their daughter in email correspondence that something just does not seem quite right in her mind. The Andersons have had the same primary care physician for more than 30 years, but these concerns have not yet been brought to their physician's attention.

Exercise 19.1: Seeking help before the diagnosis

- Where should Mr. and Mrs. Anderson turn next to discuss or get answers to their concerns?
- What or who might prompt them to schedule an appointment with their primary care physician to discuss their concerns?
- How important do you think it is for Mr. and Mrs. Anderson to find answers together? Why?

Making the diagnosis

The doctor's perspective

The pursuit of a diagnosis confronting physicians occurs against a backdrop of broader uncertainty that begins during medical training. Fifty years ago, medical sociologist Renee Fox recognized that medical uncertainty arises from a combination of the sheer volume of material that physicians-in-training are expected to digest and the gaps in scientific knowledge underlying the educational material imparted during training (Fox 1957). Examples of recent technological advances that relate directly to dementia diagnosis include (Fox 2002; Sperling *et al.* 2011):

- the rise of genetic mapping
- the development of advanced diagnostic imaging techniques, such as magnetic resonance imaging (MRI) and positron emission tomography (PET) scans
- the identification of biomarkers that are detectible in cerebrospinal fluid

Ironically, uncertainty is heightened when such technology is capable of detecting brain pathology or genes known to raise the risk of developing Alzheimer's disease in the complete absence of dementia-related symptoms. Finally, even when diagnoses are made in symptomatic individuals, the imperfect science of medical *prognosis* is another source of uncertainty (Fox 2002), reflected most clearly when persons with diagnosed dementia and their family carers ask their physician, "what will happen next?"

From a strictly clinical standpoint, the degree of uncertainty in making a diagnosis of dementia should be minimized by the availability of guidelines for primary care physicians and specialists. Most guidelines recommend that arriving at a diagnosis requires:

- a careful history of memory and other cognitive impairment symptoms
- laboratory tests to rule out potentially treatable or reversible metabolic causes of dementia such as thyroid dysfunction and infections
- neuropsychological tests of performance and interview-based tests to determine the types of and severity of cognitive impairments
- brain imaging techniques such as non-contrast computed tomography (CT scans), MRI scans, and PET scans

In the UK, the National Institute for Health and Clinical Excellence and Social Care Institute for Excellence (NICE-SCIE), under the sponsorship of the National Health Service, released evidence-based guidelines for dementia diagnosis and management in 2006. Within the past decade, a number of guidelines have been published in the USA, but unlike in the UK, these guidelines do not carry the sponsorship or sanction of the federal government. Instead, they have been sanctioned by physician specialty organizations and advocacy organizations in the voluntary sector (Small *et al.* 1997; American Geriatrics Society 2003). In Canada, the College of Family Physicians published a management guide for primary care of people with dementia (Pimlott *et al.* 2006). Other Canadian guidelines for evaluating people suspected of having dementia have also been published (Patterson *et al.* 1999). The guidelines of the American Geriatrics Society (AGS) are abstracted from practice parameters published in 2001 by Quality Standard Subcommittees of the American Neurological Association. It is noteworthy that both the AGS guidelines and the NICE-SCIE guidelines refer to the same diagnostic formulations – the National Institute of Neurologic, Communicative Disorders and Stroke-Alzheimer's Disease and Related Disorders Association Work Group – to help physicians arrive at a differential diagnosis.

Low rates of diagnosis

Despite the widely available clinical guidance to help physicians make a diagnosis, research based on medical record reviews and surveys of primary care physicians has consistently found sub-optimal levels of diagnostic performance in the UK (Audit Commission 2002), the USA (Callahan *et al.* 1995; Fortinsky and Wasson 1997; Valcour *et al.* 2000), Canada (Pimlott *et al.* 2006), and Australia (Brodaty *et al.* 1994). These poor diagnostic performance results are explained in large part by primary care physician reports of reservations about their capacity to confidently arrive at a diagnosis of dementia symptoms (Boise *et al.* 1999). Unfortunately, physician reluctance to make the diagnosis in the face of their uncertainty has the added effect of prolonging uncertainty for the patient and family. Another reaction in the face of uncertainty is to make a diagnosis that is possibly premature in order to placate the patient and family and to begin a regimen of medications to address cognitive symptoms, an approach that carries its own risks (Iliffe and Manthorpe 2004; Koch and Iliffe 2011).

Improving rates of diagnosis

Several studies with primary care physicians and other practitioners provide limited evidence regarding the value of educational interventions to improve their practice. In the UK, 35 primary care practices were randomly assigned to one of four trial arms: an electronic tutorial carried on a CD-ROM; decision support software built into the electronic medical record; in-person workshops convened at the practice site; or no intervention (Downs *et al.* 2006). Results indicated that decision support software and in-person educational workshops improved dementia detection rates. Concordance with guidelines remained low in all study arms. Preliminary but unpublished results from a more recent trial in the UK, EVIDEM-ED, indicate that the educational intervention did not measurably improve most dementia clinical management practices among primary care physicians (S. Iliffe, personal communication, 28 January 2013).

In primary care interventions in the USA, two studies employed nurses and social workers in primary care clinics to determine their effects on dementia diagnosis and dementia management practices. The first study involved 18 primary care practices in Southern California that were randomly assigned to either receive or not receive dementia guideline-based disease management led by non-physician primary care providers. Results indicated that practices with care coordinators in place did follow clinical practice guidelines in a greater proportion of patients than in practices without care coordinators (Vickrey *et al.* 2006). However, this same study did not produce improved provider self-reported knowledge about or attitudes favourable to dementia care (Chodosh *et al.* 2006). A similar primary care enhancement intervention in Indiana also found significantly improved dementia diagnosis practices concordant with clinical guidelines, but this study did not explore provider knowledge or attitudes about dementia care (Callahan *et al.* 2006).

A recent review of 15 studies that shared the goal of testing an intervention in primary care settings to improve dementia diagnosis and/or management found that most interventions did not change primary care physician behaviour. Among these 15 studies, which were conducted in several western European countries and the USA, educational interventions for physicians were most effective when they were permitted to establish their own educational agenda (Koch and Iliffe 2011). Taken together, these studies demonstrate that it is possible to introduce educational programmes directly into primary care settings and achieve modest impacts on dementia detection rates, but that much more needs to be done to improve dementia diagnostic practices in the primary care setting.

For reported barriers to adequate dementia diagnosis by primary care physicians, see Box 19.2.

Box 19.2: Reported barriers to dementia diagnosis in primary care

- Attitudes of futility towards making a diagnosis in the absence of effective drug therapies
- Concerns about consequences of making an incorrect diagnosis due to the stigma of dementia
- Limited professional training in mental health disorders of later life
- The complexity of dementia as a psychological and biological disorder with variable signs and symptoms
- The lack of specialists to confirm primary care physician suspicions, especially in rural areas
- A lack of familiarity with available community resources to which they could refer their patients with dementia and family carers

Source: Boise *et al.* (1999), Cody *et al.* (2002), Iliffe and Manthorpe (2002), Teel (2004), Fortinsky *et al.* (2010)

Two recent developments might point the way towards improved dementia diagnosis practices among primary care physicians. First, in 2011, clinical diagnostic criteria and guidelines for Alzheimer's disease were revised by an international panel of medical and scientific experts convened by the National Institute on Aging and the Alzheimer's Association in the USA. The revised clinical guideline adds mild cognitive impairment (MCI) as a clinical stage of dementia representing an intermediate stage of cognitive function between normal functioning and fulfilling diagnostic criteria for Alzheimer's disease and possibly other types of dementia (McKhann *et al.* 2011; Petersen 2011). The new MCI diagnostic guideline recommends that suspected patients undergo MRI testing in addition to cognitive status testing, and also that they undergo a thorough workup to rule out other causes for cognitive impairment such as vascular disease and depression. Moreover, this group proposed new criteria and terminology for classifying individuals with dementia caused by Alzheimer's disease (AD) (McKhann *et al.* 2011):

- probable AD dementia
- possible AD dementia
- probable or possible AD dementia with evidence of the AD brain pathology process

These new recommended guidelines acknowledge the complexity of classifying type or level of dementia while encouraging primary care and specialist physicians to conduct appropriate diagnostic workups to better fit their patients into newly recognized diagnostic categories.

The second development is a result of the 2010 Affordable Care Act (ACA) in the USA, a national law that added a new health benefit to the Medicare insurance programme, which covers nearly all Americans age 65 and older. This new benefit, known as the Medicare Annual Wellness Visit, came into effect on 1 January 2011, and it requires an assessment to detect cognitive impairment as part of the annual wellness visit. No specific cognitive impairment test was designated; in response, the Medicare Detection of Cognitive Impairment Workgroup assembled by the Alzheimer's Association recommended specific clinical guidance to primary care physicians for choosing detection tools and using practical algorithms to determine the level of assessment and follow-up required based on test findings (Cordell *et al.* 2013). It remains to be seen how widely these recommendations will be adopted by primary care physicians, and how helpful the recommended clinical practice tools and steps will be in improving their dementia diagnosis practices.

Case example 19.2: Mrs. Anderson (continued)

Dr. Knight works in a busy primary care group practice in a suburban area of New York City. One of his long-standing patients, Mrs. Anderson, visits with complaints of memory lapses that have affected her work performance and her usual social activities in negative ways. She tells Dr. Knight that her husband and daughter are also concerned, but she wanted to visit Dr. Knight alone for some reassurance and medical guidance without their interference during the visit. Dr. Knight finds that Mrs. Anderson performs quite poorly in the neuropsychological tests that he administers, and he draws blood to perform laboratory tests to rule out treatable or reversible causes of Mrs. Anderson's memory lapses. He also orders brain-imaging tests and tells Mrs. Anderson that he wants to meet again with her and her husband after the test results become available. He reassures Mrs. Anderson but makes it clear that it is important for her to schedule the brain-imaging test.

Exercise 19.2: Uncertainty and making the diagnosis

■ What might Dr. Knight be thinking about Mrs. Anderson's condition before he receives any more test results?

■ If the ordered tests reveal no treatable causes and the MRI scan shows some changes in Mrs. Anderson's brain, how should Dr. Knight respond in terms of making a diagnosis of Alzheimer's disease or related dementia?

■ What else might Dr. Knight do as he considers ways to discuss Mrs. Anderson's memory lapses at her next visit with her husband?

Disclosing the diagnosis

Numerous studies, using a variety of methodologies, have examined attitudes to disclosing the diagnosis of dementia, current practice regarding disclosure, factors influencing disclosure, the impacts of disclosure on people with dementia, and carers' views on disclosure. At first glance, it is surprising that there would be any difference in opinion or practice regarding practitioners disclosing a dementia diagnosis to persons and family carers; preference for disclosure would appear to be universal among all participants in the dementia care triad in order to relieve uncertainty about the cause of dementia symptoms and to initiate post-diagnosis treatment and early support service strategies. Empirical results, however, suggest a much more complex reality.

Bamford and colleagues (2004) published the most comprehensive review of dementia disclosure research to date, systematically summarizing methods and results of 59 studies. Carpenter and Dave (2004) published a review of dementia diagnostic disclosure, and proposed a research agenda based on identified gaps in the literature. Both reviews combined results irrespective of whether respondents were physicians, carers or persons with dementia. Both studies found wide variation in physicians' disclosure practices, preferences among carers to inform their relatives about the diagnosis, and preferences among persons with dementia to learn the diagnosis.

For reasons in favour of and against diagnostic disclosure, see Box 19.3.

Box 19.3: Reasons for and against diagnostic disclosure

Reasons for diagnostic disclosure

■ to help facilitate planning (10 studies)
■ the psychological benefit to the person with dementia and/or carers (9)
■ the person's right to know the diagnosis (6)
■ to maximize treatment possibilities (6).

Reasons against diagnostic disclosure

■ the risk of causing emotional distress (12 studies)
■ the inability of the person with dementia to understand and/or retain diagnosis (10)
■ no benefits, costs outweigh benefits (8)
■ the lack of a cure or effective treatments (6)
■ the stigma associated with dementia (6)

Source: Bamford et al. (2004)

Based on the review of Bamford *et al.* (2004), many of the reasons expressed by physicians for withholding the diagnosis are similar to reasons why physicians are reluctant to pursue diagnostic assessments, particularly due to the lack of effective therapies and perceived stigma of labelling patients with the diagnosis.

Both reviews concluded that the perspectives of people with dementia, compared with carers and professionals, appear relatively neglected in the disclosure literature, although this imbalance is slowly being rectified. From an ethical perspective, Carpenter and Dave (2004) noted that a dementia diagnosis is the "property" of the person to whom it applies, and that the individual has the right to share or withhold that information with others. Indeed, a more recent study of a small sample of people with dementia found that although they were comfortable sharing their diagnosis with family members and other loved ones, they were reluctant to do so with people beyond their immediate circle of family and close friends (Langdon *et al.* 2007).

A more recent systematic review of literature on this topic, covering 35 published studies through 2009, included views of people with dementia and family carers (Robinson *et al.* 2011). Some findings are notable:

- There is a shortage of such studies from the viewpoint of the person with dementia.
- People with dementia wish to be told their diagnosis, although the term "Alzheimer's disease" continues to carry negative connotations whereas dementia is more acceptable.
- From the perspective of both people with dementia and their family carers, diagnostic disclosure is viewed best as just one step in the process of seeking and receiving adequate support and education.
- More long-term follow-up studies with people with dementia following diagnostic disclosure are needed to learn whether immediate negative emotional consequences linger or are alleviated with the passage of time.

Case example 19.3: Mrs. Anderson (continued)

Mr. and Mrs. Anderson are meeting with Dr. Knight to discuss Mrs. Anderson's test results. They are both very anxious, and Dr. Knight explains that all of Mrs. Anderson's test results lead him to conclude that her memory lapses are likely to increase in frequency as time goes by. While he hesitates in giving her symptoms a diagnosis because he does not want to alarm them further, he does suggest that Mrs. Anderson consider reducing her work to part-time, and that Mr. Anderson get more involved in planning their social calendar so they remain actively engaged with their friends and neighbours. Dr. Knight asks them to return for another visit in three months to check on the progress of Mrs. Anderson's memory lapses. Mrs. Anderson is outwardly very disturbed at learning this news and by Dr. Knight's suggestions, and Mr. Anderson is silently angry that Dr. Knight did not provide more definitive answers about his wife's condition.

Exercise 19.3: Sharing the diagnosis

- What are the strengths and limitations of Dr. Knight's approach to discussing his diagnostic workup with Mr. and Mrs. Anderson?
- What else could Dr. Knight have offered Mr. and Mrs. Anderson in the way of guidance even if he did not pronounce a diagnosis?

■   What might account for Dr. Knight's hesitation in making and sharing a diagnosis? What would you have done if you were in his position?

Early support after the diagnosis

"Early support" refers to services designed to address the uncertainty surrounding dementia by providing information, education, and direct support as soon as possible after a dementia diagnosis is made. The most common goals of early support services include:

■   produce more knowledgeable and skilled family caregivers in managing dementia-related cognitive and behavioral symptoms exhibited by their loved ones
■   sustain and improve the mental and physical health of family caregivers
■   maximize physical function and independence for the person with dementia as long as possible
■   delay or avoid nursing or care home admissions and hospitalizations of people with dementia for both economic and quality-of-life-related reasons

Self-management of dementia and other health-related symptoms for persons with dementia is a highly sensible goal, particularly in the context of trends towards making diagnoses earlier in the disease process. However, this self-management goal of early support services has yet to be expressed as often as other listed goals in the published literature or in policy documents such as national dementia strategies that have proliferated in the past several years.

Use of early support services in the community, even those not specifically targeting dementia-related symptoms or caregiving issues, were found to lead to delayed nursing home admission in a longitudinal study of a large cohort of people with dementia and family caregivers in the USA (Gaugler *et al.* 2005). Recent studies and reviews from studies conducted in several countries have shown that primary care physicians continue to demonstrate wide variation in relation to linking their patients with dementia and their families to community-based early support services (Fortinsky *et al.* 2010; Koch and Iliffe 2011); therefore, one area requiring important action is to find creative ways to embed early support services more firmly within the existing service systems in different countries. This will allow physicians to more seamlessly refer immediately following diagnostic disclosure.

Scotland's first national dementia strategy, released in 2010, specifically identified "improved post-diagnostic information and support" as a key service delivery area in need of immediate change across the health and social care system in that country (Scottish Government 2010). Importantly, the area of self-management of the illness and its symptoms for persons with dementia is explicitly included among the objectives of an improved post-diagnostic information and support infrastructure (see Box 19.4).

Box 19.4: Post-diagnostic support: Scotland's emerging model – 2007–present

■   In 2007, the Scottish Government launched three post-diagnostic support pilot studies in local authority/health board areas.
■   In 2010, Scotland's first national dementia strategy led to the development of "five pillars of support" at the time of post-diagnosis:
   ■   help to understand the illness and manage your symptoms
   ■   support to keep up your community connections and make new ones
   ■   peer support – the chance to meet other people with dementia and their partners and families

- ■ help to plan for future decision-making
- ■ help to plan for your future support
- ■ In 2013, Scotland's second national strategy, covering the years 2013–2016, introduced a target whereby everyone newly diagnosed with dementia from 1 April 2013 is entitled to at least one year's worth of post-diagnostic support, coordinated by a named link worker employed by Alzheimer Scotland or NHS Scotland staff.
- ■ A web site is available for the general public to locate a link worker to initiate post-diagnostic support to persons and families affected by dementia

Source: http://www.alzscot.org/services_and_support/recently-diagnosed

While dementia is clearly a global issue, most published experiments to implement and test innovative community-based early support services for people with dementia and their family caregivers have occurred primarily in Australia, western Europe, the Scandinavian region, the UK, and USA. Several recent reviews of these efforts to establish an evidence base for the best practices have been published (Smits *et al.* 2007; Brodaty and Arasaratnam 2012; Gallagher-Thompson *et al.* 2012; Maslow 2013). Uptake of these early support service models from research trials to everyday practice remains scattered, requiring champions from among the investigative teams and/or health and social care providers who can envision adapting these care models to the specific health and social care systems operating in their jurisdictions. Box 19.5 provides examples of the most successful evidence-based programmes of early support for persons with dementia and/or their family carers completed in the USA.

Box 19.5: Evidence-based approaches to early support from the USA

- ■ Psycho-educational and multi-component interventions individually tailored to caregiver needs, offered for longer duration, usually six months or more (Gitlin *et al.* 2003; Mittelman *et al.* 2004, 2006; Belle *et al.* 2006; Nichols *et al.* 2008, 2011)
- ■ Supportive programmes for family carers to build peer support among group participants and share successful care strategies in groups led by peers or professionals (Ostwald *et al.* 1999; Hepburn *et al.* 2001)
- ■ Non-professional community consultants involve individuals without prior professional training who then receive specialized training in dementia and dementia care to work with persons with dementia and their families (Teri *et al.* 2005)
- ■ Occupational therapists (Gitlin *et al.* 2010)
- ■ Telephone-delivered interventions with caregivers (Tremont *et al.* 2008)
- ■ Psycho-educational interventions with both caregivers and their relatives with dementia, or dyads (Whitlatch *et al.* 2006)
- ■ Linking primary care practitioners with social workers and/or nurses to provide multi-component interventions with family caregivers (Fortinsky *et al.* 2002, 2009; Bass *et al.* 2003; Callahan *et al.* 2006; Vickrey *et al.* 2006)

Finally, in addition to the Scotland National Dementia Strategies already mentioned, the recent release in several countries of national dementia strategies or plans offers reason for optimism in moving forward with early support services. For example, England's National Dementia Strategy was published in 2009 (Department of Health 2009), the latest in a series of public policy initiatives to focus attention on the needs of people with dementia and their families. This national strategy includes 17 interrelated objectives, many of which speak directly to the need for more widely available information and services; objective #4 calls for "easy access to care, support and advice following diagnosis", adding the potential value of "dementia advisers" as members of the care team at the local level (Banerjee 2010). This national strategy is endorsed at the highest level of government in England and was reinforced in March 2012 by the Prime Minister's "Challenge on Dementia", calling for major improvements in dementia care and research by 2015.

In the USA, in May 2012, the first National Plan to Address Alzheimer's Disease was released, directing the national government to partner with leading researchers and with health and social service professionals in the public and private sectors to disseminate as widely as possible evidence-based best practices in non-pharmacological treatment and care (Maslow 2013). Additionally, the 2010 Affordable Care Act in the USA opened the way for the development of innovative dementia care models that either translate or otherwise build on successful experimental initiatives, or that represent new models. This landmark legislation focuses on efforts within the Center for Medicare and Medicaid Innovation (CMMI) to improve health, improve the quality of health care, and lower costs, for the Medicare population, which represents the vast majority of older Americans who are most likely to become diagnosed with dementia. Among new projects recently funded by CMMI is an initiative at Indiana University to provide coordinated care for Medicare beneficiaries with dementia or late-life depression, which builds directly on an evidence-based non-pharmacological treatment and on more recent work by the same investigative team to elevate the quality of dementia care throughout the greater Indianapolis metropolitan area (Callahan *et al.* 2006; Boustani *et al.* 2010, 2012; Maslow 2013).

Debates and controversies

One ongoing debate in the diagnosis of dementia is how soon after memory loss the person's symptoms are noticed by family members and friends should they discuss their concerns with the person showing symptoms. We do not have sufficient knowledge about whether it is better to diagnose dementia earlier, and if so, for whom and under what circumstances is an earlier diagnosis better.

Another debate concerns who "owns" the diagnosis. Opinions differ on whether the individual with dementia owns the diagnosis and should be told, allowing the person with symptoms to decide whether and when to share the diagnosis with family members. Others believe that family members should be told, allowing them to determine whether, when, and how the individual with dementia will be told of the diagnosis. Clearly, many providers and family members continue to keep this information from people who are showing symptoms of dementia, believing this is the right thing to do. We need to better understand the implications of disclosing, as well as the timing and method of disclosure.

There has been discussion about whether services should be tailored to specific ethnic groups, as separate from other care recipients. While opinions differ on this, at this point we simply have insufficient knowledge about the implications of either separate or integrated service delivery systems. Nor do we know how to best tailor services within a programme to respond to different ethnic groups.

Finally, we are lacking agreement on the best methods of training physicians and other health care professionals to recognize, diagnose, and manage memory problems in middle-aged and older adults. Creating effective providers will require more effective training programmes, especially those in primary care.

Conclusion

The journey from initial symptom recognition to diagnosis is characterized by uncertainty for both persons with dementia and family carers. Uncertainty about the trajectory of symptoms and impact of symptoms on loved ones and future care needs are commonly experienced. While the meanings of symptoms in early dementia are culturally determined to some extent, carers from many ethnic and cultural groups seek information from other family members and community confidantes before seeking medical counsel. Physicians also report considerable uncertainty regarding dementia diagnosis and diagnostic disclosure, and sub-optimal clinical performance revealed in research supports their reported uncertainty. Clinical trials to date have yielded modest results in improving physicians' diagnostic behaviour, and enhanced primary care trials have led to improved outcomes among persons with dementia and family carers. The degree to which these limited promising results can be widely disseminated and replicated remains unclear.

Policy initiatives in England have led to the development of dementia care partnerships across primary care, mental health, and social services sectors. Community mental health nurses with dementia care training represent potential links between persons with dementia, family carers, and physicians to improve partnerships and reduce uncertainties before and immediately after dementia diagnosis. Further research is needed to determine how professional educational programmes can be improved to provide future physicians and other practitioners with greater knowledge about memory loss and related cognitive problems to help reduce uncertainty and improve health-related outcomes in earlier stages of the dementia journey.

Further information

Alzheimer's Disease International (ADI) is a worldwide resource on progress in research and public policy regarding Alzheimer's disease and other types of dementia. A listing of available national dementia strategies and plans, all available for downloading, can be found at the ADI web site [http://www.alz.co.uk/alzheimer-plans].

Getting on With Living is a practical guide to developing early support services based on several pilot studies in England, Scotland, and Wales, and is available for download [www.knowledge.scot.nhs.uk/.../getting_on_with_living.pdf].

The Healthy Aging Brain Center (HABC) at Indiana University-affiliated Wishard Health Services has developed numerous clinically useful screening and assessment tools to assist health and social care providers improve their ability to diagnose dementia-related symptoms and determine how best to link patients and family carers with available services in the community. See the HABC resources web site [http://www.wishard.edu/our-services/senior-care/healthy-aging-brain-center/resources].

Translating Innovation to Impact. This white paper, released in September 2012, presents the findings and recommendations from a review of more than 40 state-of-the-art non-pharmacological treatments and care practices for people with Alzheimer's or other dementias and their family caregivers in the USA. Many of these programmes could be adapted as early support services in countries throughout the world. The white paper can be downloaded from the Alliance for Aging Research web site [http://www.agingresearch.org/content/article/detail/21737].

References

Alzheimer's Association (2013) *2013 Alzheimer's Disease Facts and Figures*. Chicago, IL: Alzheimer's Association.

Alzheimer's Society (2007) *Dementia UK*. London: Alzheimer's Society.

American Geriatrics Society Clinical Practice Committee (2003) Guidelines abstracted from the American Academy of Neurology's dementia guidelines for early detection, diagnosis, and management of dementia, *Journal of the American Geriatrics Society*, 51: 869–73.

Audit Commission (2002) *Forget Me Not 2002: Developing Mental Health Services for Older People in England*. London: Audit Commission.

Bamford, C., Lamont, S., Eccles, M., Robinson, L., May, C. *et al.* (2004) Disclosing a diagnosis of dementia: a systematic review, *International Journal of Geriatric Psychiatry*, 19: 151–69.

Banerjee, S. (2010) Living well with dementia – development of the national dementia strategy for England, *International Journal of Geriatric Psychiatry*, 25: 917–22.

Bass, D.M., Clark, P.A., Looman, W.J., McCarthy, C.A. and Eckert, S. (2003) The Cleveland Alzheimer's managed care demonstration: outcomes after 12 months of implementation, *The Gerontologist*, 43: 73–85.

Belle, S.H., Burgio, L., Burns, R., Coon, D., Czaja, S.J. *et al.* (2006) Enhancing the quality of life of dementia caregivers from different ethnic or racial groups, *Annals of Internal Medicine*, 145: 727–38.

Boise, L., Camicioli, R., Morgan, D., Rose, J.H. and Congleton, L. (1999) Diagnosing dementia: perspectives of primary care physicians, *The Gerontologist*, 39: 457–64.

Bond, J., Stave, C., Sganga, A., Vincenzino, O., O'Connell, B. *et al.* (2005) Inequalities in dementia care across Europe: key findings of the Facing Dementia survey, *International Journal of Clinical Practice*, 59 (Suppl. 146): 8–14.

Boustani, M.A., Sachs, G.A., Alder, C.A., Munger, S., Schubert, C.C. *et al.* (2010) Implementing innovative models of dementia care: the Healthy Aging Brain Center, *Aging and Mental Health*, 15: 13–22.

Boustani, M.A., Frame, A., Munger, S., Healey, P., Westlund, J. *et al.* (2012) Connecting research discovery with care delivery in dementia: the development of the Indianapolis Discovery Network for Dementia, *Clinical Interventions in Aging*, 7: 509–16.

Brodaty, H. and Arasaratnam, C. (2012) Meta-analysis of nonpharmacological interventions for neuropsychiatric symptoms of dementia, *American Journal of Psychiatry*, 169: 946–53.

Brodaty, H., Howarth, G.C., Mant, A. and Kurrle, S.E. (1994) General practice and dementia: a national survey of Australian GPs, *Medical Journal of Australia*, 160: 10–44.

Callahan, C.M., Hendrie, H.C. and Tierney, W.M. (1995) Documentation and evaluation of cognitive impairment in elderly primary care patients, *Annals of Internal Medicine*, 122: 422–9.

Callahan, C.M., Boustani, M.A., Unverzagt, F.W., Austrom, M.G., Damush, T.M. *et al.* (2006) Effectiveness of collaborative care for older adults with Alzheimer's disease in primary care: a randomized controlled trial, *Journal of the American Medical Association*, 295: 2148–57.

Carpenter, B. and Dave, J. (2004) Disclosing a dementia diagnosis: a review of opinion and practice, and a proposed research agenda, *The Gerontologist*, 44: 149–58.

Chodosh, J., Berry, E., Lee, M., Connor, K., DeMonte, R. *et al.* (2006) Effect of a dementia care management intervention on primary care provider knowledge, attitudes, and perceptions of quality of care, *Journal of the American Geriatrics Society*, 54: 311–17.

Cody, M., Beck, C., Shue, V.M. and Pope, S. (2002) Reported practices of primary care physicians in the diagnosis and management of dementia, *Aging and Mental Health*, 6: 72–6.

Cordell, C.B., Borson, S., Boustani, M., Chodosh, J., Reuben, D. *et al.* (2013) Alzheimer's Association recommendations for operationalizing the detection of cognitive impairment during the Medicare Annual Wellness Visit in a primary care setting, *Alzheimer's and Dementia*, 9(2): 141–50.

De Boer, M.E., Hertogh, C.M.P.M., Droes, R.M., Riphagen, I.I., Jonker, C. *et al.* (2007) Suffering from dementia – the patient's perspective: a review of the literature, *International Psychogeriatrics*, 19(6): 1021–39.

Department of Health (2009) *Living Well with Dementia: A National Dementia Strategy*. London: Department of Health [https://www.gov.uk/government/uploads/system/uploads/attachment_data/file/168220/dh_094051.pdf, accessed 29 April 2014].

Dilworth-Anderson, P. and Gibson, B.E. (2002) The cultural influence of values, norms, meanings, and perceptions in understanding dementia in ethnic minorities, *Alzheimer's Disease and Associated Disorders*, 16 (Suppl. 2): S56–S63.

Downs, M., Turner, S., Bryans, M., Wilcock, J., Keady, J. et al. (2006) Effectiveness of educational interventions in improving detection and management of dementia in primary care: cluster randomised controlled study, *British Medical Journal*, 332: 692–6.

Fortinsky, R.H. and Wasson, J. (1997) How do physicians diagnose dementia? Evidence from clinical vignette responses, *American Journal of Alzheimer's Disease*, 12: 51–61.

Fortinsky, R.H., Unson, C. and Garcia, R.I. (2002) Helping family caregivers by linking primary care physicians with community-based dementia care services: the Alzheimer's Service Coordination Program, *Dementia*, 1: 227–40.

Fortinsky, R.H., Kulldorff, M., Kleppinger, A. and Kenyon-Pesce, L. (2009) Dementia care consultation for family caregivers: collaborative model linking an Alzheimer's Association chapter with primary care physicians, *Aging and Mental Health*, 13: 162–70.

Fortinsky, R.H., Zlateva, I., Delaney, C. and Kleppinger, A. (2010) Primary care physicians' dementia care practices: evidence of geographic variation, *The Gerontologist*, 50: 179–91.

Fox, R.C. (1957) Training for uncertainty, in R.K. Merton, G. Reader and P.L. Kendall (eds.) *The Student Physician: Introductory Studies in the Sociology of Medical Education*. Cambridge, MA: Harvard University Press, pp. 207–41.

Fox, R.C. (2002) Medical uncertainty revisited, in G. Bendelow, M. Carpenter, C. Vautier and S. Williams (eds.) *Gender, Health, and Healing: The Public/Private Divide*. London: Routledge, pp. 236–53.

Gallagher-Thompson, D., Solano, N., Coon, D. and Arean, P. (2003) Recruitment and retention of Latino dementia family caregivers in intervention research: issues to face, lessons to learn, *The Gerontologist*, 43: 45–51.

Gallagher-Thompson, D., Tzuang, Y.M., Au, A., Brodaty, H., Charlesworth, G. et al. (2012) International perspectives on nonpharmacological best practices for dementia family caregivers: a review, *Clinical Gerontologist*, 35: 316–55.

Gaugler, J.E., Kane, R.L., Kane, R.A. and Newcomer, R. (2005) Early community-based service utilization and its effects on institutionalization in dementia caregiving, *The Gerontologist*, 45: 177–85.

Gitlin, L.N., Belle, S.H., Burgio, L.D., Czaja, S.J., Mahoney, D. et al. (2003) Effect of multicomponent interventions on caregiver burden and depression: the REACH multisite initiative at 6-month follow-up, *Psychology and Aging*, 18: 361–74.

Gitlin, L.N., Winter, L., Dennis, M.P., Hodgson, N. and Hauck, W.W. (2010) A biobehavioral home-based intervention and the well-being of patients with dementia and their caregivers: the COPE Randomized Trial, *Journal of the American Medical Association*, 304: 983–91.

Hepburn, K.W., Tornatore, J., Center, B. and Ostwald, S.W. (2001) Dementia family caregiver training: affecting beliefs about caregiving and caregiver outcomes, *Journal of the American Geriatrics Society*, 49: 450–7.

Hinton, L., Franz, C.E., Yeo, G. and Levkoff, S.E. (2005) Conceptions of dementia in a multiethnic sample of family caregivers, *Journal of the American Geriatrics Society*, 53: 1405–10.

Iliffe, S. and Manthorpe, J. (2002) Dementia in the community: challenges for primary care development, *Reviews in Clinical Gerontology*, 12: 243–52.

Iliffe, S. and Manthorpe, J. (2004) The hazards of early recognition of dementia: a risk assessment, *Aging and Mental Health*, 8: 99–105.

Keady, J. and Nolan, M. (2003) The dynamics of dementia: working together, working separately, or working alone?, in M. Nolan, U. Lundh, G. Grant and J. Keady (eds.) *Partnerships in Family Care: Understanding the Caregiving Career*. Maidenhead: Open University Press, pp. 15–32.

Koch, T. and Iliffe, S. (2011) Dementia diagnosis and management: a narrative review of changing practice, *British Journal of General Practice*, 61(589): e513–e525.

Langdon, S.A., Eagle, A. and Warner, J. (2007) Making sense of dementia in the social world: a qualitative study, *Social Science and Medicine*, 64: 989–1000.

Mahoney, D.F., Cloutterbuck, J., Neary, S. and Zhan, L. (2005) African-American, Chinese, and Latino family caregivers' impressions of the onset and diagnosis of dementia: cross-cultural similarities and differences, *The Gerontologist*, 45: 783–92.

Maslow, K. (2013) *Translating Innovation to Impact: Evidence-based Interventions to Support People with Alzheimer's Disease and their Caregivers at Home and in the Community*. Report for the Alliance for Aging Research, the Administration on Aging, and MetLife Foundation [http://www.aoa.gov/AoA_Programs/HPW/Alz_Grants/docs/TranslatingInnovationtoImpactAlzheimersDisease.pdf, accessed 29 April 2014].

McKhann, G.M., Knopman, D.S., Cherkow, H., Hyman, B.T., Jack, C.R. et al. (2011) The diagnosis of dementia due to Alzheimer's disease: recommendations from the National Institute on Aging and Alzheimer's Association workgroup, *Alzheimer's and Dementia*, 7(3): 263–9.

Mittelman, M.S., Roth, D.L., Coon, D.W. and Haley, W.E. (2004) Sustained benefit of supportive intervention for depressive symptoms in caregivers of patients with Alzheimer's disease, *American Journal of Psychiatry*, 161: 850–6.

Mittelman, M.S., Haley, W.E., Clay, O.J. and Roth, D.L. (2006) Improving caregiver well-being delays nursing home placement of patients with Alzheimer disease, *Neurology*, 67: 1592–9.

Moniz-Cook, E., Manthorpe, J., Carr, I., Gibson, G. and Vernooij-Dassen, M. (2006) Facing the future: a qualitative study of older people referred to a memory clinic prior to assessment and diagnosis, *Dementia*, 5: 375–95.

National Institute for Health and Clinical Excellence and Social Care Institute for Excellence (NICE-SCIE) (2006) *Dementia: Supporting People with Dementia and their Carers in Health and Social Care*. London: NICE-SCIE.

Nichols, L.O., Chang, C., Lummus, A., Burns, R., Martindale-Adams, J. et al. (2008) The cost-effectiveness of a behavior intervention with caregivers of patients with Alzheimer's disease, *Journal of the American Geriatrics Society*, 56: 413–20.

Nichols, L.O., Martindale-Adams, J., Burns, R., Graney, M.J. and Zuber, J. (2011) Translation of a dementia caregiver support program in a health care system – REACH VA, *Archives of Internal Medicine*, 171: 353–9.

Ostwald, S.K., Hepburn, K.W., Caron, W., Burns, T. and Mantell, R. (1999) Reducing caregiver burden: a randomized psychoeducational intervention for caregivers of persons with dementia, *The Gerontologist*, 39: 299–309.

Patterson, C.J., Gautheir, S., Bergman, H., Cohen, C.A., Feightner, J.W. et al. (1999) The recognition, assessment, and management of dementing disorders: conclusions from the Canadian Consensus Conference on Dementia, *Canadian Medical Association Journal*, 12 (Suppl.): S1–S15.

Petersen, R.C. (2011) Mild cognitive impairment, *New England Journal of Medicine*, 364: 2227–34.

Pimlott, N.J.G., Siegal, K., Persaud, M., Slaughter, S., Cohen, C. et al. (2006) Management of dementia by family physicians in academic settings, *Canadian Family Physician*, 52: 1108–15.

Robinson, L., Gemski, A., Abley C., Bond, J., Keady, J. et al. (2011) The transition to dementia – individual and family experiences of receiving a diagnosis: a review, *International Psychogeriatrics*, 23: 1026–43.

Scottish Government (2010) *Scotland's National Dementia Strategy*. Edinburgh: Scottish Government.

Small, G.W., Rabins, P.V., Barry, P.P., Buckholtz, N.S., DeKosky, S.T. et al. (1997) Diagnosis and treatment of Alzheimer's disease and related disorders: consensus statement of the American Association for Geriatric Psychiatry, the Alzheimer's Association, and the American Geriatrics Society, *Journal of the American Medical Association*, 278: 1363–71.

Smits, C.H., de Lange, J., Droes, R.M., Melland, F., Vermooij-Dassen, M. et al. (2007) Effects of combined intervention programmes for people with dementia living at home and their caregivers: a systematic review, *International Journal of Geriatric Psychiatry*, 22: 1181–93.

Sperling, R.A., Aisen, P.S., Beckett, L.A., Bennett, D.A., Craft, S. et al. (2011) Toward defining the preclinical stages of Alzheimer's disease: recommendations from the National Institute on Aging and Alzheimer's Association workgroup, *Alzheimer's and Dementia*, 7(3): 280–92.

Teel, C.S. (2004) Rural practitioners' experience in dementia diagnosis and treatment, *Aging and Mental Health*, 8: 422–9.

Teri, L., McCurry, S.M., Logsdon, R.G. and Gibbons, L.E. (2005) Training community consultants to help family members improve dementia care: a randomized controlled trial, *The Gerontologist*, 45: 802–11.

Tremont, G., Davis, J.D., Bishop, D.S. and Fortinsky, R.H. (2008) Telephone-delivered psychosocial intervention reduces burden in dementia caregivers, *Dementia*, 7: 503–20.

Valcour, V., Masaki, K., Curb, J. and Blanchette, P. (2000) The detection of dementia in the primary care setting, *Archives of Internal Medicine*, 160: 2964–8.

Vickrey, B.G., Mittman, B.S., Connor, K.I., Pearson, M.L., Della Penna, R.D. et al. (2006) The effect of a disease management intervention on quality and outcomes of dementia care, *Annals of Internal Medicine*, 145: 713–26.

Wackerbarth, S., Streams, M. and Smith, M. (2002) Capturing the insights of family caregivers: survey item generation with a coupled interview/focus group process, *Qualitative Health Research*, 12: 1141–54.

Weineck, R.M., Jacobs, E.A., Stone, L.C., Ortega, A.N. and Burstin, H. (2004) Hispanic health care disparities: challenging the myth of a monolithic Hispanic population, *Medical Care*, 42: 313–20.

Whitlatch, C.J., Judge, K., Zarit, S.H. and Femia, E. (2006) Dyadic intervention for family caregivers and care receivers in early-stage dementia, *The Gerontologist*, 46: 688–94.

Wilson, H.S. (1989) Family caregivers: the experience of Alzheimer's disease, *Applied Nursing Research*, 2(1): 40–5.

CHAPTER 20

Whole person assessment and care planning

Benjamin Mast

66 I took Mum to a geriatrician to see what was wrong. I said 'I think my mother has dementia' to which he said 'How did you make that assessment?' We both laughed. He was lovely. I didn't actually realize this was the assessment. I expected him to do tests, things like 'Can you remember what I told you' or to see is she could do certain things. But he just sat next to her, no notes, and chatted. It didn't look like a test of any kind. Just a nice man who she was chatting with. There were so many things she couldn't do. I just hadn't noticed. He said that I had just gotten used to it. His assessment didn't match mine at all. He asked me what my line in the sand was. I said I didn't think I had one. He said 'everyone has one.' It was half an assessment of me. So I went home and thought about it. I knew when I reached my line in the sand. I remembered what he had said. That was helpful. He was lovely. 99

—Carolyn Worth Melbourne, Australia

66 After my relative had an informal diagnosis from the GP we were referred to social services and a CPN was assigned to us. I found her extremely helpful. But the initial meeting, when my relative was introduced to the CPN, in her own home she was asked to do the Mini Mental Test, to establish how much memory loss had been sustained. My relative became anxious about the questions and kept looking at me when she could not answer some of the questions. We both found it very difficult. The CPN was very reassuring about why my relative was doing the test and told her it was not to measure her intelligence, but rather establish how much loss had been incurred. My relative's remarks to me, after the CPN left were, 'I feel so humiliated'. This was the first time that my relative had expressed her feelings about what was happening to her. I felt awful too, as I felt responsible for placing her in this situation. I've wondered since whether doing the Mini Mental Test is better done in professional surroundings – Memory Clinics. I do think that this is probably how it is done now – but I do think great care should be taken in thinking about the stress and indignity that this can create for both the patient and the carer. 99

—Vivienne Cooper Yorkshire, UK

66 When assessing someone it is important to know the person well and have all the facts. My mother had been given so many different drugs I am certain that her behaviour and hallucinations were due to them. The head psychiatric nurse in the unit told me that Mum wouldn't eat because she thought the food was poisoned. We later witnessed another patient repeatedly whispering in my mother's ear that the food was poisoned. 99

—Sue Tucker Yorkshire, UK

"I had been told how important the result of the mini mental test was to whether or not the Aricept would continue to be prescribed. We didn't know how much the Aricept was keeping the progression of the disease at bay and sustaining her current level of functioning. The test became a nightmare, it broke my heart seeing my mother struggle to answer the questions she would look across at me to answer for her. The degrading tests were stopped and she was allowed to continue with the Aricept. There has to be better ways of assessing."

—Sue Tucker Yorkshire, UK

Learning objectives

By the end of this chapter, you will be able to:

- Describe the limits of traditional deficit-focused assessments
- Explain the advantages of whole person assessment
- Explain why it is important to understand the person with dementia and what living with dementia means for them
- Describe how to conduct a whole person assessment of people with dementia
- Provide an example of how whole person assessment informs individualized care planning for an individual with dementia and their family

Introduction

The person-centred approach argues that people with dementia are more than the sum of their cognitive and functional impairments. Kitwood and others stress that a person with dementia retains personhood and deserves respect, honour, and value (Post 1995; Kitwood 1997; Sabat 2001; Woods 2001). Although understanding the nature of cognitive and functional impairments is important, there is much more we need to understand about the person in order to optimize their experience of living with dementia, reduce excess disability, and enhance quality of life.

Yet most assessment approaches focus only on the cognitive consequences of dementia and do not seek to understand other aspects of the person and their experience. Similarly, there are many person-centred activities that while they honour and respect the person, do not capture a sufficient range of information to be able to assist in diagnosis and care planning. The "whole person approach" to assessment of people with dementia provides a conceptual and practical framework for clinicians, health care providers, and family caregivers to better understand the person and their experience of living with dementia (Mast 2011, 2012).

The limitations of traditional, cognitive deficit-focused assessment

Although there are benefits to utilizing cognitive tests in the assessment and diagnosis of dementia syndromes, there are limitations to the strictly deficit-focused approach to assessment.

Dementia diagnosis has no link to long-term effective drug treatment

In the typical biomedical paradigm, a series of tests is performed with the goal of identifying deficits that suggest a diagnosis that implies a specific treatment that can either address the underlying pathology or ameliorate the symptoms. Thus far in Alzheimer's disease and other dementias, this approach has not been as successful as we would have hoped. Although a combination of tests including cognitive tests, laboratory tests, and brain scans can help accurately identify dementia and its likely causes (Knopman *et al.* 2001), these do not necessarily lead to a treatment that can address the underlying pathology and do not provide long-term relief from symptoms (Royall 2005; Birks 2006; Birks and Flicker 2006; Raschetti *et al.* 2007; Rodda and Walker 2009).

We risk frightening and devaluing the person

Dementia is often described as one of the most feared medical conditions in late life. Alzheimer's disease in particular seems to provoke much fear because its well-publicized progressive course, which begins with mild memory impairment and advances to interfere with many aspects of behaviour and cognition (Clare *et al.* 2008; French *et al.* 2011). Ultimately, dementia can result in people being unable to communicate and care for their most basic needs. As clinicians, it is important that our assessment processes and work with people with dementia do not exacerbate these feelings of fear and vulnerability. In addition, most people do not want to be characterized by their deficits but want to continue to be seen as a valuable individual who has purpose and is seeking to live a meaningful life (Moniz-Cook *et al.* 2006; Steeman *et al.* 2007; Mak 2011). Yet when people with suspected dementia undergo assessment, much of the attention is directed towards their cognitive deficits. This can result in them fearing that they will be seen through a lens of what Sabat (2001) calls "defectology". When clinicians focus too early and too often on a person's deficits, they risk reducing people to the sum of their newly developed problems, as if the truest thing about them is their memory problems. This can lead people to shut down, withdraw, or deny experiencing any sort of cognitive changes (Mast 2011).

> ❝ When clinicians put deficits first, they either neglect fears the person may be experiencing or they activate fears about what might be happening, which likely puts the person on the defensive, unable to engage in an open discussion for fear about what might happen and where the discussion is going. ❞

—Mast (2011: 73)

Living with dementia is multidimensional

Dementia is not exclusively a biomedical problem (see Chapter 8). People diagnosed with dementia can expect to live many years with cognitive impairment, and the deficit-focused approach does not provide an avenue for helping people live their remaining years well. We need to be able to address psychological, social, and spiritual aspects of living with chronic and progressive cognitive changes.

Living with dementia is unique for each person

The changes associated with dementia take place within an individual's life history (see Chapter 15) and unique social context (see Chapter 8). As such, the symptoms and care needs will be individualized. To gain a picture of the whole person, assessment must tap into the psychological, social, and spiritual aspects of their life.

The person can provide valuable information about their experience

For many years, clinicians operated under the assumption that people with dementia, and those with Alzheimer's disease in particular, lacked awareness and so could not provide useful information in the assessment process. Recent research has demonstrated retained awareness for people with dementia (see, for example, Clare 2003). Furthermore, when appropriate measures are used, the self-reports of people with dementia have good psychometric properties (Logsdon and Teri 1997; Logsdon et al. 2002; Hoe et al. 2005; Snow et al. 2005; Whitlatch et al. 2005; Burgener and Berger 2008; Judge et al. 2010; Mak 2011). As such, it is no longer acceptable to exclude the person's perspective from the process. Although reports of people with dementia and their family carers may differ, people with dementia can offer reliable and valid input into their life and care values and needs, even into moderately severe dementia (see Chapter 12). Thus, their input is essential for understanding the person, and ensuring their ongoing input will help their transition through the stages of dementia and their ongoing care planning (Manthorpe et al. 2011).

It should be noted, however, that although the deficit-focused approach to assessment has its limitations, the use of cognitive tests can be integrated into the whole person approach to assessment and care of the individual, as demonstrated in case example 20.1.

Case example 20.1: Ms. Brown – undergoing an assessment of cognitive changes

A few months after Ms. Brown's 73rd birthday, her daughter raised concerns with her mother's doctor about her mother's memory and her increasingly frequent angry outbursts. At the insistence of her daughter, Ms. Brown visited her doctor who referred her for a cognitive assessment. As part of this assessment process, a psychologist tested her memory. After the psychologist read 12 words to her, she was asked how many she could remember. She could only remember two of the words. She began to worry. The psychologist repeated the list of words two more times, and Ms. Brown recalled four and five words respectively. Twenty minutes later, the psychologist asked her to say as many of the words as she could remember from the list. Ms. Brown felt her mind go blank and her heart sank. She felt both embarrassed and afraid. Not only could she not remember any of the words on the list, she did not have *any* memory of a word list having ever being read to her. The psychologist continued to encourage her, but Ms. Brown had already given up. She found herself thinking back to her father who had died with Alzheimer's disease several years previously.

There are three aspects of this clinical encounter that are important: (1) the difficulty Ms. Brown had remembering (recalling – see Chapter 8); (2) the emotions Ms. Brown felt when failing the test of her memory; and (3) the meaning that this has for her ongoing experience.

Ms. Brown's difficulty recalling information. Ms. Brown has significant problems remembering. From a neuropsychological perspective, she has some difficulty recalling information recently presented and even more difficulty recalling that information at a later point in time. This is one of the cognitive changes characteristic of early Alzheimer's disease (Welsh et al. 1991, 1992; Grober and Kawas 1997; Bondi et al. 1999). When the psychologist compares Ms. Brown's memory performance to normative data on people in her age range (see Figure 20.1), she will conclude that her memory changes do not reflect normal ageing. Additional cognitive testing will be conducted in order to ascertain what type of dementia she is experiencing. This is often the focus of traditional dementia

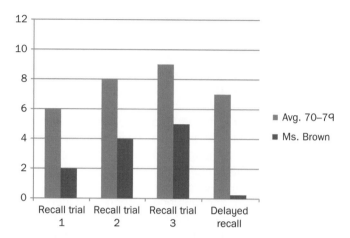

Figure 20.1: Ms. Brown's memory performance – words recalled over three learning trials and one delayed recall trial

assessment and is often considered to be a critical aspect of evaluating early dementia (Knopman *et al.* 2001; Petersen *et al.* 2001).

Exercise 20.1: A memory task

Generate a list of 15 unrelated words. Ask a friend to do the same. Take turns reading your word lists to each other, asking each other to repeat back as many words as you can remember. Before you attempt to memorize the list, imagine you are an older person with memory troubles.

■ What might be you be feeling when trying to remember this list?
■ What might be the consequences of failing to remember in this context?

After you've each completed the memory task, discuss together the range of emotions and thoughts an older person being evaluated for dementia might experience.

Ms. Brown's experience of being tested. This aspect concerns the way Ms. Brown experiences the clinical encounter in which her memory was being tested. Ideally, the clinician should use some of the assessment time to converse with her about this. For Ms. Brown, this included her feelings of embarrassment and shame. Attending to the person's feelings is an important aspect of taking care of, and understanding, them while being tested. Further questioning can sometimes reveal that the way a person responds to the experience of testing and cognitive failure may be related to past experiences. For example, the psychologist learned that Ms. Brown's father had Alzheimer's disease, she had cared for him for years after her mother died, and that this remains a painful memory. Ms. Brown has known that genetically she has had a higher risk for developing Alzheimer's disease (Jarvik *et al.* 2008). This underlying fear of developing Alzheimer's disease is activated whenever she has trouble remembering something (Cutler and Hodgson 1996; Hodgson and Cutler 2005). Her experiences with her father and the shame felt during testing may influence the extent to which she continues to engage in testing and whether she comes back to this memory clinic or hospital.

The meaning of cognitive impairment for Ms. Brown. The third aspect of this encounter reflects the overlap of the first two aspects. Ms. Brown has problems with memory, specifically recall for information presented recently, plus she has a family history of Alzheimer's disease. Her difficulty remembering combined with her fear of developing the condition led her to feel a mix of emotions. These include shame, embarrassment, and anxiety. Knowing how she feels about what is happening to her memory should influence the way we understand and seek to support her in her day-to-day life with dementia. Based on her memory tests, we can infer that she forgets a considerable amount of the moment-to-moment activity, which may leave her feeling confused and disoriented. Therefore, when we ask her about her life and experience we would want to interpret what she says in this context. We would also want to minimize the number of times we ask her, "Do you remember . . .". Her cognitive abilities and impairments will also influence the way she understands her condition. A key requirement in caring for people with dementia is to meet and communicate with them at a level that is appropriate for their cognitive ability (see Chapter 17). If during cognitive testing a person was found to be experiencing severe cognitive impairment, we would explain their condition to them differently than to a person with mild impairment. That said, in both cases the person-centred clinician would seek to explain information about the condition to the person, not just to the family. It is difficult to be person-centred without including the person in the process.

In summary, we need an approach to assessment that recognizes that a person's identity is not rooted only in her cognitive abilities, but also in other aspects of her life and being. We need to continue to develop ways to understand and support these aspects of Ms. Brown's life and identity through a deeper understanding of her and the way dementia is affecting her.

Assessing the whole person

Whole person assessment addresses three main areas:

- the dementia syndrome (including cognitive and functional changes)
- the person
- the person's experience of the dementia-related changes

The whole person approach seeks to balance the focus on cognitive impairments with an equivalent focus on the person and their experiences. This balance is achieved both in terms of the time given and the assessment approaches and instruments used. The whole person approach seeks to understand a person's history, personality, values, worldview, and needs, as well as the way these intersect with these cognitive and functional changes (labelled "Experience of dementia" in Figure 20.2). One of the key elements of the whole person approach is the recognition that in understanding the person with dementia, exclusively focusing on cognitive and functional deficits is not sufficient to guide person-centred care.

Whole person assessment encourages clinicians and health care providers to reconsider the way they think about people with dementia and the contributions they make to the assessment process. If people with cognitive impairment and dementia can provide useful information on their life and care, what should we be asking them about? What besides the cognitive symptoms should we be focusing on? How can we go about assessing these?

Assessing cognitive and functional changes

Clinicians use standardized structured tests to evaluate the nature and extent of cognitive changes and the way they impact daily functioning (Mast and Gerstenecker 2010; Mast 2011). These are not only important for the diagnostic process, but they also inform care planning in that the planned activities and care must match the person's ability level.

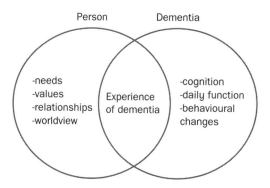

Figure 20.2: Assessment domains

Assessing the person and their experience with dementia

People with dementia can provide useful input in the assessment process and should be considered full partners in the process. Expanding the range of measures beyond cognition is necessary. Clinicians and health care providers should ensure they include sufficient time to listen to the person experiencing cognitive changes even when the referral question concerns making a dementia diagnosis. If the standardized measures only focus on cognition or are only given to caregivers, then the input of the person living with cognitive changes may be neglected even in early dementia.

Table 20.1 highlights some aspects of the person and their experience that might be assessed during the assessment process. Some of these can be assessed with structured questionnaires

Question	Aspects of the person/experience	Assessment method
What is important to the person?	Values and preferences regarding life and care	Values and Preferences Scale (Whitlatch et al. 2005)
How do they feel about their life?	Quality of life	QoL-AD (Logsdon et al. 2002)
What do they like to do? (now or in the past)	Activities	Pleasant Events Schedule-AD (Logsdon and Teri 1997)
How do they view life and the world?	Worldview and beliefs	Life review questions (see Gibson 2004; Haight and Haight 2007; Mast 2011)
Who is important? Who do they want to spend time with?	Key relationships	Life review questions
What major events influenced their life?	Major life events	Life review questions
What needs are currently being unmet?	Unmet physical and psychological needs	Behaviour observation (Algase et al. 1996; Kovach et al. 2005)
How are they experiencing dementia?	Stigma associated with dementia	Stigma Impact Scale (Burgener and Berger 2008)

Table 20.1 How are aspects of a person with dementia assessed?

(e.g. values and preferences, quality of life, activity) and others can be understood by listening to the person's story.

Exercise 20.2: Imagining daily life with dementia

- If you were diagnosed with dementia, what aspects of your daily life would be most difficult for you?
- How would you want to live the remaining chapters of your life in light of progressive memory loss and cognitive change?
- What would you want to do?
- Who would you want to spend it with?
- What are the most important aspects of your life right now?
- How could you carry them forward if you began to develop Alzheimer's disease?
- How would memory failure interfere with your ability to do these things?

As there are few structured questionnaires and measures to assess psychosocial aspects of the person, clinicians and caregivers must seek to develop understanding via other methods. Seeking to listen to and learn the person's story serves as a means for starting to understand important aspects of the person, who they feel connected to, and how they view their life and the world. The advantage is that this allows them to provide input in a way that is natural and comforting, and is helpful in communicating honour and respect for the person and their experiences. Asking another person to share their story communicates value and interest in the person and helps to build a working relationship. Moreover, although cognitive testing is a key aspect of dementia assessment, it can be distressing for people with dementia (Lai *et al.* 2008), so the sharing of one's story may help reduce some of the distress and defensiveness that can arise from testing.

Case example 20.2: Ms. Brown (continued) – whole person assessment approach

In addition to cognitive testing, Ms. Brown completed the following:

- Quality of Life Scale for people with Alzheimer's disease (QoL-AD) in which the following items were rated as fair or poor:
  - family
  - memory
  - ability to do chores around the house
- Values and Preferences Scale in which the following were highlighted as being very important:
  - avoid being physical burden
  - be with family
  - feel useful
  - be able to practise religious/spiritual beliefs
- Pleasant Events Schedule for people with Alzheimer's disease (PES-AD) in which the following were noted as activities she enjoyed:
  - going to church, attending religious services
  - laughing
  - going to museums, art exhibitions or related cultural activities

(continued)

- Experience of stigma, in which she endorsed the following items:
  - "I do not feel I can be open with others about my impairment"
  - "I feel a need to keep my impairment a secret"

Some of Ms. Brown's responses appeared to be inconsistent. For example, she noted that it is important to be with family but also that the family domain was rated as "poor" on the Quality of Life Scale. But the meaning of these responses became more apparent as the clinician asked her some questions about her life:

- "What were some of the hardest things you faced in your life?"
- "What do you hope/fear will happen as you grow older?"

Ms. Brown's story revealed two key relationships: the relationships with her daughters and with her father. She and her daughters had always been close and in the past they had shared much of their joys and sorrows together. But recently she had seemed increasingly angry with them, particularly when they tried to offer her help around her house. It was particularly difficult for them to hear their mother so angry with them – they had never envisioned that their relationship would hit this level. Her daughters were afraid and that is what had prompted this assessment.

The other key relationship Ms. Brown described shed some light on this. She had cared for her father who had lived and died with Alzheimer's disease and this was a deeply painful time for her. She did not want this experience for her daughters as she now began to realize that she was following a similar path of decline. When they pointed out her instances of forgetting, it would upset her because she did not want to think about getting Alzheimer's disease and because she was afraid of what this might mean for her daughters who would likely end up taking care of her.

Whole person care planning

Whole person assessment sets the stage for care planning that is informed not just by the person's level of cognitive impairment, but also by an understanding of the person and how they are experiencing life with cognitive impairment. It takes the opportunity to highlight previous and current chapters of the person's life and to link these to how the remaining chapters of their life could be written to help them to live the best possible life with dementia.

An approach to dementia assessment that focuses only on cognition and functioning may present the person to the family and to health care providers only as a person with moderate dementia with impaired memory and functioning. This could unintentionally communicate that these are the most important things about the person and thereby misses the opportunity to highlight how the person can remain a person of value and can continue to live a meaningful life in relationship with others.

Whole person care planning draws upon the broader understanding of the person and seeks to maintain as much continuity as possible in the face of considerable change. Care planning also regularly seeks the person's input with the goal of addressing their needs and preferences in a way that is informed by their identity and ability level.

Case example 20.3: Ms. Brown (continued) – whole person care planning

The assessment clearly laid the foundation for care planning for Ms. Brown. The results revealed not only that she was experiencing cognitive impairment consistent with Alzheimer's disease, but also that she had very real concerns about how she would live, who would take care of her, what she would do, and what was most important to her. Some important findings and themes were:

- desire for quality time with her daughters and to avoid being a burden to them
- desire to be active and to contribute
- desire to remain connected with her community of faith

The assessment helped to explain that Ms. Brown would get angry when she was frustrated with being unable to articulate her concerns during a disagreement with her daughters about her care. Based upon her prior experiences with caregiving, she felt very strongly that she did not want to be a burden on her family, while at the same time she very much wanted to be with them (the apparent contradiction or inconsistency in saying that it was "very important" to be with family, but rated this aspect of quality of life as "poor"). She wanted to spend quality time with them, enjoying them and their relationships.

Her responses on the Pleasant Events Schedule helped her daughters to identify enjoyable activities they could do together. This meant that not all of their time together was focused on care tasks. Her daughters could focus on their mother as a person, rather than on accomplishing each of the tasks on their list of caregiving duties.

The clinician also discussed ways that Ms. Brown might remain connected with her faith community. She was going to have difficulty attending church services due to the driving restrictions (due to cognitive changes). Together they came up with two ideas. First, Ms. Brown and her daughters would reach out to a group of old friends from church to ask if they could drive her to church meetings with them. This was a difficult step for Ms. Brown because she was worried about telling others about her memory problems. Together, she and her daughters talked about who they could selectively share this information with and how they would share it. Second, Ms. Brown could listen to old hymns and songs that she remembered from years of attending church services. In addition, when they were together, her daughters would read to her from her Bible which she greatly enjoyed not only because it was very meaningful to her, but also because it met her desire for quality time with her family.

Ms. Brown had expressed a desire to continue to contribute around the house. She wanted to be useful. Before initiating the assessment, her daughters had taken over much of the care of her home because they were afraid for her safety and well-being. In addition, they had wanted to take control of paying her bills and dispensing her medication. The results of the assessment helped them to see that although she needed some oversight and supervision on these tasks, it was also important for them to help her to identify which tasks she could still do.

Exercise 20.3: Focusing on the desires expressed by a person with dementia

Review Ms. Brown's three desires in the box above. Think about and write down other ways that she could maintain good relationships with her daughters, stay active, and maintain her religious and spiritual life.

Now imagine that several years have passed and Ms. Brown has continued to show cognitive and functional decline. She has difficulty remembering her daughters' names, needs much more care assistance, and is no longer able to move around as easily and therefore doesn't leave her home except for medical appointments. How would you suggest maintaining a focus on these desires in light of her progressive condition?

Debates and controversies

In the context of dementia, it is not always straightforward to determine what the person wants and then action it. When a person is experiencing cognitive decline, the things that are important to the person may not be easy to accomplish. As an example, a person may love to drive a car, but at some point it will become unsafe for them to do so. There will always be a tension in care planning between a greater need for supervision (safety) and a desire to help meet the person's needs and respect their values. The goal in care planning, even when the person may not be able to make their own decisions, is to create the care plan with an understanding of the person and their preferences in mind, while appreciating the influence that the dementia-related changes have on the ways those preferences are met.

Conclusion

More research is needed to address the extent to which changing our methods of assessment can lead to better working relationships and better care over time. The benefits of broadening the focus of dementia assessment can clearly be seen in individual accounts but further empirical evidence is needed to influence policy more broadly. In addition, the development of new methods and techniques to address a range of aspects of living with dementia are needed. For policy-makers, ongoing cost–benefit research will likely be needed to justify person-centred assessment and care.

Further information

The Pioneer Network is an organization committed to changing the culture of dementia care through person-centred principles [https://www.pioneernetwork.net/].

The Alzheimer's Society promotes better care and optimal living with dementia through advocacy and research. Their web site includes resources on "Living with Dementia" and making the most of life with cognitive impairment [http://www.alzheimers.org.uk/].

The National Dementia Initiative is a collaborative effort to better define person-centred care, to improve the quality of life of individuals with dementia, and to reduce the overuse of anti-psychotic medication in people with dementia [http://www.ccal.org/national-dementia-initiative/].

The Dementia Foundation promotes activities and training that help individuals with dementia remain valued persons in their communities. The Foundation promotes a philosophy of care that seeks to enrich the lives of people with dementia [http://www.dementiafoundation.org.au/].

References

Algase, D.L., Beck, C., Kolanowski, A., Whall, A., Berent, S. *et al.* (1996) Need-driven dementia-compromised behavior: an alternative view of disruptive behavior, *American Journal of Alzheimer's Disease and Other Dementias*, 11: 10–19.

Birks, J. (2006) Cholinesterase inhibitors for Alzheimer's disease, *Cochrane Database of Systematic Reviews*, 1: CD005593 [http://onlinelibrary.wiley.com/store/10.1002/14651858.CD005593/asset/CD005593.pdf?v=1&t=hsfyshtt&s=c51eed38370e8d29370c184d74d9fc9b403a49df]. Accessed 16th June 2014

Birks, J. and Flicker, L. (2006) Donepezil for mild cognitive impairment, *Cochrane Database of Systematic Reviews*, 3: CD006104 [http://onlinelibrary.wiley.com/store/10.1002/14651858.CD006104/asset/CD006104.pdf?v=1&t=hsfyx2nh&s=e99aa4de9f313d74aabe510809b8459e15e851fb]. Accessed 16th June 2014

Bondi, M.W., Salmon, D.P., Galasko, D., Thomas, R.G. and Thal, L.J. (1999) Neuropsychological function and Apolipo-protein E genotype in the preclinical detection of Alzheimer's disease, *Psychology and Aging*, 14: 295–303.

Burgener, S.C. and Berger, B. (2008) Measuring perceived stigma in persons with progressive neurological disease, *Dementia*, 7: 31–53.

Clare, L. (2003) Managing threats to self: awareness in early-stage Alzheimer's disease, *Social Science and Medicine*, 57: 1017–29.

Clare, L., Rowlands, J., Bruce, E., Surr, C. and Downs, M. (2008) The experience of living with dementia in residential care: an interpretative phenomenological analysis, *The Gerontologist*, 48: 711–20.

Cutler, S.J. and Hodgson, L.G. (1996) Anticipatory dementia: a link between memory appraisals and concerns about developing Alzheimer's disease, *The Gerontologist*, 36: 657–64.

French, S.L., Floyd, M., Wilkins, S. and Osato, S. (2011) The Fear of Alzheimer's Disease Scale: a new measure designed to assess anticipatory dementia in older adults, *International Journal of Geriatric Psychiatry*, 27: 521–8.

Gibson, F. (2004) *The Past in the Present: Using Reminiscence in Health and Social Care*. Baltimore, MD: Health Professions Press.

Grober, E. and Kawas, C. (1997) Learning and retention in preclinical and early Alzheimer's disease, *Psychology and Aging*, 12: 183–8.

Haight, B.K. and Haight, B.S. (2007) *The Handbook of Structured Life Review*. Baltimore, MD: Health Professions Press.

Hodgson, L. and Cutler, S. (2005) Anticipatory dementia: insights from published first-person accounts, *The Gerontologist*, 45: 129.

Hoe, J., Katona, C., Roch, B. and Livingston, G. (2005) Use of the QOL-AD for measuring quality of life in people with severe dementia – the LASER-AD study, *Age and Ageing*, 34: 130–5.

Jarvik, L., LaRue, A., Blacker, D., Gatz, M., Kawas, C. *et al.* (2008) Children of persons with Alzheimer disease: what does the future hold?, *Alzheimer Disease and Associated Disorders*, 22: 6–20.

Judge, K.S., Menne, H.L. and Whitlatch, C.J. (2010) Stress process model for individuals with dementia, *The Gerontologist*, 50: 294–302.

Kitwood, T. (1997) *Dementia Reconsidered: The Person Comes First*. Buckingham: Open University Press.

Knopman, D.S., DeKosky, S.T., Cummings, J.L., Chui, H., Corey-Bloom, J. *et al.* (2001) Practice parameter: diagnosis of dementia (an evidence-based review). Report of the Quality Standards Subcommittee of the American Academy of Neurology, *Neurology*, 56: 1143–53.

Kovach, C.R., Noonan, P.E., Schlidt, A.M. and Wells, T. (2005) A model of consequences of need-driven, dementia-compromised behavior, *Journal of Nursing Scholarship*, 37: 134–40.

Lai, J.M., Hawkins, K.A., Gross, C.P. and Karlawish, J.H. (2008) Self-reported distress after cognitive testing in patients with Alzheimer's disease, *Journals of Gerontology A: Biological Sciences and Medical Sciences*, 63: 855–9.

Logsdon, R.G. and Teri, L. (1997) The Pleasant Events Schedule-AD: psychometric properties and relationship to depression and cognition in Alzheimer's disease patients, *The Gerontologist*, 37: 40–5.

Logsdon, R.G., Gibbons, L.E., McCurry, S.M. and Teri, L. (2002) Assessing quality of life in older adults with cognitive impairment, *Psychosomatic Medicine*, 64: 510–19.

Mak, W. (2011) Self-reported goal pursuit and purpose in life among people with dementia, *Journals of Gerontology B: Psychological Sciences and Social Sciences*, 66: 177–84.

Manthorpe, J., Samsi, K., Campbell, S., Abley, C., Keady, J. *et al.* (2011) *The Transition from Cognitive Impairment to Dementia: Older People's Experiences*. Final report. NIHR Service Delivery and Organisation Programme. London: HMSO [http://www.kcl.ac.uk/sspp/kpi/scwru/pubs/2011/manthorpeetal2011transitionfinalreport.pdf, accessed 29 April 2014].

Mast, B.T. (2011) *Whole Person Dementia Assessment*. Baltimore, MD: Health Professions Press.

Mast, B.T. (2012) Methods for assessing the person with Alzheimer's disease: integrating person-centered and diagnostic approaches to assessment, *Clinical Gerontologist*, 35: 360–75.

Mast, B.T. and Gerstenecker, A. (2010) Cognitive screening and brief batteries for dementia, in P.A. Lichtenberg (ed.) *Handbook of Assessment in Clinical Gerontology* (2nd edn.). London: Elsevier.

Moniz-Cook, E., Manthorpe, J., Carr, I., Gibson, G. and Vernooij-Dassen, M. (2006) Facing the future: a qualitative study of older people referred to a memory clinic prior to assessment and diagnosis, *Dementia*, 5: 375–95.

Petersen, R.C., Stevens, J.C., Ganguli, M., Tangalos, E.G., Cummings, J.L. *et al.* (2001) Practice parameter – early detection of dementia: mild cognitive impairment (an evidence-based review). Report of the Quality Standards Subcommittee of the American Academy of Neurology, *Neurology*, 56: 1133–42.

Post, S. (1995) *The Moral Challenge of Alzheimer's Disease*. Baltimore, MD: Johns Hopkins University Press.

Raschetti, R., Albanese, E., Vanacore, N. and Maggini, M. (2007) Cholinesterase inhibitors in mild cognitive impairment: a systematic review of randomised trials, *PLoS Medicine*, 4: 1818–28.

Rodda, J. and Walker, Z. (2009) Ten years of cholinesterase inhibitors, *International Journal of Geriatric Psychiatry*, 24: 437–42.

Royall, D.R. (2005) The emperor has no clothes: dementia treatment on the eve of the aging era, *Journal of the American Geriatrics Society*, 53: 163–4.

Sabat, S.R. (2001) *The Experience of Alzhieimer's Disease: Life through a Tangled Veil*. Malden, MA: Blackwell.

Snow, A.L., Kunik, M.E., Molinari, V.A., Orengo, C.A., Doody, R. *et al.* (2005) Accuracy of self-reported depression in persons with dementia, *Journal of the American Geriatrics Society*, 53: 389–96.

Steeman, E., Godderis, J., Grypdonck, M., De Bal, N. and De Casterle, B.D. (2007) Living with dementia from the perspective of older people: is it a positive story?, *Aging and Mental Health*, 11: 119–30.

Welsh, K., Butters, N., Hughes, J., Mohs, R. and Heyman, A. (1991) Detection of abnormal memory decline in mild cases of Alzheimer's disease using CERAD neuropsychological measures, *Archives of Neurology*, 48: 278–81.

Welsh, K.A., Butters, N., Hughes, J.P., Mohs, R.C. and Heyman, A. (1992) Detection and staging of dementia in Alzheimer's disease – use of the neuropsychological measures developed for the Consortium to Establish a Registry for Alzheimer's Disease, *Archives of Neurology*, 49: 448–52.

Whitlatch, C.J., Feinberg, L.F. and Tucke, S.S. (2005) Measuring the values and preferences for everyday care of persons with cognitive impairment and their family caregivers, *The Gerontologist*, 45: 370–80.

Woods, R.T. (2001) Discovering the person with Alzheimer's disease: cognitive, emotional and behavioural aspects, *Aging and Mental Health*, 5: S7–S16.

CHAPTER 21

Living at home

Georgina Charlesworth

❝There is a notice board in the kitchen. I'm very open to telling people I have dementia. It helps me. And it helps them. So they can simplify. If I can't remember if I had breakfast I go look to see if the pots are still there. I plan the day every day. Make sure I get things out of the freezer. I start out and think what I'm gonna do. I look at the diary and say Oh yes, we're doing this, this and this. I have a pattern, a routine. Without the diary I'm lost. So I can look and see what happened the day before. Then I write what I've done. I can look at it and bring it back. It means I can bring it back. Once I have the trigger, I can remember it. ❞

—Marlene Aveyard Bradford, UK

Learning objectives

By the end of this chapter, you will be able to:

- Discuss "living with dementia" from the perspectives of the person with dementia and the family carer
- Consider the extent to which quality of life is influenced by attitudes and resources
- Understand the tensions between safety and personhood
- Describe interventions intended to meet the needs of people with dementia and family carers

Introduction

❝Most people with dementia are able to live in their own homes for most of their lives, and most care is given by families. ❞

—NCCMH (2007: 98)

Nearly two-thirds of people with dementia live at home (PSSRU 2007). The time between diagnosis of dementia and the need for nursing care is up to seven years, depending on the type of dementia and the physical health of the person, although, with improved diagnostic processes, the post-diagnosis duration may be increasing. During this post-diagnosis time, the person with dementia will need emotional support and increasing levels of assistance with activities of daily living. The increased care needs of the person with dementia affect family carers' lives, whether cohabiting with the person with dementia, living within the same locality or "at a distance". Governments around the world have begun recognizing the needs of people with dementia and their family carers and the need to meet those needs.

Support needs for both carers and people with dementia can be summarized as falling within three categories: informational (advice and knowledge), instrumental (tangible assistance, e.g. housework, shopping, transportation, and personal care), and emotional (e.g. having an available confidante). The extent to which needs can be met depends largely on the availability of resources, including family and social network, support services, finances, physical health, and psychological factors such as resilience and cognitive flexibility.

Learning to live with the diagnosis

The way in which a person learns to live with a dementia diagnosis is heavily influenced by their attitudes, and by the attitudes of their family, friends, and wider society. Emotional reactions to living with dementia can include anger, frustration, fear, confusion, sadness, and the wish to die, but can also include positive feelings and enjoyment in meaningful activities (von Kutzleben *et al.* 2012). Beliefs about, and perceptions of, dementia vary considerably, shaped by a person's current situation, past experiences, and exposure to others with dementia (Bunn *et al.* 2012). Although press headlines perpetuate the view of dementia as a "living death", there are increasing numbers of people maintaining a good quality of life post-diagnosis. Case example 21.1 provides an illustration of a person who embraces the dementia diagnosis and responds with a "fighting spirit".

Case example 21.1: David

David was a senior executive in a multinational company. He semi-retired in his late fifties but maintained an active interest in business. He started to become aware of changes in his literacy skills and short-term memory, and after thorough investigations was diagnosed with Alzheimer's disease with posterior cortical atrophy (PCA). Initially, he felt lost and uncertain about how to proceed. He and his wife searched the Internet for information and advice. Soon they had found the web sites of the PCA Support group, Innovations in Dementia, Dementia Voice, and the Dementia Advocacy and Support Network. David began to read and contribute to online support forums for people with dementia. Through connecting with others, he felt re-energized and determined to find a good quality of life "beyond the diagnosis". In addition to taking his "memory medication", he and his son set up his phone and tablet computer to act as external memory aids. He and his wife changed their diet and started to go out for walks. He sent an email to all his friends and acquaintances to explain his difficulties, also letting them know what they could do to help. He joined his national Alzheimer's Society, became a "Dementia Friend", and volunteered himself as a speaker at information and education events, giving examples of how to use technology to help maintain community involvement. Although he would never have chosen to develop Alzheimer's, he often comments on the way in which it has brought him and his wife closer together and how grateful he is to have the opportunity to work with her.

David is an example of someone who overcame his initial shock at the diagnosis to seek out information on "successful" coping. Empowered by supportive family and newly found peers, he set about finding strategies to manage his memory difficulties and found a new lease of life in sharing his new-found knowledge with others.

Not everyone has the psychological, social or financial resources that were at David's disposal, and not everyone chooses to place themselves in the public domain. The more usual goals for people learning to live with dementia are: to maintain a sense of normality; to hold on to a former sense of identity as much as possible; to maintain relationships; and to engage with meaningful activities (von Kutzleben *et al.* 2012).

The needs of those "home alone"

Around half of those living at home with dementia are living alone. Miranda-Castillo and colleagues (2010) summarized the relevant literature as follows:

- *Characteristics* People with dementia living alone are predominantly widowed women, and are less cognitively and functionally impaired than those living with others.
- *Risks* People with dementia living alone in their homes are at risk in terms of nutrition, money management, medication management, hygiene, and falls.
- *Service use* People with dementia living alone are less likely to use health services than those who co-habit with a family carer, and are more likely to get help from social services such as home-delivered meals, homecare services, and daycare.

Case example 21.2: Mrs. Franks

Mrs. Franks has always enjoyed company, and has a wide circle of friends. She has lived in the same area all her life and is well known in the local community, not least for her enthusiastic contributions to the church choir. Her husband of 55 years died five years ago, when she was 78. Mrs. Franks' daughter, Gill, lives locally and visits most days on her way home from work. Gill took her mother to their family doctor to express her concerns over Mrs. Franks losing track of dates, times, and possessions, missing occasional meals, and no longer keeping the house to her former high standard. A diagnosis of dementia was given, but Mrs. Franks does not use the term "dementia" herself. She regards her memory as normal for her age, and puts her disorientation over time down to missing her husband and "daydreaming about the past". She blames her poor eyesight for any confusion over household bills, and attributes "muddles" over dates and times to her poor hearing.

Mrs. Franks used to go out every day to get groceries, but does this less since her daughter organized a weekly delivery from the supermarket. Mrs. Franks knows that her daughter means well, and she appreciates that the deliveries save her from carrying heavy bags or going out in the rain with her arthritis, but she enjoyed the social contact with other shoppers. She is pleased when her friends and neighbours pop round, and enjoys going to various church activities and events. She was recently upset, however, when she realized that she had misidentified a doorstep sales person as someone she knew. The incident left her feeling foolish and vulnerable.

Mrs. Franks' example demonstrates the challenges faced by many people with dementia to maintain their self-identity and independence, and also highlights their vulnerability to social isolation and exploitation by unscrupulous others. An apparent denial of cognitive deficits and/or need may be a strategy to protect their sense of self. Where "lack of insight" was once considered a key component of dementia, recent research has demonstrated the range of methodological and conceptual issues that need to be considered when assessing awareness and its deficits (Clare *et al.* 2004). Mrs. Franks' example also illustrates a number of unmet needs. Studies of community dwelling people with dementia show people living alone are significantly more likely to have unmet needs than their counterparts with a co-resident carer (Meaney *et al.* 2005; Miranda-Castillo *et al.* 2010). Guidance for assessing the needs of people with dementia living at home can be gained from assessment tools such as the Camberwell Assessment of Needs in the Elderly (CANE; Orrell and Hancock 2004) or the Care Needs Assessment Pack for Dementia (CareNap-D; McWalter *et al.* 1998). The domains covered are listed in Table 21.1.

Exercise 21.1: Identifying needs and social network

1 Re-read the case example of Mrs. Franks and Table 21.1. What are Mrs. Franks' needs (met and unmet)?

2 A person's social network is characterized by proximity to kin, numbers of involved family, friends, and neighbours, and levels of interaction with family, friends, and community groups. How would you describe Mrs. Franks' social network? How would Mrs. Franks' needs differ if:

    a) her husband were still alive and well?
    b) her daughter moved to a different area?
    c) she lived in supported housing?

3 Mrs. Franks's daughter, Gill, contacted a local dementia support worker and has heard of various services that she hopes will be of interest to her mother. These include a local day centre and an alarm call pendant so that she can easily contact help in an emergency. How do you think Mrs. Franks will react to these suggestions?

Mrs. Franks' social network extends beyond her household to include local family, friends, and neighbours. She maintains involvement with her local community, and her network would fit with the pattern of "locally integrated" from Wenger's (1991) typology of social networks. Network types demonstrate some predictive power as to the demands made on health and social services with people in locally integrated support networks being more open to gaining new information and more able to adapt to a greater range of changes and pressures than people in the more restricted networks. People with dementia are most likely to remain in the community where their support networks are "locally integrated" (extends beyond tighter family or household groups to include local family, friends, neighbours – good community involvement maintained) or "family dependent" (small network and high dependency on local family). Other networks in the Wenger typology include:

- *Locally self-contained* – rely mostly on neighbours, although there may be contact with a family member; community involvement low
- *Wider community-focused* – absence of local family and high levels of community involvement
- *Private restricted* – no local family or other contacts and no community involvement

The alarm call pendant favoured by Mrs. Frank's daughter is an example of the "first-generation" telecare that is now widely available in western societies. Calls are put through to a control centre in which a call handler can organize a response of some kind, whether that be to emergency services or to a relative, neighbour or friend acting as "key holder". Advances in technology have led to the development or more sophisticated equipment. The second generation of telecare includes linking of sensors such as smoke, gas, heat, and flood to community alarm services, and can also include movement sensors and devices for monitoring the opening and closing of doors,

Domain	CANE items	CareNap-D items
Activities	Daytime activities	
Social interaction	Communication	Recognizing people
	Company	Taking part and joining in
	Intimate relationships	Understanding and informing others
	Behaviours leading to conflict with others	Talking about feelings
		Withdrawing
Thinking and memory	Memory	Making decisions
		Recognizing strangers
		Remembering routines
		Repetitive questions
Behaviour and mental state	Psychotic symptoms	Wandering or getting lost
	Psychological distress	Verbal or physical aggression
	Deliberate self-harm	Sexual disinhibition
		Agitation or anxiety
		Sleep disturbance
		Mood swings
		Unusual beliefs or hallucinations
House care	Looking after home	Housework and laundry
	Accidental self-harm	Using heating and the cooker
		Securing the home
		Safety with gas and appliances
Community living	Accommodation	Obtaining and taking medication
	Money	Shopping and making snacks
	Benefits	Using the phone and transport
	Problems with alcohol	Alcohol and smoking
		Managing finances
Health and mobility	Physical health	Physical health
	Mobility/falls	Balance and falls
	Medication	Getting up and walking
	Clear information about condition and treatment	Eyesight and hearing
		Feet and bowels
Self-care and toileting	Food	Self-washing or bathing
	Self-care	Dressing
	Continence	Dental care
		Eating
		Day or night-time wetting or soiling
Other	Vulnerable to abuse/neglect	
	Caring for another	

Table 21.1 Areas of need

the running of taps, and use of electrical appliances (Kerr *et al.* 2010). The increased availability of broadband, wireless, and audio-visual technology offers potential for "telehealth care", such as the 3 million lives project in England (www.3millionlives.co.uk).

Telecare and telehealth are intended to be "assistive technologies", that is, they are devices for personal use designed to enhance the physical, sensory, and cognitive abilities of people with disabilities to help them function more independently. Devices include "low-technology" solutions such as day/night indicators, bath and cooker monitoring and shut off devices, medicine reminders, lost item locators, automatic lights, door alarms, and programmable telephones. Evaluations of assistive technologies indicate that they can be of benefit where devices are reliable, aesthetically pleasing, meet an acknowledged need, and are easy to instal and use. Where devices are "user operated", it is also necessary that the person with dementia is both motivated and capable of operating them. Training techniques may be of benefit, such as those used within cognitive rehabilitation (see Chapter 9), but the level of awareness of the person with dementia will be an important factor in its success or otherwise. Evaluations of monitoring systems indicate that they can detect problems before they require crisis intervention and can enhance feelings of safety and security for both people with dementia and their family carers with the cost of installing systems cheaper than the costs of nursing home care (Nijhof *et al.* 2013).

Caring for a person with dementia at home

Aneshensel and colleagues (1995) referred to the stage of in-home caring as the "long haul" for carers. They highlight the development of the carer from being illness-naïve to being experientially knowledgeable, and from having pre-caring levels of resources to being socially, personally, and economically depleted. As described in Chapters 5 and 13 carers are at risk of physical exhaustion, emotional burnout, financial hardship, and social isolation. Carers of people with dementia have higher levels of stress and distress than other caring populations, and stressed and distressed carers have higher mortality and morbidity than non-carers. Although the predominant literature on carer well-being focuses on the negative aspects of caring, there is an emerging body of evidence on the positive aspects of caring (PAC). Positive aspects include satisfactions with caring, enjoyable aspects of caregiving, feeling fulfilled or important, finding a sense of companionship and meaning within the relationship, and feeling pride in one's own abilities to handle crisis. Cohen and colleagues (2002) found that 73% of carers are able to generate one or more positive aspects of caring, and Andren and Elmstahl (2005) found 51% of spouse carers and 66% of adult-offspring carers reported either a "great deal" or "quite a lot" of satisfaction. Individuals reporting higher PAC report less depression and burden and greater subjective health than those who do not endorse PAC (Cohen *et al.* 2002). Perceived uplifts are associated with lower levels of carer burden and depression. The ability to identify PAC seems to be influenced by racial or cultural factors. Roff and colleagues (2004) found that African American carers scored more highly on PAC than white Americans, with the relationship between PAC and race partially mediated by religiosity. In a systematic review of studies exploring the motivations for providing care and the meanings found in caregiving, Quinn and colleagues (2010) found evidence for carer well-being being influenced by kin relationships, cultural norms, and finding meaning. Most family carers are motivated by "emotional bonds" such as love and affection (57%), whereas only 3% say they "had no other alternative" (Triantafillou and Mestheneos 2006). In the same study, 15% of carers indicated that they were principally motivated by a "sense of duty", and 13% had a "personal sense of obligation".

Case example 21.3: Gill and Sandra

Gill and Sandra both work in the same office, and have done so for many years. Coincidentally, both Gill's mother and Sandra's mother-in-law were diagnosed with dementia around the same time. Gill has always been close to her mother, Mrs. Franks, and has always been in frequent, often daily contact. She is pleased to be able to reciprocate the care that Mrs. Franks has provided for her and for her children as they were growing up. Since Mrs. Franks has been living on her own, Gill has been concerned for her mother's well-being. Gill has agonized over what to do for the best, and wishes that she could invite her mother to move in with her. However, finances have been tight since her husband lost his job and there is no room in the house as the children (all adults) have neither found long-term employment nor moved away from home.

Sandra has often provided a "listening ear" for her work colleague, while privately "counting her blessings", as she has, to her great relief, not needed to become involved in supporting her mother-in-law. Sandra's situation changed suddenly when her father-in-law, Brian, suffered an unexpected and severe stroke one weekend. Sandra was called upon to stay with her mother-in-law, Jane, while Brian and Jane's children made arrangements to travel to be with her and with Brian during his hospital treatment. None of the family had realized quite how heavily Jane relied on Brian. She was lost without him.

Social relationships influence physical and mental well-being, and peer support is often highly valued by carers. Indeed, Aneshensel and colleagues (1995) suggest that emotional support may have a greater influence on the course of stressors than instrumental support. In the above case example, Gill has the benefit of naturally occurring peer support from her work colleague Sandra. In contrast, many spouse-carers report less social interaction and fewer friendships than do non-carers. Carers of people with dementia are at risk of experiencing a reduction in their social network due to a lack of opportunities to socialize and/or the stigma associated with dementia. Befriending and peer support services aim to meet carers' need for emotional support, but although qualitative evaluations provide positive results (Greenwood *et al.* 2013), quantitative evaluations indicate that such support is not enough to reduce depression or improve quality of life (Charlesworth *et al.* 2008).

Exercise 21.2: Planning support for family carers

" The form, content, and timing of intervention should depend to a considerable extent on where caregivers are in their [caregiving] careers, and involve an understanding of what has passed before and what is likely to lie ahead. That is, the problems encountered today should be viewed against the backdrop of yesterday and with an eye towards tomorrow" (Aneshensel *et al.* 1995: 306).

■ Gill and Sandra are both caring for a parent (in-law) with dementia. How do their situations differ? What difference will this make when planning support interventions?
■ Depending on the outcome of Brian's stroke, Sandra and her husband may become the main family supports for both Brian and Jane. This is a new situation for both of them. What will their main support needs be (informational, tangible, emotional)?

The World Health Organisation (2012) strongly recommends the following interventions for family carers of people with dementia:

■ psycho-educational interventions offered at the time of diagnosis
■ support, counselling, and/or cognitive-behaviour interventions to address carer psychological strain
■ management of depression

Training carers to cope with behavioural symptoms in people with dementia through active carer participation (e.g. role-playing of behavioural problem management) is also recommended.

There is a growing research literature on interventions to support family carers of people with dementia. Two large-scale evaluations of carer support are the Resources for Enhancing Alzheimer's Caregiver Health (REACH) initiative and Mittelman's New York University Caregiver Intervention. The primary purpose of REACH was to develop and test new ways to help families manage the daily activities and the stresses of caring for people with Alzheimer's disease or a related disorder. REACH II took the findings from REACH I to test an intervention targeting carer depression, burden, social support, and emotional self-care, plus problem behaviours in the person with dementia. Intervention strategies were largely skills-focused and included education, stress and mood management techniques, communication skills, and problem-solving delivered in 12 sessions over 6 months. In contrast, the NYU intervention had a particular emphasis on the mobilization of local family support through family counselling sessions, with the aim of enhancing the social resources of the carer.

Both interventions provided comprehensive support, and both have shown positive outcomes. In the REACH programme, carers in the intervention group improved in quality of life versus those in the control group (Belle *et al.* 2006). The NYU carer intervention also made a significant difference to participating carers. Higher levels of emotional support, more visits, and "having more network members to whom carers felt close" predicted carers' satisfaction with their social support network (Drentea *et al.* 2006). In turn, satisfaction with social support predicted better mental health outcomes (Roth *et al.* 2005).

We might hope that evidence-based interventions for carers would become part of standard service provision, but, as in other areas of health care, the translation from research to practice is slow. No single service is appropriate for all carers, and carers' needs change over their "caregiving career". The interrelationship between family care and care services is complex. Services can *supplement* family support in the early stages of dementia care, and family care *substitutes* for formal care when formal in-home care or care home provision would otherwise be required. In other words, the family "saves" the state from the need to provide formal care in the home or in care homes. As state provision of welfare services increased in some countries, concern was expressed that the introduction of services would lead to a withdrawal, or "crowding out", of family support. This concern has not been borne out. Indeed, international comparisons have found evidence for accumulation of help from statutory and family supporters, that is, a "crowding in" of support (Motel-Klingebiel *et al.* 2005). Service inputs for the person with dementia predicted higher family care inputs. In practice, this means care planners can realistically hope that by introducing new services to meet needs, they will reduce the number of unmet needs and enable families to continue caring.

The existence of services to support family carers does not mean that all services are taken up. Lack of service uptake by carers is well known for both standard services and research interventions. Although awareness of services is a vital precursor to service use (Brodaty *et al.* 2005), awareness alone does not lead to increased uptake of services. Other factors include work status, socioeconomic status, and level of burden, with burden, depression, and distress leading to increased uptake, and lack of time being linked to non-uptake. It is not unusual for carers to indicate that they believe that services should be for "others less fortunate than me", and that "knowing that they are there should I need them in the future" is in itself supportive.

The care dyad

The most successful support interventions for family carers of people with dementia have been those that are comprehensive and intensive. In an early systematic review of interventions for carers of people with dementia, Brodaty and colleagues suggested that a further characteristic of successful interventions is involving both the carer and the care recipient (Brodaty et al. 2003). Interventions do not need to involve both parties in order to have an effect on both. There is evidence to suggest that the well-being of a care recipient influences the well-being of the carer, and vice versa, and similarly the coping strategies of one influence the adjustment of the other. For example, Marriott and colleagues (2000) demonstrated that a cognitive-behavioural intervention not only reduced carer stress, but also led to a less marked increase in behavioural disturbance in the person with dementia. The reasons for the benefits of dyadic interventions have yet to be established. One possibility is that interventions involving both carer and care recipient, such as Alzheimer's cafes, meeting centres, and large group reminiscence activities offer the opportunity to enhance communication and improve relationships within care dyads. A systematic review of evidence for effects of combined interventions for both the family carer and the person with dementia demonstrated a beneficial impact on the general health of carers, the mental health of people with dementia, and a delay in admittance to long-stay care (Smits et al. 2007).

Transition from home care to care home

If a person with dementia has unmet needs, they are in a vulnerable position. Indeed, people with dementia living at home alone are 20 times more likely to move into residential or nursing care than those living with a family member (Banerjee et al. 2003). Other predictors include carer distress. The proportion of people with dementia living in care homes rises with age, from 27% for those aged between 65 and 74, to 61% for those aged over 90. This demographic is most likely due to spouses being less willing to use care homes for their partners than are adult children for their parents. Different attitudes to care homes can result in conflicts in the family. This is illustrated in Exercise 21.3, where carers are faced not only with the difficulty of making decisions on behalf of the care recipient, but also need to navigate the associated family conflicts.

Exercise 21.3: Decision to move from home care to care home

Gill's siblings think Mrs. Franks is taking too big a risk in staying at home. They want to see her move to the safety of a care home. Gill does not agree, as she fears that her mother will feel "lost".

Brian's cognitive functions are recovering well, but his physical prognosis is poor. He is shocked to find that his wife Jane is staying in respite accommodation, and horrified that none of the family could support her while he was in hospital.

Gill and Brian both feel isolated and unsupported within their respective families, making it difficult to discuss the advantages and disadvantages of care homes. How can involved workers support carers in such circumstances? How might Mrs. Franks and Jane react to any discussions?

Debates and controversies

For many years, most services were directed at family carers. For example, respite services were designed to give the carer a break and relatively little attention was paid to its impact on the person with dementia. Today, we still lack clarity as to whether such services are for persons with dementia or for carers. While we know the importance of social networks and social support, we have yet to agree on the most effective methods of assessing families and social networks.

There is considerable debate over whether services prevent or facilitate institutional care. Some argue that once carers experience some support they realize how much they need, while others argue that were services provided in a more proactive versus reactive fashion, carers would continue caring for longer. Given the influence of cultural norms on attitudes to dementia and people with dementia, it should not be assumed that "western" interventions can be generalized to low- and middle-income countries.

The nature of the relationship between positive and negative aspects of caring is not yet known. Uplifts may reduce the negative effects of caring, or distressed carers may be less likely to perceive positive aspects of caring. The finding that perceived uplifts are largely independent of objective stressors suggests that uplifts are rooted in other aspects of the carer/care recipient relationship, or related to the carer's personality or motivation (Pinquart and Sörensen 2003). More longitudinal research is needed to explore how meanings, motivations, and relationship quality change over the caregiving career (Quinn et al. 2012), and to determine whether interventions for carers are more successful if they take into account carers' differing motivations for providing care.

As described in Chapter 2, led by Belgium and Japan, initiatives to create "dementia-friendly communities" are being established throughout the UK and internationally. Time will tell whether these can counteract the ageism that makes life difficult for people affected by dementia. Similarly, we will learn to what extent there is a will to support positive risk-taking within risk-averse and litigious societies.

Conclusion

The purpose of this chapter was to explore the experiences of people living at home with dementia and those of their family carers. People with dementia are a diverse group, and responses to the dementia diagnosis range widely from a "fighting spirit" to helplessness or denial. Carer reactions are similarly diverse. Living with dementia makes demands on personal, social, and financial resources, and requires a flexibility of attitude and approach. It is often necessary to find a balance or compromise between two opposing ideals, for example maintaining personhood and ensuring safety. Although many approaches to carer support have been trialled, it is clear that development work is still required for improving interventions for people with dementia and their families. People with dementia themselves are actively shaping attitudes towards living with dementia.

Further information

There are web sites designed for people with dementia on the Alzheimer Scotland Action on Dementia web site [http://www.alzscot.org/].

The Alzheimer's Society web pages [http://www.alzheimers.org.uk/] provide direct information to both people with dementia and their carers, including the *Living with Dementia* magazine.

The Dementia Advocacy and Support Network is a worldwide organization for mutual self-help for people with a diagnosis of dementia [http://www.dasninternational.org/].

Carers UK – The Voice of Carers is a web site for carers in the UK [http://www.carersuk.org/]. It includes a range of topics from crime and education to living environment to tax questions and travel. The site is not exclusive to dementia, but more generally addresses disability.

Many countries have non-government dementia care organizations that serve as resources and advocates for people with dementia and their carers.

There are also organizations established primarily to support informal carers, such as the National Family Caregivers Association in the USA.

The Rosalynn Carter Institute for Caregiving has a searchable online database of evidence-based caregiver interventions, including descriptions of study findings and available materials.

References

Andren, S. and Elmstahl, S. (2005) Family caregivers' subjective experiences of satisfaction in dementia care: aspects of burden, subjective health and sense of coherence, *Scandinavian Journal of Caring Sciences*, 19: 157–68.

Aneshensel, C.S., Pearlin, L.I., Mullan, J.T., Zarit, S.H. and Whitlatch, C.J. (1995) *Profiles in Caregiving: The Unexpected Career*. London: Academic Press.

Banerjee, S., Murray, J., Foley, B., Atkins, L., Schneider, J. *et al.* (2003) Predictors of institutionalization in people with dementia, *Journal of Neurology, Neurosurgery and Psychiatry*, 74(9): 1315–16.

Belle, S.H., Burgio, L., Burns, R., Coon, D., Czaja, S.J. *et al.* (2006) Enhancing the quality of life of dementia caregivers from different ethnic or racial groups, *Annals of Internal Medicine*, 145: 727–38.

Brodaty, H., Green, A. and Koschera, A. (2003) Meta-analysis of psychosocial interventions for caregivers of people with dementia, *Journal of the American Geriatrics Society*, 51: 657–64.

Brodaty, H., Thompson, C. and Thompson, M.F. (2005) Why caregivers of people with dementia and memory loss don't use services, *International Journal of Geriatric Psychiatry*, 20: 537–46.

Bunn, F., Goodman, C., Sworn, K., Rait, G., Brayne, C. *et al.* (2012) Psychosocial factors that shape patient and carer experiences of dementia diagnosis and treatment: a systematic review of qualitative studies, *PLoS Medicine*, 9 (10): e1001331.

Charlesworth, G., Shepstone, L., Wilson, E., Reynolds, S., Mugford, M. *et al.* (2008) Befriending carers of people with dementia: randomised controlled trial, *British Medical Journal*, 336(7656): 1295–7.

Clare, L., Wilson, B.A., Carter, G., Roth, I. and Hodges, J. (2004) Awareness in early-stage Alzheimer's disease: relationship to outcome of cognitive rehabilitation, *Journal of Clinical and Experimental Neuropsychology*, 26: 215–26.

Cohen, C.A., Colantonio, A. and Vernich, L. (2002) Positive aspects of caregiving: rounding out the caregiver experience, *International Journal of Geriatric Psychiatry*, 17: 184–8.

Drentea, P., Clay, O.J., Roth, D.L. and Mittelman, M.S. (2006) Predictors of improvement in social support: five-year effects of a structured intervention for caregivers of spouses with Alzheimer's disease, *Social Science and Medicine*, 63: 957–67.

Greenwood, N., Habibi, R., Mackenzie, A., Drennan, V. and Easton, N. (2013) Peer support for carers: a qualitative investigation of the experiences of carers and peer volunteers, *American Journal of Alzheimer's Disease and Other Dementias*, 28(6): 617–26.

Kerr, B., Cunningham, C. and Martin, S. (2010) *Telecare and Dementia: Using Telecare Effectively in the Support of People with Dementia*. Stirling: Dementia Services Development Centre, University of Stirling.

Marriott, A., Donaldson, C., Tarrier, N. and Burns, A. (2000) Effectiveness of cognitive behavioural family intervention in reducing the burden of care in carers of patients with Alzheimer's disease, *British Journal of Psychiatry*, 176: 557–62.

McWalter, G., Toner, H., McWalter, A., Eastwood, J., Marshall, M. *et al.* (1998) A community needs assessment: the Care Needs Assessment pack for dementia (CareNap-D) – its development, reliability and validity, *International Journal of Geriatric Psychiatry*, 13(1): 16–22.

Meaney, A.M., Croke, M. and Kirby, M. (2005) Needs assessment in dementia, *International Journal of Geriatric Psychiatry*, 20: 322–9.

Miranda-Castillo, C., Woods, B. and Orrell, M. (2010) People with dementia living alone: what are their needs and what kind of support are they receiving?, *International Psychogeriatrics*, 22(4): 607–17.

Motel-Klingebiel, A., Tesch-Roemer, C. and von Kondratowitz, H.-J. (2005) Welfare states do not crowd out the family: evidence for mixed responsibility from comparative analysis, *Ageing and Society*, 25: 863–82.

National Collaborating Centre for Mental Health (NCCMH) (2007) *Dementia: The NICE-SCIE Guideline on Supporting People with Dementia and their Carers in Health and Social Care*. National Clinical Practice Guideline 42. London: British Psychological Society and Royal College of Psychiatrists.

Nijhof, N., van Germert-Pijnen, L., Woolrych, R. and Sixsmith, A. (2013) An evaluation of preventive sensor technology for dementia care, *Journal of Telemedicine and Telecare*, 19: 95–100.

Orrell, M. and Hancock, G. (2004) *CANE: Camberwell Assessment of Need for the Elderly*. London: Gaskell.

Personal Social Services Research Unit (PSSRU) at the London School of Economics and the Institute of Psychiatry at King's College London (2007) *Dementia UK: The Full Report: A Report into the Prevalence and Cost of Dementia*. London: Alzheimer's Society.

Pinquart, M. and Sörensen, S. (2003) Associations of stressors and uplifts of caregiving with caregiver burden and depressive mood: a meta-analysis, *Journals of Gerontology B: Psychological Sciences and Social Sciences*, 58 (2): 112–28.

Quinn, C., Clare, L. and Woods, R.T. (2010) The impact of motivations and meanings on the wellbeing of caregivers of people with dementia: a systematic review, *International Psychogeriatrics*, 22(1): 43–55.

Quinn, C., Clare, L. and Woods, R.T. (2012) What predicts whether caregivers of people with dementia find meaning in their role?, *International Journal of Geriatric Psychiatry*, 27: 1195–1202.

Roff, L.L., Burgio, L.D., Gitlin, L., Nichols, L., Chaplin, W. *et al.* (2004) Positive aspects of Alzheimer's caregiving: the role of race, *Journals of Gerontology B: Psychological Sciences and Social Sciences*, 59 (4): 185–90.

Roth, D.L., Mittelman, M.S., Clay, O.J., Madan, A. and Haley, W.E. (2005) Changes in social support as mediators of the impact of a psychosocial intervention for spouse caregivers of persons with Alzheimer's disease, *Psychology and Aging*, 20(4): 634–44.

Smits, C.H.M., de Lange, J., Droes, R.-M., Meiland, F., Vernooij-Dassen, M. *et al.* (2007) Effects of combined intervention programmes for people with dementia living at home and their caregivers: a systematic review, *International Journal of Geriatric Psychiatry*, 22: 1181–93.

Triantafillou, J. and Mestheneos, E. on behalf of the EUROFAMCARE Group (2006) *Summary of Main Findings from EUROFAMCARE*. Hamburg [www.uke.uni-hamburg.de/eurofamcare].

von Kutzleben, M., Schmid, W., Halek, M., Holle, B. and Bartholomeyczik, S. (2012) Community-dwelling persons with dementia: What do they need? What do they demand? What do they do? A systematic review on the subjective experiences of persons with dementia, *Aging and Mental Health*, 16(3): 378–90.

Wenger, G.C. (1991) A network typology: from theory to practice, *Journal of Aging Studies*, 5 (2): 147–62.

World Health Organization (WHO) (2012) *Dementia: A Public Health Priority*. Geneva: WHO and Alzheimer's Disease International.

CHAPTER 22

Acute care of people with dementia in the general hospital

Michael L. Malone

> ❝Three days later on Friday she was told that she could go home. I travelled down on the Saturday and found her dressed and ready to go home. She was walking with a zimmer frame and had not had an assessment as promised. I spoke to the nurse in charge and asked if she was able to go up and down stairs; she had not been assessed. And there had been no follow up of her raised blood glucose.❞

—Julia Clayton-Stead Kent, UK

> ❝When I asked for my mother to be discharged from hospital it was because I thought that she was close to dying. Her personal needs had not been met in hospital, I had been by her bedside as many hours in a day that I could since her falling in the assessment unit and breaking her hip. She had had a hip replacement and been transferred back to our local hospital. She needed 24/7 care in hospital because she didn't realise about her hip and couldn't request the toilet or feed herself. I would arrive at the hospital to have other patients complaining about her, telling me tales of how she had climbed over the cot sides and fallen. I would find the bed clothes disheveled and her lying exposing herself to the other patients on the ward. It was appalling. I wanted her home to die with dignity and respect surrounded by her family who loved her.❞

—Sue Tucker Yorkshire, UK

Learning objectives

By the end of this chapter, you will:

- Be aware of the prevalence of dementia in the general hospital
- Understand why it is important that dementia is identified early in the hospital admission
- Describe steps to prevent deterioration in health of people with dementia in hospital
- Identify strategies to improve the quality of life and safety of people with dementia in hospital settings

Introduction

People with dementia are admitted to hospitals for many reasons. High-quality care in hospitals and preparing for the transition back home requires a comprehensive and informed approach.

Excellent care in hospital for people with dementia balances thorough clinical assessment and treatment of the medical condition with attending to quality of life and maintaining cognitive and functional ability. This careful and sensitive management requires specialized knowledge about dementia as a bio-psycho-social condition (see Chapter 8), knowing how to communicate with people who have dementia (see Chapter 17), and inclusion of patients in decisions about their care (see Chapter 28). Failure to recognize that the person has dementia decreases the likelihood that the individual will receive this level of specialist attention and care.

While patients with dementia face many risks as a consequence of hospitalization, hospital admission can also provide an important opportunity to diagnose previously undiagnosed illnesses, to discuss treatment, and to establish a support structure for the person and their family. If the admission reflects a breakdown in care arrangements, a hospital stay presents an opportunity to review and create a plan to proactively address both the person's and their family's needs (see Chapters 12, 13, 20, and 21).

This chapter describes the prevalence of dementia in general hospitals; the reasons people with dementia are admitted to the hospital; risks to people with dementia in hospital, with a particular focus on delirium and extended length of stay; strategies for optimizing outcomes, including quality of life; and models that can improve the care of acutely ill individuals with dementia.

Prevalence of dementia in hospitalized older patients

Estimates from the UK and the USA suggest older patients with dementia comprise between 4% and 25% of older people in a typical general hospital (Lyketsos et al. 2000; Pearson et al. 2012; Russ et al. 2012). The biggest challenge in acute care practice is to recognize older people with cognitive impairment and to determine how the person's cognition compares to their baseline. The person's medical history should be obtained both directly from people with cognitive impairment themselves and their family carers. Best practice strategies incorporate the assessment of cognition using standardized tests (such as The Mini-Cog™: see http://www.alz.org/documents_custom/minicog.pdf) into routine evaluation of older patients.

Research has shown that dementia is often missed in older people admitted to the general hospital (Ardern et al. 1993; Harwood et al. 1997). One study documented that dementia was unrecognized half of the time. In some cases, it is unrecognized because the diagnosis has not been made, while in other cases it is known but not recorded on admission. Some hospitalized older persons have very early signs of cognitive impairment, while others may have advanced dementia (Sparks 2008). Those with early dementia may have subtle cognitive changes that are difficult to detect. Others with advanced dementia may present with pneumonia, swallowing difficulties or eating problems. These difficulties are often not recognized as end-of-life complications of dementia (Mitchell et al. 2009). Furthermore, the presence of delirium superimposed on dementia makes the cognitive assessment still more challenging (Fick et al. 2002; Fong et al. 2012).

The high rate of cognitive impairment, the possibility that cognitive impairment will affect the patient's ability to contribute accurately to their medical history, and the risk of poor outcomes from complications during hospital care make a compelling case for careful assessment of cognition of acutely ill older persons.

Box 22.1: Assessing risk for dementia

In England, the Department of Health's Commissioning for Quality and Innovation (CQUIN) rewards hospitals that offer dementia risk assessments to all over-75s admitted. As of May 2013, this had led to over 4000 people a month being referred for further investigation, such as to a memory service. This was highlighted in the Prime Minister's update on progress against his *Challenge on Dementia*. For more information, see http://dementiachallenge.dh.gov.uk/2013/05/15/progress-in-health-and-care/.

Reasons for admission to hospital

Patients with dementia are admitted to hospital for the same reasons that people without dementia are admitted, most of which are unrelated to the dementia. A large prospective study of 686 community-dwelling older persons with mild to moderate Alzheimer's disease noted the most common reasons for hospitalization were falls, fractures, and cardiovascular disorders. Eighteen per cent of people with Alzheimer's disease were hospitalized in the 21-month study period. The authors commented that the major causes of hospitalization were not direct consequences of the disease itself (Voisin *et al.* 2009).

Some older people with cognitive impairment are brought to the hospital for "safe harbour". This means that the hospital serves as a site of assessment and care for vulnerable older persons with complex bio-psycho-social needs. Examples of vulnerabilities of older people with cognitive impairment include safeguarding issues, elder abuse and neglect, self-neglect, medication non-adherence, emotional distress, behaviours that challenge, and carer stress and breakdown. In these situations, cognitive impairment is intertwined with clusters of medical, psychiatric, psychological, emotional, social, and medication needs that require attention. Focusing exclusively on the medical aspects of care is not sufficient (McCullough 2008).

While many hospitalizations are unavoidable, the availability, accessibility, and quality of primary care in the community are important determinants of hospital admissions (Hutt *et al.* 2004). This is particularly important for people with dementia. A home-based nurse practitioner and a social worker collaborating with a primary care physician may decrease emergency department visits and hospitalization among high-risk patients (Counsell *et al.* 2007). Reducing avoidable hospital admissions from care homes is receiving increasing attention (see Chapter 24).

Risks to people with dementia in hospitals

The general hospital may present a hostile and disorienting environment for the person with dementia. Older people with dementia may be particularly vulnerable to environmental changes. They may behave in ways that are difficult for staff working in a busy "acute" ward (see Chapter 6), thus requiring more nursing staff time than other patients (Erkinjuntti *et al.* 1988; Fulmer *et al.* 2001).

People with dementia are at greater risk of a cascade of unintended events during their care (Marengoni *et al.* 2011). Complications are related to:

- deterioration in both cognitive and physical functioning (Covinsky *et al.* 2011)
- psychological and emotional distress related to having unmet needs

- difficulty adjusting to, and making sense of, a change in environment
- failure of staff to recognize and address these needs (see Chapter 17)

Dementia is a risk factor for delirium, falls, use of restraints, and non-adherence with therapy (Lyons and Landefeld 2010). These complications can lead to prolonged hospital stays, increasing the likelihood of further complications, increasing the likelihood of requiring institutional care on discharge, and greatly diminishing the person's quality of life.

There is increasing evidence to suggest a higher post-discharge morbidity and mortality among people with dementia (Inouye et al. 1998; Holmes and House 2000; Lyketsos et al. 2000). One study documented a two-fold increase in death following hospitalization for hip fracture in patients with dementia compared with similar patients without dementia (Holmes and House 2000). Another study of 207 consecutive people admitted to general medicine wards of a university teaching hospital found that impairment in instrumental activities of daily living, cognitive impairment (a Mini Mental State Examination score of ≤ 20), and depressive symptoms were strongly predictive of 90-day and 2-year mortality (Inouye et al. 1998). Furthermore, another large, prospective cohort study of patients with Alzheimer's disease found that hospitalization itself was associated with a substantial increase in the risk for death and institutionalization.

A thorough history on admission increases recognition of dementia in persons previously undiagnosed and ensures an understanding of their needs early in the hospital course (Pearson et al. 2012). Listening to the concerns of caregivers may reveal cognitive problems preceding the admission that can be used to clarify the diagnosis. Assessing the patient's home situation is important. The hospital team of providers must understand the patient's former and current functional and cognitive status to assess the impact of the acute illness. Determining the patient's adherence to medications is a key component of the history. Similarly, determining if advance care planning documents are available is important. As mentioned, people with cognitive impairment who were functioning well in a familiar home environment may become profoundly disorientated within a general hospital setting. Box 22.2 outlines vulnerabilities that must be addressed to avoid agitation or distress among hospitalized patients with dementia.

Box 22.2: Factors that may contribute to emotional distress among hospitalized patients with dementia

Physical environment

- disorientation due to lack of familiarity and signage
- devices such as intravenous lines, urinary catheter, and sequential compression devices
- transfers from one nursing unit to another
- noise, bright lights, and other disturbances

Physical health, functional and communication impairments

- difficulty expressing pain
- poor food or fluid intake, related to apraxia
- constipation, urinary retention, skin irritation
- sensory deficits (hearing and vision)

Social environment

- being administered medications by unfamiliar nursing staff
- inconsistency of staff

(continued)

- poor communication among professional staff
- isolation or infrequent interaction with staff or family
- complex instructions
- lack of advance directives and lack of discussion of the patient's goals of care

Mental health

- cognitive deterioration
- depression, anxiety, loneliness
- inattention to the context of the patient's cognitive needs when formulating a care plan

Delirium

Another major risk for patients with dementia in hospital is the development of delirium (Inouye *et al.* 1993). The key clinical features of delirium are recent onset of fluctuating awareness, impairment of memory and of attention, and disorganized thinking as noted in Box 22.3 (Young and Inouye 2007). Additional features of delirium may include hallucinations and a disturbance of the sleep–wake cycle. People may have subtle features that are difficult to detect: restlessness or wandering, lack of interest, impaired ability to follow conversations, sleepiness, a poor ability to follow instructions, or a poor ability to participate in self-care.

Box 22.3: Criteria for delirium (according to the *Diagnostic and Statistical Manual of Mental Disorders*, DSM IV)

- Disturbance of consciousness with reduced ability to focus, sustain, or shift attention
- Changed cognition or the development of a perceptual disturbance
- Disturbance develops in a short period of time and fluctuates over the course of the day
- History, physical examination, and laboratory findings show that delirium can be a physiological consequence of general condition, caused by intoxication, caused by medication, or caused by more than one aetiology

---

Patients who are admitted to a hospital with symptoms of dementia may indeed have dementia or they may have delirium. The diagnosis of delirium is accomplished by using the Confusion Assessment Method (CAM), as noted in Box 22.4 (Inouye *et al.* 1990; Inouye 2003). Brief standardized cognitive testing is recommended for scoring.

Box 22.4: Confusion Assessment Method

The diagnosis of delirium requires a present or abnormal rating for criteria 1 and 2 plus either 3 or 4.

1. *Acute onset and fluctuating course*: Is there evidence of an acute change in mental status from the patient's baseline? Did this behaviour fluctuate during the past day – that is, tend to come and go or increase and decrease in severity? (Usually requires information from a family member or caregiver.)

(continued)

2. *Inattention*: Does the patient have difficulty focusing attention? For example, are they easily distracted or do they have difficulty keeping track of what is being said? (Inattention can be detected by the digit span test or asking for the days of the week to be recited backwards.)

3. *Disorganized thinking*: Is the patient's speech disorganized or incoherent, such as rambling or irrelevant conversation, unclear or illogical flow of ideas, unpredictable switching between subjects? (Disorganized thinking and sleepiness can also be detected during conversation with the patient.)

4. *Altered level of consciousness*: Overall, would you rate this patient's level of consciousness as alert (normal), vigilant (hyper-alert), lethargic (drowsy, easily aroused), stupor (difficult to arouse) or coma (cannot be roused)? All ratings except alert are scored as abnormal.

Distinguishing between delirium and dementia is difficult but important, as management depends on the underlying cause. Given the potential for poor prognosis if not treated, it is important that signs of delirium are identified early and appropriate care is provided.

Preventing delirium will decrease the need for reactive approaches, for example, the use of sedative medications, which often result in adverse events such as falls and further deterioration of cognitive function (Inouye et al. 1999, 2003). Patients with delirium may be emotionally and behaviourally distressed and staff may find this difficult on an acute medical ward. Once the underlying factors are identified and addressed, distress can be addressed with frequent contact with, and comfort from, staff and family. Providing the person with a well-lit room and with cues to help orientation will also be helpful.

Additional interventions to evaluate and treat delirium of an older patient include:

■ careful review of all medications with consideration to reduce psychoactive medications
■ continuity of location and staff (avoidance of an unnecessary move)
■ provide orientation to the environment, with the use of clocks and calendars
■ a calm and comfortable environment with familiar objects from home
■ explanation of interventions, and regular reorienting communication
■ eye glasses and hearing aids used (switched on)
■ identification and treatment of needs, e.g. pain, thirst or the need for the toilet
■ reassurance from and support for family
■ careful attention to hydration and nutrition
■ help with mobility
■ skin care to prevent pressure ulcers
■ monitoring of bowel and bladder function
■ keeping tasks simple and avoiding multiple stimuli

Delirium is a direct consequence of multi-factorial physical causes such as a medical condition, drug withdrawal or intoxication, and may be evident on or arise during admission. Dementia is the biggest single risk factor for delirium, a condition that significantly increases morbidity and mortality (Francis et al. 1990; Pompei et al. 1994; Elie et al. 1998; Inouye et al. 1999). Non-detection of delirium in the emergency department has also been associated with an increased six-month mortality rate (Kakuma et al. 2003). A prospective study of older patients undergoing cardiac surgery noted that post-operative development of delirium was a risk factor for a decline in cognitive function, as well as a prolonged period of cognitive impairment during the first year after surgery (Saczynski et al. 2012).

Overall, delirium is common among older hospitalized patients (Francis *et al.* 1990). Investigators have noted an increased risk of developing delirium among a cohort of older patients admitted to a university teaching hospital with vision impairment, severe illness, cognitive impairment, and a high blood urea nitrogen to creatinine ratio. Those patients who had more risk factors at admission to the hospital were more likely to develop delirium (Francis *et al.* 1990; Inouye *et al.* 1993).

Delirium among hospitalized patients with Alzheimer's disease is associated with an increased risk of institutionalization and of death, compared with older, community-dwelling persons with Alzheimer's (Fong *et al.* 2012). Other investigators have studied a cohort of older adults noting that there was an association between critical illness and neurocognitive impairment. Thus, there is a link between hospitalization for acute illness or critical illness and cognitive decline and dementia in older persons (Ehlenbach *et al.* 2010; Fong *et al.* 2012). Given the potential for poor prognosis if not treated, it is important that signs of delirium are identified early and appropriate care is provided.

Length of stay

Patients with dementia account for a large proportion of long-stay patients. Reasons for this include inadequate social support, lack of placement options, co-morbid psychiatric illness, co-existing medical illness, reduced activities of daily living skills, and higher incidence of complications (Erkinjuntti *et al.* 1988; Holmes and House 2000; King *et al.* 2006; Silverstein and Maslow 2006).

Several studies have shown that dementia is an independent risk factor for increased length of stay in hospital (Erkinjuntti *et al.* 1988; Holmes and House 2000; King *et al.* 2006). Patients with dementia living independently prior to admission are less likely than people without dementia to return to independent living on discharge from hospital (MacNeill and Lichtenberg 1997). Unfortunately, a longer stay in hospital may result in a decline in the ability to perform self-care and may reduce further the person's ability to return home.

Intensive rehabilitation may reduce the length of stay as shown in patients with mild to moderate dementia following a hip fracture and promote a successful return to independent living (Huusko *et al.* 2000). Applying a "social model" of care that consists of an intensive effort to identify dementia and to begin working on discharge soon after admission, may also help in reducing complications and length of admission (Lyketsos *et al.* 2000).

Optimizing outcomes for people with dementia

People with dementia have an entire spectrum of needs while in the acute care setting. Therefore, it is important that staff proactively ensure that the full spectrum of needs are met, taking care to provide person-centred care. Good hospital care includes:

- careful assessment of the medical conditions that caused the acute illness
- thoughtful review of existing medications and the need for new medications
- proper assessment of the patient's baseline and current function and cognition
- a discussion of the patient's goals of care

The complete recovery of the acutely ill older person does not occur in the hospital. Communication of the plan of care to the next site is essential to ensure optimal outcomes for the patient.

Optimizing outcomes requires attention to the following:

- nursing patients with delirium
- early discharge planning
- involving patients in decision-making
- optimizing the physical environment

Nursing patients with delirium

Given that the risk of developing delirium increases in the presence of the multiple risk factors, it would follow that good clinical practice will seek to identify and modify these risk factors wherever possible (Potter and George 2006). Experts recommend systematic case-finding of delirium in high-risk patients (Marcantonio 2012). Once delirium occurs, the main management strategy is to address all contributing factors, provide supportive care, prevent complications, and treat behavioural aspects (Inouye 2006).

Early discharge planning

Discharge planning starts on admission to the hospital. This allows time to identify difficulties the patient may have been experiencing before admission. Important information should be collected about the patient's current level of functioning. History should be gathered from the patient, relatives, caregivers, primary care physicians, and other professionals involved in the community. As noted in Box 22.5, a careful assessment of the individual's needs, and their caregiver's needs, and the available community services can facilitate a timely discharge.

Box 22.5: Information required for effective discharge planning for a hospitalized older patient with dementia

Patients' goals and wishes	Food provision and preparation
Family input concerning goals and wishes	Current housing situation
Current social contacts and supports	Sleep habits
Current level/types of care/community services	Mobility
Medications – organization and adherence	Finances
Personal care needs and home safety	Weekly structure and social outlets
Potential for getting lost when going out	Vulnerability and risk of exploitation

---

Obstacles may be overcome with the implementation of simple strategies that include: rationalization of medication to simpler regimes; increased social engagement and participation; increased home care; day-centre attendance; and meals-on-wheels. Interdisciplinary teams are the most effective way to achieve this.

Case example 22.1: Mr. D – preventing hospital-related decline

Mr. D is an 81-year-old man who lives alone and has no known history of cognitive impairment. He receives help from his granddaughter, for eight hours per day. He comes to the emergency department of his local hospital having being found on the floor after a fall at his home. He is admitted because he is unsteady on his feet and dehydrated. His initial Mini-Cog shows a poor short-term memory, but otherwise is normal. His initial Confusion Assessment Method (CAM) assessment is normal. On the first night in the hospital he becomes very restless, repeatedly leaving his bed and protesting that he is being held against his will. His repeat CAM shows that he now has difficulty shifting and sustaining his attention. In addition, it shows evidence of his having developed disorganized thinking. Before leaving for home, his visiting granddaughter describes that she has not seen Mr. D like this before. When staff try to guide him back to his bed, he starts shouting for help.

- What factors may be contributing to Mr. D's confusion? Consider both individual and environmental factors.
- What might be done to remedy the underlying causes and relieve Mr. D's distress?

In the case example above, Mr. D has been exposed to at least two unfamiliar environments and a series of unfamiliar people in his first 24 hours. The ward activity and noise may be confusing and frightening. These may cause him to be restless as he seeks to understand what is happening and where he is. In Mr. D's case, a urinary tract infection for which he is commencing treatment may be one underlying factor for his acute confusion. A diagnosis of delirium should be considered. An assessment for urinary retention and fecal impaction would also be in order.

Involving patients in decision-making

The patient should be central to decision-making. In a busy ward environment, decisions may be made without taking the time to involve the patient. Conflicts between patient and hospital staff may arise in the context of admission, treatment or in planning discharge. In 2012, the American Geriatrics Society released a patient-centred approach to the care of older adults with multiple chronic conditions. This resource helps clinicians to consider patient preferences in their care decisions. A full discussion regarding how to involve the person in decision-making can be found in Chapter 28, while the values for care people with dementia hold are discussed in Chapter 12.

Case example 22.2: Mr. D (continued) – thinking about options for the future

Mr. D has been rehydrated, has recovered from his fall, and is more settled on the ward. He remains disoriented to time and place, and history from his granddaughter suggests that he has had a gradual decline in memory over the last two years. She is concerned that he is unable to look after himself at home and needs to be discharged to a more supportive accommodation. He has not been eating properly and gets muddled with the days of the week. He has a social life that is unstructured and he sometimes forgets what he was supposed to be doing that day. On one occasion he left the house at 3 a.m. thinking it was the afternoon. On cognitive testing, he

(continued)

scores 20/30 on the Mini Mental State Examination (MMSE). Computerized tomography shows microvascular changes and he is on appropriate medication to minimize risk factors for further vascular change. Mr. D is adamant that he wants to return home because he loves his garden and his friends who live nearby.

- What factors should be considered in assessing his ability to cope at home?
- Should Mr. D make his own decisions about where he lives?
- In the event of him lacking capacity to make these decisions, how would you determine what to do next?
- How might you enable him to be discharged home?

A thorough history should be taken and further exploration of his granddaughter's concerns should be made. Objective assessment by nursing staff, occupational therapists, and physiotherapists would offer further clarification of his level of function. Some hospitals allow a trial of self-medication to assess a patient's ability to manage their own treatment routine. Ascertain what level of support he has had in his own home prior to admission. This enables you to paint a picture of how he was coping and to test his level of understanding when you assess him.

In the case example above, services may be put in place to enable Mr. D to be discharged home. These may include home care to assist with activities of daily living and to provide structure to his week. He may require help with shopping and cooking or need meals delivered. A pill box may help with medication adherence. If he is unable to manage his financial affairs, legal advice should be sought. Very close involvement of the family or supportive friends will be required.

Creating dementia-friendly hospitals

Box 22.6: Dementia-friendly hospitals

In England, there is an initiative to create dementia-friendly hospitals. Since November 2012, over 70% of acute trusts have committed to becoming dementia friendly, working in partnership with their local Dementia Action Alliance. As part of this initiative, there is a focus on how the ward environments have been designed to support the needs of patients with dementia. For example, the Bradford Teaching Hospitals NHS Foundation Trust has made a public commitment to become a dementia-friendly hospital by working with patients and their family carers to improve the quality of care and the nature of the experience for patients with dementia and their carers. This initiative includes improving way-finding and orientation, as well as development of outside environments. The Trust has recently been awarded "Improving the environment of care for people with dementia" capital funding.

Models of care

Over the last several decades, innovative models of care have been created to improve hospital care for older people. The three main types of specialist geriatric services for acute care of older people, found in several countries, are:

- specialist geriatric wards
- specialists in geriatric medicine working with physicians on a ward
- admission to wards based on complexity or frailty (Metz and Labrooy 2005)

In the UK, these approaches are derived from the multidisciplinary models first described in the 1940s (Parker 2005). In the USA, nurses have been used as acute care specialists for geriatric patients. Specialty nurses with advanced skills and knowledge initiate clinical protocols and follow patients throughout their hospital stay and after discharge. Their roles often interface with specialized units similar to those in the UK, such as the Acute Care for Elders (ACE) unit and Geriatric Evaluation and Management (GEM) unit. Founded in the 1990s, Nurses Improving Care for Health System Elders (NICHE) offers a range of resources for both individual nurses and hospitals to develop, use, and evaluate best practice care (Boltz *et al.* 2008). Some models of care have been integrated into the electronic health record, resulting in an improved ability to identify vulnerable elders and to prevent complications (Malone *et al.* 2010). In Australia, dementia clinical nurse consultants were created to provide expert advice, education, and support to families and staff on acute care wards of hospitals.

In the UK, service models such as Proactive care of Older People undergoing Surgery (POPS) and Older Persons' Assessment and Liaison team (OPAL), created by geriatricians, use the comprehensive geriatric assessment (CGA) approach to screen older people admitted under the care of acute surgical (Harari *et al.* 2007a) and medical teams (Harari *et al.* 2007b), respectively. The OPAL team (consisting of a nurse, a senior physiotherapist, and a geriatrician) screens all acute medical patients over 70 years of age within 24 hours of admission in a pre-admission unit and facilitates a plan of care for these patients. Early assessment by the OPAL team identifies those patients who require intensive geriatric care, leading to improved care and decreased length of stay (Harari *et al.* 2007b).

Models of specialist psychiatric care

Psychiatric services play an important role in caring for people with dementia. They assist with diagnosis and management and they offer advice on placement options. Brindle and Holmes (2005) described the roles that psychiatric services play in assessing capacity: education of other professionals; provision of specialist input in more complex cases; and provision of information on the range of services available to support older people with dementia so that options may be fully understood.

Models of psychiatric care for patients with dementia in the general hospital involve varying degrees of integration between acute and mental health staff (Royal College of Psychiatrists 2005). One promising model uses a liaison mental health nurse, which enables a rapid response and ongoing input when a patient needs follow-up of their mental health problems during admission. The role of a liaison mental health nurse covers several domains: expert practice, professional leadership, education, and practice and service development. In the clinical settings, the liaison nurse focuses on practical and care-oriented interventions.

In Australia, the impact of the consultation-liaison nursing role demonstrates improved access to specialist mental health care and expert assistance to staff (Sharrock *et al.* 2006). Liaison psychiatric nurses and psychiatrists also improve effectiveness of care and facilitate appropriate discharge options.

The liaison multidisciplinary team brings expertise from occupational therapy, social work, and medical and nursing input. This allows all aspects of a patient's care to be addressed within one team. The liaison model promotes more referrals and improved diagnostic accuracy compared with the consultation or reactive models (Swanwick *et al.* 1993).

Case example 22.3: Mr. D (continued) – a turn for the worse

Mr. D developed pneumonia, prolonging his stay in hospital. He has become withdrawn and has stopped drinking liquids. He has told staff that he does not feel like eating or watching the television.

- What do you think is the problem?
- How would you proceed?

Possible diagnoses include delirium, further deterioration in cognitive function secondary to prolonged admission or recent infection. He also presents with reduced appetite and has stopped doing an activity that he previously enjoyed. This may be due to a loss of interest, an inability to concentrate or sensory impairment. Some of these symptoms may be indicative of a depressive episode. Depression is prevalent among older hospital inpatients and, in combination with cognitive impairment, further increases the length of stay.

The medical team should carefully assess Mr. D to identify and treat the underlying cause of any delirium. Nursing staff should monitor food and fluid intake, as Mr. D is at risk of dehydration and electrolyte disturbance.

International comparisons

It is difficult to compare the effectiveness of various specialist nurses and care models across the world, as there are marked differences in training curricula of nurses and doctors, health care costs, provision and systems, resources, culture, and practices. It is, however, a common global theme that the general hospital staff require enhanced skills and knowledge to look after the complex needs of older people with dementia. A recent report from the UK has recommended the initiation of an Older Person's Nurse specialist, noting the failure of nurses in some hospitals to understand the basics of care for older adults (Francis 2013). This report parallels the Institute of Medicine's recent findings that many health care providers are ill prepared to care for older adults.

Globally, there are an abundance of guidelines on best practice and government frameworks to improve the care of older people with dementia in a general hospital. The common themes are comprehensive assessment, appropriate skills, training, and attitudes, and person-centred care. These principles were not intended to be implemented in isolation (Young *et al.* 2003).

In the UK, the Royal College of Psychiatrists' document *Who Cares Wins* (2005) and the *National Service Framework: Older People* (Department of Health 2001) highlighted the importance of a skill mix necessary to meet the complex needs of older people. In Australia, the government initiative advocated care in the right place at the right time for people with dementia and has published the *National Framework for Action on Dementia 2006–2010* (NSW Department of Health 2006), which highlighted workforce training as one of its five key priorities. Box 22.7 outlines workforce competencies in caring for hospitalized patients with dementia.

Box 22.7: Knowledge and skills needed to work with patients who have dementia

- identifying symptoms and signs of dementia
- identifying delirium
- identifying depressive or psychotic symptoms
- understanding the trajectory of the illness
- providing cognitive stimulation
- providing person-centred communication and care
- understanding how to optimize care in older people
- understanding how to maintain fluid balance and prevent infection
- understanding how to communicate with someone who has dementia
- understanding how to manage the environment to prevent agitation
- understanding the judicious use of psychotropic medication
- being comfortable working in an interdisciplinary team
- participating in early discharge planning
- understanding how to assess risks of hospitalization for someone with dementia

---

Debates and controversies

There are several key debates and controversies related to acute care for people with dementia. Some relate to specific treatment decisions and others to the general organization of hospital care and services. For example, there is continuing debate over the most effective general approach to hospital care of people with dementia. Some suggest that the most effective approach is specialist units for older adults or people with dementia, while others suggest promoting a general "dementia-friendly" hospital environment. This has important implications for the design of training programmes, whether all hospital staff should be trained to care for people with dementia or whether it would be more effective to focus the development of expertise in designated units.

Increasingly, hospital caregivers and administrators are concerned about the development of delirium in hospitalized older people. While delirium affects many older people, not only those with dementia, the consequences are particularly serious for people with an underlying dementia. Many hospitals have adopted the development of delirium as a quality measure, and have developed training programmes for staff to promote prevention, early asessment, and early intervention with people showing signs of delirium.

Another ongoing debate is the use of feeding tubes in people with dementia. Increasingly, feeding tubes are not viewed as appropriate for people with advanced dementia, although there are some who disagree. The American Geriatrics Society has recently issued a recommendation for the use of oral assisted feeding rather than percutaneous feeding tubes in patients with advanced dementia.

Conclusion

Many hospitalized older people have dementia, but this may be missed as hospital staff focus their attention on other, more acute problems. Accurate diagnosis early in hospital admission is important, as it sets the course for appropriate intervention and discharge planning. People with dementia are at increased risk of developing complications and experiencing a prolonged hospital stay, often leading to long-term disability. In particular, failure to detect and manage delirium appropriately can lead to serious negative outcomes. Much is known about ways to decrease hospital risks for people with dementia, although widespread implementation of these risk-reduction processes has not yet been achieved.

Further information

The American Psychiatric Association provides guidance and identifies published research for psychiatrists on diagnosing and treating dementia [http://www.psych.org/].

The Mental Capacity Act 2005 (UK) includes discussion of dementia. It addresses decision-making capacity in people with dementia, including decisions made in acute care settings.

Bradford Teaching Hospitals' dementia-friendly hospital wards demonstrate ways to adapt the environment to better suit the needs of people with dementia and families [http://www. bradfordhospitals.nhs.uk/about-us/news-and-media/news-and-press-releases/bradford-teaching-hospitals2019-dementia-wards-win-national-award].

"This is me" is a simple and practical tool that people with dementia who are receiving professional care can use to tell staff about their needs, preferences, likes, dislikes, and interests. It can be downloaded from the Alzheimer's Society web site [http://alzheimers.org.uk/thisisme].

The Butterfly Scheme is an opt-in scheme offering appropriate care for people with dementia while in hospital. It is based on easy-to-learn, quickly delivered skills-based education for all staff who come into contact with patients [http://www.rcn.org.uk/development/practice/dementia/best_practice_examples/barbara_hodkinson].

References

American Geriatrics Society (2012) Patient-centered care for older adults with multiple chronic conditions: a stepwise approach from the American Geriatrics Society, *Journal of the American Geriatrics Society*, 56: 1–12.

Ardern, M., Mayou, R., Feldman, E. and Hawton, K. (1993) Cognitive impairment in the elderly medically ill: how often is it missed?, *International Journal of Geriatric Psychiatry*, 8: 929–37.

Boltz, M., Capezuti, E., Bower-Ferres, S., Norman, R., Secic, M. *et al.* (2008) Changes in the geriatric care environment associated with NICHE (Nurses Improving Care for HealthSystem Elders), *Geriatric Nursing*, 29(3): 176–85.

Brindle, N. and Holmes, J. (2005) Capacity and coercion: dilemmas in the discharge of older people with dementia from general hospital settings, *Age and Ageing*, 34: 16–20.

Counsell, S.R., Callahan, C.M., Clark, D.O., Tu, W., Buttar, A.B. *et al.* (2007) Geriatrics care management for low-income seniors: a randomized controlled trial, *Journal of the American Medical Association*, 298: 2623–33.

Covinsky, K.E., Pierluissi, E. and Johnston, B. (2011) Hospitalization-associated disability: "She was probably able to ambulate, but I'm not sure", *Journal of the American Medical Association*, 306: 1782–93.

Department of Health (2001) *National Service Framework: Older People*. London: Department of Health [https://www.gov.uk/government/uploads/system/uploads/attachment_data/file/198033/National_Service_Framework_for_Older_People.pdf, accessed March 2013].

Ehlenbach, W.J., Hough, C.L., Crane, P.K., Haneuse, S.J.P.A., Carson, S.S. et al. (2010) Association between acute care and critical illness hospitalization and cognitive function in older adults, *Journal of the American Medical Association*, 303: 763–70.

Elie, M., Cole, M.G., Primeau, F.J. and Bellavance, F. (1998) Delirium risk factors in elderly hospitalized patients, *Journal of General Internal Medicine*, 13: 204–12.

Erkinjuntti, T., Autio, L. and Wistrom, J. (1988) Dementia in medical wards, *Journal of Clinical Epidemiology*, 41: 123–6.

Fick, D.M., Agostini, J.V. and Inouye, S.K. (2002) Delirium superimposed on dementia: a systematic review, *Journal of the American Geriatrics Society*, 50: 1723–32.

Fong, T.G., Jones, R.N., Marcantonio, E.R., Tommet, D., Gross, A.L. et al. (2012) Adverse outcomes after hospitalization in persons with Alzheimer disease, *Annals of Internal Medicine*, 156: 848–56.

Francis, J., Martin, D. and Kapoor, W.N. (1990) A prospective study of delirium in hospitalised elderly, *Journal of the American Medical Association*, 263: 1097–101.

Francis, R. (2013) *Report of the Mid Staffordshire NHS Foundation Trust Public Inquiry*. London: The Stationery Office [https://www.gov.uk/government/publications/report-of-the-mid-staffordshire-nhs-foundation-trust-public-inquiry, accessed 29 April 2014].

Fulmer, T., Foreman, M., Walker, M. and Montgomery, K. (2001) *Critical Care Nursing of the Elderly*. New York: Springer.

Harari, D., Hooper, A., Dhesi, J., Babic-Illman, G., Lockwood, L. et al. (2007a) Proactive care of older people undergoing surgery ("POPS"): designing, embedding, evaluating and funding a comprehensive geriatric assessment service for older elective surgical patients, *Age and Ageing*, 36(2): 190–6.

Harari, D., Martin, F., Buttery, A., O'Neill, S. and Hopper, A. (2007b) The older persons' assessment and liaison team: evaluation of comprehensive geriatric assessment in acute medical inpatients, *Age and Ageing*, 36(6): 670–5.

Harwood, D.M.J., Hope, T. and Jacoby, R. (1997) Cognitive impairment in medical inpatients. II: Do physicians miss cognitive impairment?, *Age and Ageing*, 26: 37–9.

Holmes, J. and House, A. (2000) Psychiatric illness predicts poor outcome after hip fracture: a prospective cohort study, *Psychological Medicine*, 30: 921–9.

Hutt, R., Rosen, R. and McCauley, J. (2004) *Case-managing Long-term Conditions: What Impact does it have in the Treatment of Older People?* London: King's Fund [http://www.kingsfund.org.uk/pdf/casemanagment.pdf, accessed 25 March 2013].

Huusko, T.M., Karppi, P., Avikainen, V., Kautiainen, H. and Sulkava, R. (2000) Randomised, clinically controlled trial of intensive geriatric rehabilitation in patients with hip fracture: subgroup analysis of patients with dementia, *British Medical Journal*, 321(7269): 1107–11.

Inouye, S.K. (2003) *The Confusion Assessment Method (CAM): Training Manual and Coding Guide*. New Haven, CT: Yale University School of Medicine.

Inouye, S.K. (2006) Delirium in older persons, *New England Journal of Medicine*, 354: 1157–65.

Inouye, S.K., van Dyck, C.K., Alessi, C.K., (1990) Clarifying confusion: confusion assessment method, *Annals of Internal Medicine*, 113(12): 941–8.

Inouye, S.K., Viscoli, C.M., Horwitz, R.I., Hurst, L.D. and Tinetti, M.E. (1993) A predictive model for delirium in hospitalized elderly medical patients based on admission characteristics, *Annals of Internal Medicine*, 119: 474–81.

Inouye, S.K., Peduzzi, P.N., Robinson, J.T., Hughes, J.S., Horwitz, R.I. et al. (1998) Importance of functional measures in predicting mortality among older hospitalized patients, *Journal of the American Medical Association*, 279(15): 1187–93.

Inouye, S.K., Bogardus, S.T., Charpentier, P.A., Leo-Summers, L., Acampora, D. et al. (1999) A multicomponent intervention to prevent delirium in hospitalised older adults, *New England Journal of Medicine*, 340: 669–76.

Inouye, S.K., Bogardus, S., Vitagliano, G., Desai, M., Williams, C. et al. (2003) Burden of Illness Score for Elderly Persons: risk adjustment incorporating the cumulative impact of diseases, physiologic abnormalities, and functional impairments, *Medical Care*, 41(1): 70–83.

Kakuma, R., Galbaud du Fort, G., Arsenault, L., Perrault, A., Platt, R. et al. (2003) Delirium in older emergency department patients discharged home: effect on survival, *Journal of the American Geriatrics Society*, 51(4): 443–50.

King, B., Jones, C. and Brand, C. (2006) Relationship between dementia and length of stay of general medical patients admitted to acute care, *Australasian Journal on Ageing*, 25: 20–3.

Lyketsos, C.G., Sheppard, J.-M.E. and Rabins, P.V. (2000) Dementia in elderly persons in a general hospital, *American Journal of Psychiatry*, 157: 704–7.

Lyons, W.L. and Landefeld, C.S. (2010) Hospital care, in J.T. Pacala and G.M. Sullivan (eds.) *Geriatrics Review Syllabus: A Core Curriculum in Geriatric Medicine* (7th edn.). New York: American Geriatrics Society, pp. 134–44.

MacNeill, S. and Lichtenberg, P. (1997) Home alone: the role of cognition in return to independent living, *Archives of Physical Medicine and Rehabilitation*, 78: 755–8.

Malone, M.L., Vollbrecht, M., Stephenson, J., Burke, L., Pagel, P. *et al.* (2010) Acute Care for Elders (ACE) Tracker and e-Geriatrician: methods to disseminate ACE concepts to hospitals with no geriatricians on staff, *Journal of the American Geriatrics Society*, 58: 161–7.

Marcantonio, E.R. (2012) Postoperative delirium: a 76-year-old woman with delirium following surgery, *Journal of the American Medical Association*, 308(1): 73–81.

Marengoni, A., Corrao, S., Nobili, A., Tettamanti, M., Salerno, F. *et al.* (2011) In-hospital death according to dementia diagnosis in acutely ill elderly patients: the REPOSI study, *International Journal of Psychiatry*, 26(9): 930–6.

McCullough, D. (2008) *My Mother, Your Mother: Embracing "Slow Medicine". The Compassionate Approach to Caring for Your Aging Loved Ones*. New York: HarperCollins.

Metz, D.H. and Labrooy, S.J. (2005) The future of geriatric medicine in an era of patient choice, *Age and Ageing*, 34: 553–5.

Mitchell, S.L., Teno, L.M., Kiely, D.K., Shaffer, M.L., Jones, R.N. *et al.* (2009) The clinical course of advanced dementia, *New England Journal of Medicine*, 361: 1529–38.

New South Wales Department of Health (2006) *National Framework for Action on Dementia 2006–2010*. North Sydney, NSW: NSW Department of Health [http://www.health.gov.au/internet/wcms, accessed 29 March 2013].

Parker, S.G. (2005) *Do Current Discharge Arrangements from Inpatient Hospital Care for the Elderly Reduce Admission Rates, the Length of Inpatient Stay or Mortality, or Improve Health Status?* Health Evidence Network Report. Copenhagen: WHO Regional Office for Europe. [http://www.euro.who.int/Document/E87542.pdf, accessed March 29 2013].

Pearson, K., Jeffrey, D. and Rogers, D. (2012) *Delivering Dignity*. London: Commission on Dignity in Care, Local Government Association, NHS Confederation and Age UK.

Pompei, P., Foreman, M., Rudberg, M.A., Inouye, S.K., Braund, V. *et al.* (1994) Delirium in hospitalized older persons: outcomes and predictors, *Journal of the American Geriatrics Society*, 42: 809–15.

Potter, J. and George, J. (2006) The prevention, diagnosis and management of delirium in older people: concise guidelines, *Clinical Medicine*, 6 (3): 303–8.

Royal College of Psychiatrists (RCP) (2005) *Who Cares Wins: Improving the Outcome for Older People Admitted to the General Hospital*. Report of a Working Group for the Faculty of Old Age Psychiatry. London: RCP.

Russ, T.C., Shenkin, S.D., Reynish, E., Ryan, T., Anderson, D. *et al.* (2012) Dementia in acute hospital inpatients: the role of the geriatrician, *Age and Ageing*, 41(3): 282–4.

Saczynski, J.S., Marcantonio, E.R., Quach, L., Fong, T.G., Gross, A. *et al.* (2012) Cognitive trajectories after postoperative delirium, *New England Journal of Medicine*, 367: 30–9.

Sharrock, J., Grigg, M., Happell, B., Keeble-Devlin, B. and Jennings, S. (2006) The mental health nurse: a valuable addition to the consultation–liaison team, *International Journal of Mental Health Nursing*, 15: 35–43.

Silverstein, N. and Maslow, K. (eds.) (2006) *Improving Hospital Care for Persons with Dementia*. New York: Springer.

Sparks, M.B. (2008) Inpatient care for persons with Alzheimer's disease, *Alzheimer's Care Today*, 9(3): 204–10.

Swanwick, G.R.J., Lee, H., Clare, A.W. and Lawlor, B.A. (1993) Consultation–liaison psychiatry: a comparison of two service models for geriatric patients, *International Journal of Geriatric Psychiatry*, 9: 495–9.

Voisin, T., Sourdet, S., Cantet, C., Andrieu, S. and Vellas, B. (2009) Descriptive analysis of hospitalizations of patients with Alzheimer's disease: a two-year prospective study of 686 patients from the REAL.FR study, *Journal of Nutrition, Health and Aging*, 13(10): 890–2.

Young, J. and Inouye, S.K. (2007) Delirium in older people, *British Medical Journal*, 334 (7598): 842–6.

Young, J., Sturdy, D. and Bhattacharjee, G. (2003) *Approaches to Improving General Hospital Care of Older People*. London: Department of Health [http://www.dh.gov.uk, accessed 29 March 2012].

CHAPTER 23

The role of specialist housing in supporting older people with dementia

Simon Evans, Sarah Vallelly and Karen Croucher

> ❝In her case, her surroundings were incredibly important. Lovely art, lovely antiques. She cared deeply about her surroundings. As you progress it seems you lose the right to have the surroundings you choose. The apartments get smaller ... she was very aware that she was in a tiny little room. We were stunned, how tiny these rooms are. I would not want a postage stamp room ... give them space for; another chair, a place for their favorite books.
>
> The worst case, in a nursing home, you have to share the room with someone else. The idea of putting two people in the same room is, I just can't imagine that.. It's as if the builders of these places think these people are reverting back to their childhood. For Heaven's sake respect these people's humanity. They retain their humanness right up to the very end.
>
> (Where she is now) The lobby looks like a living room. We can bring our family there. The activity director puts the grandchildren onto an activity. For her 100th birthday, the grandchildren took cake around to everyone. The nurse seems very knowledgeable about health matters, is kind, has a good relationship with my mother's doctor, all those things make us very comfortable. We feel like family. Would you like a cup of coffee? Would you like to eat with your mother? When you visit you need to feel comfortable. The caregivers take a delight in my mother and she takes delight in them. She is really close to them. I would recommend to anyone that they move their parent to a small town in Wisconsin. ❞
>
> — Earl and Shirley Barnes Wisconsin, USA

Learning objectives

By the end of this chapter, you will be able to:

- Discuss the changing social policy discourse that has underpinned the development of specialist housing settings for older people
- Understand the key differences between the main models of specialist housing for older people
- Identify the key challenges involved in providing specialist housing for people with dementia and their family carers

Introduction

The latter half of the twentieth century and the early years of the twenty-first century have been marked by a number of key socio-demographic trends that have profound implications for housing. In particular, the increase in life expectancy, decrease in household size, and growth in owner-occupation are having a considerable impact. Over this same period, the emphasis of public policy has shifted from caring for frail older people in institutional settings to providing care and support for them in their own homes or other environments that are as "domestic" or "homely" as possible. This shift towards "care in the community" has led to rapid growth in the provision of housing with care in many European countries, although there are questions about how long such settings are able to support people with dementia (Bernard et al. 2004; Means 2007).

There has often been a lack of understanding of the needs of people with dementia among housing, social care, and health professionals, and an over-emphasis on the potential levels of risk associated with supporting people in the community. Together, these can lead to the exclusion of people with dementia from community-based care and housing services and pressures to moving to institutional care settings instead, particularly as their condition progresses (Evans et al. 2007). Housing is about more than bricks and mortar and the notion of "home" is an important framing concept in cultural theory about identity. Home is the repository of memories, the place where we literally represent our private selves through photographs, ornaments, and possessions (Darke 1994). The concept of home is therefore key to individual identity when the processes of memory are impaired and the self is fragmented, as can be the case for people living with dementia.

In many nations, dementia has become an increasingly important issue for government and a priority area for national policy development. This was acknowledged in the UK through the National Dementia Strategy (Department of Health 2009). The strategy was developed with three main goals in mind: to improve awareness of dementia; to improve early diagnosis and intervention; and to improve the quality of care for people with dementia, their carers and families. The success of the strategy is contingent on a whole systems approach, which has a broader focus than health and social care. The dementia strategy recognizes the value of the housing sector to promoting the well-being of people with dementia, and its approach has been given increased impetus through the Prime Minister's Challenge on Dementia (Department of Health 2012). This report acknowledges that dementia is the biggest health concern for people over 55. The Dementia Challenge has three main aims: to promote dementia-friendly communities, to drive health and social care improvements, and to improve and support dementia research. The role of housing in supporting older people, including those with dementia, is also an important element in a range of international initiatives, including the World Health Organisation's age-friendly cities initiative (WHO 2007).

This chapter provides an overview of housing with care, including the people it is for, the identifying features of different models, and their key aims and objectives. It also explores how well specialist housing settings can meet these broad aims for people with dementia. The chapter begins by describing the most common forms of housing with care and comparing their key features. It then goes on to consider the social and policy context in which housing with care has become increasingly popular in recent years and the importance of the concept of "home" for people with dementia. A third section considers how appropriate and achievable these aims are for people with dementia by reviewing the existing evidence and identifying gaps in the knowledge base. Finally, the reader is offered a summary of the key issues and some further debating points.

Models of housing with care

In recent years, there has been increasing recognition of the role that housing can play in promoting quality of life, health, independence, and well-being for older people. However, the terminology associated with older people's housing often lacks clarity and can be confusing for the public and professionals. International variations in provision and terminology can only add to the challenges in this respect (Howe *et al*. 2013).

In the mid-1990s in the UK, "extra care" or "very sheltered" housing began to emerge as a new model, largely due to a growing focus on the needs of an ageing and increasingly frail population and the search for alternatives to institutional settings for care. Extra care housing is now firmly established as a popular form of housing with care provision for older people. Extra care housing has been a key plank of UK Government policy in terms of its aims to promote choice, independence, and well-being for older people. Many different models of extra care have been developed and the flexibility of this form of provision is one of its key strengths. However, this flexibility also makes extra care hard to define. Put simply, extra care offers housing that has the full legal rights associated with being a tenant or home owner, along with 24-hour care that can be delivered flexibly according to a person's changing needs. In the USA, this type of housing (referred to as "assisted living") has also experienced an explosion in growth. In some cases, they stand alone while in others they are formally linked to either retirement communities, residential aged care (nursing homes) or both, providing a continuum of care and support (Sikorska-Simmons and Wright 2007). Many states have produced guidelines for developers and care providers in these settings, some of which are dementia-specific. One of the most pressing challenges for assisted living is how to provide a safe environment for people with dementia (Rasin and Kautz 2007; Zimmerman *et al*. 2007; Bellantonio *et al*. 2008).

Extra care housing and assisted living aim to support independence and well-being for residents for as long as possible in this setting. Different provider organizations have placed varying emphasis on the housing or care element of their provision, depending on whether they position their schemes as alternatives to residential care or as a replacement for traditional sheltered housing. Key features of extra care housing are that it is less institutional than residential care and is fundamentally about "quality of life" not just "quality of care". This type of housing can be for rent, outright sale or part-ownership; some developments are mixed-tenure, offering homes for sale and for rent.

Retirement villages are another increasingly popular housing option for older people, driven by a range of factors, including the ageing population, changing older age lifestyle aspirations, and recognition of the need for greater choice and flexibility in later life housing options (Heywood *et al*. 2002). Retirement villages are usually bigger than other forms of housing with care. In the UK, they tend to accommodate 200–300 residents, while in the USA and Australia (where they are often known as "lifestyle villages") they range from under 100 residents to several thousand. Such economies of scale allow for the provision of a wide range of facilities and social and recreational activities. Flexible care is typically available, including home help, personal care, health care, home maintenance, eating facilities, and transport.

Table 23.1 summarizes the key features of each of these models of housing with care and compares them with the more traditional form of "residential care".

	Extra care housing	Retirement village	Residential care
Also known as:	Very sheltered housing; serviced housing; close care; flexicare	Continuing care retirement village; retirement community	Category 3; care home; rest home; elderly mental infirm (EMI) unit; nursing home
Key features	Typically 40 or more self-contained flats with ensuite facilities; inclusive design standards. Some schemes include specialist dementia clusters or units.	100 or more houses, apartments or bungalows. Many have a care home on site; some have dementia units	Have individual rooms, some with private bathrooms and kitchenettes, on-site catering facilities, and resident lounges
Provided By	Mostly housing associations, some local authorities. Increasingly, private sector developers are building extra care "villages"	Not-for-profit organizations, housing associations, and private developers	Mostly private care companies
Tenure options	Social rent, shared ownership, outright sale, and mixed-tenure. Assured tenancy rights	Private ownership, market rental, some mixed-tenure. Assured tenancy rights	Most "placements" are paid for by local authorities or privately. No tenancy rights
Typical facilities	Communal lounge; catering; shop; beauty salon; day centre; activities room; Internet room	Communal lounge; catering; shop; activities room; beauty salon; Internet room; gym; swimming pool; jacuzzi	Communal lounges; catering
Care and support	Emergency alarm system. 24/7 care and support	Emergency alarm system. Most have flexible packages that can be purchased from care team and out-of-hours emergency provision	On-site care staff 24 hours a day, 7 days a week. Registered with Commission for Social Care Inspection
Provision in England	39,000 units in 2008	About 600 schemes in 2010	453,00 registered care home places in 2010

Table 23.1 Models of housing with care and residential care

Exercise 23.1: The benefits of housing with care

One of the key features of extra care housing/assisted living has been 24/7 on-site care for residents. Consider how realistic it is to deliver care flexibly to support people with dementia outside planned hours and what are the main facilitators and challenges to doing so.

■   What evidence could be collected to measure success in this respect?

Role of housing with care for people with dementia

This section explores what we currently know about housing with care for people with dementia. It draws largely on the research evidence but is also based on the experiences of people with dementia and their carers.

Few studies have focused on the role and capacity of different models of "specialist" housing for later life with regard to the needs and preferences of people with dementia (O'Malley and Croucher 2005). Vallely *et al.* (2006) found that the benefits of extra care housing were recognized by people with dementia, especially in relation to the care and support provided, relationships with other residents, feeling safe, and being able to choose how they spent their time. The relatives of residents with dementia felt that extra care housing offered them reassurance that help was readily available when needed, particularly in a crisis. Most residents with dementia received frequent visits from family members who provided much informal support. Brooker *et al.* (2011) explored the impact of a whole-scheme approach to supporting people with dementia that included specialist staff, leadership, staff training, individualized care work, community liaison, and the provision of appropriate activities. They reported that those receiving the service were less likely than residents in the control sites to move to a care home or to be admitted to hospital. They were also more likely to be seen by a range of community health professionals. Summarizing the findings from a number of studies in this area, Dutton (2010) found strong evidence that certain aspects of extra care have a positive impact on the well-being of residents with dementia. These included person-centred care, maximization of dignity and independence, effective communication, and meaningful social interactions. Research from the Netherlands, where there has been a move towards small-scale group accommodation for people with dementia, suggests that key elements in the provision of care are facilitating the involvement of family carers, the use of technology, and modifications to the living environment (Hoof *et al.* 2009).

Croucher *et al.* (2006) explored a range of models of housing with care and concluded that they do not easily accommodate people with dementia. This was largely because although the independence and security that these models aim to provide are greatly valued by older people, the provider organization's understanding of the concept of independence was different to that of the older people themselves. As a result, some residents had expected more assistance and support than was available.

It is crucial to include the voice of people with dementia in housing with care, in terms of both strategic decisions and day-to-day issues and activities. However, their views have been largely absent, while other people, particularly professionals and families, often speak for them (Bowers *et al.* 2009). Some housing providers are now making efforts to address this situation, as demonstrated by the dementia self-help group run by the Mental Health Foundation with extra care housing residents (www.mentalhealth.org.uk/our-news/blog/121109dementiaselfhelp/).

The overall aim of housing with care is to promote quality of life for older people by supporting independence, maximizing health and well-being, and providing opportunities for ageing in place. Let us now examine the evidence for the extent to which these can be achieved for people with dementia.

Promoting independence

By providing residents with their own front door and self-contained accommodation, the most recent models such as extra care housing/assisted living and retirement villages offer an environment that has the potential to maximize independence. Other features that are key to independence include flexible care packages, accessible design, and an active social life. However, there are a number of specific challenges to supporting independence for people with dementia in this setting.

One such challenge is providing the right care in the most appropriate way. There is evidence that good-quality person-centred care can be effective in managing the behavioural symptoms of people with dementia in residential care (Fossey *et al.* 2006). Work by Croucher and Bevan (2012) extended this finding to housing with care settings and emphasized the importance of establishing an atmosphere of tolerance and respect. Vallely *et al.* (2006) found that the skills and experience of managers in terms of dementia were also one of the main determinants of the extent to which extra care housing/assisted living residents with dementia were integrated. The model of care in operation was also central to supporting independence. The flexible care packages were found to be particularly important for meeting the needs of people with dementia, which can change frequently.

Case example 23.1: Albert

An extra care housing tenant with mild dementia, whom we will call Albert, had previously lived in a maisonette (duplex). He began to find the stairs difficult to manage, which prevented him from going out much and put him at increased risk of isolation. His ground floor flat in an extra care housing scheme was much more suitable. As Albert put it: "They put me on a level that was much more convenient for me and I can get out of the door quick." He appreciated the independence that this gave him and he spent a lot of time walking in the local area. Albert got on all right with the other tenants but he placed great value on having the privacy of his own flat. "Oh yes, if I know anybody I'll stop and talk but I am a bit of a loner. I stay here nodding off, go for a walk and then it's time for dinner."

The attitudes and behaviour of other residents also has an impact on the quality of life of those with dementia. Evans and Vallely (2007) highlighted the need for greater insight and understanding in this respect, while a Swedish study (Ericsson *et al.* 2011) found that awareness in people with dementia seemed to be greater than others perceived, which often meant that interaction was adversely affected by frequent well-intentioned corrections and comments. Another important consideration is how staff perceive and manage risk. People who live in extra care housing have the legal right as tenants to come and go as they please and to decide who visits them. However, for staff supporting people with dementia this can present challenges in terms of maintaining a balance between autonomy and security. Evans and Means (2006) reported that extra care staff often considered people with dementia to be more at risk than other tenants. A number of potential risks were identified by care staff, such as so-called "wandering". This was perceived by care staff as a significant challenge to supporting people with dementia in extra care housing, although there were few actual examples of its being a problem. This highlights the importance of providing care and support staff with the appropriate training to support people with dementia. Vallely *et al.* (2006) found that few staff had received dementia-specific training and that this limited the effectiveness of the support they provided. There are currently no statutory dementia training and qualification guidelines in the UK for housing with care settings, although many providers have developed their own standards. Equally important for people with dementia is the continuity of care and support staff (NICE-SCIE 2006). This is a major challenge in a range of settings, including housing with care, where a lack of job status and low pay are often associated with high levels of staff turnover.

There is considerable evidence that the built environment is a major factor in the extent to which a housing with care environment can promote independence (e.g. Parker *et al.* 2004). There has also been much debate about what aspects of building design can support people with dementia, particularly in terms of maximizing independence, enhancing self-esteem, and reinforcing personal identity (Wright 2010; Barnes *et al.* 2012). Many good practice viewpoints and checklists have been developed, listing principles and features for designing home and care environments in a way that supports people with dementia (Judd *et al.* 1998; Utton 2007). The research evidence base regarding design for dementia remains relatively small, but there is considerable "commonsense" consensus on the overall principles of design that can be effective. These include:

■ creating small, familiar environments
■ incorporating unobtrusive safety features
■ providing different rooms for different functions
■ good signage
■ the use of colour, lighting, and architectural landmarks to aid orientation and way-finding
■ the appropriate use of assistive technology

Vallelly *et al.* (2006) have highlighted the importance of good design. They concluded that many extra care housing schemes incorporated features that supported residents with dementia in terms of orientation and way-finding. This included the use of indoor streets or malls, which provide an environment that is dry, level, and secure. This enables access for people with dementia to a range of facilities that are crucial to their independence, such as shops, restaurants, and communal areas.

Promoting health and well-being

Many residents with dementia in housing with care settings also have complex health care needs. Vallelly *et al.* (2006) found that these needs were more likely to be met where service provision was part of an overall strategy across housing, health, and social care. Housing with care has a major preventative role to play in terms of maximizing health. For example, there is growing research into the potential for people with dementia to benefit from rehabilitative activities (Jorm 1994; Evans 2008), and considerable scope for these to be provided in housing that includes care, although Vallelly *et al.* (2006) found limited evidence of this happening to date.

There is much evidence to suggest that personal relationships and social interaction are important factors in quality of life for older people (Phillipson 1997; Age Concern 2006). Social well-being was found to be important in housing with care settings by Evans and Vallelly (2007), who interviewed staff and residents in six extra care schemes across England. They found that people with dementia were particularly at risk of social exclusion in this setting and identified six key factors that can impact on social well-being:

■ friendship and social interaction
■ engaging with the wider community
■ the importance of design
■ the role of family carers
■ staffing and the culture of care
■ providing appropriate facilities

Evans and Vallelly's respondents valued the opportunity to mix with other tenants and it was therefore important to provide opportunities for developing and maintaining social networks. The provision of appropriate facilities and activities was particularly important in this respect, and the schemes that took part in the study offered a range of activities for residents, including exercise classes, memory groups, art and craft projects, games, and trips. However, there were significant variations in the number and scope of activities, often due to the systems and funding mechanisms in operation.

Vallelly et al. (2006) identified prejudice among other residents as a potential barrier to social integration for residents with dementia, largely due to lack of information and understanding. Kitwood et al. (1995) found that people with dementia were often a focus for resentment and tended to be scapegoats for a range of problems. They suggested that residents were more supportive of others that had developed dementia since moving into a scheme, compared with those who had dementia when they moved in. This was largely because they had already become part of social networks and were therefore less disadvantaged by their reduced social skills. Croucher et al. (2006) reported that the old and frail, and particularly those with dementia, were consistently on the margins of social networks and were excluded from many social activities. It is also important to recognize that some people who are aware of their illnesses chose to withdraw from social interaction to preserve their dignity (Croucher and Bevan 2012).

Exercise 23.2: Variations in housing and services

Pick a few communities in your country and in other countries. Explore the levels of housing with care provision they offer and the extent to which this appears to meet the needs of people with dementia.

- Do they specifically address care of people with dementia?
- What indication do they give about whether they might provide a home for life?

You might want to start with some web resources: in the UK (www.eac.org.uk); in the USA (http://www.assistedlivinglocators.com/facilities/; http://www.assistedlivinginfo.com/); in Canada (http://assisted-living-directory.com/canada.cfm)

Ageing in place and a home for life

In recent years, much emphasis has been placed on providing housing options for older people and their right to "age in place". This contrasts with traditional models where older people are required to move to a different housing setting, often a residential home, in order to have their care needs met. This is often referred to as "a home for life" or "ageing in place". However, this has proved to be a major challenge, particularly for residents with dementia, and some commentators have suggested that it can be problematic and even unrealistic (e.g. Oldman 2000; Bernard et al. 2004; Croucher et al. 2006). Croucher et al. (2006) concluded that while the evidence seems to suggest that housing with care can accommodate people with mild to moderate cognitive impairment, there is no evidence to suggest that these residents can be supported over the full course of their illness. Similarly, Vallelly et al. (2006) reported that worsening dementia was recorded as a factor for 41% of residents who moved to nursing care. However, the average length of tenancy was very similar for all tenants, whether they had dementia or not, at just over two years. The complexities of long-term care funding also present a challenge to achieving a home for life, as shown by the case study in case example 23.2.

Case example 23.2: An elderly woman referred to a housing scheme

An 87-year-old woman who had been diagnosed with dementia was referred to a housing scheme by social services so that she could have her health needs met while being close to her family. She moved into the scheme, which was part sheltered and part extra care.

She was later diagnosed as being terminally ill with cancer and was thought to have only a few weeks to live. At this point, the local authority was keen to refer her to a hospice so that responsibility for funding would transfer from the social services budget to "continuing care".

The resident's GP, her family, and the court manager all felt that an enforced move was not in her best interests because, although her physical health had deteriorated, her quality of life had improved since she moved into the scheme. Negotiations between health and social care providers and the housing association led to her staying in the scheme, supported by Macmillan nurses, until she died later that year.

This case study illustrates the difficulties of implementing a complex continuing care policy across housing, health, and social care. However, achieving this can be crucial to providing dignity and choice for older people with dementia in housing with care settings.

A number of larger housing with care developments incorporate specialist dementia services. For example, Westbury Fields retirement village in Bristol, England, has a dementia unit within its on-site care home. Evans and Means (2007) found that this was greatly valued by the spouses of village residents who developed dementia because it meant that they could continue living in the village while supporting their partners in the specialist unit. It is also important to emphasize that, while extra care residents do have the legal protection of assured tenancies, it is still possible for the landlord to evict them under certain circumstances, including "anti-social" behaviour.

Although most extra care housing schemes aim to integrate people with dementia within the overall scheme, one extra care housing scheme in the study of Vallelly et al. (2006) included a specialist dementia unit. While acknowledging the potential benefits of this arrangement in terms of targeting specialist services, the study identified a number of challenges, which are outlined in case example 23.3.

Case example 23.3: Oak House

Oak House, an extra care housing scheme run by Housing 21, has 38 self-contained flats, eight of which are in a separate unit designed to meet the specific needs of people with dementia. This unit is accessed from the main building via a keyfob-protected door and has its own dining area and residents' lounge. The "Opening Doors" study identified a range of issues that created challenges for the specialist unit:

- When a couple move in and one partner has dementia but not the other, should they live in the main scheme or the dementia unit?
- It is not easy to assess who should live in the unit because many residents have cognitive impairment but no diagnosis of dementia.
- What happens when someone living in the scheme develops dementia – do they stay in their flat or move into the dementia unit?
- Does a specialist unit increase stigma and prejudice in relation to dementia by reducing contact with other residents?

Debates and controversies

A number of issues remain unresolved in terms of the best ways of supporting people with dementia in housing and care settings. These include the following:

- Some developments support people with dementia within the main housing scheme (an integrated approach), while others have dementia clusters, units or wings. Which works best in terms of quality of life, quality of care, and cost-effectiveness?
- Given economic austerity and changes to commissioning practices brought about by personalization and the pressures on social care budgets, it is increasingly difficult to provide flexible, 24/7 care and support. This is likely to be especially detrimental to the well-being of people with dementia and may impact on their ability to live independently in housing with care settings.
- Mixed-tenure – there is a conflicting ethos between "active lifestyle" for the increasing number of leaseholders or shared owners who buy apartments compared with the growing number of people with advanced dementia in rented accommodation. Fair Access to Care (FAC) criteria used by most local authorities for referrals is now at critical/substantial rather than moderate or lower level needs. For the scheme operators, there is a challenge around the duty of care to all residents and balancing different expectations and dependencies.

Conclusion

Recognition of the need to provide a range of housing options for the increasing number of older people has led to the development of new models of housing with care. However, there is a lack of detailed evidence for the extent to which these meet the needs of people with dementia. Research to date suggests that housing with care settings can support quality of life and independence for people with mild to moderate dementia, as long as a range of factors are taken into account. These include design of the built environment, models of care, staff training, the provision of facilities, social well-being, a balanced approach to risk, and the appropriate use of assistive technologies. However, challenging questions have been posed about the ability of housing with care to support residents as their dementia becomes more advanced.

Further information

The Housing Learning and Information Network (LIN) web site for housing and dementia addresses housing and disabilities and has a specific section on housing and dementia. The focus is on extra care housing [http://www.housinglin.org.uk/].

The Elderly Accommodation Counsel provides information about housing, care, and support for older people [http://www.eac.org.uk/].

The Alzheimer's Society has a web site that includes information on housing adaptations, design improvements, and repairs for people with dementia [http://www.alzheimers.org.uk/].

References

Age Concern (2006) *Promoting Mental Health and Well-being in Later Life*. London: Age Concern.

Barnes, L., Torrington, J., Darton, R., Holder, J., Lewis, A. *et al.* (2012) Does the design of extra care housing meet the needs of residents? A focus group study, *Ageing and Society*, 32(7): 1193–1214.

Bellantonio, S., Kenny, A., Fortinsky, R., Kleppinger, A., Robison, J. *et al.* (2008) Efficacy of a geriatrics team intervention for residents in dementia specific assisted living facilities: effect on unanticipated transitions, *Journal of the American Geriatrics Society*, 56(3): 523–8.

Bernard, M., Bartlam, B. and Biggs, S. (2004) *New Lifestyles in Old Age: Health, Identity and Well-being in Berryhill Retirement Village*. Bristol: Policy Press.

Bowers, H., Clark, A., Crosby, G., Easterbrook, L., Macadam, A. *et al.* (2009) *Older People's Vision of Long Term Care*. York: Joseph Rowntree Foundation.

Brooker, D., Argyle, E., Scally, A. and Clancy, D. (2011) The Enriched Opportunities Programme for people with dementia: a cluster-randomised controlled trial in 10 extra care housing schemes, *Aging and Mental Health*, 15 (8): 1008–17.

Croucher, K. and Bevan, M. (2012) *Promoting Supportive Relationships in Housing with Care*. York: Joseph Rowntree Foundation.

Croucher, K., Hicks, S.L. and Jackson, K. (2006) *Housing with Care in Later Life: A Literature Review*. York: Joseph Rowntree Foundation.

Darke, J. (1994) Women and the meaning of home, in R. Gilroy and R. Woods (eds.) *Housing Women*. London: Routledge, pp. 11–30.

Department of Health (2009) *Living Well with Dementia: A National Dementia Strategy*. London: Department of Health [https://www.gov.uk/government/publications/living-well-with-dementia-a-national-dementia-strategy, accessed 29 April 2014].

Department of Health (2012) *The Prime Minister's Challenge on Dementia*. London: The Stationery Office.

Dutton, R. (2010) People with dementia living in extra care housing: learning from the evidence, *Working with Older People*, 14(1): 8–11.

Ericsson, I., Hellström, I. and Kjellström, S. (2011) Sliding interactions: an ethnography about how persons with dementia interact in housing with care for the elderly, *Dementia*, 10(4): 523–38.

Evans, S. (2008) Providing rehabilitation services for people with dementia through intermediate care, *Nursing Older People*, 20(2): 33–5.

Evans, S. and Means, R. (2006) Perspectives on risk for older people with dementia in extra care housing in the UK: findings from a longitudinal study, *International Journal of Disability and Human Development*, 5(1): 77–82.

Evans, S. and Means, R. (2007) *Balanced Retirement Communities? A Case Study of Westbury Fields Mixed Tenure Retirement Village*. Bristol: St. Monica Trust.

Evans, S. and Vallelly, S. (2007) Never a dull moment? Promoting social well-being in extra care housing, *Housing Care and Support*, 10(4): 14–20.

Evans, S., Fear, T., Means, R. and Vallelly, S. (2007) Supporting independence for people with dementia in extra care housing, *Dementia*, 6(1): 144–50.

Fossey, J., Ballard, C., Juszczak, E., James, I., Alder, N. *et al.* (2006) Effect of enhanced psychosocial care on anti-psychotic use in nursing home residents with severe dementia: cluster randomised trial, *British Medical Journal*, 332(7544): 756–61.

Heywood, F., Oldman, C. and Means, R. (2002) *Housing and Home in Later Life*. Philadelphia, PA: Open University Press.

Hoof, J., Kort, H.S.M. and Waarde, H. (2009) Housing and care for older adults with dementia: a European perspective, *Journal of Housing and the Built Environment*, 24(3): 369–90.

Howe, L.A., Jones A.E. and Tilse, C. (2013) What's in a name? Similarities and differences in international terms and meanings for older people's housing with services, *Ageing and Society*, 33(4): 547–78.

Jorm, A.F. (1994) Disability in dementia: assessment, prevention, and rehabilitation, *Disability and Rehabilitation*, 16(3): 98–109.

Judd, S., Marshall, S. and Phippen, P. (1998) *Design for Dementia*. London: Hawker Publications.

Kitwood, T., Buckland, S. and Petre, T. (1995) *Brighter Futures: A Report on Research into Provision for Persons with Dementia in Residential Homes, Nursing Homes and Sheltered Housing*. Oxford: Anchor Trust.

Means, R. (2007) Safe as houses? Ageing in place and vulnerable people in the UK, *Social Policy and Administration*, 41(1): 65–85.

National Institute for Health and Clinical Excellence and Social Care Institute for Excellence (NICE-SCIE) (2006) *Dementia: Supporting People with Dementia and their Carers in Health and Social Care*. London: NICE-SCIE.

Oldman, C. (2000) *Blurring the Boundaries: A Fresh Look at Housing and Care Provision for Older People*. York: Joseph Rowntree Foundation.

O'Malley, L. and Croucher, K. (2005) Housing and dementia care – a scoping review of the literature, *Health and Social Care in the Community*, 13(6): 570–7.

Parker, C., Barnes, S., McKee, K., Morgan, K., Torrington, J. *et al.* (2004) Quality of life and building design in residential and nursing homes for older people, *Ageing and Society*, 24: 941–62.

Phillipson, C. (1997) Social relationships in later life: a review of the research literature, *International Journal of Geriatric Psychiatry*, 12(5): 505–12.

Rasin, J. and Kautz, D. (2007) Knowing the resident with dementia: perspectives of assisted living facility caregivers, *Journal of Gerontological Nursing*, 33(9): 30–6.

Sikorska-Simmons, E. and Wright, J. (2007) Determinants of resident autonomy in assisted living facilities: a review of the literature, *Care Management*, 8(4): 187–93.

Utton, D. (2007) *Designing Homes for People with Dementia*. London: Hawker Publications.

Vallelly, S., Evans, S., Fear, T. and Means, R. (2006) *Opening the Doors to Independence: A Longitudinal Study Exploring the Contribution of Extra Care Housing to the Care and Support of Older People*. London: Housing Corporation and Housing 21.

World Health Organization (WHO) (2007) *Global Age-friendly Cities: A Guide*. Geneva: WHO [http://www.who.int/ageing/publications/Global_age_friendly_cities_Guide_English.pdf, accessed 18 May 2012].

Wright, F. (2010) What is the extra in extra care housing?, *British Journal of Social Work*, 40(7): 2239–54.

Zimmerman, S., Mitchell, C., Chen, C., Morgan, L., Gruber-Baldini, A. *et al.* (2007) An observation of assisted living environments: space use and behavior, *Journal of Gerontological Social Work*, 49(3): 185–203.

CHAPTER 24

Care homes

Jane Fossey

"Here's a place. Don't be shocked when you go there. You have to look beyond the building. This is the best place for Peter but how will we explain it to the relatives? The care was in a completely different league than anywhere else. Their philosophy was 'any excuse for a party ... Australia Day, someone's birthday, Italian Republic Day, Christmas, whatever. Every week they had outside people in. People would go and play to residents in their rooms, who were too ill to participate in the group. They encouraged costumes and colors. People loved the color and the glamour. They had a safe environment but not weighed down by bureaucracy. The new home is very bureaucratic. They put out edicts like 'It has come to our notice that some families take trays off the trolley themselves! This presents all sorts of health and safety issues.' I think they would like families to disappear into the sunset."

—Frances Annal Melbourne, Australia

"My Mum became friends with another lady on the EMI wing. She could not speak very much and was very bent over. She was a kind lady. My Mum had a stroke and became blind and although she could walk stayed in a chair. This lady came up one day and held Mum's hand. I was very moved and touched by this but was also shocked at myself because I had been surprised at this lady's action. I had assumed she did not have the mental capacity for such an act."

—Brenda Smith Yorkshire, UK

"A very good nurse explained to me that the EMI unit is the person's home and the last home they will have. All carers and managers should have this as an important fact when they are caring for residents."

—Brenda Smith Yorkshire, UK

Learning objectives

By the end of this chapter, you will:

- Understand what it is like to live in a care home
- Understand the factors which influence how a person with dementia experiences a care home
- Understand different approaches to care that can meet residents' physical, psychological, and social needs
- Understand how consultation can enhance care practices

Introduction

Although many people with dementia continue to live in their own homes (see Chapter 21) and improvements in planning and coordination for social support can be found in a number of countries (WHO 2012), a significant number of people still live in some type of care home. In the UK, this is approximately a third of people with dementia (Knapp *et al.* 2007). In nursing homes, where the majority of residents are over age 85 in most countries (AIHW 2010), the percentage of residents with dementia varies significantly by country. Percentage estimates are: 80% in the UK (Quince 2013), 60% in Germany, 50% in the USA, and 30% in Australia, Denmark, and Japan (Knapp *et al.* 2007).

In most instances, the decision to move to a care home is distressing for both the person with dementia and their family carers (Caron and Bowers 2003; Davies and Nolan 2003). Family members often look after their relatives until there is a crisis or they feel they have reached "breaking point" (O'May 2007). This is especially difficult when the person with dementia requires, but does not recognize the need for, more assistance than a family carer alone can provide. Until recently, little help has been available to family carers when thinking about whether moving to a care home is the best option (Baldwin *et al.* 2005). However, charities and regulators have started to provide resources to support relatives in choosing a care home (for the Alzheimer's Society, SCIE, and Department of Health in the UK, Trinity College Dublin web site in Ireland, ABC Health & Wellbeing guides in Australia, and Alzheimer's Association in the USA, see "Further information").

Families aspire to find homes that will provide a high "quality of life" for their relatives. Although quality of life is difficult to define, it generally includes physical, social, and psychological dimensions (Gerritson *et al.* 2004). Being recognized as a unique individual, maintaining independence, being able to make choices, having friends, having privacy and dignity, participating in leisure and community activities, and being able to assess and take risks in a supported way, all continue to be important (Alzheimer's Society 2010; Cahill and Diaz 2010). It is important to remember that people with dementia retain many abilities and sensitivities and place similar importance on values that are reflected in the general population. A study of over 300 people with dementia living in care homes revealed considerable "capacity for retained awareness" of self, relationship, and environment (Clare *et al.* 2008: 2366).

One way of maintaining quality in care homes is through standard setting. In many nations, governmental standards for care homes have been developed and systems established to investigate whether standards are being met. However, as Briggs and Bachelor (2004) point out, it is important not to define care only by what is measurable but also to address what is important from the perspective of individuals with dementia. This has been reflected more recently in policy through the concept of "co-production" of services by professionals directly engaging with users of services in the design and development of their own care (Care Services Improvement Partnership 2007; Boyle and Harris 2009).

Moving into a care home

Research on the impact of moving into a care home has focused on three main areas: the experience of relocation for the person with dementia; the impact of the decision-making process for relatives and carers of the person with dementia; and the role of professionals in supporting and guiding the process. It is also the case that moving into care is not always a one-off event, in that some people move from one type of care home to another as their needs change. For example, further relocation may be necessary if they require more nursing, move closer to their family, or relocate when a care home closes. It is important to consider the impact on the person at each point of transition, as relocation can be physically and psychologically disruptive.

Relocation has been shown to have a negative effect on the abilities and well-being of people with dementia. Studies investigating the impact of moves between homes have indicated that people who move by themselves experience higher rates of mortality and depression than those who move as part of a group, together with the staff who care for them (Day *et al.* 2000). This highlights the need to maintain familiarity and continuity of social support networks when considering a move (Shippee 2009).

Research also suggests that it is helpful for the new resident if staff understand what the move means for that person in terms of losses, fears, hopes, and expectations. This allows staff to help residents cope with the move and to maintain existing positive relationships (Reed *et al.* 2003; Glasby *et al.* 2012). A biographical "life-history" approach to understanding what matters to individuals, their values, and wishes is now common in admission assessment procedures and development of care plans (see Chapter 15). It is a means for staff to get to know the person and their preferences and can be a key to establishing relationships through sharing past and present experiences (McKee *et al.* 2005). Understanding a person's life history also provides an opportunity to engage with family members and a means by which families can contribute to ongoing care as their role in direct care delivery changes (Davies and Nolan 2006).

A plan of care can be made jointly with the person and their family. Places to start include developing a life story (Thompson 2010) and life-history boxes, which contain personally significant items. These can provide important links to meaningful experiences and people. Knowing about an individual is a good starting point in helping to maintain their identity. However, it is important to consider how this knowledge can be used on a day-to-day basis to influence the routines and lifestyle. For example, recognizing that someone has worked night shifts throughout their life suggests that they may be awake and need to be occupied at night, sleeping in the afternoons.

Exercise 24.1: Recognizing the importance of individual habits

Think of an older person you know, someone you are close to and care about. Make a list of the things that you would do for them if they became unable to tell you what was important.

- What do you know about them that would be useful in providing their care?
- What might be missed if suddenly they were being cared for by strangers? What important things would they lose?
- What do you know about their personal history that would be important? How would that affect their life or their care?

Factors that influence a person's experience of care

Research in several countries and in all types of care homes confirms that there are widespread problems with the quality of care (WHO 2012). Several governments have published national dementia plans addressing treatment, care, and research emphasizing the importance of better treatment and care for people with dementia in care home settings. National dementia strategies in France and England and care home regulators in the USA prioritize improvement in the quality of care and development of an informed, effective workforce (Menard 2008; Department of Health 2009; Centres for Medicare and Medicaid Services 2012).

Basic principles of care

Person-centred dementia care principles provide a good starting point for high-quality care (NICE 2011). These principles reflect the increasing evidence that people with dementia continue to experience a range of emotions in response to their interactions and environment (Quince 2013). Brooker (2007) refers to the core principles as VIPS because they include:

■ **V**aluing the person and their family
■ treating the person as an **I**ndividual
■ taking the **P**erspective of the person when planning and providing care
■ ensuring that a positive **S**ocial environment exists in which the person can experience relative well-being

Exercise 24.2: Engagement in activities

Think about how you might engage someone with advanced dementia in activities, using the principles outlined above:

■ How would you learn what is important to them? What are some of the sources you would use?
■ How would you design an activity that acknowledges these things?
■ How would you build such activities into the person's day?
■ What are some of the common care home activities that might not be appropriate?
■ How often do you think people should be supported in these activities? Once a day? Once a week? How often are you engaged in meaningful activities? Would this be often enough for you or someone you cared about?

The answers to these questions can provide some insight into basic quality of life issues for residents.

Resonant with Kitwood's (1997) work on psychological needs in person-centred care, Nolan *et al.* (2001) have developed the "Senses Framework" as a way to think about the psychological needs of people with dementia, family carers, and staff in care homes. The six senses are those of:

■ security
■ continuity
■ belonging
■ purpose
■ achievement
■ significance

Checklists of how these principles may appear in practice have become available through a number of web portals, with factors such as environmental design, availability of activities, and staff understanding all being important considerations. In a recent Alzheimer's Society report (Quince 2013), the top five areas carers and family members felt were important and demonstrated good care were (in order of importance):

- staff understanding of dementia
- friendliness of staff
- cleanliness of the home
- activities offered to residents
- quality of food in the home

In the USA, culture change initiatives such as the Eden Alternative, Greenhouse, and Pioneer programmes are based on person-centred principles and reflect efforts to change care homes from "health care institutions" to "person-centered homes that also offer long-term care services" (Koren 2010: 312). Architectural innovations such as smaller, more homelike environments and care practices such as consistent assignment, family style dining, and organization of routines around resident preferences are believed to improve both quality of life and quality of care. Small-house care homes have been in use across Europe for many years, particularly for people with dementia (Verbeek et al. 2009). Research confirms greater resident and family quality of life in such environments (Lum et al. 2008/9; Willemse et al. 2011).

Promoting positive interpersonal relationships

The importance families place on staff understanding of dementia and friendliness is supported in the professional literature, which suggests that relationships are the most important features maintaining well-being (Zgola 1999; Werezak and Morgan 2003; Robinson and Banks 2005). Consistent assignment of staff helps to achieve this. It also maximizes people's ability to build trusting relationships. People with dementia are often faced with increasing dependency and therefore need dependability and reliability in care staff who can individualize care. However, if consistent assignment is not possible, similar outcomes can be achieved if care leaders are able to ensure that all staff develop a knowledge of people's individual stories and preferences and how these unique preferences can be used in daily care (Fossey and James 2008).

Simple everyday interaction that supports friendships is a vital component in sustaining well-being for people in care homes. Staff introducing residents to each other, helping with phone calls and letter writing to maintain existing relationships, and making time to chat, all are useful interventions in maintaining well-being (Edvardsson et al. 2010).

Many people with dementia also have sensory disabilities that affect their ability to form relationships. For example, people with cognitive or sensory perceptual impairment (such as reduced ability to understand what is said to them due to dysphasia or hearing impairment) may find their ability to participate in activities restricted, leading to social isolation and a reduced sense of self-worth (Flannery 2002). Staff can modify the way they communicate to enhance their ability to interact effectively with residents. This can be done, for example, by ensuring that they face a resident and have light on them rather than behind them, so their face is not in shadow and can be more easily seen; by using gestures that are consistent with their verbal message; and by presenting information simply – one idea at a time – so that the recipient is not overwhelmed (see Chapter 17). These simple strategies used in daily care routines or in single-activity sessions such as reminiscence can improve communication with residents (Vasse et al. 2010).

Exercise 24.3: Recognizing the power of social interaction

■ List all of the people you meet or speak to today. Now think of a person with dementia whom you know, and list who they have met or spoken to today.

■ Are there differences in the types of contact you and they have with other people?

Intimate relationships and sexuality are often neglected in care homes. The public nature of care home living space makes intimacy difficult and poses challenges to privacy and dignity. Care homes can address this by considering how couples can have privacy during visits, or share rooms that provide sofas to allow for affectionate contact. However, many staff find it difficult to openly discuss sexuality with residents and their families. The UK Royal College of Nursing has produced a helpful paper about practical ways care homes can respond to this (RCN 2011), taking into account both individual rights and wishes and the concerns care staff may have about approaching the topic with residents and family members.

Opportunities to create relationships that enable residents to give as well as receive care also have a positive impact on well-being. This can involve interaction between residents and between residents and staff. For example, homes can actively engage residents in arranging activities as well as being recipients of them, have a residents' forum, or work alongside other organizations such as schools, nurseries or community groups where older people's skills and views can be offered to maintain a sense of identity and esteem. In addition, companion animals can provide an opportunity to provide affection and attention and can provide purpose and comfort beyond that of human visitors (Perkins et al. 2008).

Encouraging family involvement in care home life

Good practice requires family involvement in the development and review of the person's care plan (Gaugler 2005). However, in many homes, working with family members is rarely acknowledged as part of the role of care staff. Consequently, family carers often feel they have to take the initiative if they wish to remain involved in the care of their relative (Train et al. 2005). Having open discussions about concerns and areas of potential risk can be particularly helpful in keeping the person's best interests at the fore.

One common issue is how to respond to residents who enjoy walking but are at risk of falling. Discussions around the extent to which they are accompanied, areas of the home and grounds that may reduce the risk, and the use of aids such as hip protectors to reduce the possible impact should a fall occur, all can facilitate the individual in having a greater freedom of movement around the home than might otherwise be immediately possible.

Case example 24.1: John – recognizing the value of supportive relationships

John had just moved into the care home. On the first visit from his family, his daughter found John sitting alone in his room, crying out for someone to help him. Mary began trying to comfort her father, taking him outside in a wheelchair, wandering around the grounds, talking softly to him about what she had been doing at home, what his grandchildren were doing, and pointing out things in the garden that were of interest to him. He eventually became quite calm and fell asleep in his room soon after she brought him inside. Not wanting to upset the staff, she expressed her concern but did not show her anger. The staff reassured her that he would eventually adjust to the

(continued)

care home and would be fine, that she should not worry. On her next visit, she found him agitated, alone, and shouting. The care attendant told her that he was "a bit of a problem", as he was disturbing other residents and that nothing seemed to calm him.

Considering the 'Senses' framework described earlier:

- What do you think might be going on?
- What do you think might be done for John?

Supporting personal identity of the resident

Helping people to maintain their identity is closely linked to self-esteem and quality of life in care homes (McKee *et al.* 2005). To address this, biographical approaches such as reminiscence, life-story work, and oral history can act as a basis for personally meaningful activity that will affirm the person's identify. This enables people to engage in previously enjoyed activities or link new activities to significant events or aspirations from the past (see Chapter 15).

Specific psychosocial and creative therapies (see Table 24.1 for examples of these) can also be used to promote meaningful occupation for the person, affirming identify, increasing self-expression, improving communication skills, and providing opportunities to enhance a person's identity and self-esteem. Individualized assessments can identify activities that reflect individual preferences and effectively increase engagement in activities that are meaningful to the individual (Brooker and Woolley 2006; Cohen-Mansfield *et al.* 2010a).

Culture and ethnicity can be basic to a person's identity. Therefore, cultural awareness is important for all aspects of dementia care, both to provide overseas staff with knowledge of everyday practices concerning food and drink, local customs and sayings, and important historical and current events to which clients might relate. Some homes provide language tuition for their staff. This provides the opportunity to ensure that useful vocabulary is identified, and to support all staff in meeting the needs of minority ethnic residents for whom Mold and colleagues' (2005) systematic review of care has shown that there are a number of difficulties in delivering culturally appropriate care and that language and communication difficulties arise that need to be addressed. A recent study examining the views of people with dementia from three cultural groups documented significant differences in how dementia is perceived and how related losses are experienced (Lawrence *et al.* 2010).

Knowing an individual's story and beliefs also enables homes to support their spiritual life, through prayer areas and practices such as providing or avoiding food consistent with the person's faith, recognizing days of celebration, and enabling residents to participate in particular seasonal activities and rituals.

Providing an enabling physical environment

Evidence suggests that the design of a home can improve the living experience of people with dementia, such as by increasing participation in activities and reducing time spent alone, and by providing safe space for residents to walk, meaning less restriction on their freedom (Reimer *et al.* 2004). A review of the design of therapeutic environments for people with dementia recommended that environments be small in size with separate facilities for people with cognitive impairment, be non-institutionalized in décor, and provide environmental stimulation such as ornaments, plants, and varied furnishings (Fleming *et al.* 2008).

Approach	Comments
Reality orientation See Spector *et al.* (2002) and Verkaik *et al.* (2006)	Uses rehearsal and physical prompts to improve cognitive functioning related to personal orientation
Cognitive stimulation therapy See Spector *et al.* (2008)	Derived from reality orientation, focuses on information processing rather than rehearsal of factual knowledge
Reminiscence therapy and life review See Woods *et al.* (2005)	Involves discussion of past experiences individually or in a group setting. Photographs, familiar objects, music, or sensory items prompt recall
Validation therapy See Neal and Barton Wright (2003, updated 2009)	Based on the general principle of acceptance of the reality of the person and validation of their experience; incorporates a range of specific techniques
Behavioural management techniques See Moniz-Cooke *et al.* (2012)	Based on learning theory, utilizes the antecedents and consequences of behaviour to elicit change in an individual
Music/music therapy See Vink and Birks (2003)	Includes playing and listening to music as a way of generally enhancing well-being, or can be more goal-directed with specific activities being used for a clearly defined therapeutic purpose
Creative therapies See Wilkinson *et al.* (1998) and James *et al.* (2006)	Drama, art, toys, dance – all offer creative ways of communicating; they facilitate verbal and non-verbal self-expression with the aim of improving well-being
Snoezelen/multisensory stimulation See Chung *et al.* (2002, updated 2009) and Buettner and Fitzsimmons (2009)	Stimuli such as light, sound, and tactile sensations, often in specially designed rooms, increase the opportunity for communication and improved quality of experience
Simulated presence therapy See Zetteler (2008)	An audio-tape of positive memories and experiences compiled in a conversational style by family members or friends is played to the person to provide reassurance, information, and stimulation
Structured activity/interaction programmes See Cohen-Mansfield (2001) and Cohen-Mansfield *et al.* (2010b)	Formal sessions of interaction using a structured conversational format, photos and pictures as discussion items with the aim of improving engagement and involvement
Exercise See Rolland *et al.* (2007)	Walking or group activities have been used to address depression and behavioural difficulties
Environmental manipulation See Fleming *et al.* (2008)	Cues such as colour and textural coding in rooms and furnishings, clear signage to private, communal and outdoor areas, planned furniture and building layout, all facilitate communication, exercise and pleasure, and reduce disorientation
Animal-assisted activity or therapy See Perkins *et al.* (2008)	Involves animals visiting people (or vice versa) to provide opportunities for social, motivational, recreational or therapeutic benefits to enhance quality of life
Psychotherapies See Miller (2009) and James (2010)	Cognitive-behavioural therapy for anxiety or depression for carers and clients in early stages of illness. Personal construct and brief psychotherapy to address emotional adjustment and self-esteem
Psycho-education with paid and family caregivers See Kuske *et al.* (2007) and Teri *et al.* (2005)	Promotes understanding of medical and non-medical factors, communication skills, behaviour management strategies, environmental modification, ethical issues, ways of involving families, stress management, practical and legal issues

Table 24.1 Psychosocial approaches to care

A similar level of reflection is needed in planning outside environments for people with dementia by providing opportunities for increased personal space, fresh air, exercise, stimulation for conversation, contact with nature, and the chance to engage with neighbours (Chalfont 2005). Paths to guide residents around areas of interest, clear focal points, and planting that enables a stimulation of the senses through scent or edibility of the plants, all promote well-being (van Hoof *et al.* 2010).

Practices such as locking doors to prevent people from wandering off are still used in many homes, despite the ethical concerns this practice has raised. In some instances, modification of the environment through the use of signs, the use of patterned floor coverings to create a visual guide for people, and the use of cloth barriers can overcome the need for more restrictive interventions to ensure physical safety (Feliciano and Vore 2004). Modifying the environment to curtail freedom often appears to "solve" the immediate concern of staff, but in doing so discourages care practice that takes the resident's perspective and seeks to understand the reasons they may have for acting in a certain way, their needs, and wishes. This may in turn limit the range of potential activities a resident can engage in and the possibility of building relationships. The debate generally focuses on the rights of the individual and the right to take risks (Welsh *et al.* 2003).

The use of deceptive practices when interacting with residents is controversial but appears to be widespread. A survey of care staff showed that "lying" was a common strategy, often intended kindly, to ease the distress of residents (James *et al.* 2003). Care staff perceived situations in which lying could be an appropriate therapeutic response in which "the ends justify the means" (Tuckett 2004), such as to gain compliance or immediately pacify a person in distress. Whether this approach is of benefit or of harm to recipients in the longer term is yet to be ascertained. Guidance regarding a care home's policy and detailed individual care plans will help staff to clarify how they are expected to behave when residents are distressed. Reaching a decision about an acceptable way to keep people safe requires a good understanding of what they are trying to achieve. Knowing this will allow care staff, in collaboration with the family and the person with dementia, to determine an appropriate course of intervention (Hughes and Louw 2002; see also Chapter 4).

Supporting staff practice

Within long-term care settings, there are both qualified (licensed) staff, usually nurses, and direct care staff. There are often poor pay structures and limited opportunities for staff to specialize (Hussein and Manthorpe 2011). Providing long-term care requires staff to be able to work at an emotional level as well as addressing physical care needs. It can be stressful, as staff have to deal with residents' distress, confusion, and styles of communication that may not be easy to interpret. This requires staff to have knowledge about dementia care, a positive attitude to their work, and also to develop communication skills to support their practice. For many care staff, the relationship with residents is the most important aspect of their work and a major reason for staying in their job (Parsons *et al.* 2003). Lack of opportunity to build personal attachments and reciprocal relationships with residents is a strong predictor of staff burnout and turnover (Duffy *et al.* 2009).

Training staff about dementia, ways to understand the factors that contribute to people's expressions of need, and supporting their independence can reduce resident distress (James 2011). Sometimes staff undertake tasks that individuals are still capable of engaging with because of the focus on efficiency and "getting the job done" (Jirovec 1991). This can result in "learned helplessness" for the resident, an induced dependency in which it becomes easier to be a recipient of care than to try to maintain independence (Flannery 2002). Letting go of independence in this way poses a risk to self-concept and autonomy (Kitwood 1997). A recent review of qualitative literature highlights the importance of staff "seeing beyond the illness" and their knowledge of the individual as foundational requirements for the successful implementation of psychosocial care (Lawrence *et al.* 2012).

There is growing recognition of the need for specialist training for care workers. For example, in Australia many states have mandatory competency-based dementia training for dementia care workers (Brodaty and Cummings 2010). Guidelines have been produced in a number of countries such as Sweden, the Netherlands, and UK (WHO 2012). However, implementing this in practice can be difficult to achieve. In the USA and UK, for example, despite the requirement for staff certification and training, there is considerable evidence that staff are not receiving sufficient training for their work (Spilsbury and Meyer 2004).

Working with the wider health care team

People with dementia often receive less effective medical and mental health services than those in the community (Fahey *et al.* 2003). For example, the ability to recognize pain in people with cognitive impairment has been found to be poor, despite evidence that simple pain management strategies can be effective in reducing signs of distress (Husebo *et al.* 2011; Gilmore-Bykovskyi and Bowers, 2013). Given that a person with dementia may have reduced abilities to communicate their specific needs, it is important that care staff are aware of the signs to look out for. Among care homes, there is considerable variability in relationships with local medical practices and physical and mental health teams.

There is evidence to suggest that good practice requires multidisciplinary consultation and that liaison services should extend advice and treatment to care homes (Glendinning *et al.* 2002; Hancock *et al.* 2006). Physical and occupational therapists have an important role in maintaining ambulation and reducing falls, as people with dementia have almost twice the risk of falling than people without dementia (van Doorn *et al.* 2003). A study of the Evercare programme demonstrated a significantly lower hospitalization rate for people in nursing homes with advance practice nurses than in comparison populations. This held for both those with and without dementia (Kane *et al.* 2003).

Debates and controversies

From a philosophical point of view, there has been a significant shift in the approach to care for people with dementia in care homes. However, in practice the change in approach has continued to develop much more slowly. One of the key areas of debate both at a clinical and political level is the methods that will best facilitate the implementation of knowledge of person-centred principles in practice in routine care. While regulation and standards are a starting point, there continue to be cases of abuse and neglect of older people reported that must be prevented in the future.

Allied to the debate about skill-mix is training needs of staff and how this can best be provided both in-service and through formal educational routes. The role of management practices and leadership style have also been identified as key to influencing resident outcomes (Rokstad *et al.* 2013) but have only begun to receive attention from academics and policy-makers.

An ongoing debate is how people can be helped to remain in their own homes for longer and avoid the need for care home provision. There has been a growing provision of supported/sheltered/extra care schemes – termed differently in different countries – that aim to promote independence for as long as possible, with people moving to more supported provision as their condition progresses. This in itself raises issues about the way transitions in care are managed, but may establish a clearer expectation at the outset which can ameliorate the potential distress of moving.

Conclusion

Despite an increasing focus on therapeutic interventions for people with dementia, the integration of these practices is by no means universal. For care practices to improve and more adequately meet the needs of people with dementia, greater clarity concerning key skills and care practices is needed. There is also evidence that people in care homes are not receiving the same levels of health care service as those in the community, despite having significant and complex health care needs. Well-organized liaison services between care homes and community-based service providers, particularly rehabilitative services, could help support the remaining independence of people with dementia. There is also scope for policy within individual care home organizations to be proactive and address the ways that homes engage with local health care providers.

Research on how care practices and models of care can improve quality of life has provided some insights into improving life in care homes. Though much is known of effective care practice, much is still to be learned. Standards to guide support for person-centred care have been created, but more work is needed to accurately reflect the experiences of people with dementia.

Long-term care for older people with dementia is a diverse and complex service. In several countries, clear frameworks for person-centred principles and standards of care have been developed alongside expectations for staff training. However, these standards do not adequately address quality of life. There have been positive changes in the way in which people with dementia themselves are being consulted about their views about care and the need for them to be explicitly involved in planning their own care. The expectation that family members continue to be involved in the care of their relatives is also a welcome development. However, this has not been widely implemented.

Although the principles of person-centred care have been developing over the last 10–15 years, research has lagged behind in taking the person with dementia's perspective on their experience of care home life, focusing instead on symptom reduction and the observable outcomes of a variety of different practices. For research to adopt person-centred principles in a way that is encouraged in care practice, questions that address the individual's personal experience need to be explored. An obvious starting point is the experience of people with dementia, for whom there continues to be a paucity of information compared with family carers.

In increasingly multicultural societies, there is also a need for research to address the effects that the different cultural perspectives of both staff and residents have on the quality of care and quality of life in order to inform future education and training of the workforce to deliver excellence in dementia care.

Further information

The Alzheimer's Society in the UK and the Alzheimer's Association in the USA have web sites covering a range of topics. Several reports are available that address various aspects of living in and working in a care home [http://www.alzheimers.org.uk/; http://www.alz.org/].

The Royal National Institute of Blind People has a web site that includes reports and discussions about working with people who are blind and have dementia [http://www.rnib.org.uk].

Action on Hearing Loss (formerly the Royal National Institute of Deaf People) has a web site addressing hearing loss in general. As hearing loss is common in older adults, this information will pertain to many people with dementia [http://www.actiononhearingloss.org.uk].

Age UK has a web site that includes a wide array of topics relevant to older people. This includes pensions, lifelong learning, and a number of papers and discussion related to dementia. This web site would be useful to people with dementia, carers, and professionals [http://www.ageuk.org.uk/].

The National Institute for Health and Clinical Excellence (NICE) maintains a web site that addresses many health issues, including dementia. It is primarily for those working in the field [http://www.nice.org.uk/].

See also:

- ABC Health & Wellbeing [http://www.abc.net.au/health/].
- The UK Department of Health [https://www.gov.uk/government/organisations/department-of-health].
- The Social Care Institute for Excellence [http://www.scie.org.uk].
- Trinity College Dublin [http://www.socialwork-socialpolicy.tcd.ie/livingwithdementia/].

References

Alzheimer's Society (2010) *My Name is not Dementia*. London: Alzheimer's Society.

Australian Institute of Health and Welfare (AIHW) (2010) *Residential Aged Care in Australia 2008–09: A Statistical Overview*. Aged Care Statistics Series No. 31. Canberra, ACT: AIHW [https://www.aihw.gov.au/WorkArea/DownloadAsset.aspx?id=6442472719, accessed 3 March 2013].

Baldwin, C., Hope, T., Hughes, R., Jacoby, R. and Ziebland, S. (2005) *Making Difficult Decisions: The Experience of Caring for Someone with Dementia*. London: Alzheimer's Society.

Boyle, D. and Harris, M. (2009) *The Challenge of Co-production: How Equal Partnerships between Professionals and the Public are Crucial to Improving Public Services*. London: NESTA.

Briggs, K. and Bachelor, J. (2004) What are the core values of care?, *Journal of Dementia Care*, 12: 14–15.

Brodaty, H. and Cummings, A (2010) Dementia services in Australia, *International Journal of Geriatric Psychiatry*, 25: 887–95.

Brooker, D. (2007) *Person-centred Dementia Care: Making Services Better*. London: Jessica Kingsley.

Brooker, D. and Woolley, R. (2006) *Enriching Opportunities. Unlocking Potential: Searching for the Keys. Summary of a Developmental Evaluation*. Bradford: Extra Care Charitable Trust and Bradford Dementia Group.

Buettner, L. and Fitzsimmons, S. (2009) *NEST Approach: Needs, Environment, Stimulation, Techniques. Dementia Practice Guidelines for Disturbed Behaviors*. Palo Alto, CA: Venture Publishing.

Cahill, S. and Diaz, A. (2010) *Living in a Nursing Home: Quality of Life, The Priorities of Older People with a Cognitive Impairment*. Dublin: Trinity College Dublin, School of Social Work and Social Policy [http://livingwithdementia.tcd.ie/assets/pdf/Quality%20of%20Life%20in%20Nursing%20Homes.pdf, accessed 29 April 2014].

Care Services Improvement Partnership (2007) *Strengthening the Involvement of People with Dementia Toolkit*. London: Department of Health.

Caron, C. and Bowers, B. (2003) Deciding whether to continue, share, or relinquish caregiving: caregiver views, *Qualitative Health Research*, 13: 1252–71.

Centres for Medicare and Medicaid Services (2012) *CMS 2012 Nursing Home Action Plan*. Baltimore, MD: Department of Health and Human Services.

Chalfont, G. (2005) *Architecture, Nature and Care: The Importance of Connecting to Nature with Reference to Older People and Dementia*. Sheffield: School of Architecture, University of Sheffield.

Chung, J.C., Lai, C.K., Chung, P.M. and French, H.P. (2002) Snozelen for dementia, *Cochrane Database of Systematic Reviews*, 4: CD003152.

Clare, L., Rowlands, J., Bruce, E., Surr, C. and Downs, M. (2008) "I don't do like I used to do": a grounded theory approach to conceptualising awareness in people with moderate to severe dementia living in long-term care, *Social Science and Medicine*, 66: 2366–77.

Cohen-Mansfield, J. (2001) Nonpharmacologic interventions for inappropriate behaviours in dementia: a review, summary and critique, *American Journal of Geriatric Psychiatry*, 9: 361–81.

Cohen-Mansfield, J., Marx, M., Thein, K. and Dakheel-Ali, M. (2010a) The impact of past and present preferences on stimulus engagement in nursing home residents with dementia, *Aging and Mental Health*, 14(1): 67–73.

Cohen-Mansfield, J., Marx, M., Dakheel-Ali, M., Reiger, N. and Thein, K. (2010b) Can persons with dementia be engaged with stimuli?, *American Journal of Geriatric Psychiatry*, 18(4): 351–62.

Davies, S. and Nolan, M. (2003) "Making the best of things": relatives' experiences of decisions about care home entry, *Ageing and Society*, 23: 429–50.

Davies, S. and Nolan, M. (2006) "Making it better": self-perceived roles of family caregivers of older people living in care homes – a qualitative study, *International Journal of Nursing Studies*, 43(3): 281–91.

Day, K., Carreon, D. and Stump, C. (2000) Therapeutic design of environments for people with dementia: a review of the empirical research, *The Gerontologist*, 40: 397–416.

Department of Health (2009) *Living Well with Dementia: A National Dementia Strategy.* London: Department of Health [https://www.gov.uk/government/publications/living-well-with-dementia-a-national-dementia-strategy, accessed 29 April 2014].

Duffy, B., Oyebode, J. and Allen, J. (2009) Burnout among care staff for older adults with dementia: the role of reciprocity, self-efficacy and organizational factors, *Dementia*, 8(4): 515–41.

Edvardsson, D., Fetherstonhaugh, D. and Nay, D. (2010) Promoting a continuation of self and normality: person-centred care as described by people with dementia, their family members and aged care staff, *Journal of Clinical Nursing*, 19 (17/18): 2611–18.

Fahey, T., Montgomery, A.A., Barnes, J. and Prothero, J. (2003) Quality of care for elderly residents in nursing homes and elderly people living alone: controlled observational study, *British Medical Journal*, 326: 580–3.

Feliciano, L. and Vore, J. (2004) Decreasing entry into a restricted area using a visual barrier, *Journal of Applied Behaviour Analysis*, 37: 107–10.

Flannery, R.B. (2002) Treating learned helplessness in the elderly dementia patient: preliminary enquiry, *American Journal of Alzheimer's Disease and Other Dementias*, 17: 345–9.

Fleming, R., Crookes, P. and Shum, S. (2008) *A Review of the Empirical Literature on the Design of Physical Environments for People with Dementia.* Research Online Repository for the University of Wollongong [research-pubs@uow.edu.au].

Fossey, J. and James, I. (2008) *Evidenced Based Approaches to Improving Dementia Care in Care Homes.* London: Alzheimer's Society.

Gaugler, J.E. (2005) *Promoting Family Involvement in Long-term Care Settings: A Guide to Programs that Work.* Baltimore, MD: Health Professions Press.

Gerritson, D.L., Steverink, N., Ooms, M.E. and Ribbe, M.W. (2004) Finding a useful conceptual basis for enhancing the quality of life of nursing home residents, *Quality of Life Research*, 13: 611–24.

Gilmore-Bykovskyi, A.L. and Bowers, B.J. (2013) Understanding nurses' decisions to treat pain in nursing home residents with dementia, *Research in Gerontological Nursing*, 6(2): 127–38.

Glasby, J., Robinson, S. and Allen, K. (2012) *Achieving Closure: Good Practice in Supporting People during Residential Care Closure.* A joint publication by the Health Service Management Centre, University of Birmingham and The Association of Directors of Adult Social Services in association with the Social Care Institute for Excellence. Birmingham: University of Birmingham.

Glendinning, C., Jacobs, S., Alborz, A. and Hann, M. (2002) A survey of access to medical services in nursing and residential homes in England, *British Journal of General Practice*, 52(480): 545–8.

Hancock, G., Woods, B., Challis, D. and Orrell, M. (2006) The needs of older people with dementia in residential care, *International Journal of Geriatric Psychiatry*, 21: 43–9.

Hughes, J.C. and Louw, S.J. (2002) Electronic tagging of people with dementia who wander, *British Medical Journal*, 325: 847–8.

Husebo, B.S., Ballard, C., Sandvik, R., Nilsen, O.B. and Aarsland, D. (2011) Efficacy of treating pain to reduce behavioural disturbances in residents of nursing homes with dementia: cluster randomised clinical trial, *British Medical Journal*, 343: d4065.

Hussein, S. and Manthorpe, J. (2011) The dementia social care workforce in England: secondary analysis of a national workforce dataset, *Aging and Mental Health*, 16(1): 110–18.

James, I. (2010) *Cognitive Behavior Therapy with Older People: Interventions for Those With and Without Dementia.* London: Jessica Kingsley.

James, I. (2011) *Understanding Behavior in Dementia that Challenges.* London: Jessica Kingsley.

James, I.A., Powell, I., Smith, T. and Fairbairn, A. (2003) Lying to residents: can the truth sometimes be unhelpful for people with dementia?, *PSIGE Newsletter*, 82: 26–8.

James, I.A., MacKenzie, L. and Mukaetova-Ladinska, E. (2006) Doll use in care homes for people with dementia, *International Journal of Geriatric Psychiatry*, 21: 1093–8.

Jirovec, M.M. (1991) Effects of individualised prompted toileting on incontinence in nursing home residents, *Applied Nursing Research*, 4: 188–91.

Kane, R., Keckhafer, G., Flood, S., Bershadsky, B. and Siadaty, S. (2003) The effect of Evercare on hospital use, *Journal of the American Geriatrics Society*, 51(10): 1427–34.

Kitwood, T. (1997) *Dementia Reconsidered: The Person Comes First.* Buckingham: Open University Press.

Knapp, M., Comas-Herrera, A., Somani, A. and Banerjee, S. (2007) *Dementia: International Comparisons.* Summary Report for the National Audit Office. London: PSSRU.

Koren, M. (2010) Person-centered care for nursing home residents: the Culture Change Movement, *Health Affairs*, 29(2): 312–17.

Kuske, B., Hanns, S., Luck, T., Angermeyer, M., Behrens, J. *et al.* (2007) Nursing home staff training in dementia care: a systematic review of evaluated programs, *International Psychogeriatrics*, 19: 818–41.

Lawrence, V., Samsi, K., Banerjee, J., Morgan, C. and Murray, J. (2010) Threat to valued elements of life: the experience of dementia across three ethnic groups, *The Gerontologist*, 51(1): 39–50.

Lawrence, V., Fossey, J., Ballard, C., Moniz-Cook, E. and Murray, J. (2012) Improving quality of life for people with dementia in care homes: making psychosocial interventions work, *British Journal of Psychiatry*, 201: 344–51.

Lum, T., Kane, R., Cutler, L. and Yu, T. (2008/9) Effects of Green House® nursing homes on residents' families, *Health Care Financing Review*, 30(2): 35–51.

McKee, K., Downs, M., Gilhooly, M., Gilhooly, K., Tester, S. *et al.* (2005) Frailty, identity and the quality of later life, in A. Walker (ed.) *Understanding Quality of Life in Older Age.* Maidenhead: Open University Press.

Menard, J. (2008) *Commission nationale chargée de l'élaboration de propositions pour un plan national concernant la maladie d'alzheimer et les maladies apparentées, Alzheimer's Plan* [http://www.alzheimer-europe.org/Policy-in-Practice2/National-Dementia-Plans/France#fragment-1, accessed 29 April 2014].

Miller, M. (2009) *Clinician's Guide to Interpersonal Psychotherapy in Late Life: Helping Cognitively Impaired or Depressed Elders and their Caregivers.* Oxford: Oxford University Press.

Mold, F., Fitzpatrick, J.M. and Roberts, J.D. (2005) Minority ethnic elders in care homes: a review of the literature, *Age and Ageing*, 34(2): 107–13.

Moniz-Cook, E.D., Swift, K., James, I., Malouf, R., De Vugt, M. *et al.* (2012) Functional analysis-based interventions for challenging behaviour in dementia, *Cochrane Database of Systematic Reviews*, 2: CD006929.

National Institute for Health and Clinical Excellence (NICE) (2011) Dementia: Supporting People with Dementia and their Carers in Health and Social Care. Clinical Guideline No. 42. London: NICE [http://publications.nice.org.uk/dementia-cg42, accessed 29 April 2014].

Neal, M. and Barton Wright, P. (2003) Validation therapy for dementia, *Cochrane Database of Systematic Reviews*, 3: CD001394.

Nolan, M., Davies, S. and Grant, G. (2001) *Working with Older People and their Families: Key Issues in Policy and Practice.* Buckingham: Open University Press.

O'May, F. (2007) Transitions into a care home, in Help the Aged (ed.) *My Home Life: Quality of Life in Care Homes – A review of the Literature.* London: Help the Aged [http://www.scie.org.uk/publications/guides/guide15/files/myhomelife-litreview.pdf, accessed 29 April 2014].

Parsons, S., Simmons, W., Penn, K. and Furlough, M. (2003) Determinants of satisfaction and turnover among nursing assistants: the results of a statewide survey, *Journal of Gerontological Nursing*, 29: 393–410.

Perkins, J., Bartlett, H., Travers, C. and Rand, J. (2008) Dog-assisted therapy for older people with dementia: a review, *Australasian Journal on Ageing*, 27(4): 177–82.

Quince, C. (2013) *Low Expectations: Attitudes on Choice, Care and Community for People with Dementia in Care Homes.* London: Alzheimer's Society.

Reed, J., Cook, G., Sullivan, A. and Burridge, C. (2003) Making a move: care-home residents' experiences of relocation, *Ageing and Society*, 23(2): 225–41.

Reimer, M.A., Slaughter, S., Donaldson, C., Currie, G. and Eliasziw, M. (2004) Special care facility compared with traditional environments for dementia care: a longitudinal study of quality of life, *Journal of the American Geriatrics Society*, 52(7): 1085–92.

Robinson, J. and Banks, P. (2005) *Care Services Enquiry: The Business of Caring*. London: King's Fund.

Rokstad, A.M.M., Vatne, S., Engedal, K. and Selbaek, G. (2013) The role of leadership in the implementation of person centred care using Dementia Care Mapping: a study in three nursing homes, *Journal of Nursing Management*, 1: 1–12.

Rolland, Y., Pillard, F. and Klapouszczak, A. (2007) Exercise program for nursing home residents with Alzheimer's disease: a 1-year randomized, controlled trial, *Journal of the American Geriatrics Society*, 55: 158–62.

Royal College of Nursing (RCN) (2011) *Older People in Care Homes: Sex, Sexuality and Intimate Relationships*. An RCN discussion and guidance document for the nursing workforce. London: RCN.

Shippee, T.P. (2009) "But I am not moving": residents' perspectives on transitions within a continuing care retirement community, *The Gerontologist*, 49(3): 418–27.

Spector, A., Orrell, M., Davies, S. and Woods, B. (2002) Reality orientation for dementia, *Cochrane Database of Systematic Reviews*, 3: CD001119.

Spector, A., Woods, B. and Orrell, M. (2008). Cognitive stimulation for the treatment of Alzheimer's disease, *Expert Review of Neurotherapeutics*, 8(5): 751–7.

Spilsbury, K. and Meyer, J. (2004) Use, misuse and non-use of health care assistants: understanding the work of health care assistants in a hospital setting, *Journal of Nursing Management*, 12: 411–18.

Teri, L., Huda, P., Gibbons, L., Young, H. and van Leynseele, J. (2005) STAR: a dementia-specific training program for staff in assisted living residences, *The Gerontologist*, 45(5): 686–93.

Thompson, R. (2010) Realizing the potential: developing life story work in practice, *Foundation of Nursing Studies Dissemination Series*, 5(5). [http://www.dementiauk.org/assets/files/info_and_support/Realising_the_potential, accessed 2 June 2014].

Train, G., Nurock, S., Kitchen, G., Manela, M. and Livingston, G. (2005) A qualitative study of the views of residents with dementia, their relatives and staff about work practice in long term care settings, *International Psychogeriatrics*, 17: 237–51.

Tuckett, A. (2004) Truth-telling in clinical practice and the arguments for and against: a review of the literature, *Nursing Ethics*, 11: 500–13.

Van Doorn, C., Gruber-Baldini, A., Zimmerman, S., Hebel, J.R., Port, C. *et al.* (2003) Dementia as a risk factor for falls and fall injuries among nursing home residents, *Journal of the American Geriatrics Society*, 51(9): 1214–18.

Van Hoof, J., Kort, H., van Waarde, H.and Blom, M. (2010) Environmental interventions and the design of homes for older adults with dementia: an overview, *American Journal of Alzheimer's Disease and Other Dementias*, 25(3): 202–32.

Vasse, E., Vernooij-Dassen, M., Spijker, A., Olde-Rikkert, M. and Koopmans, R. (2010) A systematic review of communication strategies for people with dementia in residential and nursing homes, *International Psychogeriatrics*, 22(2): 189–200.

Verbeek, H., van Rossum, E., Zwakhalen, S.M., Kempen, G.I. and Hamers, J.P. (2009) Small, homelike care environments for older people with dementia: a literature review, *International Psychogeriatrics*, 21(2): 252–64.

Verkaik, R., van Weert, J. and Franke, A. (2006) The effects of psychosocial methods on depressed, aggressive and apathetic behaviours of people with dementia: a systematic review, *International Journal of Geriatric Psychiatry*, 20: 301–14.

Vink, A.C. and Birks, J.S. (2003) Music therapy for people with dementia, *Cochrane Database of Systematic Reviews*, 3: CD003477.

Welsh, S., Hassiotis, A., Mahoney, G. and Deahl, M. (2003) Big brother is watching you – the ethical implications of electronic surveillance measures in the elderly with dementia and in adults with learning difficulties, *Aging and Mental Health*, 7: 372–5.

Werezak, L.J. and Morgan, D.G. (2003) Creating therapeutic psychosocial environments in dementia care: a preliminary framework, *Journal of Gerontological Nursing*, 29: 18–25.

Wilkinson, N., Srikumar, S., Shaw, K. and Orrell, M. (1998) Drama and movement therapy in dementia: a pilot study, *Arts in Psychotherapy*, 25(3): 195–201.

Willemse, B.M., Smit, D., de Lange, J. and Pot, A.M. (2011) Nursing home care for people with dementia and residents' quality of life, quality of care and staff well-being: design of the Living Arrangement for people with Dementia (LAD) study, *BioMed Central Geriatrics*, 11(1): 11 [http://www.biomedcentral.com/1471-2318/11/11, accessed 29 April 2014].

Woods, B., Spector, A., Jones, C., Orrell, M. and Davies, S. (2005) Reminiscence therapy for dementia, *Cochrane Database of Systematic Reviews*, 2: CD001120.

World Health Organization (WHO) (2012) *Dementia: A Public Health Priority*. Geneva: WHO [http://www.who.int/mental_health/publications/dementia_report_2012/en/, accessed 29 April 2014].

Zetteler, J. (2008) Effectiveness of simulated presence therapy for individuals with dementia: a systematic review and meta-analysis, *Aging and Mental Health*, 12(6): 779–85.

Zgola, J.M. (1999) *Care that Works: A Relationship Approach to Persons with Dementia*. Baltimore, MD: Johns Hopkins University Press.

CHAPTER 25

Palliative care

Katherine Froggatt and Claire Goodman

> ❝I remember when she got to the stage in her illness when it was no longer possible to take her out of the care home, I would visit and used this time to sit and talk with Nana, brush her hair or give her a hand massage. These activities always seemed to have a calming effect on her, we would sit in a quiet room and although I'm sure she no longer understood what I was talking about, I used a calm softly spoken voice, a genuine smile and eye contact to help reassure and sooth Nana.❞
>
> —Shelley Angelique Cooper, Yorkshire, UK

> ❝David died on a sunny morning at home, 12 years after being diagnosed, the doors to the garden open to let in the sound of the birds singing as he had always loved nature.❞
>
> —Gillian Watson, Yorkshire, UK

> ❝When my mother eventually died, which was early one morning, I was called to the home and went with my daughter. I had never in my life at the time seen any person dead. The sister on duty said to me would I like to see my mother. I quickly said 'no' to which she said, and very kindly, 'I think you ought.' I will always be grateful to that nurse.❞
>
> —Geoff Redman, Yorkshire, UK

Learning objectives

By the end of this chapter, you will:

- Recognize that people living with dementia also die with dementia, even if this is not the primary cause of death
- Understand what we mean by palliative care for people with dementia and their families in different places of care, and its links with person-centred dementia care
- Recognize the relatively underdeveloped evidence base that guides palliative care
- Appreciate the challenges associated with advanced planning for care towards the end of life
- Critically review the evidence base for palliative pain assessment and treatment

Introduction

People can live many years with dementia, eventually dying from the consequences of dementia or from other causes. Palliative care is an appropriate way to ensure optimal care for people with dementia and their families from diagnosis until the end of life. In this chapter, we describe experiences of dying for people with dementia and their families in different settings where care is provided (domestic homes, care homes, hospitals). We provide a working definition of palliative care, distinguishing it from end-of-life care and terminal care, and identify ways in which optimal palliative care is provided. We provide an overview of two key aspects of palliative care for people with dementia: (1) advance care planning and (2) the detection and management of pain.

Dying with dementia

A diagnosis of dementia for a person will result in them dying with dementia, regardless of the primary cause of death. The length of survival from diagnosis to death varies by gender and age, with a population median survival time of 4.1 years (Xie *et al.* 2008). While dementia has been identified as one of the leading causes of death, it is difficult to ascertain exact figures for the numbers of deaths from dementia, as it is under-reported on death certificates. Estimates from the UK suggest that approximately 100,000 people with dementia die each year (Bayer 2006), and one in three people over 65 years die with dementia in the USA (Alzheimer's Association 2013).

Cox and Cook (2002) identify three ways in which people with dementia can die. First, there are people who have a diagnosis of dementia, but their death is caused by another medical condition, for example, cancer or heart disease. Second, people may die from the interplay of another illness and dementia, where the dementia has not affected their functioning. Third, there are people who are described as having end-stage dementia, where the associated consequences of the dementia impact all domains of their life and they ultimately die of the complications of this condition. For example, with increased immobility and the loss of a swallowing reflex, there is a greater incidence of infections, which may ultimately be fatal.

Each of these different ways will directly influence the place and experience of death for an individual and their family members. People with dementia will live and die in a range of settings: hospitals, nursing or residential care homes (long-term care settings), and domestic homes. As the illness progresses for people with dementia, so the increased need for physical care and greater accommodation of behavioural changes may necessitate a change in the place of residence and care. Some people with advanced dementia may need to move into long-term care facilities such as nursing homes or residential care homes (Milne and Dening 2011). People with dementia may sometimes be transferred to hospital following an exacerbation of a chronic condition or an accident, leading to their death in an acute setting. The place of death varies greatly between European countries, with the greatest proportion of people with dementia dying in nursing homes (Houttekier *et al.* 2010), a pattern also seen in the USA (Mitchell *et al.* 2005).

Domestic homes

Even as they become frailer and more cognitively impaired, some individuals may be able to remain in their own homes. They are increasingly reliant on the availability of formal and informal sources of community support. The provision of palliative care for older people with dementia in primary care is provided by a range of nursing services working in collaboration with general practitioners and consultants in palliative medicine. We know relatively little about family provision of palliative care at home, as it is not reported in the academic literature (Diwan *et al.* 2004). Few studies to date have addressed carers' needs and assessed carers' input, issues of the environment, the possibilities and experiences with home care, and overall decision-making processes in this setting.

> ## Case example 25.1: Gracie
>
> Gracie was a lady in her seventies with multi-infarct dementia. When her husband was no longer able to cope, she was admitted to a nursing home from her own home. She did not settle, began to lose weight, and showed signs of distress in the setting. Her wider family decided to move her from the nursing home to their home, where she lived for eight years before she died. Using a team of carers, alongside the introduction of specific appliances to assist with lifting, washing, toileting, and feeding, a committed family were able to care for their mother/mother-in-law over many years until her death.
>
> *Source*: Treloar (2006)

Care homes

In care homes, whether they provide on-site nursing care or rely on off-site nursing support, while dying is an expected final outcome, it is not the reason for receiving care and support. Care homes rely on primary health care services for medical support and specialist nursing care. Yet older people in care homes have variable and often inequitable access to state health services such as allied health support, including physiotherapy and occupational therapy (Gage *et al*. 2012). There are also regional variations with regard to hospice and palliative care services for this population, often reflecting differences in local policies and funding. The need for a more strategic proactive approach when providing palliative care in these settings has been highlighted (Goodman *et al*. 2010). This approach to providing palliative care in these settings is being developed in many countries through the introduction of nationally supported palliative care frameworks such as the Gold Standards Framework in the UK (Department of Health 2008).

Hospitals

Hospital care for people with dementia is not always appropriately delivered People with dementia with palliative care needs do not receive the same level of support as people without dementia with the same palliative care needs (Sampson *et al*. 2006). Staff on general hospital wards often lack dementia awareness knowledge leading to inappropriate care for the person with dementia and their family (see Chapters 22 and 29).

   Given the challenges of supporting people as they die with dementia, wherever they live and are cared for, a clear understanding of palliative care and what it offers in terms of care is important. Recognizing dementia as a terminal condition is the beginning of identifying and addressing future issues (van der Steen *et al*. 2013).

Defining palliative care

Palliative care focuses upon the support of people as they live and die with life-limiting illnesses. The origins of palliative care lie with the modern hospice movement. Since the 1960s in the UK, a range of hospice and palliative care services have developed, including inpatient, day, and home care services. The hospice movement initially addressed the needs of people with cancer. Recent expansion and diversification in the specialty have sought to address the needs of people dying with other conditions, including dementia, as illustrated in the World Health Organization (WHO) definition for palliative care, which is not disease specific:

> ❝An approach that improves the quality of life of patients and their families facing the problems associated with life-threatening illness, through the prevention and relief of suffering by means of early identification and impeccable assessment and treatment of pain and other problems, physical, psychosocial and spiritual.❞
>
> —Sepulveda *et al.* (2002: 91)

Palliative care is often associated with care as a person is dying. Yet for effective palliative care, intervention and support need to be considered early on and throughout a person's life with any life-limiting condition. For the person with dementia, this could begin at diagnosis (Small *et al.* 2007). For example, future planning about care preferences can begin to be raised then.

We use the term "palliative care" in this chapter to mean an approach to care over a long period. We recognize that different understandings for this term exist between health care and social care professionals, both within and between countries (Radbruch and Payne 2009). This can lead to different emphases in care provision.

General and specialist palliative care

There is a distinction between general palliative care and specialist palliative care (Radbruch and Payne 2009). General palliative care is provided by health and social care professionals to individuals in whatever care setting they find themselves. This is the type of palliative care that all people living with dementia could expect to receive, as their needs change, from their usual care providers. For people with dementia, this may include mental health professionals and health and social care staff supporting them at home or in a long-term care setting. It will also include their general practitioner who provides the medical advice and guide treatments.

Specialist palliative care teams can support these generalist staff to deliver this care. These professionals provide specialist palliative care for people with unresolved symptoms, or complex psychosocial, end-of-life or bereavement issues. Specialist palliative care may be provided in dedicated settings such as hospices, but also in hospitals, people's homes, and long-term care facilities. Historically, people with dementia have had limited access to specialist palliative care services, with some exceptions in the USA. Increasingly, the engagement between specialist palliative care practitioners and the usual providers of care to people with dementia is on a partnership model. The expertise of both parties is required to ensure that the needs of a person with dementia when dying are addressed appropriately (Small *et al.* 2007).

The terms "end-of-life care" and "terminal care" are also used. End-of-life care is a term used in the USA and UK to mean care provided in the final one to two years of life, but in other countries is used to mean the care provided in the last few days of life when an individual is actively dying, and is synonymous with the term "terminal care" (Radbruch and Payne 2009).

The principles of whole person treatment, comfort, support, and person-directed care promoted by the palliative care movement align closely with person-centred dementia care. Both approaches share similar concerns: care for the whole person, encompassing their physical, emotional, social, and spiritual needs; quality of life and quality of living until a person dies; and the people with whom the person has close relationships, be they family, friends, or care staff (Downs *et al.* 2006).

Exercise 25.1: Providing information to family members about palliative care

As a manager you are writing a leaflet for family members about the care you provide for people with dementia. Your care home wants to provide good palliative care for all its residents, recognizing this approach to care can support people with dementia with their physical, emotional, and spiritual needs. However, recent press coverage about care for dying people in institutions has confused palliative care interventions with treatments to hasten death.

■   How would you describe the care you provide to help explain the benefits for people with dementia and their families?

Limited evidence base to guide care

There is limited robust, high-quality research on palliative care interventions to guide care for people with dementia (Goodman *et al.* 2010; van der Steen 2010). Most research has been conducted in specialist units and hospice settings, to which few people with dementia have access. A recent review of palliative care for community-dwelling older people with dementia noted that the identification of good-quality outcome indicators for this population is problematic (Goodman *et al.* 2010). The most robust measures available were in the areas of symptoms and symptom control (particularly pain), quality of life and satisfaction. Significant gaps existed in the evidence base on continuity of care, advance care planning, spiritual needs, and caregiver well-being. A large number of outcome measures are used in research but not used consistently across studies, so comparisons are difficult and the relevance for care providers is not clear. Their appropriateness for this population needs further examination.

The evidence for effective care interventions is not yet strong for people with dementia towards the end of life. Reliance solely on evidence about individual patients' experiences, while important, may avoid addressing wider system issues of care provision, policy, and funding. Evidence for culture change of care environments and wider health and social care systems is also required.

The methodological challenges of researching palliative care mean that evaluations usually rely on post-bereavement views of relatives and secondary analysis of patient notes. Prognostication and the management of specific symptoms appear to be given greater weight than a focus on a holistic process and care planning for a good ending. An emphasis on survival analysis and prognostication has also meant that little is known about how individuals themselves engage with the anticipation of dying.

Although there are significant ethical and methodological challenges of undertaking research with people with dementia, the scope and range of evidence that is able to directly influence practice are disappointing. There are a lack of intervention-based studies, lack of consistency across studies as to definitions of palliative care, and very few examples of evidence from people with dementia themselves with an over-reliance on proxy or retrospective accounts and data. Palliative care for someone with dementia is as likely to involve decision-making about not doing things, such as aggressively treating certain conditions, as acting upon specific symptoms. Although this is discussed extensively in practice and professional literature, there is little research that makes explicit how this is addressed and the consequences for patients and carers. This ambiguity may lead to unclear pathways for care and sub-optimal distribution of resources. The consequences of a lack of evidence may contribute to a poor quality of life for people with dementia and their carers, and inappropriate and costly responses to the problems that emerge at the end of life, which can then result in hospital admissions and further disablement. To ensure that the needs and expectations of people with dementia and their families are met, and that good-quality palliative care is provided, there is a need for further research and staff training across and between dementia and specialist palliative care.

Advance care planning for end of life and dying

A key element in the national End of Life Care Strategy (Department of Health 2008) and National Dementia Strategy (Department of Health 2009) for England is that people should be involved in planning their care and in decisions about their place of care and ultimately death. In England, advance care planning within the health and social care context focuses upon three types of care planning:

- information about personal wishes and preferences (for guidance but with no legal status)
- a legally binding advanced decision to refuse treatment
- the nomination of proxy decision-makers

These processes are all undertaken and enacted under the guidance of country-specific mental capacity legislation (Henry and Seymour 2008). For example, in England and Wales, the Mental Capacity Act 2005 came into force in 2007 and provides:

> a statutory framework for people who lack capacity to make decisions for themselves, or who have capacity and want to make preparations for a time when they may lack capacity in the future. It sets out who can take decisions, in which situations, and how they should go about this.

—Department for Constitutional Affairs (2007: 1)

The well-documented delays and difficulties in making and conveying a diagnosis of dementia to the person and their family (see Chapter 19), however, mean that timely discussion and planning for future treatment and care often cannot take place (Robinson *et al.* 2012). Leaving discussions until people are in need of greater support and care, such as a move into a long-term care setting, may be too late to fully involve the person with dementia (Small *et al.* 2007; Robinson *et al.* 2012). As such, facilitating people with dementia to retain autonomy and to exercise choice about their care, treatment, and place of death needs to be undertaken while they still retain capacity to be fully involved.

Advance care planning not only requires early diagnosis, it also requires a degree of comfort and facility with having conversations about the options at end of life. All care workers who engage with people with dementia need to be aware of dementia as a terminal illness. For people with dementia, everyday preferences and identification of significant family carers can and should inform how advance care plans are reviewed and updated (Goodman *et al.* 2013). At any point in the illness, people with dementia and their family members may need information about, and support for, dying and end-of-life issues. Health and social care staff need to feel able to initiate conversations about dying, and be comfortable with the topic, to ensure that adequate support and care is provided at the time, or later on, as the person's health deteriorates. As the person with dementia becomes more cognitively disabled, the emphasis will be upon discussions with family members, who may have legal authority to make decisions, and wish to be included in discussion and medical decision-making that will affect end-of-life care practices, especially in times of crisis.

Case example 25.2: Family discussions in care homes

Professionals working in and together with care homes support people with dementia to die in those homes through discussions with care home staff and family members about what they can do.

One family member noted how the district nurse's involvement had been instrumental in enabling their mother to die in the care home: "They knew my mother didn't want to go into hospital, they knew what the situation was, um and they . . . the home felt . . . When she spoke to me about, when [the deputy manager] spoke to me about mother going to hospital, I said 'can you care for her in the home? Have you got enough you know' . . . and she said 'yes, we have, with the district nurses coming in'."

One outcome of these discussions was described by a care home manager: "Yeah, basically, he [family member] doesn't want his mum to go to hospital, so it's not so much a 'Do Not Resuscitate' [as a] 'Don't Call Paramedics – Call GP'."

Exercise 25.2: Planning end of life with a person with dementia you work with

Think of someone with dementia with whom you work or who you know. Thinking over your various conversations and interactions with them, has there ever been a time where they discussed or introduced the idea of their own death? What was it they said? How did you feel? What did you say in reply? What did you do?

You may find when you think about these conversations that people with dementia think about their own death more than you had realized. How difficult was it for you as a member of staff or other colleagues to engage with the person about these issues?

Pain assessment and management

The dementia illness trajectory is one of progressive deterioration with acute episodes of care (Lunney *et al.* 2003), and patients at the end of their life frequently require 24-hour care either in long-stay hospital wards or in nursing homes (Hall *et al.* 2011).

The prevalence of pain in elderly nursing home residents is estimated to be 40–80% (Zwakhalen *et al.* 2006). Pain assessment in people with dementia can be complicated by memory loss, personality changes, and loss of judgement, abstract thinking and communication skills. Additionally, behaviours commonly associated with pain may be absent or difficult to interpret. However, aggressive behaviours may be a response by people with dementia who are not able to articulate their pain verbally (Regnard *et al.* 2003).

There is evidence that pain assessment is inadequate and that people with dementia are being under-treated (Sampson *et al.* 2006; McAuliffe *et al.* 2009). In a study of people with dementia at home, Hirakawa *et al.* (2006) compared symptom experience and palliative care received by home patients based on cognitive function. After controlling for age and other differences in baseline characteristics, dementia was determined to be a significant independent predictor of incontinence or uncontrolled pain. People with dementia may be unable to inform nurses and professionals about levels of pain, or discomfort, as illustrated in case example 25.3.

Case example 25.3: Joe

"We knew that Joe was in pain, he tensed when we moved him in the bed and he grimaced and shouted and tried to push the care staff away. He could not settle and that was not like him. Even though he could not speak he could answer 'yes' or 'no' to simple questions. So I took a long hard look at him, at how he was lying in the bed and it seemed to me that one shoulder was hunched and his head was more on one side than normal. So I gently touched his neck and asked him if it hurt there. He grunted 'yes'. I think he may have been lying in one position too long. So we tried a heat pack on his neck, and started a pain chart that noted his reactions. He seemed to like the pad and the GP prescribed a stronger painkiller and in about an hour afterwards you could see he was more relaxed, his body less tense, and we were able to move him without him protesting."

—Care home carer

Studies have also pointed to what appears to be a lack of adequate professional training for pain management, leading to experiences as described in the case study above. In a survey of 68 UK nursing homes, 69% of homes did not have a written policy regarding pain management and 75% did not use a standardized pain assessment tool. In addition 40% of qualified staff and 85% of care assistants had no specialist knowledge regarding the management of pain in older people (Allcock *et al.* 2002).

The optimal pain assessment would be self-report but this is not always possible with people with dementia and proxy accounts from carers are often used. A recent systematic review to ascertain which behavioural pain assessment tools are available to assess pain in elderly people with dementia and what the psychometric qualities of these tools are (Zwakhalen *et al.* 2006), identified 12 observational pain assessment scales (see Box 25.1).

Box 25.1: Pain assessment scales for use with cognitively impaired adults

- DOLOPLUS-2
- L'Echelle Comportementale pour Personne Agées (ECPA) [Behavioural Scale for the Elderly]
- L'échelle Comportementale simplifiée (ECS) [Simplified Behavioural Scale]
- The Observational Pain Behavior Tool
- Checklist of Non-verbal Pain Indicators (CNPI)
- Pain Assessment Checklist for Seniors with Limited Ability to Communicate (PACSLAC)
- Pain Assessment in Advanced Dementia (PAINAD)
- Pain Assessment in Dementing Elderly (PADE)
- Rating Pain in Dementia (RaPID)
- The Abbey Pain Scale
- The Non-Communicative Patient's Pain Assessment Instrument (NOPPAIN)
- Pain Assessment Tool for Use with Cognitively Impaired Adults

Source: Zwakhalen *et al.* (2006)

Zwakhalen *et al.* (2006) found that most observational scales are still under development. Based on psychometric qualities, together with their sensitivity and clinical usefulness, the authors concluded that PACSLAC and DOLOPLUS2 were the most appropriate scales currently available. Further research is needed to improve these scales through further testing of their validity, reliability, and clinical utility.

Although such assessment tools exist for people with dementia, people are still suffering unnecessarily (Sampson *et al.* 2006) and clear treatment guidelines and training in pain management are required. Research and development is being undertaken internationally in this area (ee www.cost.eu/domains_actions/isch/Actions/TD1005).

Exercise 25.3: Pain in people with dementia towards the end of life

You have just taken the post of training manager in a long-term care facility for older people. Like many other facilities, many of your residents have dementia and differing levels of cognitive impairment. You are determined that residents' pain will be adequately assessed and that residents in your care home will have their pain effectively managed.

- How would you go about finding out how pain is currently being assessed and managed?
- What are three things you would do to improve the pain assessment and management of residents?

Debates and controversies

This chapter has addressed two issues related to palliative care for people with dementia: advance care planning and pain management. An underlying issue that threads through advance care planning, pain management, and other aspects of palliative care provision is the recognition that living and dying with dementia is characterized by uncertainty. There are accounts of people who were identified as dying who then lived for several more years, as well as those that document inappropriate hospital admissions when someone has only a few days left to live. The challenge for carers and professionals is finding ways to limit the uncertainty and make decisions according to what appears to be best for the person at the time. Therefore:

- *Is it appropriate to be raising issues of mortality and dying when a person is only just coming to terms with a diagnosis of dementia?* Not raising and addressing the implications of living and dying with a life-limiting illness can ultimately result in the person with dementia and their family carers receiving a poorer quality of care when dying, and care that is less likely to reflect that person's values and wishes. Knowing that uncertainty is present can act as a catalyst to prepare and have discussions in a timely way.
- *Is prognostication a central element of quality end-of-life care? Could some treatment and care decisions be made without the prognostication process?* Similarly, knowing when someone will die is often a key factor in determining palliative care treatment decisions. For people with dementia, whose disease progression is often long term and slow, this may detract from assessment of current needs and meeting them, regardless of whether a person is deemed to be "palliative" because it can be estimated they will die within a certain time span.

Conclusion

The recognition that people with dementia can benefit from palliative care is dependent upon an acknowledgement that people living with dementia will die with dementia. While this understanding is more widely accepted, there are still policy and practice challenges that lead to variable standards in the quality of care people with dementia receive, wherever they live and die. Advance care planning and pain management both exemplify the challenges around palliative care provision for people with dementia and support for family members. They both illustrate the importance of good communication, and the challenges of doing this early on and throughout the illness journey.

Current evidence falls short of describing, assessing, and responding to the experiences and expectations of people with dementia and their family carers for end-of-life care. The limited evidence available from professionals about care provision, and the lack of evidence from family carers requires further research to develop the provision of good-quality support for people with dementia who are coming to the end of their lives.

Further information

Age UK provides a useful factsheet on advance decisions, advance statements, and living wills [http://www.ageuk.org.uk/Documents/EN-GB/Factsheets/FS72_Advance_decisions_advance_statements_and_living_wills_fcs.pdf?dtrk=true].

The Alzheimer's Society provides a helpful overview of the Mental Capacity Act 2005, covering its five main principles, as well as best interests decision-making, planning for the future (including lasting power of attorney and advance decisions), Deputies and the Court of Protection, and safety measures (including independent mental capacity advocates and public guardians) [http://www.alzheimers.org.uk/site/scripts/documents_info.php?documentID=354].

The National Council for Palliative Care initiated a dementia project in 2007. Their reports on dementia can be found on their web site. This organization also sponsors workshops on palliative care and has speakers' presentations available to view. Publications about dementia include: *Out of the Shadows: End of Life Care for People with Dementia*, *The Power of Partnership: Palliative Care for People with Dementia*, and *How Would I Know, What Can I Do?* [www.ncpc.org.uk/dementia].

The Hospice Foundation of America provides general support and information regarding hospice care for people of all ages. They have published a report that is exclusively about hospice care for someone with dementia [www.hospicefoundation.org].

The Dying Well organization provides general advice on living to the fullest until the end of life. It is operated by Dr. Byock, MD, and includes a collection of his articles. Dr. Byock has been involved in hospice care since 1978. He is known for founding a hospice for indigent people in Fresno, California. He has received many awards for his work in hospice care [www.dyingwell.org]. Canadian Virtual Hospice provides information and resources for people and their family members facing life-limiting illnesses, including dementia [www.virtualhospice.ca].

The Social Care Institute for Excellence (SCIE) Dementia Gateway provides resources for people working in social care around all aspects of dementia including end-of-life care [http://www.scie.org.uk/publications/dementia/]. It includes SCIE information on pain experienced by people with advanced dementia plus resources and exercises. [www.scie.org.uk/publications/dementia/endoflife/pain.asp].

References

Allcock, N., McGarry, J. and Elkan, R. (2002) Management of pain in older people within the nursing home: a preliminary study, *Health and Social Care in the Community*, 10(6): 464–71.

Alzheimer's Association (2013) 2013 Alzheimer's disease facts and figures, *Alzheimer's and Dementia*, 9 (2).

Bayer, A. (2006) Death with dementia – the need for better care, *Age and Ageing*, 35(1): 1–12.

Cox, S. and Cook, A. (2002) Caring for people with dementia at the end of life, in J. Hockley and D. Clark (eds.) *Palliative Care for Older People in Care Homes*. Buckingham: Open University Press, pp. 86–103.

Department for Constitutional Affairs (2007) Mental Capacity Act 2005: Code of Practice. Norwich: TSO [http://www.direct.gov.uk/prod_consum_dg/groups/dg_digitalassets/@dg/@en/@disabled/documents/digitalasset/dg_186484.pdf, accessed 29 April 2014].

Department of Health (2008) *End of Life Care Strategy: Promoting High Quality Care for All Adults at the End of Life*. London: Department of Health [https://www.gov.uk/government/publications/end-of-life-care-strategy-promoting-high-quality-care-for-adults-at-the-end-of-their-life, accessed 29 April 2014].

Department of Health (2009) *Living Well with Dementia: A National Dementia Strategy*. London: Department of Health [https://www.gov.uk/government/publications/living-well-with-dementia-a-national-dementia-strategy].

Diwan, S., Hougham, G. and Sachs, G. (2004) Strain experienced by caregivers of dementia patients receiving palliative care: findings from the Palliative Excellence in Alzheimer Care Efforts (PEACE) program, *Journal of Palliative Medicine*, 7(6): 797–807.

Downs, M., Small, N. and Froggatt, K.A. (2006) Explanatory models and end of life care for people with dementia, *International Journal of Palliative Nursing*, 12(5): 209–13.

Gage, H., Dickinson, A., Victor, C.R., Williams, P., Cheynel, J. et al. (2012) Integrated working between residential care home and primary care: a survey of care homes in England, *BMC Geriatrics*, 12: 71.

Goodman, C., Evans, C., Wilcock, J., Froggatt, K., Drennan, V. et al. (2010) End of life care for community dwelling older people with dementia: an integrated review, *International Journal of Geriatric Psychiatry*, 25: 329–37.

Goodman, C., Amador, S., Elmore, N., Machen, I. and Mathie, E. (2013) Preferences and priorities for ongoing and end-of-life care: a qualitative study of older people with dementia resident in care homes, *International Journal of Nursing Studies*, 50(12): 1639–47.

Hall, S., Petkova, H., Tsouros, A.D., Costantini, M. and Higginson, I.J. (eds.) (2011) *Palliative Care for Older People: Better Practices*. Copenhagen: WHO.

Henry, C. and Seymour, J. (2008) *Advance Care Planning: A Guide for Health and Social Care Staff*. London: Department of Health.

Hirakawa, Y., Masuda, Y., Kuzuya, M., Kimata, T., Iguchi, A. et al. (2006) End-of-life experience of demented elderly patients at home: findings from DEATH project, *Psychogeriatrics*, 6(2): 60–7.

Houttekier, D., Cohen, J., Bilsen, J., Addington-Hall, J., Onwuteaka-Philipsen, B.D. et al. (2010) Place of death of older persons with dementia: a study in five European countries, *Journal of the American Geriatrics Society*, 58(4): 751–6.

Lunney, J.R., Lynn, J., Foley, D.S., Lipson, S. and Guralnik, J.M. (2003) Patterns of functional decline at the end of life, *Journal of the American Medical Association*, 289: 2387–92.

McAuliffe, L., Nay, R., O'Donnell, M. and Fetherstonhaugh, D. (2009) Pain assessment in older people with dementia: literature review, *Journal of Advanced Nursing*, 65(1): 2–10.

Milne, A. and Dening, T. (eds.) (2011) *Mental Health and Care Homes*. Oxford: Oxford University Press.

Mitchell, S.L., Teno, J.M., Miller, S.C. and Mor, V. (2005) A national study of the location of death for older persons with dementia, *Journal of the American Geriatrics Society*, 53(2): 299–305.

Radbruch, L., Payne, S. and EAPC Board of Directors (2009) White paper on standards and norms for hospice and palliative care in Europe: part 1, *European Journal of Palliative Care*, 16(6): 278–89.

Regnard, C., Mathews, D., Gibson, L., Clark, C. and Watson, B. (2003) Assessing distress in people with severe communication problems: piloting the Northgate DisDAT, *International Journal of Palliative Nursing*, 9: 173–6.

Robinson, L., Dickinson, C., Rousseau, N., Beyer, F., Clark, A. *et al.* (2012) A systematic review of the effectiveness of advance care planning interventions for people with cognitive impairment and dementia, *Age and Ageing*, 41(2): 263–9.

Sampson, E., Gould, V., Lee, D. and Blanchard, M. (2006) Differences in care received by patients with and without dementia who died during an acute hospital admission: a retrospective case note study, *Age and Ageing*, 35: 187–9.

Sepulveda, C., Marlin, A., Yohida, T. and Ullrich, A. (2002) Palliative care: the World Health Organization's global perspective, *Journal of Pain and Symptom Management*, 24(2): 91–6.

Small, N., Froggatt, K.A. and Downs, M. (2007) *Living and Dying with Dementia: Dialogues about Palliative Care.* Oxford: Oxford University Press.

Treloar, A. (2006) Hope for home: the terminal care of people with dementia at home, in *Palliative Care for People with Dementia*, Leveson Paper No. 12. West Midlands: The Foundation of Lady Katherine Leveson, Temple Balsall, pp. 10–15.

van der Steen, J.T. (2010) Dying with dementia: what we know after more than a decade of research, *Journal of Alzheimer's Disease*, 22(1): 37–55.

van der Steen, J., Radbruch, L., Hertogh, C.M.P.M., de Boer, M.E., Hughes, J.C. *et al.* (2013) White paper defining optimal palliative care in older people with dementia: a Delphi study and recommendations from the European Association for Palliative Care, *Palliative Medicine* [DOI: 10.1177/0269216313493685].

Xie, J., Brayne, C., Matthews, F.E. and the Medical Research Council Cognitive Function and Ageing Study Collaborators (2008) Survival times in people with dementia: analysis from population based cohort study with 14 year follow-up, *British Medical Journal*, 336: 258–62.

Zwakhalen, S.M., Hamers, J.P., Abu-Saad, H.H. and Berger, M.P. (2006) Pain in elderly people with severe dementia: a systematic review of behavioural pain assessment tools, *BMC Geriatrics*, 27(6): 3.

CHAPTER 26

Grief and bereavement

Jan Oyebode

> ❝I think that after the loss of someone you have cared for who has dementia, there are a lot of suppressed emotions, particularly as you have little or no verbal communication with the patient. I am sure that bereavement counselling is important for carers, and their families, in the aftermath of the loss of their relative.❞
>
> —Vivien Cooper Yorkshire, UK

> ❝The photograph album was a great success, as she recognized the faces in them even when she could not say who they were – particularly those of her four sons. But, some photographs upset her – these were often photographs of relatives that had died, or were from difficult episodes in her life.❞
>
> —Vivien Cooper Yorkshire, UK

> ❝On one of our regular visits to (name of town) pottery Nana managed to wander off without us realising (it happened very quickly). After searching for her in the shopping area and alerting the staff and police, I took the car to see if she had left the pottery and I eventually found her heading into town. I stopped the car, got out and attempted to persuade Nana to get in the car. She resisted at first, she was frightened and clearly couldn't remember who I was. Eventually I managed to gently convince her that I was her granddaughter and that her daughter-in-law was looking for her back at the shopping centre. Once we got back to (name of town) Pottery and just before we got out of the car, Nana grabbed my hand and looked at me, she had tears in her eyes. She said I hope you never get what I have, it is frightening to not remember anything. It was like her memory had suddenly allowed her a moment of clarity and she could see what was happening to her. She looked so sad and frightened in those few minutes and then just as quickly I saw the confusion appear in her eyes once again and she had forgotten once again.❞
>
> —Shelley Angelique Cooper Yorkshire, UK

Learning objectives

By the end of this chapter, you will:

- Be aware of the ways in which impaired cognitive functioning may affect responses to bereavement
- Know about ways to support people with dementia who are bereaved
- Be aware of the influences of anticipatory grief, chronic sorrow, caregiving, and separation through institutional care on those who experience the death of a relative with dementia
- Know about strategies that that may promote good adaptation and ways to help those who are most vulnerable

Introduction

The purpose of this chapter is to address how the best possible care and support can be provided to people with dementia who experience bereavement, and people who are bereaved of a relative with dementia.

The first part addresses the responses and needs of people with dementia and goes on to consider how we can support people with dementia who are bereaved. The second part considers the nature of bereavement when it is someone with dementia who has died, and includes a discussion about the ways people may react, the factors that influence reactions, and the role of professionals in providing support or care for families.

The experience of bereavement for people with dementia

The reactions of people with dementia who are bereaved of someone close to them are influenced by how their cognitive impairment affects their understanding and ability to process the event and its consequences. In responding, a primary goal is to enable the person to feel secure and supported. This primary goal informs (1) whether and how we work to enable the person to take in the news, (2) whether we facilitate expression of feelings, and (3) how we help the person to establish a new routine.

Issue	Mechanism	Consequence for person with dementia
Failure to take in the loss	Natural denial made worse by poor memory	Responds with renewed grief each time bereavement is rediscovered
		Invents an alternative explanation for absence (e.g. the person is at work or has been kidnapped)
Mistakes someone else for the deceased relative	Natural wish to restore the person compounded by poor memory and poor visual recognition	Mistakes, for example, son for husband or fellow resident for spouse
		Can be upsetting for person and awkward and embarrassing for others
Dwells on certain events or conversations, especially in early dementia	Natural rumination made worse by perseveration caused by impaired brain function	Focuses on and keeps repeating an account of one event, e.g. something said or done
		May involve self-blame or blame of others
Difficulty regulating and modulating emotions	Inhibition that is usually exercised is not maintained due to frontal lobe damage	Sorrow or anger may be openly and deeply expressed rather than restrained
Difficulty verbalizing feelings	Natural difficulty in voicing intimate feelings exacerbated by brain impairment in vocabulary and word-finding	Distress may be acted out in disturbed behaviour or expressed in metaphor

Source: Rentz *et al.* (2005) and Grief and Myran (2006)

Table 26.3 Responses to bereavement observed in people with dementia

This area has not been well researched but there is a good deal of clinical knowledge. As recently as 2010, Gataric and colleagues published a paper entitled "Reflections on the under-researched topic of grief in persons with dementia", yet they found that just over half the dementia professionals who attended their symposium reported that they frequently encountered a grieving person with dementia.

Rentz *et al.* (2005) and Grief and Myran (2006) provide a series of descriptions from cases in clinical practice about ways in which people with dementia respond to bereavement. Most are similar to how any of us might respond to the loss of someone close to us, but with the complicating layer of cognitive impairment. These are summarized in Table 26.1.

Supporting people with dementia who are bereaved

Worden's (1991) grief work hypothesis suggests that there are four tasks to be addressed in adjusting to bereavement: taking in the reality of the loss, experiencing the pain of separation, learning to live without the deceased, and emotionally relocating the deceased so as to be able to move on with life. The first three are considered below in relation to dementia, while consideration of the fourth is integrated throughout the discussion.

Taking in the reality of the loss

Whether and how to tell a person with dementia that their friend or relative has died is a difficult decision. Caregivers may be anxious about giving the news because they will be concerned about causing distress to the person with dementia or fear they will be unable to take it in (Rentz *et al.* 2005). It needs to be borne in mind that if the person is not informed, they will not be able to attend the funeral, wake or other rituals. If rituals are not attended, the person will not have the chance to take in the reality of the death, thus blocking the start of the usual process of grieving. This is therefore a decision that needs to be carefully thought through. It has been suggested that, in some cases, we disenfranchise those with dementia from grieving by not including them in the family and societal response to the death. It is worth noting that the experience of professionals in Gataric and colleagues' (2010) study was that people with dementia found being involved in discussions about funeral preparations to be soothing rather than distressing.

Generally, in early dementia, it is appropriate to tell the person and then judge whether or not they absorb the news. The issue becomes more acute if the person appears to forget, as we risk exposing them and ourselves to repeated distress every time we bring the loss to their attention (Grief and Myran 2006). Rentz and colleagues (2005) suggest it may be more important to consider the relief of sorrow at the expense of truth. In later dementia, it is unlikely the person will be able to take in the news, so it may not be appropriate for them to be told. Professionals involved in the person's care may be able to help families to think through these dilemmas and accept that there is only a reasonable – not a perfect – solution.

When it is important for the person to recognize and absorb that they have been bereaved, techniques used to address learning in dementia can be used (see case example 26.1 and Chapter 9). Reminders of the funeral, such as the order of service, shown and discussed in a supportive and sympathetic atmosphere, or talking about the person in the past tense, may be helpful.

> ## Case example 26.1: Helping an elderly woman take in that her niece had died
>
> Lewis and Trzinski (2006) describe an 87-year-old woman with mild dementia who was highly anxious as she knew "someone" had died. Her therapist used a spaced retrieval paradigm to help her understand it was her niece who had passed away. This involved reminding her who had died at gradually increasing intervals of time during two hour-long appointments. This helped her to take in the information. This reduced her high anxiety levels, and enabled her to grieve rather than keep re-experiencing initial grief.

Experiencing the pain of separation

Painful feelings are common after bereavement, accompanying emotional separation from the deceased. Professionals report that openly talking about the deceased, and simply "being there", can assist with expressions of sorrow and provide comfort (Gataric et al. 2010). However, the notion that *everyone* needs to grieve has been questioned (Bonanno et al. 2002; Rentz et al. 2005). Where someone with dementia is not grieving, do we have any justification for trying to prompt them to express their emotions? On the other hand, a person with dementia may show distress through problematic behaviour, due to an inability or lack of opportunity to express their feelings verbally. Where this is the case, it may be helpful to carry out systematic observation to determine whether there are particular factors triggering or maintaining grief (Rentz et al. 2005; see also Chapter 11). Identification of such factors might allow changes to be made to avoid the triggering of painful grief or to enable a more appropriate expression of grief (see case study 26.2). As well as behavioural/problem-solving approaches, psychotherapeutic or spiritually based approaches may also be helpful.

> ## Case example 26.2: Helping a distressed care home resident with severe dementia
>
> A care home resident screams whenever her son comes to see her, upsetting other residents, disturbing her son, and leaving herself distressed. Staff observe that this started after her husband died. They wonder if her screams are triggered because the sight of her son, looking so much like his father, reminds her of her bereavement. The staff and her son decide between them how they might help her to express her grief in a more beneficial way. They decide to make sure she knows when he is going to visit by showing her his photo just before visits and reminding her who he is. They invite her to move into her own room before he arrives, so the two of them have a private space. When he arrives, he is ready to talk with her about her husband, thus allowing both of them space to reminisce and to grieve should they feel the need.

People with advanced dementia may not be able to benefit from support groups or counselling but it may be possible to use creative techniques to enable expressions of sadness and loss. One such technique involves using "group buddies", which are soft toys used in therapeutic play. Lewis and Trzinski (2006) observed that following bereavement, group members gained comfort from hugging their soft toy and seemed more able to express their feelings. Other creative techniques could include the use of art or music, though there do not seem, to date, to be any reports on evidence for their effectiveness. It may also be important to consider how to enable the person to find alternative ways of meeting their attachment needs whether through the use of substitute relationships, comfort objects or spiritual means such as prayer.

Learning to live without the deceased

Learning to live without the deceased can be understood using the "dual process model" (Stroebe and Schut 1999). This model suggests that as we make sense of bereavement, we move between loss-oriented and restoration-oriented processes. Loss-oriented processes focus on the emotional consequences of losing the relationship and restoration-oriented processes focus on the practicalities of living life without the deceased; so not only do we need to look back to the lost relationship but we also need to look ahead and learn new ways of living. This is a useful and necessary focus of work with people with dementia who have been bereaved, particularly those in the community. For those who lived with a carer who has now died, there may be a complete change in their living situation. They will need to develop a new structure in their day-to-day life (Rentz *et al.* 2005), possibly in a new living situation, and will require assistance and guidance to achieve this.

It is hoped that Exercise 26.1 prompts you to think clearly about the pros and cons of telling people with dementia about the death of someone close. It may help you to realize that there is no single correct way to proceed. It may also help you to think empathically about the positions of both Dorothy and her daughter, while also considering how to tackle an emotional issue in a sensitive way.

Exercise 26.1: Deciding what and how much to tell someone with dementia

Dorothy is a 73-year-old woman with moderate Alzheimer's disease. She has been living at home with support from her husband. She manages daily life quite well with his assistance, although she has not shopped alone or cooked independently for quite some time. She has always recognized her husband but sometimes gets mixed up about the identity of her two sons and her daughter. Her husband was admitted to hospital with an acute illness two days ago and died on the same day. Although her daughter told her what had happened, the following day she was shocked to find her mother asking when he would be home. The family asks your advice about what to do.

- Bearing this in mind, write down three points indicating issues or advice you would discuss with the family to help them find a way forward.
- Think of two possible advantages of the family sensitively repeating to her that her husband will not be coming home and that he has died.
- Think of two possible barriers or risks associated with telling her.
- Now think of two possible advantages of *not* repeating to Dorothy that her husband has died, and then think of two possible disadvantages.

Family bereavement of a person with dementia

People whose relative dies of dementia may be at no greater risk of difficulty adapting than those accommodating to other deaths, yet a minority may be more vulnerable. There is some evidence that those who do not acknowledge or express grief during dementia caregiving may be vulnerable, as are those who have become very exhausted or depressed. Lack of social support during caregiving also predicts a struggle after bereavement. Preventive interventions to address these areas may be helpful.

One of the early studies of loss and grief among family caregivers of people with dementia points out that this is a unique and complex situation (Collins et al. 1993). In this section, I will try to provide some explanation of why this is, and suggest ways in which, as service providers, we can be aware of and respond to relatives' needs.

This section starts with a description of what is known about the way people respond to the death of a relative with dementia. It then considers the influence of four particular issues: anticipatory grief, chronic sorrow, caregiving, and institutionalization. The chapter concludes with a summary of the implications for service provision.

Responses to bereavement of a relative with dementia

The death of a person with dementia, especially after a lengthy period of caregiving, is a major turning point for relatives. Paradoxically, bereavement often brings improvements in quality of life and functioning if there has been a period of prior intensive caregiving (see comprehensive review by Schulz et al. 1997). Skaff et al. (1996) note that the death may provide a renewed opportunity for those who were providing care to reaffirm or rediscover their own identity and achieve personal growth. Skaff and colleagues quote from a daughter who said: "[I am] at a turning point, crossroads . . . But whatever, I am going to be doing things I want at my pace. Because for the last six years I lost control" (1996: 255); and from a wife: "My life at this point is a real learning experience because I have never before been totally independent" (1996: 255).

Despite this relatively optimistic picture, however, a significant minority find the period following bereavement very difficult. Schulz et al. (2006) found that one in five bereaved caregivers had high levels of grief and depression 15 weeks after the death, although these rates decreased dramatically over the following 6–12 months. By contrast, however, two studies have reported elevated levels of depression in caregivers up to four years after bereavement (Kiecolt-Glaser et al. 1991; Bodnar and Kiecolt-Glaser 1994). It has been found that between 11.5% (Bradley et al. 2004) and 30% (Schulz et al. 2003) of bereaved caregivers experience depression 12 months after the death. Table 26.2 shows factors drawn from research findings that give some indication of those who may be at risk of difficulty adjusting.

Spouses are more likely to experience a sense of grief during caregiving that continues after the person has died, whereas adult children report feeling worn down and may experience an initial sense of relief after bereavement, although this can give way to a resurgence in grief over the following months (Mullan 1992; Meuser and Marwit 2001). Collins and colleagues (1993) and Almberg et al. (2000) also note an additional theme of guilt/regret.

In summary, the results of research indicate differences in the bereavement responses dependent on the relational and care context prior to death. Following bereavement, there are likely to be gains in some aspects of life for bereaved relatives compared with the strains of caregiving. Yet a substantial minority of those whose relative with dementia dies finds it hard to adjust to living without them.

There are four aspects in particular that make losing a person with dementia distinctive. These are anticipatory grief, chronic sorrow, caregiving, and institutionalization. Each of these is defined and its impact described in Table 26.3, along with the implications for service provision.

Exercise 26.2 is intended to help you think about influences of anticipatory grief, ongoing sorrow, and caregiving on reactions to bereavement.

- Being a spouse rather than an adult child (Boerner *et al.* 2004; Schulz *et al.* 2006; Givens *et al.* 2011)
- Being co-resident with the person with dementia, including prior to a move to a nursing home (Givens *et al.* 2011)
- Having a relative with more severe dementia (Schulz *et al.* 2006)
- Having poor physical or mental health, especially depression, prior to bereavement (Almberg *et al.* 2000; Boerner *et al.* 2004; Schulz *et al.* 2006)
- Having higher levels of pre-loss grief (Givens *et al.* 2011)
- Gaining benefit and satisfaction from caregiving (Boerner *et al.* 2004; Schulz *et al.* 2006)
- Having poorer perceived support prior to bereavement (Bass *et al.* 1991)
- Being dissatisfied with aspects of nursing home care (Bass *et al.* 1991)
- Not being able to think about, plan for or grieve for the death in advance (Owen *et al.* 2001)
- Not being able to acknowledge pre-death losses or associated grief (Mullan 1992; Collins *et al.* 1993)
- Being unable to say goodbye (Almberg *et al.* 2000)
- Having a shorter time since the death (Boerner *et al.* 2004)
- Being unable to access any positive memories (Almberg *et al.* 2000)

Table 26.2 Factors shown to be associated with, or to predict, complicated grief after bereavement of a person with dementia

Exercise 26.2: When someone with dementia dies – helping carers to adjust

Pauline cared for her husband, Jack, who had increasingly severe dementia over about eight years before his recent death a few days after admission to hospital with a chest infection. She was at his side when he died.

Pauline and Jack had a long and close marriage. Although exhausted by the physical effort involved in 24-hour care, Pauline took pride in looking after Jack. She liked to show visitors a photo of them together at their golden wedding and felt she continued to ensure he looked just as smart as he had done in that photo. The couple's only son has a responsible job and when talking to him Pauline has always minimized Jack's problems and her own "caregiving burden", feeling her son should not have to worry about them.

- Think about and list factors that may predispose Pauline to finding adjustment to the death of her husband difficult.
- Think about and list factors that may help Pauline to adjust.

Implications for services

There appear to be few services for caregivers of people with dementia following bereavement (Murphy *et al.* 1997) and little research into best practice. Nonetheless, it is possible to suggest some interventions that can be helpful to all who are bereaved of a relative with dementia, and other interventions that are indicated for those vulnerable to complicated grief. The two sections below outline these possibilities.

Issues in relation to having a relative with dementia	Findings in relation to dementia	Implications for service provision
Anticipatory grief, i.e. grieving in advance of a death through anticipating it		
Hard to grieve when heavily involved in personal care	Anticipatory grief in dementia carers lessened grief after bereavement (Owen *et al.* 2001)	Give relatives space and permission to express feelings of grief. This can lessen grief later (Ott *et al.* 2010)
Chronic sorrow, i.e. grieving for losses in the person with dementia or relationship (Lindgren *et al.* 1999)		
Illustrated in moving accounts by Meuser and Marwit (2001)	Those who experience chronic sorrow nonetheless feel able to cope (Johansson *et al.* 2013), and experience personal growth (Ott *et al.* 2007).	Remember that experiencing sorrow does not mean someone is not coping
Between 66% (Sanders and Corley 2003) and 71% (Diwan *et al.* 2009) of carers report grieving for losses		Distinguish grief from depression so that depression can be addressed
Grief is provoked by diagnosis (Diwan *et al.* 2009), loss of intimacy and past roles of person with dementia (Sanders and Corley 2003)	Chronic sorrow may lessen degree of grief after bereavement (Mullan 1992; Collins *et al.* 1993)	
	Those with high levels of depression before bereavement are more likely to have sustained depression after (Schulz *et al.* 2006)	
Caregiving		
Caregiving can be understood using a stress-process model (see Chapter 5)	Bereavement decreases the direct stress of caring and frees the person to pick up other areas of life.	Carer support that develops resilience, that maintains social networks, and gives enough help to avoid exhaustion can result in lower levels of complicated grief after bereavement (Schulz *et al.* 2006)
	Caregivers may have developed resilience that helps them face bereavement (Skaff *et al.* 1996; Wells and Kendig 1997)	
	But some carers may be exhausted by the point of bereavement (Bass and Bowman 1990; Almberg *et al.* 2000; Schulz *et al.* 2006)	Drawing families together to formulate care plans may be helpful in mobilizing family resources post-bereavement (Almberg *et al.* 2000)
	And those who invested a lot in caring suffer from loss of identity and purpose (Mullan 1992; Boerner *et al.* 2004; Schulz *et al.* 2006)	
	Support from family and friends may be helpful (Almberg *et al.* 2000) but caring may have decreased the person's social network	
Institutionalization, i.e. move into nursing home care		
A move into care for the person with dementia provokes sadness and guilt for spouses (Rudd *et al.* 1999; Ott *et al.* 2010)	Where relatives have concerns about quality of care, distress levels are higher after bereavement (Bass *et al.* 1991)	Try to assist with resolution of feelings and concerns about nursing home care
Nursing home placement frees adult-children to re-establish life (Meuser and Marwit 2001)		

Table 26.3 Processes that make bereavement of a relative with dementia unique

Interventions for all who are bereaved

During caregiving

Caregiver interventions that pay attention to grieving and promote skills and resources prior to bereavement are outlined in Table 26.3.

At the time of death

Around the time of death, research shows that it is helpful for subsequent well-being for relatives to have a chance to say goodbye. The more services can recognize and offer this, the better the outcome is likely to be for carers (Almberg *et al.* 2000).

Following bereavement

Almberg *et al.* (2000) found that almost a third of caregivers in their Swedish sample spoke of missing professional support after the death of their relative with dementia, a view echoed in findings by Collins *et al.* (1993). In view of this, it would seem appropriate that professionals who have been involved in the person's care offer to meet with relatives at least once after the death. This might provide an opportunity for the family to talk with someone who knew their relative in his or her last days and knew the circumstances of their death. It would also give the opportunity to ask questions that might dispel misconceptions and guilt, and it would mark the end of contact by design rather than by circumstance, allowing relatives to feel cared for rather than abandoned.

Almberg *et al.* (2000) were surprised to find, in the largely secular society of Sweden, that a number of their participants reported spiritual support as being very helpful after bereavement. This reminds us to consider spiritual well-being as well as secular practical and emotional support.

Preventative interventions for those at risk of complicated responses to bereavement

Caregivers who are isolated or whose resources are depleted may struggle following bereavement. Almberg *et al.* (2000) suggest that drawing the family together to formulate care plans during the period of caregiving may mobilize family resources and be helpful after bereavement.

Those who do not acknowledge or express loss during caregiving have greater emotional distress after bereavement and it may be that if professionals can offer the opportunity to caregivers to talk about ongoing and anticipated losses during caregiving, this would be helpful afterwards (Collins *et al.* 1993).

We have also seen how carers who have been depressed are at risk of being depressed after bereavement. Thus distinguishing depression from grief and offering interventions to alleviate depression may also make a difference (Schulz *et al.* 2006).

Exercise 26.3: Teaching staff to support families in bereavement

You are asked to provide a two-hour training session for staff working in a nursing home for people with dementia on how to support families whose relative has died there.

Give three learning objectives you might have for this session, along the lines of:

- for staff to _____
- for staff to _____
- for staff to _____

List three pieces of information you might include to address one of these learning objectives.

Describe a discussion point or interactive exercise you could use to address another of your three learning objectives.

Thinking about teaching others forces us to think clearly about our understanding of a topic. This exercise was intended to help you consolidate what you have learned about how to provide excellent care for relatives who have lost a loved one from dementia.

Debates and controversies

In relation to bereaved people with dementia, perhaps the greatest dilemma is whether to try to enable them to understand that someone has died. Telling may provoke upset in ourselves and in the person with dementia, yet not telling may add to their social exclusion and cheat them of the chance to grieve.

With regard to those whose relative dies with dementia, one dilemma is whether services can justify input for family members after the death of the "identified patient". However, if we can provide good family and relationship-centred support and care during the dementia journey, relatives are less likely to be left with severe and lasting distress.

Conclusion

Adaptation to bereavement for someone with dementia is greatly complicated by cognitive impairment. Knowing how to help a bereaved person with dementia challenges us to think carefully about the ethical and moral basis of how we respond. We need to bear in mind a primary goal of enabling the person to feel secure and supported, letting this inform whether we work to enable the person to take in the death, whether we facilitate expression of emotions, and how we help the person to establish a new routine.

For the relative of someone with dementia, chronic sorrow, anticipatory grief, caregiving, and institutionalization are intertwined with what happens after the person with dementia dies. Overall, bereaved relatives may be at no greater risk of difficulty adapting than those accommodating to other deaths, yet a minority are more vulnerable. The chapter suggests strategies during dementia care, at the time of death, and post-bereavement that may help to promote good adaptation. It also suggests ways of intervening that may be helpful to those who are more vulnerable.

To inform better support, there is a need for further research on the nature and effectiveness of interventions that are being used, both with bereaved people with dementia and those bereaved of a relative with dementia.

Further information

The BBC website provides a wide range of information on bereavement [http://www.bbc.co.uk/]. The main organization in the UK concerned with bereavement care is Cruse Bereavement Care.

CRUSE provides counselling and support and offers information, advice, education, and training services [http://www.cruse.org.uk/].

The Alzheimer's Society provides a factsheet on grief and bereavement [http://www.alzheimers.org.uk/site/scripts/download_info.php?fileID=1796].

References

Almberg, B.E., Grafstrom, M. and Winblad, B. (2000) Caregivers of relatives with dementia: experiences encompassing social support and bereavement, *Aging and Mental Health*, 4(1): 82–9.

Bass, D. and Bowman, K. (1990) The transition from caregiving to bereavement: the relationship of care-related strain and adjustment to death, *The Gerontologist*, 30: 35–44.

Bass, D., Bowman, K. and Noelker, L. (1991) The influence of caregiving and bereavement support on adjusting to an older relative's death, *The Gerontologist*, 31: 32–42.

Bodnar, J. and Kiecolt-Glaser, J. (1994) Caregiver depression after bereavement: chronic stress isn't over when it's over, *Psychology and Aging*, 9: 372–80.

Boerner, K., Schulz, R. and Horowitz, A. (2004) Positive aspects of caregiving and adaptation after bereavement, *Psychology and Aging*, 19: 668–75.

Bonanno, G.A., Wortman, C.B., Lehman, D.R., Tweed, R.G., Haring, M. *et al.* (2002) Resilience to loss and chronic grief: a prospective study from preloss to 18-months postloss, *Journal of Personality and Social Psychology*, 83: 1150–64.

Bradley, E.H., Prigerson, H., Carlson, M.D., Cherlin, E., Johnson-Hurzeler, R. *et al.* (2004) Depression among surviving caregivers: does length of hospice enrollment matter?, *American Journal of Psychiatry*, 161: 2257–62.

Collins, C., Liken, M., King, S. and Kikinakis, C. (1993) Loss and grief among family caregivers of relatives with dementia, *Qualitative Health Research*, 3: 236–53.

Diwan, S., Hougham, G.W. and Sachs, G.A. (2009) Chronological patterns and issues precipitating grieving over the course of caregiving among family caregivers of persons with dementia, *Clinical Gerontologist*, 32: 358–70.

Gataric, G., Kinsel, B., Currie, B.G. and Lawhorne, L.W. (2010) Reflections on the under-researched topic of grief in persons with dementia: a report from a symposium on grief and dementia, *American Journal of Hospice and Palliative Medicine*, 27: 567–74.

Givens, J.L., Prigerson, H.G., Kiely, D.K., Shaffer, M.L. and Mitchell, S.L. (2011) Grief among family members of nursing home residents with advanced dementia, *American Journal of Geriatric Psychiatry*, 19: 543–50.

Grief, C. and Myran, D. (2006) Bereavement in cognitively impaired older adults: case series and clinical considerations, *Journal of Geriatric Psychiatry amnd Neurology*, 19: 209–15.

Johansson, A.K., Sundh, V., Wijk, H. and Grimby, A. (2013) Anticipatory grief among close relatives of persons with dementia in comparison with close relatives of patients with cancer, *American Journal of Hospice and Palliative Medicine*, 30: 29–34.

Kiecolt-Glaser, J., Dura, J., Speicher, C., Trask. J. and Glaser, R. (1991) Spousal caregivers of dementia victims: longitudinal changes in immunity and health, *Psychosomatic Medicine*, 53: 345–62.

Lewis, M. and Trzinski, A. (2006) Counseling older adults with dementia who are dealing with death: innovative interventions for practitioners, *Death Studies*, 30: 777–87.

Lindgren, C., Connelly, C. and Gaspar, H. (1999) Grief in spouse and children caregivers of dementia patients, *Western Journal of Nursing Research*, 2: 521–37.

Meuser, T. and Marwit, S. (2001) A comprehensive stage-sensitive model of grief in dementia caregiving, *The Gerontologist*, 41: 658–70.

Mullan, J. (1992) The bereaved caregiver: a prospective study of changes in well-being, *The Gerontologist*, 5: 673–83.

Murphy, K., Hanrahan, P. and Luchins, D. (1997) A survey of grief and bereavement in nursing homes: the importance of hospice grief and bereavement for the end-stage Alzheimer's disease patient and family, *Journal of the American Geriatrics Society*, 45: 1104–7.

Ott, C.H., Sanders, S. and Kelber, S.T. (2007) Grief and personal growth experience of spouses and adult–child caregivers of persons with Alzheimer's disease or related dementias, *The Gerontologist*, 47: 798–809.

Ott, C.H., Kelber, S.T. and Blaylock, M. (2010) "Easing the way" for spouse caregivers of individuals with dementia: a pilot feasibility study of a grief intervention, *Research in Gerontological Nursing*, 3: 89–99.

Owen, J., Goode, K. and Haley, W. (2001) End of life care and reactions to death in African-American and white family caregivers of relatives with Alzheimer's disease, *Omega*, 43: 349–61.

Rentz, C., Krikorian, R. and Keys, M. (2005) Grief and mourning from the perspective of the person with a dementing illness: beginning the dialogue, *Omega*, 50: 165–79.

Rudd, M., Viney, L. and Preston, C. (1999) The grief experienced by spousal caregivers of dementia patients: the role of place of care of patient and gender of caregiver, *International Journal of Aging and Human Development*, 48: 217–40.

Sanders, S. and Corley, C. (2003) Are they grieving? A qualitative analysis examining grief in caregivers of individuals with Alzheimer's disease, *Social Work in Health Care*, 37: 35–53.

Schulz, R., Newsom, J., Fleissner, K., Decamp, A. and Nieboer, A. (1997) The effects of bereavement after family caregiving, *Aging and Mental Health*, 1: 269–82.

Schulz, R., Mendelsohn, A.B., Haley, W.E., Mahoney, D., Allen, R.S. *et al.* (2003) End of life care and the effects of bereavement among family caregivers of persons with dementia, *New England Journal of Medicine*, 349: 1936–42.

Schulz, R., Boerner, K., Shear, K., Zong, S. and Gitlin, L. (2006) Predictors of complicated grief among dementia caregivers: a prospective study of bereavement, *American Journal of Geriatric Psychiatry*, 14: 650–8.

Skaff, M., Pearlin, L. and Mullan, J. (1996) Transitions in the caregiving career: effects of sense of mastery, *Psychology and Aging*, 11: 247–57.

Stroebe, M. and Schut, H. (1999) The dual process model of coping with bereavement: rationale and description, *Death Studies*, 23: 197–224.

Wells, Y.D. and Kendig, H.L. (1997) Health and well-being of spouse caregivers and the widowed, *The Gerontologist*, 37: 666–74.

Worden, W. (1991) *Grief Counselling and Grief Therapy: A Handbook for the Mental Health Practitioner*. New York: Springer.

CHAPTER 27

Supporting persons with dementia through transitions in care

Amy Kind and Andrea Gilmore-Bykovskyi

❝My mother deteriorated rapidly. She was out of her comfort zone and background and now depressed. It taught me a lesson that I had put my value judgements to use rather than being in her mind so to speak and it exacerbated a deteriorating situation.❞

—Geoff Redman Yorkshire, UK

❝We had always been a very close family and when the time came for my father to be taken into residential care – he became a danger to both himself and my mother – it was a traumatic time for the entire family. How would he cope without us? How would we cope with releasing him into the care of strangers? The only way that I could cope was to decide which EMI Nursing Home I would like him to go into and so I researched those available to us both on line and by visiting.

I made my choice, but there was a long waiting list. More worryingly, the home of my choice was concerned at the disruptive effect my physically fit and sometimes aggressive father might have on the status quo of the nursing home, and were not at all sure they would accept him.

I communicated with everyone: his consultant, the nursing home and social services, that I would only be at peace if he was admitted to the home I had chosen. The response was marvellous. The consultant allowed him to remain for the necessary period of time on the NHS assessment ward. When a room became available at the nursing home, the consultant and his team, and my father's social worker, helped him to settle in by frequently visiting him in the first few weeks in his new home, and providing advice and guidance remotely on his more difficult days, until he had transitioned successfully and was no longer frightened and confused by the change.

My dad was obviously unaware of the degree of care which was being taken on his behalf. But we, as his loving family, were able to go on with our own lives due to the care and team working of the professionals who ultimately met not only my dad's, but also his family's, needs.❞

—Fiona Hardy Yorkshire, UK

Learning objectives

By the end of this chapter you will be able to:

- Describe what a care transition is and identify different types of care transitions experienced by persons with dementia
- Identify consequences of poor transitions and how they affect persons with dementia

- Understand how health system fragmentation contributes to poor-quality care transitions
- Describe features of existing transitional care interventions
- Appreciate the need for inclusion of persons with dementia in transitional care research
- Recognize that effective communication lies at the core of safe transitions, especially for persons with dementia
- Recommend strategies for improving the quality of care transitions for persons with dementia

Introduction

Transitions in care refer to people's movement between different levels or sites of care. Transitions can be difficult for vulnerable older persons, particularly those with dementia and other cognitive impairments. In many countries, fragmented care systems exacerbate existing poor communication within and between care systems, leaving patients and family members to bridge the gaps between care settings on their own. However, most health systems do not empower patients and their families or care partners to succeed in this role or prepare them adequately for the next setting of care that they will encounter. This lack of empowerment together with system fragmentation leads to poor quality transitions, which may result in medication errors, care plan discontinuity, patient and family dissatisfaction, and avoidable re-hospitalizations. Older persons with dementia are at particularly high risk for experiencing poor care transitions because their cognitive limitations make it more difficult for them to compensate for system fragmentation or to advocate for themselves during care transitions. Older persons with dementia are also more likely to experience transitions into indefinite long-term care placement, such as nursing homes, which present unique challenges for both the person with dementia and their care partners.

Interventions that support transitions into or out of acute care, whether for a few weeks before or after hospital discharge, have been shown to improve the quality of care and reduce negative outcomes. However, persons with dementia have been largely excluded from transitional care intervention research, which presents challenges to informing best practice. Interventions have, however, been developed to support care partners of persons with dementia during transitions to long-term care that have demonstrated positive outcomes for care partners. This chapter discusses the factors that contribute to transitional care challenges for persons with dementia and discusses key features of transitional care interventions.

Case example 27.1: The experience of multiple care transitions for the person with dementia

Transition from community to acute care

Stephan was diagnosed with early-onset Alzheimer's disease at age 62. Three years ago, Stephan moved in with his daughter's family for additional support. The transition was challenging because Stephan lost contact with his home health nurses and had to try to establish new relationships with different providers. In the past month, Stephan became increasingly agitated and occasionally aggressive. His daughter, Vera, had previously identified several strategies to reduce Stephan's agitation but recently, none were working. Stephan's GP suggested admitting him to the local hospital after Stephan struck out at his son-in-law. During the hospital stay, Stephan was

(continued)

diagnosed with a urinary tract infection. With treatment, Stephan's behaviours only improved slightly. The care staff identified that Stephan's agitation greatly increased after he received his evening anti-anxiety medication. This care team decided to discontinue the anti-anxiety medicine and the family came into the hospital to coach care staff on the strategies they used at home that were effective with Stephan. After several days, Stephan's agitation greatly reduced and he began to demonstrate a more positive mood and to participate in activities on the unit. Stephan's daughter recently had been feeling overwhelmed by Stephan's needs, and during his hospital stay made the decision to have Stephan move into a care home in their neighbourhood.

Transition from acute care to care home

Before Stephan's transition, the family dropped off personal belongings at the care home so that Stephan would feel safer and more comfortable in his new environment. The nurse in the hospital who was preparing Stephan's discharge orders and transfer had just returned from vacation. She hadn't previously worked with Stephan and wasn't able to talk to the other nurse about his care plan before preparing his discharge paperwork. She noticed that he was on an anti-anxiety medication when at home that had been discontinued during the hospital stay. She assumed that because his primary problem was agitation, the care home would be better off giving him the anti-anxiety medication to reduce his agitation. She did not have time to read previous nursing or social work notes about interventions that care staff implemented with Stephan to avoid agitated behaviours. The nurse faxed just the medication orders, including the anti-anxiety medication, to the care home and called the care home to provide a verbal report, during which she communicated that Stephan had received antibiotics for a urinary tract infection that relieved all of his behaviours.

Stephan's family went to visit him at the care home that evening. They learned that Stephan had hit a nursing aide during evening rounds, and found him in his room, where he was crying and pacing back and forth and repeatedly asking for his things to be returned to him. They noticed that none of his belongings had been placed in his room and learned that Stephan was very confused about where he was. During his care conference the next day, they learned that the hospital hadn't shared any information about the effective strategies they used when providing care to Stephan. Vera waited several days for the care home to get orders to discontinue Stephan's anti-anxiety medication and spent several days staying in the care home to help Stephan cope with the transition.

Understanding the need for high-quality transitional care

Transitional care is defined as a set of actions designed to ensure the coordination and continuity of health care as patients transfer between different locations or different levels of care in the same location (Coleman 2003). Transitions in care are points of heightened vulnerability for all patients and can be dangerous (see Table 27.1).

There are numerous negative patient and system outcomes associated with poor-quality transitional care. Poor-quality care transitions between levels of care and across settings can result in a range of negative outcomes, including (Coleman 2003; Coleman *et al.* 2006; Medicare Payment Advisory Commission, 2007; King *et al.* 2013):

- heightened patient vulnerability
- medication errors

Outcomes follow:	Prevalence	Source
Adverse events	19%	Forster *et al.* (2003)
Anxiety and dissatisfaction		Coleman (2003)
Communication failures	*	King *et al.* (2013)
▪ missing and incomplete information	*	
▪ conflicting information	*	
▪ inaccurate information	*	
Re-hospitalization or re-admission	12–25%	Medicare Payment Advisory Commission (2007)
Discharged with pending laboratory test that is not communicated to next site of care	32%	Walz *et al.* (2011)
Medication errors	49%	Moore *et al.* (2003)

*Reported in a qualitative study to occur frequently.

Table 27.1 Negative outcomes associated with transitions in care following hospitalization

- decreased patient satisfaction
- care fragmentation
- unnecessary resource utilization, including avoidable re-hospitalizations

Thirty-day re-hospitalization, which occurs when a patient is re-admitted to an acute care setting within 30 days of discharge, has been identified in several countries as a serious health system problem (Medicare Payment Advisory Commission 2007; Clarke *et al.* 2012; Nuffield Trust 2012). In the USA, one in five patients over the age of 65 experiences a re-hospitalization within 30 days of discharge, which accounts for over US$17.4 billion in health care spending annually (Medicare Payment Advisory Commission 2007; Jencks *et al.* 2009). In the UK, approximately 8% of all patients discharged from the hospital are re-admitted within 30 days, costing the NHS an estimated £1.6 to £2.2 billion a year (NuffieldTrust 2012). Whether a patient is receiving acute care for medical or surgical reasons, the majority of re-hospitalizations are due to chronic medical issues such as heart failure or pneumonia (Jencks *et al.* 2009). Research suggests that nearly half of these re-hospitalizations could be avoided, if better care were provided during transition periods.

In the UK, the government has made shifts in payment for care costs to motivate improved transitional care quality. Beginning in 2010, hospitals in England began to no longer receive reimbursement for some emergency hospital readmissions. Substantial efforts to develop strategies for identifying patients most at risk for short-term re-admissions have since taken place in the UK. Among these are efforts by the Nuffield Trust, who developed the Patient At Risk of Re-hospitalization (PARR) algorithm to assist care providers in "flagging" patients who are at higher risk for 30-day readmission (Billings *et al.* 2012). This tool has demonstrated strong potential and identifies a large proportion of patients who are re-hospitalized; however, at the time of writing, the model still requires additional development and testing before it is reliable enough for use in practice.

Similar efforts to address re-hospitalization were included in the US 2010 Patient Protection and Affordable Care Act. The Affordable Care Act included provisions that mandate financial penalties for hospitals with higher than projected re-hospitalization rates. The legislation also provided funding for the development of new care models aimed at reducing re-hospitalization and associated care, such as accountable care organizations (ACOs). Accountable care organizations consist of a group of providers who assume responsibility for the health of a population of patients across settings of care. There are additional financial incentives available to ACOs that succeed in keeping patients out of acute care hospitals, as a way to encourage increased coordination across settings of care. In addition to ACOs, other innovative models of care organization, payment, and delivery are being tested as a result of the Affordable Care Act. This legislation represents a sweeping change in the payment system for health care in the USA with its ultimate results yet to be determined. Nevertheless, these legislative changes have directly led many US health systems to explore and adopt transitional care interventions as a way to improve care coordination and decrease negative post-hospital outcomes.

Exercise 27.1: Reflecting on the transition experience

Recall Stephan and Vera's experience transitioning from home to acute care, and then from acute care to a care home. Reflect on the following:

- Try to place yourself in Vera's position. Considering what you know about the stress that caregivers experience, how might the lack of support for Stephan during the transition have affected Vera's health and well-being?
- What type of communication between the hospital staff and care home staff could have improved the transition experience for Stephan and Vera?
- How might this experience have been different if Stephan did not have Alzheimer's disease?
- What are some other negative outcomes that resulted from the lack of information-sharing between the hospital and care home?

Barriers to providing high-quality transitional care

Transitional care is a relatively new concept/practice in health care made necessary by fundamental changes that have spread widely throughout health systems over the last 40 years. In the mid twentieth century and earlier, it was common for physicians to follow and care for their patients across all settings of care, by providing care in the hospital, nursing home, outpatient clinic, and the patient's home. However, with the advent and rapid spread of single-site physician specialists, like hospitalists, at the end of the twentieth century, typical physician practice changed. It became (and is now) much more common for physicians to practise in single sites (such as a clinic), rarely accompanying their patients to other settings. From the patient's perspective, this cultural change resulted in large gaps in care – time between discharge at one setting and before being seen in the next – when it was unclear who was responsible for the patient's care. Additionally, system infrastructures and leadership were slow to adapt to meet the needs of patients in this new fragmented health system, but are now starting to recognize the importance of care to support patients during these system gaps (i.e. transitional care). Some systems are better poised to deliver high-quality transitional care than others.

Many factors have been identified that pose barriers to the provision of high-quality transitional care, but one of the most important is health system fragmentation (see Figure 27.1). Care

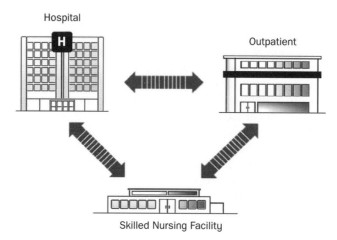

Figure 27.1: Care settings provided by health systems

settings within fragmented health systems tend to be organized in distinct "silos" that emphasize specialized health care, and result in patients receiving care from multiple site-specific providers across a variety of settings. These care settings often have limited formal relationships, inconsistent communication, and little or no medical record integration. Care staff trying to bridge these settings may not have a clear, standardized process to effectively communicate important pieces of information about a patient's care plan such as medications, emotional/behavioural needs, or care preferences (King *et al*. 2013).

Other factors are also barriers to high-quality care transitions. Until recently, transitional care has not been widely recognized by clinical training programmes as an important area, so clinical staff are usually unprepared to successfully manage care transitions. In addition, clinical staff are rarely trained in care settings other than the hospital or outpatient clinic. This limited exposure may contribute to a poor understanding of the resources or delivery of care in non-hospital settings, which may contribute to inadequate transitional care services and communication of care plans following acute hospital stays (Callahan *et al*. 2012). It is difficult for patients, particularly those with multiple health conditions and cognitive impairments, to compensate for the effects of health system fragmentation (Jencks *et al*. 2009; Callahan *et al*. 2012). Patients are often not well educated about the next setting of care, and there is often little patient empowerment in the hospital to prepare them for the next setting of care.

Exercise 27.2: Communicating between settings of care

Although health system fragmentation is a reality in many countries, it is vital that providers seek innovative ways to help vulnerable patients, including those with dementia, bridge the gaps between different settings in care. Reflect on:

■ Different settings of care where you live and the extent of communication between these settings.
■ Strategies that patients, families, and care providers can use to enhance communication between these settings.

Consider whether the strategies you came up with would be readily accessible for a person with dementia. If they might not be, what additional type of support or adaptation would support the person with dementia?

The experience of transitions in care for persons with dementia

Transitions are commonly experienced by persons with dementia and their care partners, and are fundamentally challenging experiences. Persons with dementia have a limited capacity to adapt to stressors and frequent change. This is believed to be both a result of the neuro-degeneration that occurs in dementia and the individual's diminished capacity to communicate their resultant needs and to anticipate and respond to changes in environment, people, and situations. People with dementia are very sensitive to their surroundings and generally benefit from standard routines and similar physical and social environments (caregivers). Loss of familiar surroundings and people presents a substantial change that can contribute to the manifestation of behavioural symptoms, increased depression or withdrawal (Knopman *et al*. 1999) (see Chapter 16).

Persons with dementia are more likely than non-cognitively impaired individuals to experience a transition into permanent care, such as a long-term care home or nursing home. In fact, dementia is the strongest predictor of risk for institutionalization (i.e. placement in a nursing home for long-term services) (Luppa *et al*. 2010). In the USA, about 60% of people with dementia who live alone are placed into nursing homes earlier than those who live with family, although overall estimates of the rate of institutionalization for persons with dementia are around 20%. Transitions into nursing homes for permanent care can also pose cross-cultural challenges if the cultural norms in the facility are not congruent with the norms and values of an individual's culture (Kong *et al*. 2010). However, most people with dementia spend most of their life and often die in community settings, where they are likely to receive care informally from family members and care partners. Transitions between different care settings are common in this population and are often temporary.

Persons with dementia experience more transitions within the last three months of life than those without dementia (Aaltonen *et al*. 2012; Callahan *et al*. 2012). Research has shown that individuals with dementia who live in nursing home settings are likely to experience burdensome and likely unnecessary transitions in the last 90 days of life, including transitions into intensive care and acute care within the last few days of life and frequent transitions between different nursing home settings (Gozalo *et al*. 2011) (see Chapter 25). This is widely considered to reflect poor quality of life for persons with dementia, since these transitions in care are understood to be both stressful and disruptive to the patient. See case example 27.2 to gain an understanding of transitions between care settings experienced for someone with dementia.

Case example 27.2: Sandra

Sandra, an only child, had spent most of her life living and working on her father's dairy farm. Sandra and her husband took over management of the farm until five years ago when her husband passed away. Sandra began to have difficulty with her memory about seven years ago and three years ago was placed in a care home. In the past two years, Sandra has been hospitalized on five separate occasions for exacerbations of her congestive heart failure and pneumonia. During her most recent hospital admission, Sandra was found to have trouble swallowing and was placed on

(continued)

a special diet with thickened liquids to avoid her aspirating on food – which is likely to have contributed to her recurrent pneumonia infections. Sandra was discharged back to her care home but when the physician wrote the discharge order she did not consult with the speech language pathologist who made the recommendation to change Sandra's diet. The care home starts Sandra back on her regular diet, which she has previously seemed to enjoy and tolerate well. Five days later, after choking on some food during breakfast, Sandra develops pneumonia and has to be sent back to the hospital for oxygen therapy and antibiotics. During the hospital stay she develops delirium, and is transferred to an intensive care unit for a week. After several more days in the hospital, she is transferred back to the care home.

As a result of their diminished capacity to adapt to change and their limited ability to advocate on behalf of their own care needs, individuals with dementia are particularly vulnerable to breakdowns in care and thus have an increased need for high-quality transitional care. Dementia has been shown to increase re-hospitalization risk by an alarming 40%, although little research has addressed the role of dementia in re-hospitalizations.

Very few studies have explored the experience of transitioning to different care settings from the perspective of the person with dementia. In an interview study conducted by Thein and colleagues (2011), persons with dementia communicated hopes and fears for the transition to permanent care (Table 27.2). They also had a desire to be meaningfully involved in the transition process. This research demonstrates that persons with dementia would appreciate and perceive benefit from the opportunity to express their expectations for the transition. They also expressed a desire to have their family members continue to be involved during the transition process to offer additional support (Thein *et al.* 2011). Research also suggests that individuals who have the opportunity to provide input into the decision to transition into a nursing home for permanent care are more likely to be accepting of the decision (Tyrrell *et al.* 2006). (See the vignette in case study 27.1 and Exercise 27.1 to gain an understanding of the experience of care transitions from the perspective of the person with dementia.)

Individual with dementia	
Pre-care transition	"I don't think I can manage at home anymore. You see I live alone and it can get quite difficult sometimes." (Thein *et al.* 2011: 11)
Post-care transition	"It's nice to have people around. I feel I don't have to try and manage doing things on my own now." (Thein *et al.* 2011: 14)
Family/carer	
Post-care transition	"Yeah, and they know I'm all right and that helps them a lot. Whereas when I was miles away, they worried about me." (Thein *et al.* 2011: 14)

Source: Quotations from study conducted by Thein and colleagues examining expectations and experiences of moving into a care home from the perspective of older people with dementia (2011: 7–18)

Table 27.2 What persons with dementia have reported about transitioning into a care home

Exercise 27.3: Your experiences of transition

Reflect on transitions you have experienced in your life that were challenging for you.

- What made them challenging?
- Did you have adequate time to prepare for the transition and was it something you were able to control?
- How might you have experienced the transition differently if you received more support during the process?

Thinking about these questions can help you gain an understanding of the emotional challenges persons with dementia face during marked transitions, such as those in care that they may not have much control over.

It is critical to understand the role of the care system in facilitating transitions in care for persons with dementia. Important points to remember are:

- Although a person with dementia may be transferred from an acute care hospital to home, they ultimately rely on a system or combination of systems and the care workers therein to facilitate an effective transition.
- Persons with dementia are uniquely vulnerable to care system fragmentation and inadequate communication surrounding transitional care because they have a limited ability to recall and communicate their own health needs.
- As a result of this weakened compensation, they are likely to be at increased risk for adverse outcomes following transitions.

The experience of transitions in care for care partners

A large body of research has focused on the experience of transitions to permanent care for care partners of persons with dementia, but limited research is available to understand care partners' experience during post-hospital transitions. People with dementia and their care partners function as a unit (dyad) (see Chapter 12) and care partners are often essential to the relative's success. As such, the care partner's needs for information and support must be considered in any care transition. As discussed in Chapter 5, caregiving for someone with dementia is often stressful and burdensome. Often, new conflicts arise for care partners following certain transitions, such as those to nursing homes, wherein care partners may experience feelings of guilt or frustration or may encounter conflicts with staff (Nikzad-Terhune *et al.* 2010). Despite these challenges being well documented, few care partners plan for nursing home placement, and as a result, they are often not prepared to address the emotional conflicts that arise during the transition (Gaugler *et al.* 2001).

A small study of carers in Ireland found that they often experienced conflicting emotions during transitions, met challenges while trying to adapt to their new role, and often felt bereft during the transition process (Argyle *et al.* 2010). Care partners also generally desired to continue to participate in the care of their loved one and felt that this would be most effectively facilitated by ongoing communication and emotional support from staff. Recently, interventions have been developed to provide care partners with support following nursing home placement. Enhanced support provided by a practitioner with advanced counselling training, including individual and family counselling, support groups, and ad hoc counselling has been shown to benefit care partners in both the short and long term (Gaugler *et al.* 2008; Davis *et al.* 2011).

Exercise 27.4: Engaging care partners

Return to case example 27.2 and consider the following:

■ How could a care partner be involved in the frequent transitions between settings?
■ What would the benefits of care partner involvement be in this situation?

Evidence-based interventions to improve hospital-to-community transitional care quality

Transitional care interventions are clinical programmes that support patients as they move from the hospital to the community to improve medication management, self-care, and satisfaction. However, only two transitional care interventions have been shown to decrease re-hospitalizations in randomized controlled trials – Coleman's Care Transitions Intervention and Naylor's Transitional Care Model (Naylor *et al.* 2004; Coleman *et al.* 2006). These interventions reduce re-hospitalizations by about one-third in older patients discharged to home by using a series of post-hospital in-home visits with a nurse practitioner to teach patients about their medications, medical follow-up, signs of condition worsening, and provider contact information (Bourgeois *et al.* 2003). Even though they only contact patients for four weeks, the re-hospitalization reduction effects of these transitional care interventions can last up to 180 days, likely because enrolled patients gain a lasting empowerment and increased skills to better manage their own health (Naylor *et al.* 2004; Coleman *et al.* 2006). Home visit-based transitional care interventions typically find that up to one-half of enrolled patients have medication discrepancies (i.e. taking medications in a way different from that which is prescribed) within two to three days of hospital discharge (Coleman *et al.* 2005; Kind *et al.* 2012). These interventions work with the patient to correct medication discrepancies, many of which are very serious. However, both of these programmes excluded patients with dementia in their trials.

Supporting persons with dementia through transitions in care

Few existing transitional care programmes reported in the literature currently target patients with dementia. The Coordinated-Transitional Care (C-TraC) Program (Kind *et al.* 2012) is a telephone-based programme that specifically targets patients with dementia and their care partners. It uses a nurse case manager to coordinate the patient's transitional care through a series of protocol-driven in-hospital visits, intensive post-hospital phone calls, and coordination of communications between in-hospital and post-hospital clinical teams. The C-TraC uses methods of spaced retrieval to tailor teachings and explicitly engages caregivers to ensure applicability to patients with dementia. In preliminary testing at a US Department of Veterans Affairs Hospital, C-TraC enrollees experienced one-third fewer 30-day re-hospitalizations than a comparable baseline group (Kind *et al.* 2012). However, additional more rigorous, multi-site testing of this intervention is needed. Another programme that purposefully includes persons with dementia is the Intervention to Reduce Acute Care Transfers (INTERACT). INTERACT II is a nursing home focused quality improvement intervention designed to help nursing home staff to identify, assess, and communicate changes in resident status soon after the change occurs (Ouslander *et al.* 2011). INTERACT II has tools to improve communications and transitions that occur from the nursing home to the hospital, and can reduce re-hospitalizations in nursing home facilities that fully engage in the programme.

Key components of successful transitional care efforts include the following:

- Educate and empower the patient and care partner in medication management, ideally through a patient-/care partner-led medication reconciliation during the post-hospital period.
- Ensure medical follow-up is in place and the patient and care partner are ready to participate in that follow-up.
- Educate patient and care partner in red flags or signs of a worsening condition.
- Ensure they understand who to contact and how to make contact with questions.
- The four key components above should be reinforced through a series of contacts over time during the post-hospital period.

Providers should consider the unique needs of patients with dementia as they tailor transitional care services. Research has consistently documented that patients and caregivers who are engaged and activated to fully participate in their care demonstrate better outcomes (Hibbard *et al.* 2013). Traditional evidence-based transitional care programmes are designed to empower the patient to better manage their own medical needs; however, in the case of dementia it is critical that care partners are also included in this empowerment and activation process. Additionally, transitional care support for persons with dementia should emphasize the remaining abilities of the person with dementia, facilitating and empowering their participation in choices about the timing, nature, and manner in which transitions evolve. Identifying an individual's response to past transitions, and strategies that eased these past transitions can also be informative. Educational approaches need to be adapted to the specific needs of the patient with dementia. Persons with earlier stages of dementia are capable of learning new information, and research has shown that they can benefit from educational approaches that use spaced-retrieval strategies. Spaced-retrieval is a method of learning information by practising recalling that information over increasingly longer periods of time (Bourgeois *et al.* 2003). Care partners of persons with dementia may also be struggling with the impending transition, and may require adapted educational approaches to be fully activated for the transition period.

In summary, the following strategies may be helpful in providing transitional care support for persons with dementia:

- Actively engage the person with dementia in decision-making about care transitions.
- Identify and advocate for services to address the psychosocial needs of care partners during transitions.
- Apply patient/care partner education strategies that are responsive to the capabilities, existing knowledge base, and needs of the individual.
- For persons with dementia, patient education that utilizes spaced-retrieval methods may be most effective.
- Emotional support/services for care partners struggling with the transitions to permanent care placement are beneficial and may ultimately help the person with dementia.

Debates and controversies

Persons with dementia have been excluded from most evidence-based transitional care services, resulting in limited evidence-based interventions for this patient group. Although not fully explained in the original studies, this systematic exclusion may have been prompted by the impression that all persons with dementia are unable to learn new information, which Sabat has shown (Chapter 8) is not true. Furthermore, many existing evidence-based transitional care interventions do not automatically include care partners in their protocols, even though care partners are key participants in the post-hospital care plan. Further work is needed to overcome these limitations to ensure that more services are designed specifically for the needs of cognitively impaired persons. Some early work has begun in this area (see above) but more rigorous studies are needed.

It may be unclear which health system or staff are responsible for a patient during a care transition. Systematic care fragmentation often creates myopia, in that clinical staff within a particular health care setting have difficulty seeing beyond that setting. In such an environment, staff in one setting may not understand the limitations and complexities of care in other settings. This creates problems of poor communication, intra-setting conflict, and a lack of accountability during care transitions. Additionally, discharging staff may be unaware of the issues that patients may encounter in their first days at home. In such environments, patients and care partners can be unsure of who is ultimately responsible for their care or who to turn to if questions/problems arise. This issue of accountability is very contentious and often a point of debate in health policy.

Future directions (implications)

Additional research, clinical practice changes, and policy developments are needed to improve the quality and safety of care transitions for persons with dementia. Some of these steps could include:

- more rigorous testing/development of transitional care models for persons with dementia and their care partners
- inclusion of persons with dementia in future transitions of care research
- developing more clinical interventions and optimal communication strategies to improve system-to-system transitions (no evidence-based transitional care interventions currently exist to support hospital-to-nursing home transitions)
- educating all types of health staff/practitioners about the safety risks inherent in care transitions, the resources/limitations of other settings patients may encounter, and the basic principles of high-quality transitional care
- policy and payment changes to encourage health systems to integrate and coordinate care more effectively, and to support clinical transitional care interventions

Conclusion

Transitions between care settings can be dangerous for patients, especially those with dementia or other cognitive impairments. Health system fragmentation exacerbates this risk. Clinical transitional care interventions can help to make transitions safer, but few of them have been designed to meet the needs of persons with dementia and their care partners. Much more research, clinical and policy work is needed in this area to improve care.

Acknowledgements

The authors would like to acknowledge Brock Polnaszek and Jacquelyn Porter for assistance with formatting/graphics and Lydia Lemmenes for assistance with the review of literature that contributed to this chapter.

Further information

HIPxChange hosts the Coordinated-Transitional Care (C-Trac) programme, a telephone-based initiative aimed at improving patient safety and post-discharge outcomes. The web site provides a toolkit that includes protocols that can be obtained upon free registration [http://www. hipxchange.org/].

INTERACT II is a quality improvement programme created to manage rapid changes in resident condition and includes clinical and educational tools for use in everyday practice. The resource can be found online [http://www.interact2.net/tools.html].

The National Transitions of Care Coalition provides tools and resources to address challenges in the process of transition between care settings. The tools and resources can be found on their web site [http://www.ntocc.org/].

The Care Transitions Intervention (CTI) is a transitional care intervention that utilizes a coaching model to support patients and families during transitions across settings. Information regarding the intervention and training is available on the web site [http://www.caretransitions.org/caregiver_resources.asp].

The Transitional Care Model (TCM) is a transitional care model that emphasizes coordination and continuity as well as prevention of complications using active engagement of patients and caregivers. Resources and more information about the TCM are available on the web site [http://www.nursing.upenn.edu/media/transitionalcare/Pages/default.aspx].

References

Aaltonen, M., Rissanen, P., Forma, L., Raitanen, J. and Jylha, M. (2012) The impact of dementia on care transitions during the last two years of life, *Age and Ageing*, 41(1): 52–7.

Argyle, E., Downs, M. and Tasker, J. (2010) *Continuing to Care for People with Dementia: Irish Family Carers' Experience of their Relative's Transition to a Nursing Home*. Bradford: Bradford Dementia Group, The Alzheimer Society of Ireland and St. Luke's Home.

Billings, J., Blunt, I., Steventon, A., Georghiou, T., Lewis, G. et al. (2012) Development of a predictive model to identify inpatients at risk of re-admission within 30 days of discharge (PARR-30), *BMJ Open*, 2(4) [http://bmjopen.bmj.com/content/2/4/e001667.full.pdf+html, accessed 3 June 2014].

Bourgeois, M.S., Camp, C., Rose, M., White, B., Malone, M. *et al.* (2003) A comparison of training strategies to enhance use of external aids by persons with dementia, *Journal of Communication Disorders*, 36(5): 361–78.

Callahan, C.M., Arling, G., Tu, W., Rosenman, M.B., Counsell, S.R. *et al.* (2012) Transitions in care for older adults with and without dementia, *Journal of the American Geriatrics Society*, 60(5): 813–20.

Clarke, A., Blunt, I. and Bardsley, M. (2012) PS18 analysis of emergency 30-day readmissions in England using routine hospital data 2004–2010: is there scope for reduction?, *Journal of Epidemiology and Community Health*, 66 (Suppl. 1): A45.

Coleman, E.A. (2003) Falling through the cracks: challenges and opportunities for improving transitional care for persons with continuous complex care needs, *Journal of the American Geriatrics Society*, 51(4): 549–55.

Coleman, E.A., Mahoney, E. and Parry, C. (2005) Assessing the quality of preparation for posthospital care from the patient's perspective: the care transitions measure, *Medical Care*, 43(3): 246–55.

Coleman, E.A., Parry, C., Chalmers, S. and Min, S.J. (2006) The care transitions intervention: results of a randomized controlled trial, *Archives of Internal Medicine*, 166(17): 1822–8.

Davis, J.D., Tremont, G., Bishop, D.S. and Fortinsky, R.H. (2011) A telephone-delivered psychosocial intervention improves dementia caregiver adjustment following nursing home placement, *International Journal of Geriatric Psychiatry*, 26(4): 380–7.

Forster, A.J., Murff, H.J., Peterson, J.F., Gandhi, T.K. and Bates, D.W. (2003) The incidence and severity of adverse events affecting patients after discharge from the hospital, *Annals of Internal Medicine*, 138(3): 161–7.

Gaugler, J.E., Pearlin, L.I., Leitsch, S.A. and Davey, A. (2001) Relinquishing in-home dementia care: difficulties and perceived helpfulness during the nursing home transition, *American Journal of Alzheimer's Disease and Other Dementias*, 16(1): 32–42.

Gaugler, J.E., Roth, D.L., Haley, W.E. and Mittelman, M.S. (2008) Can counseling and support reduce burden and depressive symptoms in caregivers of people with Alzheimer's disease during the transition to institutionalization? Results from the New York University caregiver intervention study, *Journal of the American Geriatrics Society*, 56(3): 421–8.

Gozalo, P., Teno, J.M., Mitchell, S.L., Skinner, J., Bynum, J. *et al.* (2011) End-of-life transitions among nursing home residents with cognitive issues, *New England Journal of Medicine*, 365(13): 1212–21.

Hibbard, J.H., Greene, J. and Overton, V. (2013) Patients with lower activation associated with higher costs: delivery systems should know their patients' "scores", *Health Affairs (Millwood)*, 32(2): 216–22.

Jencks, S.F., Williams, M.V. and Coleman, E.A. (2009) Rehospitalizations among patients in the Medicare fee-for-service program, *New England Journal of Medicine*, 360(14): 1418–28.

Kind, A.J.H., Jensen, L., Barczi, S., Bridges, A., Kordahl, R. *et al.* (2012) Low-cost transitional care with nurse managers making mostly phone contact with patients cut rehospitalization at a VA hospital, *Health Affairs (Millwood)*, 31(12): 2659–68.

King, B.D., Gilmore-Bykovskyi, A., Roiland, R., Polnaszek, B., Bowers, B. *et al.* (2013) The consequences of poor communication during hospital-to-skilled nursing facility transitions: a qualitative study, *Journal of the American Geriatrics Society*, 61(7): 1095–1102.

Knopman, D., Berg, J., Thomas, R., Grundman, M., Thal, L. *et al.* (1999) Nursing home placement is related to dementia progression: experience from a clinical trial, *Neurology*, 52(4): 714–18.

Kong, E.H., Deatrick, J.A. and Evans, L.K. (2010) The experiences of Korean immigrant caregivers of non-English-speaking older relatives with dementia in American nursing homes, *Qualitative Health Research*, 20 (3): 319–29.

Luppa, M., Luck, T., Weyerer, S., König, H.-H., Brähler, E. *et al.* (2010) Prediction of institutionalization in the elderly: a systematic review, *Age and Ageing*, 39(1): 31–8.

Medicare Payment Advisory Commission (2007) *Report to the Congress: Medicare Payment Policy* [http://www.medpac.gov/documents/Mar07_EntireReport.pdf, accessed 24 February 2011].

Moore, C., Wisnivesky, J., Williams, S. and McGinn, T. (2003) Medical errors related to discontinuity of care from an inpatient to an outpatient setting, *Journal of General Internal Medicine*, 18(8): 646–51.

Naylor, M.D., Brooten, D.A., Campbell, R.L., Maislin, G., McCauley, K.M. *et al.* (2004) Transitional care of older adults hospitalized with heart failure: a randomized, controlled trial, *Journal of the American Geriatrics Society*, 52(5): 675–84.

Nikzad-Terhune, K.A., Anderson, K.A., Newcomer, R. and Gaugler, J.E. (2010) Do trajectories of at-home dementia caregiving account for burden after nursing home placement? A growth curve analysis, *Social Work in Health Care*, 49(8): 734–52.

Nuffield Trust (2012) *Predicting Risk of Hospital Readmission with PARR-30*. London: Nuffield Trust [http://www. nuffieldtrust.org.uk/our-work/projects/predicting-risk-hospital-readmission-parr-30, accessed 3 June 2013].

Ouslander, J.G., Lamb, G., Tappen, R., Herndon, L., Diaz, S. *et al.* (2011) Interventions to reduce hospitalizations from nursing homes: evaluation of the INTERACT II collaborative quality improvement project, *Journal of the American Geriatrics Society*, 59(4): 745–53.

Thein, N.W., D'Souza, G. and Sheehan, B. (2011) Expectations and experience of moving to a care home: perceptions of older people with dementia, *Dementia*, 10(1): 7–18.

Tyrrell, J., Genin, N. and Myslinski, M. (2006) Freedom of choice and decision-making in health and social care: views of older patients with early-stage dementia and their carers, *Dementia*, 5(4): 479–502.

Walz, S.E., Smith, M., Cox, E., Sattin, J. and Kind, A.J. (2011) Pending laboratory tests and the hospital discharge summary in patients discharged to sub-acute care, *Journal of General Internal Medicine*, 26(4): 393–8.

PART 5

Making sustainable change happen in dementia care (changing the culture of care)

CHAPTER 28

Involving people with dementia in service development and evaluation

Rachael Litherland and Andrea Capstick

> ❝If service users are to be involved it needs to be at the centre of services and not as a 'bolt on' in order to comply with a tick box exercise, which is tokenism. ❞
>
> —Keith Oliver Canterbury, UK

Learning objectives

By the end of this chapter, you will:

- Know about a range of approaches to elicit views of people with dementia
- Recognize the challenges involved in seeking the views of people with dementia
- Have an understanding of service user involvement for people with dementia

Introduction

Considering people with dementia as "users of services", with an active role to play in their design and delivery, is a recent but growing phenomenon. Until relatively recently, it was more common to think of people with dementia as passive *recipients* rather than active *users* of services. Recently, there has been a move away from seeing dementia as the "complete annihilation of self" (Beard 2004: 806) to a position that acknowledges the awareness that many people with dementia have about their situation (Clare *et al.* 2005), including the services they use.

The voices of people with dementia can now be heard in research on the experience of dementia (e.g. Wilkinson 2002; Bryden 2005), increasingly in terms of their experience of health and social care (e.g. Barnett 2000; Lorentzon and Bryan 2007). People with dementia are acting together to have collective influence on the world around them through local, regional, and national user involvement initiatives such as the Scottish Dementia Working Group (Weaks *et al.* 2011), the Open Door Network (Howorth *et al.* 2011), and the PROP (People Relying on People) group (Chaston *et al.* 2004). Narratives about the experience of people with dementia who have been involved in campaigning and dementia activism have also been presented (Clare *et al.* 2008; Bartlett and O'Connor 2010). The Dementia Engagement and Empowerment Project (DEEP) (Williamson 2012) is supporting these user involvement groups and providing networking and mentoring opportunities between local groups to further their collective voice and to have national influence. Additionally, there are international initiatives that promote the voices of people with dementia, for example, "I can! I will!" – a website of ideas by Alzheimer's Disease International.

Together with this emerging user voice are legislative and policy frameworks that vigorously promote user involvement. In 2004, a position paper by the Social Care Institute for Excellence

(Carr 2004) summarized the impact and benefits of service user participation for social care services. A useful framework is the Mental Capacity Act 2005, which establishes a set of principles to support people with dementia making their own decisions. The purpose of this chapter is to provide an overview of user involvement with particular emphasis on user involvement of people with dementia. This chapter will draw on practice and research to provide guidance on approaches to and principles of involving people with dementia. Some of the challenges involved in this work will be highlighted. Ironically, discussions of service user involvement often shift the perspective of service users back to the periphery, focusing instead on the experiences of professionals who *choose* to involve people who use the services. I will therefore attempt to keep the voices of people with dementia central to this discussion by drawing on my early work through the Alzheimer's Society's "Living with Dementia" programme (2000–2005).

What does service user involvement mean?

" Service user" has become the recognized term in health and social care to describe people in receipt of services. The term "service user" suggests that the user is central to shaping service development and delivery, shifting power away from the provider towards the consumer. It suggests that the recipients of services have the right to choose and change services, to better meet their needs.

Involvement has been an objective for a range of groups for many years. The mental health field has seen a change in landscape from the individual achievements of the mental health activists of the 1970s and 1980s to a degree of permanence within the field that acknowledges users as experts (see Sainsbury Centre for Mental Health 2005). Similarly, self-organized groups of older people are influencing decisions at the highest level [e.g. Older Persons Advisory Group (OPAG) and older persons forums supported by Help the Aged] with a move away from just consulting with older people towards active partnerships to influence decisions (Reed *et al.* 2006).

Robson *et al.* (2003) distinguished between management-centred and user-centred user involvement. In management-centred user involvement, the service user is involved by responding to agendas set by the organization, for example, giving views on an organization's strategic plan. User-centred user involvement, on the other hand, refers to circumstances where service users' objectives and priorities become the organization's objectives and priorities. An example of this is the operation of the Scottish Dementia Working Group, an independent campaigning group formed by people with dementia. The group is supported by a paid coordinator to identify its own objectives and develop a work plan to meet those objectives, which have included giving views on a range of health and community care issues such as medication, national templates for dementia services, and stem cell research. As members of the Dementia Working Group describe, this approach can result in important outcomes for service users: "It's actually great to feel part of something with someone else who has the same problems as you and nobody understands this illness more than someone else with the illness, that's the truth" (Williamson 2012: 44).

Management-centred user involvement has been criticized for resulting in a form of "moral coercion" (Small and Rhodes 2001) where users feel obliged to be involved – maybe as a condition of receiving a service or because of how they perceive the authority of those in charge of services. Research with people who are seriously ill or approaching the end of their lives concludes that user involvement is not a priority for this group and that such people often have other agendas and more pressing concerns than to be involved in service development or evaluation (Small and Rhodes 2001).

An additional criticism of user involvement is the potential for it to be a tokenistic exercise. A common experience of service users participating in a management-centred user approach is to be asked for views and then to feel their knowledge is not valued or taken seriously by professionals and policy-makers (Branfield and Beresford 2006):

> 66 People think the only thing we know is how to moan. But they are not listening. We know what needs changing; we know what works and what doesn't work. We know this because we live it 24/7, 52 weeks a year with no days off. 99

—Branfield and Beresford (2006: 3)

Exercise 28.1: Approaches to involving service users

Research and practice within other fields have been critical of user involvement initiatives based on the agendas of organizations rather than defined and developed directly by service users.

- Why do you think management-centred approaches to user involvement have been criticized?
- What do you think are the challenges in applying a purely user-centred approach to the involvement of people with dementia?

Involving people with dementia in service development and evaluation

There is now a growing recognition that people with dementia are able to provide accurate and valid reports about services, whether verbally (Bamford and Bruce 2000) or behaviourally (see Chapter 16). Bamford and Bruce (2000) conducted a small study to determine the feasibility of consulting people with dementia about desired service outcomes. In common with their carers, people with dementia discussed a range of outcomes that were significant to them, including access to social contact, company, meaningful activity and stimulation, having a sense of social integration, and maximizing a sense of autonomy. Sometimes people with dementia expressed different views to their carers. For example, maintaining a sense of personal identity, "a sense of oneself as a competent and valued person" (Bamford and Bruce 2000: 556) was seen as important by service users but was rarely identified as important by carers.

Dementia Advocacy Support Network International (DASNI) (http://www.dasninternational.org/) successfully lobbied Alzheimer's Disease International (ADI) – the international federation of Alzheimer associations – to consider ways to become more inclusive of people with dementia. Achievements to date include:

- representatives with dementia on the executive council of ADI
- a conference fund to support people with dementia and their care partners to attend ADI conferences
- a strategic commitment to giving people with dementia greater voice in decision-making at ADI

In theory, service user involvement should be expected throughout the illness. That said, for many people with dementia there is a "window of opportunity" (Litherland 2003) – a short period of time before the impact of dementia reduces one's ability to respond to opportunities, and the window is closed. As one person with dementia described:

> **❝**I have a short time to make a difference. I know this and it is frustrating that things take so long to change. **❞**

This accelerates the need to support involvement, testing an organization's commitment to user involvement, where organizational structures are complex and decision-making is lengthy and management centred. This challenge is highlighted in *Engaging People with Early Stage Alzheimer's Disease in the Work of the Alzheimer's Society* (Alzheimer's Society Canada 2006), a research report commissioned by the Alzheimer Society Canada where urgency to act and adapt is counterbalanced by funding cutbacks, the impact of cognitive decline, and the need for internal policies and regulations that support involvement.

Involving people with dementia in a national organization

As a starting point, it is useful to consider lessons from initiatives in other fields. However, the specific and variable impact of dementia on people's capacity to be involved relies on developing new practices. The Living with Dementia Programme, launched by the Alzheimer's' Society in 2000, is instructive in how to involve people with dementia, by doing just that, by emphasizing the expert role of people with dementia in working out the "how" of user involvement.

A first challenge was to find people with dementia who wanted to get involved in a national programme. People with dementia were contacted through local support groups and dementia practitioners were asked to identify people they thought might like to get involved. As the programme was advertised more widely, people with dementia began to make direct contact. Initially, most of the concerns presented were very individual:

> **❝**Support is the key to me leading as normal a life as possible. People knowing and treating me as the person I still am. Giving me room to live. **❞**

But as I travelled to meet more people, in their own environments, a critical mass of people who wanted to be part of the programme began to develop. They believed that the views of people with dementia should be heard within the Alzheimer's Society and externally:

> **❝**You need to focus on the ability and contribution that we can make, rather than what we can no longer do. **❞**

"User involvement" was not a meaningful way of explaining the purpose of the Living with Dementia programme. Similarly, a user-centred approach (Robson *et al.* 2003), with people with dementia setting their own objectives and priorities, was not an option as a starting point. Most contacts were not used to having their experience listened to, had little confidence in their ability to be involved, and had never met anyone else with dementia – "meeting people in the same boat, it makes you feel better about yourself and what you can achieve". Instead, we discussed activities that people might like to be involved in. The following are concrete examples:

- writing a booklet
- giving views on making supermarkets easier to use
- keeping a photographic diary
- recruiting a new member of staff
- talking about day support opportunities
- speaking at a conference

The skills and interests of individuals with dementia were matched with available opportunities: a former GP began to give presentations about life with dementia to the medical profession; a former architect discussed the changes that could be made to an office environment to make it more accessible for people with dementia. Alongside emerging activists was the growth of a movement of people and groups of people with dementia who connected with the aims of the Living with Dementia programme and began to feel supported to "come out" about their experiences and wishes.

People with dementia said the following practices helped them to get involved:

- being respected and listened to
- a welcoming attitude
- being given encouragement
- a clear and prompt response to questions and concerns
- early diagnosis (leaving more time to be involved)
- acknowledging the diagnosis (not pretending "we don't have dementia")
- varied opportunities to get involved
- opportunities to take part without it involving "consultation"

They said that the following made involvement more difficult:

- fear that I will not be taken seriously
- lack of time for people to listen and make relationships
- lack of money
- poor access to transport
- lack of diagnosis
- negative attitudes about the abilities or rights of people with dementia
- being asked about issues that are not relevant
- lack of feedback about what has happened as a result of being involved
- lack of personal identification with issues of "dementia" or "Alzheimer's"

Involvement approaches – ideas from research and practice

Cantley et al. (2005) looked at how to involve people with dementia in service planning and development by reviewing the practice experience of 16 projects and groups. Four projects acted as development sites for the study, where staff and service users were helped to develop specific involvement activities. The focus was on consultation approaches – about home care, services, methods of involvement, and quality of life – and a range of involvement methods were used, including individual and group discussions, questionnaires, observation, and consultation events. Together with some useful pointers to best support involvement activities (e.g. selecting a venue for a consultation event, questions to consider when planning involvement activities and developing a reflective diary), common features that underpin involvement approaches emerged across project sites. Well-thought-through plans, prior to any involvement activity, are essential to enable people with dementia to fully participate; ethical practice should be paramount. Project success relied on the willingness of staff to be innovative and responsive in their approach. In one case, pre-planned consultation questions were abandoned when it became clear that people with dementia could not recollect the topic they were questioned about (information at a local memory clinic). Instead, a word – "information" – was written on a large sheet of paper that then triggered other words and discussion and ultimately reminded people of their experiences at the memory clinic (Cantley et al. 2005: 37).

Allan (2001) explored how staff could encourage people with dementia to express views and preferences. Allan worked with 40 practitioners in 10 dementia care settings to consider appropriate techniques for engaging with people with dementia. She found that enabling people to express their views took many forms, with individuals responding to different approaches at different times in different ways. The communication needs of individuals, the person's background and interests, and their relationships with staff needed to be taken into account before identifying the most appropriate consultation approach. Approaches were tested by staff and included observation, verbal exchanges as a part of other activities, the use of pictures to stimulate discussion, and indirect discussion where the service user was encouraged to think about what another person's opinions might be. Part of Allan's work was to support staff in recognizing their existing skills and becoming more confident about knowing how and when to apply these skills. In the service environment, this meant care staff being more alert to everyday situations when consultation might be possible, for example, during personal care tasks. Allan also notes the organizational systems that need to be in place to support practitioners to take on this role, including enough workplace time to allow for reflection and discussion.

Finally, Hubbard *et al.* (2003) suggested we develop a repertoire of strategies to use with different individuals. They used interviews or observations to determine the experiences of new residents of a care home. Observations removed the constraints of an interview situation, allowing residents to converse in their own way within the context of their immediate environment, while interviews provided an opportunity for residents to discuss their past and shape the conversation. Sometimes, however, the interview presented difficulties such as when people became embarrassed because they could not recall something, suggesting that combining observation with interviewing may have been more appropriate.

These studies highlight the considerable skills required: good preparation, ability to identify appropriate involvement method, being responsive and sensitive, and allocating time for review and reflection. It is also important to be mindful of the organizational context within which user involvement occurs. Promoting creativity and innovation requires recognition and development of staff skills and the creation of an environment where service user involvement is valued and achievable (Cantley *et al.* 2005).

In thinking about Exercise 28.2, you may want to identify attributes that a worker could bring to a user involvement situation, such as enthusiasm, patience, creativity, and good communication skills. There may also be relevant, practical approaches such as strategic thinking and the ability to form good relationships with other services. Consider whether the skills are inbuilt or can be learned. You may want to think about the emotional impact of this specialist work on individual workers and how an organizational environment might help or hinder a worker to implement a user involvement approach.

Exercise 28.2: Skills for involving users

The skills of workers have been highlighted as an important component of a good user involvement approach.

- What skills do you think are necessary to support involvement of people with dementia?
- How do you think this might affect the workers?

Policy context

In recent years, the government has emphasized empowering patients to have a greater say in the services they use. As a result, health and social care practitioners increasingly expect and are expected to work alongside people with dementia as stakeholders.

Finding out what people with dementia think of the service they use

If we think of involvement as a process rather than a one-off event, then the techniques and approaches we choose are just one step on the journey. Answering the following questions will help to ensure the most appropriate approach is chosen:

- How will you identify people who wish to be involved?
- How can you best support people to identify their own needs and set their own priorities?
- Know your purpose: Why do you want to involve people with dementia? What is it you want to know/what activities do they want to engage in?
- What might be the best techniques for finding out? Is it relevant to people with dementia?
- What issues might emerge during involvement activities? What measures can you put in place to deal with these issues? Do you have a contingency plan?
- Do you have the right skill set to support a particular involvement initiative? If not, who could you ask to support the initiative?
- Are there lessons you can draw on from other practice examples? If so, what adaptations would you need to make?

Direct approaches: talking to people

Interviews

Successful interviews are dependent on successful communication between the interviewer and interviewee. As we have seen in the chapter on communication and relationships (see Chapter 17), there is much that the interviewer can do to enable effective communication. Dewing (2002: 165) suggests that the complexity of the questions needs to be set at a comprehensible level and recommends "dementia-specific interview methods". These might include a photograph of someone being interviewed or using a tape-recorder or video camera for play-back. Participants' ability to communicate verbally can vary from day to day, within the same day, and from one week to the next (Hubbard *et al.* 2003). Therefore, multiple interviews over time can be useful (Pratt 2002).

The flexible interview approach illustrated in case example 28.1, adapted in response to individual need, yields a wealth of information about the topic under discussion. The interviewer is initially directive, using questions, prompts, and analogies. This seemed to help by keeping people focused on the web site and aware of the purpose of their involvement, with the interviewer acting as a memory aid and facilitator.

> ### Case example 28.1: Interviewing about the Alzheimer's Society web site
>
> People with dementia were asked their views on the content and design of the Alzheimer's Society's web site. The interviewer showed them the web site and asked them to think about it as a giant library containing all the information in the world. People were then invited to think of questions they had about dementia. A variety of techniques were used depending on individual need – using the web site as a visual tool, using pre-prepared headings written on sheets of paper to help prompt questions and open-ended discussion with the interviewer about issues that were important to them. The interviewer was well known to many of the participants and used her knowledge of people's communication styles to support people to express their views.

Group discussions

One-to-one interviews can sometimes feel pressurized and people may worry about the impact of what they say. Group discussions can overcome this by generating a group rather than individual response. Hearing the views of others can help people articulate their own thoughts. Bamford and Bruce (2002), running focus groups with people with dementia, noted some difficulties, including: lack of respect of viewpoint among participants, constraints of existing social relationships preventing people expressing their viewpoints, and parallel conversations.

> ### Case example 28.2: Living with Dementia meetings
>
> The people attending Living with Dementia meetings in London came up with the following terms of conduct:
>
> - Distribute easy-to-understand agendas before meetings. This gives us a chance to prepare and write down our thoughts.
> - Meetings should be short, with only one or two agenda points. We get tired and find it difficult to concentrate after a while.
> - It helps if you give us some ideas. But sometimes we will want to talk about things that are important to us.
> - Slow down the pace of discussion to give people time to say what they want to say. Don't talk too much!
> - Take turns so that everyone can have their say, even if this is not in words.
> - Refreshments are essential. They help us to relax and make our journey worthwhile.
> - Send us an easy-to-understand record of the meeting as soon as possible.
> - Send us a reminder just before the next meeting.

There was clear agreement within the group when setting ground rules. Some are common to all group situations; many, however, are particular to being a group member with dementia. They recognized the requirement for meetings to be adapted so that everyone was able to participate as fully as possible, expressing a desire for equity within the group, particularly making sure that those who had more significant communication difficulties were given time and support to contribute. The importance of the individual within this new group was paramount. As one group member describes: "We are not all talkative, some of us need space and time but we've still got a lot to say!"

Use of props and prompts

Physical cues and prompts can aid communication during interviews and focus groups, helping people focus on the discussion. Pictures or cards with single emotions written on them have been successfully used to stimulate discussion (Allan 2001). Talking Mats, a low-tech communication tool using simple picture symbols, has been shown to improve the ability of people at all stages of dementia to communicate (Murphy *et al.* 2007). Dewing (2002) suggests that interactions involving the handling of props can enable the person to feel more confident and therefore respond less hesitantly.

Indirect approaches

Discussion as part of other activities

Focusing exclusively on talking may be intimidating for some people with dementia. Conversations can be facilitated through other activities such as going for a walk (Allan 2001). It may be necessary to approach involvement activities in a much more fluid way, "talking around the research" (Dewing 2002: 12) in an effort to engage the person, or responding to "intermittent conversation" (Hubbard *et al.* 2003), which can be less demanding for the person with dementia.

Case example 28.3: A voluntary organization

"I think we approach user involvement differently to other areas. We maybe don't do it so formally. We do it by listening to the groups, during lunch or whatever . . . so we don't really sit down and say, 'What would everyone like to do?' because you don't get a direct answer because no one wants to say, 'This is what we want to do.' We try to listen to the conversations, ask all the workers involved what they think we should be going, and go out and try it. If it is successful we know we've done the right thing. If it is not successful, then that's also telling us it's not the right thing they want. So we try and learn from those sorts of things. It is not really a formal way of approaching it and I don't know if that is right or not . . ."

—Voluntary organization providing day care, quoted in Cantley *et al.* (2005: 18)

Service user involvement and social inclusion

Since dementia has been such a latecomer to the field of service user involvement, there is no question that all initiatives to include the voices of people with dementia should be welcomed. A lot has been achieved in this respect in a relatively short time. Currently, however, there is still a long way to go in making service user initiatives truly representative of the population with dementia at large. There is significant over-representation, in demographic terms, of the relatively young, those with milder cognitive impairments, those living in their own homes, and white, former professionals. While women are more likely to be diagnosed with dementia than men and, once diagnosed, to find themselves in long-term care (Bamford 2011), this gender divide is also not well represented in the make-up of many current service user groups.

There is some irony about this current situation, particularly when we consider that it is the experiences and views of people with more severe dementia – those who are most likely to be socially isolated and subject to stigmatization – that most need to be heard if anything is to change. It is, of course, easy to conclude that the nature of dementia itself makes service user involvement for people who have more pronounced cognitive impairments, or are in longer-term care, unfeasible. Unfortunately, we then run the risk of this becoming a self-fulfilling prophecy (Downs 1997). If we do not elicit the views of people who experience at first-hand the practices that we seek to change, then there is a danger of overlooking key dimensions of the lived experience of dementia, and also of failing to acknowledge the extremes of social and cultural diversity among those who are affected.

The client groups encountered by many direct care practitioners – in the community, in day care, intermediate or longer-term care, on acute and general hospital wards – have very different needs and priorities from those of service-user representatives who are not themselves actually using those services (Thompson *et al.* 2007). And it is in these same contexts of service delivery that improvement is both most needed and most difficult to achieve. So how do we come up with a model of service user involvement in which the voices of all people with dementia can be heard? How do we involve in service user consultations representatives of the vast and largely voiceless constituency of people already experiencing formal dementia care "from the inside"? The following subsection highlights some conceptual changes that are needed in thinking about what genuinely inclusive service user involvement might mean for people with dementia, and some strategies for eliciting the views of those who communicate using less orthodox means.

Broadening the context: participatory methods and principles

We might tend to think immediately about conference platforms, formal meetings, or the completion of measures such as surveys and questionnaires as the stuff of service user involvement. In reality, however, it need not take these forms at all, and the fact that some people with dementia would find it difficult to cope with such activities should not be used as a reason for excluding them. Given the concurrent physical health and mobility problems many people with dementia experience, in addition to their difficulties with short-term memory, it is incumbent upon anyone who wants to do service user involvement in anything other than a tokenistic way to consult people at a time and place convenient to them. Over the last five years, for example, Bradford Dementia Group has implemented a service user involvement strategy that involves outreach work to involve people with dementia in the environments where they normally spend their time, rather than restricting service user involvement to on-site activities at the University of Bradford (Capstick 2011).

There is, moreover, a wide range of approaches that can be used to facilitate the views of people who have difficulties with verbal communication. There is currently a tendency to assume that people with dementia who are not able or willing to take part in formal sit-down interviews cannot therefore be involved in research at all. In reality, however, this is a challenge to our own methodological ingenuity, rather than a legitimate reason for excluding people.

Here are a few examples of methods we have used to involve "experts by experience" (Katz *et al.* 2000) in practitioner education and practice development in dementia care:

1 *Walking interviews.* Some people with dementia prefer to be on the move, and movement may also facilitate their communication. One man who attended a day centre we visited was often slumped in a chair when we arrived with the appearance of being disengaged and unapproachable. In reality, he was merely bored, and happily accompanied us on a circular walking route, where he became animated and articulate. Among other things, we found out that he thought the garden needed improvement, and that he felt somewhat excluded from activities in the lounge. We also learned a lot about the values-base he brought with him from his previous career and community work. This interaction was filmed and has been used in practitioner education (Capstick and Chatwin 2011).

2 *Elicitation techniques using pictures, music or objects.* If a walking interview might be thought of as the use of movement to elicit service-user voices, similar outcomes can be achieved using other elicitation techniques, depending on a person's preferred way of communicating. For example, a practitioner-student on one of our degree programmes used the reactions of people with dementia to pictures of different kinds of table setting in order to improve their mealtime experience. In another study, practitioners used an exploration of clients' favourite music as way of finding out what was important to them, and informing care planning (Capstick 2012a). These small local studies also provide a model for broader service user involvement initiatives.

3 *Participatory video.* Media coverage of dementia tends to rely on negative visual imagery that contributes to the "no cure/no hope/no help" view of dementia identified by Kitwood (1995) almost 20 years ago. Various studies have involved people with dementia talking on film about their experiences of dementia, and while these can be useful for education and public awareness raising, the person involved can also sometimes be positioned by the camera in a passive role (the object of the "gaze" of others). It is rare to find a person with dementia taking control of either the film-making process or its content. Participatory video is intended to reverse power relationships in film-making by giving those whose voices are traditionally stifled a direct role in making films about subjects that are of importance to them (Lunch and Lunch 2006). The first research trial of participatory video is currently taking place in a care centre for people with dementia in the north of the UK. Interim findings suggest that participatory video enhances self-esteem and status within and between peer groups for the people with dementia taking part (Capstick 2012b). In the longer term, participatory video may prove to have significant potential for enabling those people with dementia who are relatively socially invisible to get their views into public arenas in the form of service-user-directed film.

4 *Observations of day-to-day life, including conversations and comments that arise spontaneously.* People with dementia tell us about their experience of receiving services all the time through their verbal and non-verbal communication. The problem isn't always that people have nothing to say, but that their first-hand testimony is not taken seriously. For example, Bryce and colleagues' (2010) analysis of care home narratives includes numerous extracts similar to the following one from a woman with dementia, who had herself earlier in life been a housekeeper in a large hotel:

> 66 The way that waitress [actually a staff member] talks to me . . . she swears . . . it's just not the thing. I told the lady last night that she didn't have to go just because they said it's time to go to bed [. . .] I said I don't want to go to bed. I can go to bed on my own, thank you very much [. . .] They never laugh and they don't speak to you and they more or less throw the food at you [. . .] *You don't really know until you stay here what it's like.* 99

> —Bryce *et al.* (2010: 189; emphasis added)

In his Introduction to the anthology by Bryce and colleagues, David Clegg, who initially collected the narratives, notes that the director of a major private care company dismissed such feedback on the quality of its service as "gossip". From the perspective offered by narrative health care, however, it can be framed quite differently as the amplification of voices that would otherwise have been lost (Frank 2010).

All such consultative approaches can help to elicit valuable information about how people with dementia experience the services they receive. They may also help to establish the uncomfortable truth that what still tends to be described as "challenging behaviour" is, in fact, often legitimate customer complaint about standards of care: the kind of feedback that would have be taken seriously in a hotel, but rarely is in a nursing home. The findings from such exercises can be fed back in a variety of formats to more formal meetings of established service user groups for their consideration and action. This may require a transitional stage in which the current service user involvement agenda is troubled and unsettled, but this seems necessary if we genuinely wish to ensure that everyone has a voice.

Exercise 28.3: User involvement in practice

Imagine you are organizing an event for 30 people with dementia, to learn their views on how best to design accommodation for people with dementia.

- What would you consider when planning the event?
- How would you decide which involvement approaches to use?
- What practical adjustments would you make to ensure everyone could be involved?

Guiding principles for involving people with dementia in service development and evaluation

Key principles to successful involvement of people with dementia in service development and evaluation include: building trust; deciding whose views to seek; providing enough time and being flexible; providing a supportive physical and social environment; and having a commitment to acting on the feedback received.

Building trust

Being questioned can be perceived as threatening to someone with dementia, since they often make mistakes when asked questions (Stalker *et al.* 1999). When there is an imbalance of power between people using a service and people providing the service, building trust is essential.

Deciding whose views to seek

Gatekeepers such as a social worker, community psychiatric nurse, care home manager, or family carer, are sometimes relied upon to access service users or to aid communication. Although someone the person knows and trusts can play a role in supporting them to understand a process, potential biases should be considered. For example, Bamford and Bruce (2000) noted that, when asked for advice on participants for their focus group, staff excluded people with severe cognitive impairment, those with communication difficulties, and those who disliked being sedentary.

Having sufficient time and being flexible

The experience of dementia is unique to each person. As discussed in Chapter 14, people with dementia process information at a slower rate than those without dementia, need more time to complete tasks, and may become anxious if put under undue pressure:

> ❝There are times of course when it is simply impossible for me to take part in anything. Apart from the gradual mental deterioration associated with Alzheimer's I often succumb to sporadic episodes of confusion which may last for just a day, or as much as a week, and to varying degrees of intensity . . . On my good days I will give all I've got. ❞
>
> —Robinson (2002: 104–5)

Providing a supportive social environment

Ignoring social cues can damage involvement approaches. Hubbard *et al.* (2003) noted the feelings of an interviewee with dementia as she struggled to remember facts and reflected that interjecting or prompting could have reduced her embarrassment. Public perceptions of dementia can undermine a person's willingness to get involved in decisions or activities. Sharing positive messages and demonstrating the achievements of people with dementia can help to provide a more positive social context for involvement activities.

> ❝I went to the Newcastle convention a while ago and was totally amazed at what I saw. It was the first time I had seen people with dementia giving talks about the illness and their lives. Being there made me realise that I was certainly not alone and if other people could do this sort of thing then perhaps I should get involved. My wife said the change in me after this was remarkable . . .❞
>
> —*Living with Dementia* (June/July 2006: 2)

Providing a supportive physical environment

Many people with dementia need environmental cues to understand what is being discussed (Dewing 2002). Some people find it easier to talk in a quiet, private place while others may be uncomfortable with this level of intensity. Allan (2001) suggests a flexible approach to finding an environment that suits the person.

Having a commitment to acting on the feedback received

People need to know when they have taken the time and trouble to contribute their perspective and be involved that it will be taken into account. The time needed for follow-up action, evaluation, and feedback can easily be underestimated in the face of pressing organizational agendas (Cantley *et al.* 2005).

What does user involvement achieve?

Providers and researchers have begun to ask what evidence there is that user involvement improves services (Branfield and Beresford 2006), and service users have been questioning the usefulness of getting involved ("what difference does it actually make?"). Meanwhile, for people with dementia, it is a new experience to have their voice "privileged" (Wilkinson 2002), to be listened to, and to be influential. For example, within the Living with Dementia project, one participant said: "It is nice to speak up for yourself instead of having professionals do it for you." And staff often find their sense of meaning in the work they do with people with dementia is reinforced: "You have a better understanding with the client and now have built a better relationship with them" (Allan 2001). There is a growing body of evidence about the impact of user involvement for service users in general, including resources collated by the national advisory group Involve.

Debates and controversies

When seeking to involve people with dementia in service development and evaluation, there is a danger that we will assume that all people with dementia have the same experience of a service, what Reid *et al.* (2001) refer to as an assumed "uniformity of experience". In addition, we are in danger of relying on those who are more articulate or more able to represent that experience. It is important to acknowledge that different service users will have different experiences of different services. The most effective way to do this is not always clear.

Working with people with dementia as service users can be difficult if people are unaware they have dementia or do not have insight into their condition. However, this can be overcome by using terms preferred by the service user, such as "memory problems", and by discussing a "representation" (Reid *et al.* 2001) of the aims of the involvement process – for example, in Reid and colleagues' case, asking about what it is like "being here" rather than discussing the day centre. Any opinions expressed are still credible and valid regarding the issue at hand.

Sometimes we are unsure as to the meaning of what is being communicated (Dewing 2002). Bamford and Bruce (2002) have cautioned against interpreting metaphors in storytelling, especially as participants did not always recall comments or stories they had told. They also suggest that participation in a focus group or interview may provide a welcome distraction from usual routines and activities and so may result in the expression of predominantly positive views. Group settings can also result in people giving idealized "public" accounts of their feelings, which are sometimes contradicted in subsequent contributions by the same participant. Using proxies to gain important information must be done cautiously and skilfully. The extent to which proxies are used, and determining the point at which they should be consulted, remain controversial.

Although we have said that involvement should be expected throughout the experience of dementia, the reality is that a lot of involvement activity is with people who are in the earlier stages. There is still much work to be done to ensure that the voice of people throughout their whole experience of dementia is accessed in practice. There remains disagreement about the most effective ways to involve people throughout the course of dementia.

Conclusion

The involvement of people with dementia as service users has developed a momentum that is seeing the appearance of a growing amount of innovative practice, led to some extent by people with dementia. Now that the "voice" of the person with dementia has emerged, and there are methods available to ensure that voice is heard, the key will be to take action with or on behalf of those voices. Although the experience of dementia is unique to each individual, there is a collective voice emerging, which expects to be listened to and is beginning to set its own agendas and priorities. Many researchers and practitioners are enthused by the possibilities this presents and will continue to chart new waters, with people with dementia as our teachers: "Like Columbus, I am on a voyage of discovery. My route is not exact and I must make adjustments as I go along."

Further information

The Dementia Engagement and Empowerment Project (DEEP) is a national initiative led by Innovations in Dementia in partnership with the Mental Health Foundation. DEEP supports the development of user involvement groups for people with dementia across the UK, sharing ideas and approaches in order to develop a national network of the collective voices of people with dementia [www.dementiavoices.org.uk].

I can! I will! is a web site of ideas from Alzheimer's Disease International. It provides resources that support people around the world to stand up and raise awareness about dementia. There are dedicated resources for people with dementia [www.alz.co.uk/icaniwill].

Involve is a national advisory group that supports greater public involvement in NHS, public health, and social care research. They provide a range of ideas and evidence about the impact of user involvement [www.invo.org.uk].

The Alzheimer's Society is a membership organization that is working to improve the lives of people affected by dementia. It has 25,000 members including people with personal experience of dementia and professionals who provide or design services for people with dementia and their carers. The organization provides local support in the form of information to people and communities that are affected by dementia. There are similar organizations in most countries and many regions [http://alzheimers.org.uk].

References

Allan, K. (2001) *Communication and Consultation: Exploring Ways for Staff to Involve People with Dementia in Developing Services*. Bristol: Policy Press.

Alzheimer's Society Canada (2006) *Engaging People with Early Stage Alzheimer's Disease in the Work of the Alzheimer's Society*. Toronto: Imagine Canada.

Bamford, C. and Bruce, E. (2000) Defining the outcomes of community care: the perspectives of older people with dementia and their carers, *Ageing and Society*, 20: 543–70.

Bamford, C. and Bruce, E. (2002) Successes and challenges in using focus group with older people with dementia, in H. Wilkinson (ed.) *The Perspective of People with Dementia: Research Methods and Motivations*. London: Jessica Kingsley.

Bamford, S.-M. (2011) *Women and Dementia – Not Forgotten*. London: International Longevity Centre (ILC-UK).

Barnett, E. (2000) *Including the Person with Dementia in Designing and Delivering Care – "I Need to Be Me!"* London: Jessica Kingsley.

Bartlett, R. and O'Connor, D. (2010) *Broadening the Dementia Debate: Towards Social Citizenship*. Bristol: Policy Press.

Beard, R. (2004) Advocating voice: organisational, historical and social milieux of the Alzheimer's disease movement, *Sociology of Health and Illness*, 26(6): 797–819.

Branfield, F. and Beresford, P. (2006) *Making User Involvement Work: Supporting Service User Networking and Knowledge*. York: Joseph Rowntree Foundation.

Bryce, C., Capstick, A., Clegg, D., Cinamon, G., Davis, P.E.H. *et al*. (2010) *Tell Mrs. Mill her Husband is Still Dead: More Stories from the Trebus Project*. London: Trebus Publishing.

Bryden, C. (2005) *Dancing with Dementia: My Story of Living Positively with Dementia*. London: Jessica Kingsley.

Cantley, C., Woodhouse, J. and Smith, M. (2005) *Listen to Us: Involving People with Dementia in Planning and Developing Services*. Northumbria: Dementia North.

Capstick, A. (2011) Travels with a Flipcam: bringing the community to people with dementia in a day care setting through visual technology, *Visual Studies*, 26(2): 142–7.

Capstick, A. (2012a) Dancing to the music of time: an experiential learning exercise in dementia care, *Journal of Applied Arts and Health*, 3(2): 117–31.

Capstick, A. (2012b) Participatory video and situated ethics: avoiding disablism, in E.-J. Milne, C. Mitchell and N. de Lange (eds.) *Handbook of Participatory Video*. New York: Alta Mira.

Capstick, A. and Chatwin, J. (2011) *Bay Tree Voices*. Bradford: University of Bradford/Visible Research.

Carr, S. (2004) *Has Service User Participation Made a difference to Social Care Services?* Position Paper No. 3. London: Social Care Institute for Excellence.

Chaston, D., Pollard, N. and Jubb, D. (2004) Young onset of dementia: a case for real empowerment, *Journal of Dementia Care*, 12(6): 24–6.

Clare, L., Roth, I. and Pratt, R. (2005) Perceptions of change over time in early Alzheimer's disease, *Dementia*, 4(4): 487–520.

Clare, L., Rowlands, J. and Quin, R. (2008) Collective strength: the impact of developing a shared social identity in early stage dementia, *Dementia*, 7(1): 9–30.

Dewing, J. (2002) From ritual to relationship: a person-centred approach to consent in qualitative research with older people who have a dementia, *Dementia*, 1(2): 157–71.

Downs, M. (1997) The emergence of the person in dementia research, *Aging and Society,* 17: 597–607.

Frank, A. (2010) *Letting Stories Breathe: A Socio-narratology*. Chicago, IL: University of Chicago Press.

Howorth, M., Riley, C., Drummond, G. and Keady, J. (2011) The Open Doors network: a pioneering scheme, *Journal of Dementia Care*, 19(3): 20–1.

Hubbard, G., Downs, M. and Tester, S. (2003) Including older people with dementia in research: challenges and strategies, *Aging and Mental Health*, 7(5): 351–62.

Katz, A.M., Conant, L., Inui, T., Baron, D. and Bor, D. (2000) A council of elders: creating a multi-voiced dialogue in a community of care, *Social Science and Medicine*, 50: 851–60.

Kitwood, T. (1995) Cultures of care: tradition and change, in T. Kitwood and S. Benson (eds.) *The New Culture of Dementia Care*. London: Hawker Publications, pp. 7–11.

Litherland, R. (2003) Listen to us, *Working with Older People*, 7(4): 17–20.

Lorentzon, M. and Bryan, K. (2007) Respect for the person with dementia: fostering greater user involvement in service planning, *Quality in Ageing*, 8(1): 23–9.

Lunch, N. and Lunch, C. (2006) *Insights into Participatory Video: A Handbook for the Field*. Oxford: Insightshare.

Murphy, J., Gray, C.M. and Cox, S. (2007) The use of talking mats as a communication resource to improve communication and quality care for people with dementia, *Journal of Housing, Care and Support*, 10(3): 21–7.

Pratt, R. (2002) Nobody's ever asked how I felt, in H. Wilkinson (ed.) *The Perspective of People with Dementia: Research Methods and Motivations*. London: Jessica Kingsley.

Reed, J., Cook, G., Bolter, V. and Douglas, B. (2006) *Older People "Getting Things Done": Involvement in Policy and Planning Initiatives*. York: Joseph Rowntree Foundation.

Reid, D., Ryan, T. and Enderby, P. (2001) What does it mean to listen to people with dementia?, *Disability and Society*, 16(3): 377–92.

Robinson, E. (2002) Should people with Alzheimer's disease take part in research?, in H. Wilkinson (ed.) *The Perspective of People with Dementia: Research Methods and Motivations*. London: Jessica Kingsley.

Robson, P., Begum, N. and Locke, M. (2003) *Developing User Involvement: Working towards User Centred Practice in Voluntary Organisations*. Bristol: Policy Press.

Sainsbury Centre for Mental Health (2005) *Beyond the Water Towers: The Unfinished Revolution in Mental Health Services 1985–2005*. London: Sainsbury Centre for Mental Health.

Small, N. and Rhodes, P. (2001) *User Involvement and the Seriously Ill*. York: Joseph Rowntree Foundation.

Stalker, K., Gilliard, J. and Downs, M. (1999) Eliciting user perspectives on what works, *International Journal of Geriatric Psychiatry*, 14: 120–34.

Thompson, R., Capstick, A., Heyward, T., Pulsford, D. and Hope, K. (2007) Involving people with dementia and carers in educating professionals: how are we doing?, *Journal of Dementia Care*, 15(4): 26–8.

Weaks, D., Wilkinson, H., Houston, A. and McKillop, J. (2011) *Challenging Attitudes, Challenging Ourselves: Exploring the Benefits and Struggles of Ten Years of the Scottish Dementia Working Group*. Edinburgh: Scottish Dementia Working Group.

Wilkinson, H. (ed.) (2002) *The Perspective of People with Dementia: Research Methods and Motivations*. London: Jessica Kingsley.

Williamson, T. (2012) *A Stronger Collective Voice for People with Dementia*. York: Joseph Rowntree Foundation.

CHAPTER 29

A trained and supported workforce

Barbara Bowers

> &&After yet another visit from health professionals to our home my mother who had been diagnosed with Alzheimer's disease some time previously commented "What a lot of good friends we have. I treasure that remark for it showed that those people with whom we were in touch, simply because my mother had dementia, she felt were our friends.&&
>
> —Doug Jenks London, UK

Learning objectives

By the end of this chapter, you will:

- Know the characteristics of people who work as paid caregivers for people with dementia
- Understand the influence of training on work life and care quality
- Understand the components of effective dementia training programmes

Introduction

The preceding chapters clearly demonstrate the importance of skills, knowledge, and commitment in providing high-quality care for people with dementia. Recruiting and training skilled and compassionate workers has become a serious challenge across the world (Mathers and Leonardi 2000). In addition to chronic worker shortages, there is evidence that many health and social care practitioners who work with people with dementia are inadequately prepared for their work (All-Party Parliamentary Group on Dementia 2009). This chapter will outline the characteristics of workers caring for people with dementia and what is known about recruiting, developing, supporting, and retaining competent staff.

Dementia care: crossing settings and specialties

The focus of this chapter is on workers employed in settings specifically designated to care for older adults. However, contrary to common assumptions, understanding how to care for people with dementia is relevant to health care providers in all care settings. Health care workers, whether in generic (hospitals, clinics, home care, and hospices) or specialty settings (emergency, orthopaedics, surgery, etc.), care for people who have dementia.

Dementia care across settings

Older people comprise a large and growing percentage of hospitalized patients. For example, in the USA, over 50% of hospital days are used by older people, half of whom are estimated to have some degree of dementia (Silverstein and Maslow 2006; NHPCO 2007), while in the UK estimates suggest that at any one time at least 25% of hospital beds are occupied by people with dementia (Alzheimer's Society 2009).

Most research on paid care for people with dementia has been conducted in nursing home settings. Recent estimates suggest that the rate of dementia in residential aged care (nursing homes, high care) settings is between 40% and 85%, and is expected to increase significantly (Cipher *et al.* 2006; Feldman *et al.* 2006; Kuske *et al.* 2007; Lithgow *et al.* 2012). The recent report on long-term care by Alzheimer's Disease International (2013) argues that institutional settings will continue to provide a much needed service for people with advanced dementia.

While we know little about care provided in assisted living or extra care housing (see Chapter 23), this is the fastest growing choice of housing for older people in developed as well as developing countries (AIHW 2004; Teri *et al.* 2005; Hyde *et al.* 2007) and is expected to eventually surpass the number of people living in nursing homes (Teri *et al.* 2005). Current estimates are that more than half of the people in assisted living have some degree of dementia (Rosenblatt *et al.* 2004). Little is known about the workers who provide care in this setting, such as their level of education, their knowledge of dementia, their attitudes towards people with dementia, their training opportunities after taking the job, or their care practices.

Most people with dementia live at home, with a family carer or alone. Although there are only estimates of the prevalence of dementia among recipients of home care services, the majority of those receiving home care are over 65 (NCHS 2004; Tarricone and Tsouros 2008; Genet *et al.* 2011). Increasingly, governments around the world are encouraging older people, including people with dementia, to remain at home, cared for primarily by family, for as long as possible (Korczyk 2004; Tarricone and Tsouros 2008; Alzheimer's Disease International 2013). Understanding how to care for people with dementia is vital for home care workers, as they are a major resource for family caregivers.

Aged care/dementia care workers

The characteristics of aged care workers are quite consistent across the world. They tend to be older, poorer, and less well educated than other health care workers, primarily female (generally 90–95%), often employed part-time with unpredictable work hours (Crown *et al.* 1995; Spratley *et al.* 2000; GAO 2001; Korczyk 2004; Colombo *et al.* 2011; Hussein and Manthorpe 2012), and have extremely complicated and stressful personal lives (Tellis-Nayak and Tellis-Nayak 1989; Colombo *et al.* 2011). In the USA, they are less likely than other service workers to have health cover (Stone *et al.* 2005).

Developing and supporting a high-quality workforce

Aged care workers overall have lower educational levels and receive less formal training for their work than do other workers in health-related fields (Beck *et al.* 1999; Korczyk 2004; Colombo *et al.* 2011; Hussein and Manthorpe 2012). Specific competencies needed by dementia care workers have been identified by international organizations such as Alzheimer's associations and in the UK by Skills for Health and Skills for Care. They generally include: basic knowledge of dementia, person-centred care and quality of life for people with dementia, communicating with someone who has dementia, and responding to distressing or aggressive behaviour (MDC 2006).

While some nations, such as Sweden, the Netherlands, and Germany are attempting to increase the basic educational requirements for aged care workers, many nations continue to recruit workers who have been "economically inactive" for many years, with recent experience as a housewife being their primary skill base (Korczyk 2004). Minimal or no supplementary training in dementia care is common. For example, in the USA, nurse aides (who provide 80–90% of direct care in nursing homes and most of the direct care in assisted living and home settings) complete a 75-hour general aged care training programme (varying somewhat by state). The federal government currently mandates that "some portion" of this time be devoted to communicating with people who have cognitive impairments (Federal Regulations 2005). In the UK, there is no specified level of training required to work with people with dementia. This lower level of training both reflects and contributes to the perception that workers in this field are insufficiently skilled, which in turn works to keep wages and worker respect low.

Exercise 29.1: Finding and developing competent dementia care workers – dementia care as an employment programme

You have recently taken a post with responsibility for developing a dementia training programme for workers in assisted living residences across your region. The workers currently providing care in assisted living are primarily mothers who have recently re-entered the workforce after many years at home raising children, workers from a clothing factory that has recently closed, and immigrants who have had some difficulty finding work. The immigrant group is comprised of relatively highly educated, professional women who have not been able to engage in their professions since arriving in the country. What is your assessment of this situation and how will you proceed to prepare the workers?

The importance of education

It is important to understand that many direct care workers and supervising nurses in long-term care are insufficiently prepared for the work they are doing (Menne *et al.* 2007; Bourbonniere and Strumpf 2008). Although the lack of sufficient skills and knowledge in aged care workers has been well documented, staff and management in long-term care are slow to recognize and address the problem. For example, a study of staff recognition of resident pain in two Dutch nursing homes revealed a high level of staff satisfaction with pain recognition and management despite considerable deficits in relevant knowledge (Zwakhalen *et al.* 2007). This suggests a lack of awareness regarding the necessary knowledge base.

Caring for people with dementia can be highly stressful, particularly for workers who are not well prepared. The pervasiveness of worker stress is reflected in long-term care research. The focus of research has been on staff stress, job satisfaction, and worker turnover. This is not surprising, since the "behaviour" of people with dementia has been repeatedly identified as a major source of worker stress, low job satisfaction, and high turnover (Nagatomo *et al.* 2001; Roper *et al.* 2001; Brodaty *et al.* 2003; Pekkarinen *et al.* 2004; Kim 2006; Ruiz *et al.* 2006; Coogle *et al.* 2007; Davison *et al.* 2007; Gleckman 2010). It is estimated that 28% of residents engage in behaviours staff consider "seriously" problematic, while an additional 31% engage in "mildly problematic" behaviours (Nametz and Jesudason 1990; Heponiemi *et al.* 2006). Staff with limited education working within a person-centred, psychosocial approach are less likely to resort to the use of anti-psychotic medication (Fossey *et al.* 2006).

Staff education has been shown to reduce worker stress and improve worker performance (Edvardsson *et al.* 2009). A review of research on "behaviour management" training programmes concluded that effective educational programmes have significant "secondary benefits" (Kuske *et al.* 2007; McCabe *et al.* 2007), including increased staff satisfaction, reduced staff stress, and decreased staff turnover. Perception of behaviour as challenging is amenable to change. There is increasing evidence that perceptions of residents as displaying "distressing behaviour" is often the result of staff members' inability to communicate effectively with people who have dementia and that worker stress strongly influences the quality of interactions between residents and staff (Sourial *et al.* 2001).

Research has repeatedly documented that high-quality dementia care training programmes have a positive impact on staff knowledge, attitude, and self-efficacy, while reducing stress, improving overall performance (as assessed by supervisors), and reducing residents' behaviours that staff find distressing (Sloane *et al.* 2004; Teri *et al.* 2005; Chrzescijanski *et al.* 2007; Davison *et al.* 2007; Chenoweth *et al.* 2009). Significantly, staff education was found to improve the ability of staff to identify indicators of resident distress, and to respond accordingly (Chrzescijanski *et al.* 2007).

In a study of three nursing homes, workers' ability to read emotional cues, both body language and facial expression, greatly enhanced the communication between the person with dementia and the caregiver (Magai *et al.* 2002). One of the most significant findings from this research is the ability of staff, following a carefully designed training programme, to more effectively interpret and respond to resident behaviour, resulting in less aggressive behaviour on the part of people with dementia, improved quality of life, and lower worker stress.

What makes a successful educational programme?

Unfortunately, many educational programmes have resulted in minimal or no improvement in quality of life or quality of care, highlighting the importance of designing effective educational programmes (Noel *et al.* 2000; Sveinsdottir *et al.* 2006; McCabe *et al.* 2007). It is well documented that new knowledge, by itself, rarely results in sustained practice change (Broad 1997; Baumbusch *et al.* 2008). Sustained practice change requires an effective training programme, learner preparation prior to the training, and sustained, targeted support following educational sessions (Cromwell and Kolb 2004). While learner characteristics are often assumed to be the primary determinant of whether new learning is applied in the practice setting, research suggests otherwise (Cromwell and Kolb 2004). Cromwell and Kolb (2004) suggest that worker intent to use the new knowledge, worker confidence, voluntariness of attendance at the training programme, and support from supervisors and peers, collectively, determine the eventual use of knowledge gained.

While intent-to-use new knowledge, worker confidence, and voluntariness of attendance at the educational programme might appear to reflect individual worker motivation and ability, they are largely determined by the worker's direct supervisor and the work environment. For example, a review conducted by Cromwell and Kolb demonstrated how support and encouragement of supervisors positively influenced both worker intent to use new knowledge and worker confidence (which influences actual use). Voluntariness of attendance is also related to supervisor effectiveness in that sending the right worker to the right training programme, matching worker interests with opportunities, increases the voluntariness of attendance and subsequently the likelihood that new learning will be used to improve practice (Cromwell and Kolb 2004).

A review of research on the effectiveness of staff development programmes in long-term care revealed that many training programmes, both dementia-specific and others, were not designed to maximize the transfer of learning back to the practice setting. A review of dementia-specific staff development programmes found that lack of preparation or follow-up significantly diminished success (Aylward *et al.* 2003; Stolee *et al.* 2005; Kuske *et al.* 2007). Although critical of the general quality of research on staff development in long-term care, Kuske *et al.* (2007) confirmed that preparation of the learner, the use of adult education principles, supervisor support, and worksite reinforcement of learning and support for subsequent application, all contribute to the effectiveness and longevity of training impact. Lack of supervisor involvement, poorly designed educational programmes, failure to address the context of application, and lack of follow-through, all undermine the application and sustainability of new practices (Yeatts *et al.* 2010). Successful educational programmes were those with ongoing reinforcement, supervisor support, and careful attention to learning styles.

Supporting and retaining dementia care workers

Turnover and retention of workers

Staff turnover is a serious challenge to maintaining an adequate and competent workforce (Chou *et al.* 2002; Moyle *et al.* 2003; Kiata *et al.* 2005; Sung *et al.* 2005). In the USA, turnover rates for nurse aides in residential aged care commonly reach 60–70%, sometimes surpassing 100% annually (Institute of Medicine 2001). For supervising nurses, the rate of annual turnover averages around 50%. Even managers in residential aged care settings leave their jobs at relatively high rates, around 40% annually (Castle 2005), leading to chaotic environments and the undermining of care quality and worker morale. Quality of life for people with dementia is highly dependent on worker familiarity with the person's preferences, fears, and routines. Turnover interferes with this and also undermines the development of relationships between residents and staff. Both are extremely important for resident quality of life (Foner 1994; Bowers *et al.* 2006). High turnover also makes it difficult to maintain a workforce with sufficient skill.

Aggression and assaults

According to the US Government Occupational Safety and Health Office (Michael 2002), aged care work has one of the highest rates of worker injury and has been established as one of the most dangerous worksites in the USA (Michael 2002). Data compiled by the Canadian Government have also documented a high rate of worker injuries in long-term care settings (Yassi *et al.* 2004). Repeated exposure to aggressive and/or demanding behaviour, from both residents and family, is common in long-term care (Vinton and Mazza 1994; Morrison and Siu 2000; Secrest *et al.* 2005) and has a negative impact on both job satisfaction and job performance (Chappel and Novak 1992). Staff training has been shown to decrease resident aggression and assaults on workers. For example, in a study examining the impact of a training programme to teach nurse aides to prevent and deal effectively with aggression, Maxfield *et al.* (1996) documented a reduction in resident aggression following the intervention. The researchers provided two one-hour training sessions with follow-up visits and instruction to improve care, particularly during bathing and grooming. Consequently, two hours of training had a significant impact on improving quality of care and reducing injuries related to resident aggression. Other studies have reported similar results (Palmer and Withee 1996; Chrzescijanski *et al.* 2007).

Assaults on workers are also less frequent in specialty dementia care units where workers are likely to be trained in care of people with dementia (Vinton and Mazza 1994; Morgan *et al.* 2005). Both worker stress and lack of training were correlated with a higher incidence of assaults from residents.

Depression

Caring for people with depression is stressful. As depression is common among nursing home residents, estimated to be somewhere between 10% and 40% (Burgio *et al.* 1988; Nametz and Jesudason 1990), this is probably a significant source of stress for staff. A study in Japan demonstrated a high correlation between dementia and depression, and that people with dementia who are depressed are more likely to engage in behaviours that are stressful for workers (Nagatomo *et al.* 2001). This would indicate that educational programmes for dementia care workers should include the development of skills to identify and respond to depression and that better general treatment of depression would lead to lower levels of stress among workers.

Daily care

Daily care is a common source of difficulty for inadequately trained staff, especially when working with people who have dementia. Several studies have examined the impact of training on bathing, feeding, and daily care of residents with dementia. Collectively, these studies show a reduction in aggression, and better resident nutrition when workers are skilled in communicating with people who have dementia (Chang and Lin 2005; Chang and Madigan 2006; Hoeffer *et al.* 2006). Another study (Stevens *et al.* 1998) demonstrated the effectiveness of combined nurse aide training and improved supervision by nurses for increasing resident self-care. This same study demonstrated that a combination of formal training and structured self-monitoring can improve the quality of nurse aides' responses to resident anxiety and distress (Stevens *et al.* 1998). Effective training can clearly reduce the distress experienced by people with dementia and, as a consequence, their caregivers.

Staffing

Inadequate staffing has been consistently correlated with high levels of stress among workers (Bowers and Becker 1992; Chappel and Novak 1992; Institute of Medicine 2001) and has been correlated with higher worker injury rates (Trinkoff *et al.* 2005). Many aged care staff find the workload to be extremely heavy, often finding it impossible to complete their assigned work in the time allotted (Bowers 1987; Bowers *et al.* 2001). As a consequence, workers often leave at the end of their shift feeling bad about the care they were able to provide (Bowers 1987; Foner 1994). Inadequate staffing has an impact on care quality (Harrington *et al.* 2000) and is a particularly important issue in dementia care settings where rushing residents and maintaining rigid schedules can distress residents and, as a consequence, staff. The relatively older age of the workforce in aged care, compared with workers in other health care environments, compounds the stress of heavy physical work.

Not feeling valued or respected: the importance of good supervision

Many aged care workers feel unsupported and devalued, particularly by the professional staff and managers in their work settings and by families of the people they care for (Foner 1994; Bowers *et al.* 2003; Noelker *et al.* 2006; Brannon *et al.* 2007; Ryzin 2007). Not feeling supported or valued by their supervisors is the main reason workers in aged care settings decide to leave their jobs (Bowers *et al.* 2003; McGillis *et al.* 2005; McGilton *et al.* in press). While aged care workers around the world have identified this as a major source of dissatisfaction, licensed staff and managers in the same environments often speak about the respect and admiration they have for the carers (Bowers *et al.* 2003; Brannon *et al.* 2007; Castle *et al.* 2007). This apparent contradiction seems to be a reflection of the difference between carers and their supervisors about what constitutes a positive work environment and positive relationships between carers and their supervisors.

Managers play a pivotal role in creating a supportive work environment, sustaining practice change, and facilitating practice innovation (Yeattes and Seward 2000). Good supervisory practices can be learned but are unfortunately overlooked or incorrectly assumed to be determined exclusively by innate personality traits (McDonald and Kahn 2007).

Not having a say

While the importance of including front-line workers (carers, nurse aides) in care planning conferences is widely recognized, nurse aides are often not invited to or, more frequently, are unable to attend because of heavy work demands and failure to factor care conferences into their work routine (Stone *et al.* 2002; Gurnik and Hollis-Sawyer 2003; McDonald and Kahn 2007). Consequently, such invitations can be perceived by carers as disingenuous, thus creating resentment. In response to this, involving carers more actively and consistently in care decisions is a core goal of the nursing home culture change movement (Kane *et al.* 2007; Bowers and Nolet 2014), which has been designed to improve quality of care and quality of work life (see Chapter 26).

Emotional distress

Aged care workers experience a high level of emotional distress. One reason for this is that caring for, and becoming bonded to, people who are at the end of life means that workers experience continual loss of people they have become attached to. Workers have described particular emotional turmoil when they believe an older person is dying, not wanting the person to die alone (Parks *et al.* 2005). Seeing residents with untreated pain is also a source of great emotional stress for workers (Cipher *et al.* 2006).

Exercise 29.2: Developing programmes to keep staff

You have just accepted a position as Director of Education for an organization that operates several care homes, mostly for people with dementia. This new position was created to develop training programmes for staff at all levels. How will you decide where to start? How will you determine priorities? What information do you need to collect? Who do you need to talk to?

The suggestion has been made that its mostly the carers (nurse aides) who need training, as the nurses are quite competent care providers and have a good knowledge base about care of people with dementia. How will you respond to this suggestion?

What workers say about working with people with dementia

Many workers come to think of the people they care for as family, finding great rewards in the relationship and their ability to make a difference in their lives (Foner 1994; Secrest *et al.* 2005). Studies from several countries have validated that workers in long-term care settings, caring for people with dementia, are highly satisfied with their work, even when they are unhappy with their working conditions (Stone *et al.* 2002; Moyle *et al.* 2003). Workers with prior experience caring for family or friends with dementia are most likely to find their work rewarding, particularly when sufficiently supported (Bowers 1987; Maas *et al.* 1994; Coogle *et al.* 2007). An important finding, however, is that workers with previous rewarding experience caring for friends or family are less likely to remain in their job (Coogle *et al.* 2007). A study of how nurse aides think about their work (Bowers 1987) suggests that it is the inability to provide high-quality care under adverse working conditions that drives these workers away.

A survey conducted in Sweden across care environments found that while nurses working in dementia care environments perceived greater emotional conflicts and greater knowledge demands than did nurses in other environments, they also reported feeling greater support from colleagues than did nurses in other elderly care environments (Josefsson *et al.* 2007).

Debates and controversies

Providing effective education and support for workers in dementia care will result in high-quality care and workers who are likely to enjoy their work and remain in their jobs. This requires effective educational programmes and effective supervision of dementia care workers. Dementia care educational programmes are too often uninformed by what we know is successful, wasting valuable resources and raising expectations that are not subsequently met.

One of the most important influences on the quality of work life is the quality of supervision. Despite this, there are few serious efforts to develop the skills of supervisory staff or to hold them accountable for effective supervision. Maintaining a competent, stable workforce will require much greater commitment to the improvement of working conditions, such as effective, supportive supervisors.

The level of compensation for workers caring for older people and people with dementia continues to be inadequate. This workforce continues to be paid less than other workers, despite the demanding and stressful working conditions, the emotional and physical challenges of the work, and the difficult home lives of many people in this workforce.

Finally, one of the most contentious issues, worldwide, is the level of staffing in residential settings despite the convincing documentation that inadequate staffing hurts both workers and the people they care for.

Conclusion

Dementia care workers will be needed in increasing numbers around the world. The international competition for health workers, along with high turnover rates, has created workforce instability with negative consequences for both workers and the people they care for. There are reasons to believe that the instability of the workforce can be effectively addressed with high-quality educational programmes, improved skills of supervisors, and other consistently favourable working conditions. In particular, research has demonstrated the effectiveness of well-designed educational programmes in improving many of the work-related situations that workers find most stressful. Dementia care workers are generally satisfied with their work, find it rewarding, and are motivated to remain by strong bonds with the people they care for.

Further information

The Pioneer Network is a network of care homes committed to improving the culture of nursing homes, improving care quality and working conditions. It has created a loose affiliation among homes from all over the USA that work together to promote person-centred values in resident care and respect for care providers. It is a grass roots organization started in the 1980s [http://www. pioneernetwork.net/].

The Paraprofessional Healthcare Institute is an organization operated by care workers. It provides a forum for discussing issues, and disseminates reports that are relevant to the working conditions in care homes [http://www.phinational.org/].

Better Jobs/Better Care was a national initiative in the USA funded by the Robert Wood Johnson Foundation, which is committed to enhancing both work life for care workers across settings and for the people receiving services. The initiative, housed in the American Association of Homes and Services for the Aging, managed a four-year initiative that included innovative demonstration projects as well as research [http://www.rwjf.org/].

The WHO Global Workforce Alliance is a WHO-sponsored alliance of worker organizations and governments to track working conditions, need for workers, and the movement of workers around the world. The web site keeps up-to-date information from many countries around the world as well as historical reports on workforce changes over time [http://www.who.int/workforcealliance/en/].

The UK Higher Education in Dementia Network is a network of universities in the UK interested in promoting dementia education at university level. Most recently, they have agreed a curriculum for dementia education in this sector [https://www.dementiauk.org/what-we-do/networks/hedn/].

Skills for Care and Skills for Health (2011) has produced a guide to training the social and health care workforce called *Common Core Principles for Supporting People with Dementia* [https://www. gov.uk/government/publications/common-core-principles-for-supporting-people-with-dementia].

References

All-Party Parliamentary Group on Dementia (2009) *Prepared to Care: Challenging the Dementia Skills Gap*. London: Alzheimer's Society.

Alzheimer's Disease International (2013) *Long Term Care*. London: Alzheimer's Disease International.

Alzheimer's Society (2009) *Counting the Cost: Caring for People with Dementia on Hospital Wards*. London: Alzheimer's Society.

Australian Institute of Health and Welfare (AIHW) (2004) *The Impact of Dementia on the Health and Aged Care Systems*. Canberra: AIHW [http://www.aihw.gov.au/publications/index.cfm/title/10011, accessed 15 January 2008].

Aylward, S., Stolee, P., Keat, N. and Johncox, V. (2003) Effectiveness of continuing education in long-term care: a literature review, *The Gerontologist*, 43(2): 259–71.

Baumbusch, J., Kirkham, S., Khan, K., McDonald, H., Semeniuk, P. *et al.* (2008) Pursuing common agendas: a collaborative model for knowledge translation between research and practice in clinical settings, *Research in Nursing and Health*, 31: 130–40.

Beck, C., Ortigara, A., Mercer, S. and Shue, V. (1999) Enabling and empowering certified nursing assistants for quality dementia care, *International Journal of Geriatric Psychiatry*, 14(7): 197–212.

Bourbonniere, M. and Strumpf, N. (2008) Enhancing geriatric nursing competencies for RNs in nursing homes, *Research in Gerontological Nursing*, 1(3): 171–75.

Bowers, B. (1987) Intergenerational caregiving: adult caregivers and their aging parents, *Advances in Nursing Science*, 9(2): 20–31.

Bowers, B. and Becker, M. (1992) Nurse aides in nursing homes: the relationship between organization and quality, *The Gerontologist*, 32(3): 360–6.

Bowers, B. and Nolet, K. (2014) Developing the Green House® nursing care team: variations on development and implementation, *The Gerontologist*, 54(Suppl. 1): S53–S64.

Bowers, B.J., Lauring, C. and Jacobson, N. (2001) How nurses manage time and work in long-term care facilities, *Journal of Advanced Nursing*, 33(4): 484–91.

Bowers, B., Esmond, S. and Jacobson, N. (2003) Turnover reinterpreted: CNAs talk about why they leave, *Journal of Gerontological Nursing*, 29(3): 36–43.

Bowers, B., Esmond, S., Norton, S. and Holloway, E. (2006) The consumer/provider relationship as care quality mediator, in S. Kunkel and V. Wellin (eds.) *Consumer Voice and Choice in Long Term Care.* New York: Springer.

Brannon, D., Barry, T., Kemper, P., Schreiner, A. and Vasey, J. (2007) Job perceptions and intent to leave among direct care workers, *The Gerontologist*, 47(6): 820–7.

Broad, M. (1997) Overview of transfer of training: from learning to performance, *Performance Improvement Quarterly*, 10(2): 7–21.

Brodaty, H., Draper, B. and Low, L. (2003) Nursing home staff attitudes towards residents with dementia: strain and satisfaction with work, *Journal of Advanced Nursing*, 44(6): 583–90.

Burgio, D., Jones, L., Butler, F. and Engel, B. (1988) Behavior problems in an urban nursing home, *Journal of Gerontological Nursing*, 14: 31–4.

Castle, N. (2005) Turnover begets turnover, *The Gerontologist*, 45(2): 186–94.

Castle, N., Engberg, J. and Men, A. (2007) Nursing home staff turnover: impact on nursing home compare quality measures, *The Gerontologist*, 47(5): 650–61.

Chang, C. and Lin, L. (2005) Effects of a feeding skills training programme on nursing assistants and dementia patients, *Journal of Clinical Nursing*, 14: 1185–92.

Chang, C. and Madigan, A. (2006) The effect of a feeding skills training program for nursing assistants who feed dementia residents in Taiwanese nursing homes, *Geriatric Nursing*, 27(4): 229–36.

Chappel, N. and Novak, M. (1992) The role of support in alleviating stress among nursing assistants, *The Gerontologist*, 32: 351–9.

Chenoweth, L., King, M., Jeon, Y., Brodaty, H., Stein-Parbury, J. *et al.* (2009) Caring for Aged Dementia Care Resident Study (CADRES) of person-centred care, dementia-care mapping, and usual care in dementia: a cluster-randomised trial, *Lancet Neurology*, 8: 317–25.

Chou, S., Boldy, D. and Lee, A. (2002) Measuring job satisfaction in residential aged care, *Journal for Quality in Health Care*, 14(1): 49–54.

Chrzescijanski, D., Moyle, W. and Creedy, D. (2007) Reducing dementia-related aggression through a staff education intervention, *Dementia*, 6(2): 271–86.

Cipher, D., Clifford, A. and Roper, K. (2006) Behavioral manifestations of pain in demented elderly, *Journal of the American Medical Directors' Association*, 7: 355–65.

Colombo, F., Llena-Nozal, A., Mercier, J. and Tjadens, F. (2011) Long term care workers: needed but often undervalued, in *Help Wanted? Providing and Paying for Long Term Care*. OECD Health Policy Studies. Paris: OECD Publishing.

Coogle, C., Parham, A. and Young, K. (2007) Job satisfaction and career commitment among nursing assistants providing Alzheimer's care, *American Journal of Alzheimer's Disease and Other Dementias*, 22: 251.

Cromwell, S. and Kolb, J. (2004) An examination of work–environment support factors affecting transfer of supervisory skills training to the workplace, *Human Resource Development Quarterly*, 13(4): 449–71.

Crown, W., Ahlburg, D. and MacAdam, M. (1995) The demographic and employment characteristics of home care aides, hospital aides, and other workers, *The Gerontologist*, 35: 162–70.

Davison, T.E., McCabe, M.P., Visser, S., Hudgson, C., Buchanan, G. *et al.* (2007) Controlled trial of dementia training with a peer support group for aged care staff, *International Journal of Geriatric Psychiatry*, 22: 868–73.

Edvardsson, D., Sandman, P., Nay, R. and Karlsson, S. (2009) Predictors of job strain in residential dementia care nursing staff, *Journal of Nursing Management*, 17: 59–65.

Federal Regulations (2005) *Code of Federal Regulations*, Title 42, Vol. 3. Washington, DC: US Government.

Feldman, H., Clarfield, A., Bdodsky, J., King, Y. and Tzvi, D. (2006) An estimate of the prevalence of dementia among residents of long term care geriatric institutions in the Jerusalem area, *International Psychogeriatrics*, 18(4): 643–52.

Foner, N. (1994) Nursing home aides: saints or monsters?, *The Gerontologist*, 34: 245–50.

Fossey, J., Ballard, C., Juszczak, E., James, I., Alder, N. *et al.* (2006) Effect of enhanced psychosocial care on anti-psychotic use in nursing home residents with severe dementia: cluster randomised trial, *British Medical Journal*, 332: 756–61.

General Accounting Office (GAO) (2001) *Nursing Workforce: Emerging Nurse Shortages Due to Multiple Factors* (GAO-01–944). Washington, DC: GAO.

Genet, N., Boerma, W., Kringos, D., Bouman, A., Francke, A. *et al.* (2011) Home care in Europe: a systematic literature review, *BMC Health Services Research*, 11: 207.

Gleckman, H. (2010) The faces of homecare: report from the field, *Health Affairs*, 29(1): 125–9.

Gurnik, M. and Hollis-Sawyer, L. (2003) Empowering assisted living front line staff to better care for Alzheimer's and dementia residents, *Ageing International*, 28(1): 82–97.

Harrington, C., Kovner, C., Mezey, M., Kayser-Jones, J., Burger, S. *et al.* (2000) Experts recommend minimum nurse staffing standards for nursing facilities in the United States, *The Gerontologist*, 40(1): 5–16.

Heponiemi, T., Elovainio, M., Pekkarinen, L., Noro, A., Finne-Soveri, H. *et al.* (2006). The moderating effect of employee hostility on the association of long-term elderly care unit's negative resident characteristics to employee stress and well-being, *Journal of Occupational Health Psychology*, 11(2): 157–68.

Hoeffer, B., Talerico, K.A., Rasin, J., Mitchell, M., Stewart, B.J. *et al.* (2006) Assisting cognitively impaired nursing home residents with bathing: effects of two bathing interventions on caregiving, *The Gerontologist*, 46 (4): 524–32.

Hussein, S. and Manthorpe, J. (2012) The dementia social care workforce in England: secondary analysis of a national workforce data set, *Aging and Mental Health*, 16(1): 110–18.

Hyde, J., Perez, B. and Forester, B. (2007) Dementia and assisted living, *The Gerontologist*, 47 (Special Issue III): 51–67.

Institute of Medicine (2001) *Quality of Care in Nursing Homes*. Washington, DC: National Academy Press.

Josefsson, K., Sonde, L., Winblad, B. and Wahlin, T.-B.R. (2007) Work situation of registered nurses in municipal elderly care in Sweden: a questionnaire survey, *International Journal of Nursing Studies*, 44: 71–82.

Kane, R., Lum, T., Culter, L., Dagenholtz, H. and Yu, T. (2007) Resident outcomes in small house nursing homes: a longitudinal evaluation of the initial GREEN HOUSE program, *American Journal of Geriatrics*, 55: 832–9.

Kiata, L., Kerse, N. and Dixon, R. (2005) Residential care workers and residents: the New Zealand story, *New Zealand Medical Journal*, 118(1214): 1–11.

Kim, J. (2006) Effects of gerontological nursing practicum on attitudes toward elders with dementia and elders among Korean nursing students, *Taehan Kanho Hakhoe*, 36(4): 645–51 [in Chinese].

Korczyk, S. (2004) *Long-Term Workers in Five Countries: Issues and Options*. Washington, DC: AARP Public Policy Institute [http://assets.aarp.org/rgcenter/health/2004_07_care.pdf, accessed 2 June 2014].

Kuske, B., Hanns, S., Luck, T., Angermeyer, M.C., Behrens, J. *et al.* (2007) Nursing home staff training in dementia care: a systematic review of evaluated programs, *International Psychogeriatrics*, 19(5): 818–41.

Lithgow, S., Jackson, G. and Browne, D. (2012) Estimating the prevalence of dementia: cognitive screening in Glasgow nursing homes, *International Journal of Geriatric Psychiatry*, 27(8): 785–91.

Maas, M., Buckwalter, K., Swanson, E. and Mobily, P. (1994) Training key to job satisfaction, *Journal of Long Term Care Administration*, Spring, pp. 23–6.

Magai, C., Cohen, C.I. and Gomberg, D. (2002) Impact of training dementia caregivers in sensitivity to nonverbal emotion signals, *International Psychogeriatrics*, 14(1): 25–38.

Mathers, C. and Leonardi, M. (2000) *Global Burden of Dementia in the Year 2000: Summary of Methods and Data Sources*. The Lancet Global Mental Health Series [http://www.who.int/healthinfo/statistics/bod_dementia.pdf, accessed 15 February 2008].

Maxfield, M., Lewis, R., and Cannon, S (1996) Training staff to prevent aggressive behavior of cognitively impaired elderly patients during bathing and grooming. *Journal of Gerontological Nursing,* 22: 37–43.

McCabe, M., Davison, T. and George, K. (2007) Effectiveness of staff training programs for behavioral problems among older people with dementia, *Aging and Mental Health*, 11(5): 505–9.

McDonald, I. and Kahn, K. (2007) Respectful relationships, *Future Age*, 6(2): 12–16.

McGillis, L., McGilton, K., Krejci, J., Pringle, D., Johnston, E. *et al.* (2005) Enhancing the quality of supportive supervisory behavior in long term care facilities, *Journal of Nursing Administration*, 35(4): 181–7.

McGilton, K., Boscart, V., Brown, M. and Bowers, B. (in press) Making tradeoffs between the reasons to leave and reasons to stay, *International Journal of Nursing Studies*.

Menne, H., Ejaz, F., Noelker, L. and Jones, J. (2007) Direct care workers' recommendations for training and continuing education, *Gerontology and Geriatrics Education*, 28(2): 91–108.

Michael, R. (2002) OSHA continues nursing home focus occupational safety and health, *Ergonomics Today* [www.osha.gov, accessed 10 March 2008].

Michigan Dementia Coalition (MDC) (2006) *Knowledge and Skills Needed for Dementia Care: A Guide for Direct Care Workers*. Lansing, MI: MDC.

Morgan, D., Stewart, N., D'Arcy, C., Forbes, D. and Lawson, J. (2005) Work stress and physical assault of nursing aides in rural nursing homes with and without special care units, *Journal of Psychiatric and Mental Health Nursing*, 12: 347–58.

Morrison, R. and Siu, A. (2000) A comparison of pain and its treatment in advanced dementia and cognitively intact patients with hip fracture, *Pain and Symptom Management*, 19: 240–8.

Moyle, W., Skinner, J., Rowe, G. and Gork, C. (2003) Views of job satisfaction and dissatisfaction in Australian long-term care, *Journal of Clinical Nursing*, 12: 168–76.

Nagatomo, I., Akasaki, Y., Tominaga, M., Hashiguchi, W., Uchida, M. *et al.* (2001) Abnormal behavior of residents in a long-term care facility and the associated stress of care staff members, *Archives of Gerontology and Geriatrics*, 33: 203–10.

Nametz, P. and Jesudason, V. (1990) Behavioral problems among nursing home residents: data from the 1988 Wisconsin annual survey of nursing homes, *Health Data Review*, 4: 1–7.

National Center for Health Statistics (NCHS) (2004) *Home Health Care Patients: Data from the 2000 National Home and Hospice Care Survey* [http://www.cdc.gov/nchs].

National Hospice and Palliative Care Organization (NHPCO) (2007) *Facts and Figures: Hospice Care in America* [http://www.nhpco.org/files/public/public_policy/advocacy/key-facts-figures.pdf, accessed 10 February 2008].

Noel, M.A., Pearce, G.L. and Metcalf, R. (2000) Front line workers in long-term care: the effect of educational interventions and stabilization of staffing ratios on turnover and absenteeism, *Journal of the American Medical Directors Association*, November/December, pp. 241–7.

Noelker, L., Ejaz, F., Menne, H.I. and Jones, J. (2006) The impact of stress and support on nursing assistant satisfaction with supervision, *Journal of Applied Gerontology*, 25(4): 307–23.

Palmer, A.C. and Withee, B.M. (1996) Dementia care: effects of behavioral intervention training on staff perceptions of their work in veterans' nursing home, *Geriatric Nursing*, 17(3): 137–40.

Parks, S.M., Haines, C., Foreman, D., McKinstry, E. and Maxwell, T.L. (2005) Evaluation of an educational program for long-term care nursing assistants, *Clinical Experience,* January/February, pp. 61–5.

Pekkarinen, L., Sinervo, T., Perala, M.L. and Elovainio, M. (2004) Work stressors and the quality of life in long-term care units, *The Gerontologist*, 44(5): 633–64.

Roper, J., Shapira, J. and Beck, A. (2001) Nurse caregiver feelings about agitation in Alzheimer's disease, *Journal of Gerontological Nursing*, 27: 32–9.

Rosenblatt, A., Samus, Q., Steele, C., Baker, A., Harper, M. *et al.* (2004) The Maryland Assisted Living Study: prevalence, recognition, and treatment of dementia and other psychiatric disorders in the assisted living population of Central Maryland, *Journal of the American Geriatrics Society*, 52(10): 1618–25.

Ruiz, J., Smith, M., van Zuilen, M., Williams, C. and Mintzer, M. (2006) The impact of a computer-based training tutorial on dementia in long term care for licensed practice nursing students, *Gerontology and Geriatrics Education*, 26(3): 67–9.

Ryzin, J. (2007) Workplace interventions for retention, quality, and performance, *Future Age*, 6(2): 16–19.

Secrest, J., Iorio, D. and Martz, W. (2005) The meaning of work for nursing assistants who stay in long term care, *Journal of Clinical Nursing*, 14(8b): 90–7.

Silverstein, N. and Maslow, K. (2006) *Improving Hospital Care for Persons with Dementia*. New York: Springer.

Sloane, P.D., Hoeffer, B., Mitchell, C.M., McKenzie, D.A., Barrick, A.L. *et al.* (2004) Effect of person-centered showering and the towel bath on bathing-associated aggression, agitation, and discomfort in nursing home residents with dementia: a randomized, controlled trial, *Journal of the American Geriatrics Society*, 52: 1795–1804.

Sourial, R., McCusker, J., Cole, M. and Abrahamowicz, M. (2001) Agitation in demented patients in an acute care hospital: prevalence, disruptiveness and staff burden, *International Psychogeriatrics*, 13: 183–97.

Spratley, E., Johnsom, A., Spchalski, J., Fritz, M. and Spencer, W. (2000) *The Registered Nurse Population: Findings from the National Sample Survey of Registered Nurses*. Washington, DC: US Department of Health and Human Services.

Stevens, A., Burgio, L., Bailey, E., Burgio, K., Paul, P.L. *et al.* (1998) Teaching and maintaining behavior management skills with nursing assistants in a nursing home, *The Gerontologist*, 38: 379–84.

Stolee, P., Esbaugh, J., Aylward, S., Cathers, T., Harvey, D. *et al.* (2005) Factors associated with the effectiveness of continuing education in long term care, *The Gerontologist*, 45(3): 399–409.

Stone, R., Reinhard, S., Bowers, B., Zimmerman, D., Phillips, C. *et al.* (2002) *Evaluation of the Wellspring Model for Improving Nursing Home Quality*. Commonwealth Fund [http://cmwf.org, accessed 3 March 2008].

Stone, R., Lipson, D., Barbaratta, L., Bryant, N. and Mosely, N. (2005) Family care and paid care: separate worlds or common ground?, *Better Jobs, Better Care Issue Brief*, 5 [http://www.bjbc.org/content/docs/BJBCIssueBriefNo5.pdf, accessed 5 December 2007].

Sung, H., Chang, S. and Tsai, C. (2005) Working in long term care settings for older people with dementia: nurses' aides, *Journal of Clinical Nursing*, 14(5): 587–93.

Sveinsdottir, H., Biering, P. and Ramel, A. (2006) Occupational stress, job satisfaction and working environment among Icelandic nurses: a cross-sectional questionnaire survey, *International Journal of Nursing Studies*, 43: 875–89.

Tarricone, R. and Tsouros, A.D. (eds.) (2008) *The Solid Facts: Home Care in Europe*. Copenhagen: WHO Regional Office for Europe.

Tellis-Nayak, V. and Tellis-Nayak, M. (1989) Quality of care and the burden of two cultures: when the world of the nurse aide enters the world of the nursing home, *The Gerontologist*, 29: 307–13.

Teri, L., Huda, P., Gibbons, L., Young, H. and van Leynseele, J. (2005) STAR: a dementia-specific training program for staff in assisted living residences, *The Gerontologist*, 45(5): 686–93.

Trinkoff, A., Johantgen, M., Muntaner, C. and Rong, L. (2005) Staffing and worker injury in nursing homes, *American Journal of Public Health*, 95(7): 1220–5.

Vinton, L. and Mazza, N. (1994) Aggressive behavior directed at nursing home personnel by residents' family members, *The Gerontologist*, 34(4): 528–33.

Yassi, A., Cohen, M., Cvitkovich, Y., Park, I., Ratner, P. *et al.* (2004) Factors associated with staff injuries in intermediate care facilities in British Columbia, Canada, *Nursing Research*, 53(2): 87–98.

Yeatts, D. and Seward, R. (2000) Reducing turnover and improving health care in nursing homes: the potential effects of self-managed work teams, *The Gerontologist*, 40(3): 358–63.

Yeatts, D., Cready, C., Swan, J. and Shen, Y. (2010) The perception of "training availability" among certified nurse aides: relationship to CAN performance, turnover, attitudes, burnout and empowerment, *Gerontology and Geriatrics Education*, 31: 115–32.

Zwakhalen, S., Hamers, J., Peijnenburg, R. and Berger, M. (2007) Nursing staff knowledge and beliefs about pain in elderly nursing home residents with dementia, *Pain Research and Management*, 12(3): 177–84.

CHAPTER 30

Leadership in dementia care

Kimberly Nolet and Tonya Roberts

66 There was enormous care in recruiting. They found people who were warm and welcoming, who really liked older people. They had very good staff ratios and were multi-skilled. Sometimes the manager did the barbeque and the music therapist helped in the kitchen. They genuinely welcomed family, like 'how's your son with the broken arm? And 'would you like me to make you a cup of tea?' It was a heavy emphasis on creating a real family environment. 99

—Frances Annal Melbourne, Australia

Learning objectives

By the end of this chapter, you will be able to:

- Identify the roles of leaders in influencing dementia care delivery
- Recognize key skills for health and social care leaders, including strategic planning, supporting employees, and systems thinking
- Apply strategic planning skills and systems thinking to health and social care delivery

Introduction

Effective leaders are recognized as being essential to achieving and embedding excellence in dementia care (National Audit Office 2010). Gershon and colleagues (2004) found leaders are responsible for defining organizational culture (e.g. values, expected behaviours, rituals) by communicating and reinforcing goals and expectations over time. Organizational culture has been shown to influence the success of companies, including their ability to adapt and compete in turbulent times (Collins and Hansen 2011). In fact, some suggest that failures in implementing organizational change occur because leaders have not properly tended to organizational culture (Prajogo and McDermott 2005; Cameron and Quinn 2011).

The culture that leaders create within an organization has been shown to be particularly important in person-centred dementia care. Many of the organizations that have undergone changes to implement person-centred care have described the role of leadership as vital to the continued success of efforts. Morgan and colleagues (2005) elicited first-hand accounts of creating and sustaining dementia special care units from Directors of Care in Canada to understand key factors in their success. The success of these units was dependent on nurse leaders' determination to create and foster a shared vision, empower staff to make decisions, and act as role models and teachers on the units. Effective leadership in person-centred care organizations reduces resistance, produces opportunities for staff to obtain and use new skills and knowledge, and provides clarity of the concepts and values underpinning the organization's model of dementia care.

As you read this chapter, it will be clear that successful leadership requires investment of effort. Leaders need to role model quality care practices and clearly articulate employee expectations while providing appropriate coaching and resources. Leaders utilize several strategies to successfully shape organizational culture, thereby ensuring services align with the goals of person-centred care. These include (Yukl 2006):

- strategic planning and embedding a shared vision
- systems thinking
- supporting and empowering employees

These are skills that can be learned and should continually be refined. This chapter discusses these key domains and their implications for overcoming the challenges facing an organization providing evidenced-based, person-centred dementia care.

Vision and mission

Vision and mission should be used to guide daily activities in an organization. However, there is a lack of clarity about what visions and missions are and how to execute them. Vision and mission statements are often inaccurately used interchangeably. Vision statements push an organization towards a future achievement, while mission statements guide current organizational behaviour. Championing the vision and mission is a key leadership practice.

In dementia care, focusing on individual needs and personhood is at the core of both vision and mission statements. For example, a vision statement might be "Smith Home will become a national exemplar for providing person-centred dementia care." A related mission statement is, "Smith Home recognizes the individual lives and needs of residents and strives to create a homelike environment for each person. By showing respect, sharing in their past, present and future, developing significant relationships, and nurturing interests, staff will nurture residents in maintaining meaningful lives."

Exercise 30.1: Understanding links between mission/vision and practice

Use the Internet to search for the Alzheimer's Association's web site in your country. Review the Association's mission and vision statements, often found in the "About Us" section of the web site. Review how the Association carries out their mission and vision through focused initiatives.

Once a vision is created and a mission statement produced, leaders must then bring the vision and mission alive in the organization. Shared vision can foster innovation and increase employee commitment. To achieve these benefits, a leader must move to spread and operationalize vision and mission throughout the organization. If communicated and modelled effectively, employees should be able to explain the vision and mission to outsiders and new employees, further driving the vision into the organization. Dolak (2001) outlines several steps leaders can take to infuse vision and mission throughout the organization:

- create a simple statement called a "strategic principle" (Gadiesh and Gilbert 2001) that is simple and memorable to employees (for example, coffee brand Starbucks' is to "never stop pursuing the perfect cup of coffee")

- insist all managers model behaviours consistent with the vision
- share the vision at every opportunity, internally and externally
- design communication (email footer, newsletters, advertising, etc.) to always include elements of the vision
- set the expectation that all employees will share the vision (e.g. incorporate into job descriptions and evaluations)
- consistently act in accordance with the behaviour expected of others

Additionally, there may be systems (e.g. redesign of supply procurement systems that allow staff to respond quickly to a person's requests), investments (e.g. staff education or adding additional staff), and/or policies that need to be examined to carry out vision and mission, particularly when these are necessarily aligned with quality dementia care practices and principles. For example, a facility policy may be established that supports and encourages staff to dine with residents during their break time, allowing natural opportunities for relationship development between staff and residents. Creating new systems and policies leads into the next topic of creating a plan to progress towards the mission and vision.

Exercise 30.2: Developing mission and vision

Lakeview is a 98-bed nursing home that has seen an increase in persons with dementia over the last five years. The director of nursing's father in another city recently was diagnosed with dementia, and upon choosing a long-term care facility for him, she found herself drawn to facilities with special dementia care units. She brought this up in a meeting with the administrator, inquiring if she could explore the idea of having a specialized unit at Lakeview. She'd like to provide other residents and families with the same comfort she had, knowing staff were well trained for caring for dementia residents. The administrator and director of nursing visit a few other facilities with this type of unit and gather some readings. They agree it is the right direction for Lakeview to go, but have some concerns about implementing such a change. How will they decide which staff to assign to the unit? Can the facility afford minor remodelling for a special unit? What might residents with dementia expect or want from a special care unit? Will they have enough dementia residents on a consistent basis to fill the unit? Staff at the facilities visited appear to need more time with residents in dementia care units, yet Lakeview's staffing budget is already stretched thin.

According to the stages of strategic planning, how might they proceed? What types of information might they need to gather as part of strategic planning? What might a mission and vision statement look like for the facility?

Strategic planning

Strategic planning has an important impact on how the overall organization operates and determines the priorities that drive decision-making and resource allocation. In dementia care, where resources are scarce, regulation is tight, and personhood is being increasingly valued, the importance of strategic planning cannot be understated. Strategic planning helps organizations understand where they are, where they want to be, and how to get there (Bryson 2011).

Strategic planning is proactive, long-range planning that addresses an issue of concern for the entire organization by:

- addressing internal and external factors during times of change and turbulence
- using staff and other resources most effectively and efficiently
- focusing the organization's culture and its customer base
- building consensus about where an organization is going

Strategic planning creates an opportunity to influence organizational culture through proactive leadership (Zuckerman 2006). Involving multiple levels of staff in the planning phase maximizes communication, buy-in and dissemination of efforts across the organization. For example, if providing state-of-the-art dementia care is part of an organization's mission, formulating strategy around the mission can provide an opportunity for leaders to bring together nursing, engineering, dietary and communications staff, physical therapists, and social workers, as well as patients' families, forming an inclusive strategy. Sharing in strategy creation increases the likelihood that the strategy will be appreciated and comprehensively disseminated across the organization.

Models of strategic planning

Traditional models of strategic planning, which ensure the achievement of an organization's vision, involve some basic steps (Mintzberg 2000) (see Figure 30.1). Volatility in an organization's environment and the general market context influences the selection and use of a strategic planning model (see examples in Table 30.1).

Many health care organizations have adopted tools that support these models to assist with strategic plan implementation and performance monitoring once the plan has been identified. The Institute for Healthcare Improvement (IHI) recommends the Model for Improvement (Langley *et al.* 2009). The model uses a "plan–do–study–act" cycle to implement strategic changes, focusing on testing

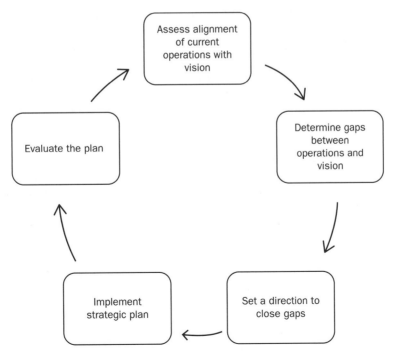

Figure 30.1: Basic process of strategic planning

Strategic planning model	Description	Common use
Issue-based strategic planning	Emphasizes a one-year plan in the context of a long-term strategic plan	Turbulent or competitive markets
Goals-based strategic planning	Focuses on goals to carry out the organization's vision	Stable markets
Alignment planning	Examines "what works well" and what does not; how they can be adjusted to create vision and strategy	Organizations facing widespread internal problems
Scenario planning	Uses systems thinking to thoroughly evaluate how a variety of strategies could best and worst impact an organization	Large corporations facing change
Strategy making or organic planning	Uses continuing dialogue with stakeholders to identify what is successful in the organization, focusing on retaining and expanding this, as well as identifying improvements	Interconnected, multi-stakeholder organizations where future may be unpredictable

Table 30.1 Sample strategic planning models

changes prior to widespread implementation. The Balanced Scorecard (BSC), popular in health care and across other industries, is an evidence-based performance management tool that helps leaders monitor success in implementing strategy. Kaplan and Norton (1996) warn that many organizations rely only or primarily on financial data to drive strategy, and suggest the BSC approach as a more balanced, multi-perspective look at the past, present, and future. The BSC approach emphasizes linking individual performance to vision and goals, and using learning and feedback (in addition to objective data) to evaluate and adjust strategy. While no single model is as popular as the BSC in most North American and European countries (Paranjape *et al.* 2006), the Performance Prism is another example of an implementation strategy and performance management model that focuses on implementing and measuring stakeholder needs and preferences. The creators argue that the method more effectively identifies appropriate strategies and measures for success that matter most (Neely *et al.* 2002).

Unfortunately, health care organizations often see strategic planning as a project rather than a constant management process (Zuckerman 2006). Bryson (2011) emphasizes that strategic planning is only successful when people think, act, and learn strategically along the entire process. It is important to consider the uniqueness of every organization and marketplace (see Table 30.1) prior to selecting a strategic planning model and appropriate tools to support implementation and monitoring.

Components of strategic planning

Although forms of strategic planning have differences, the common components include organizational assessment, vision and mission alignment, and creating and evaluating a plan.

Assessment

The SWOT Analysis (Strengths, Weaknesses, Opportunities, and Threats; developed by Stanford professor Albert Humphrey in the 1970s) and Environmental Scan (groundwork laid by Francis Aguilar in the 1960s and refined over decades) are two common tools used to assess the state of an organization. Items such as consumer perception of the organization, position in the marketplace relative to competition, strengths and weaknesses within the organization, and areas for growth can be assessed using these models. It should be noted that these models are ways to organize information for analysis, but will not tell an organization the best way to collect the data.

Employee surveys and interviews, consumer surveys and interviews, marketplace data (e.g. number of competitors, consumer demand, and specialized services available), the organization's financial information, and other performance indicators (e.g. health outcomes used to assess quality, employee retention statistics) can be used to inform the assessment. The SWOT and Environmental Scan models are valuable, yet some have argued they are too simplistic, cumbersome and time-consuming, and are reliant on self-perception (Helms and Nixon 2010). The importance of obtaining multiple perspectives, both internal and external from the organization, must be underscored. Alternative methods for assessing and strategic planning are emerging but none have replaced the SWOT and Environmental Scan as gold standard models.

Creating and implementing the plan

While vision and mission guide the "big picture" in an organization, developing goals and objectives are steps to action. Developing goals and objectives, and the strategies to meet those, are at the heart of the strategic plan. Goals are statements of what will be achieved and should be aligned with the mission and vision of the organization. Objectives are sub-units of how goals will be achieved. Table 30.2 contrasts goals and objectives.

Effective leaders will approach developing goals, objectives, and strategies with a diverse team of employees. The process of strategic planning will, at minimum, need to include willing individuals who share a vision across levels, including (Sullivan and Decker 2001): (1) top-level administrators, (2) representatives of those closest to the work (e.g. frontline caregivers, social workers), and (3) staff to collect data and distribute information. Sullivan and Decker highlight the importance of including staff in the early stages of planning who "buy in" to the vision and mission, To increase buy-in, naysayers "can be included once some parts of the plan are formulated" (Sullivan and Decker 2001: 27).

Vision and mission alignment

Strategic planning provides an opportunity to review and assess the adequacy of your vision and mission statements. If, during the prior steps of strategic planning, you recognize a key need your

	Focus	**Level of focus**	**How measured**	**Example:**
Goals	Outcomes	Organizational	"Met"/"Not met"	"Each person with dementia receiving our services will have a medication dispensing system in their homes to allow for better tracking and management of their medications"
Objectives	Processes	Individual or unit	Quantified measure of progress (e.g. 7 out of 10 people)	"Monthly totals of persons with dementia owning a medication dispensing system will increase"

Table 30.2 Goals and objectives

organization can fill in the community, or a core value that is important to uphold, you may want to revise your mission and vision accordingly.

It is also important to do a "vision check" to ensure each goal and strategy you select during strategic planning is congruent with your vision and mission. If alignment is not achieved, barriers to implementation may arise and employees may become confused about how they are to accomplish the mission when goals that influence practices are at odds with what the organization has already stated it wants to achieve.

Evaluating the plan

Success of the strategic plan must be evaluated at multiple levels. Evaluating individual strategies requires clear objectives. Input at multiple levels (data, interviews with staff and consumers) is important to include (Zuckerman 2006). However, it is important to have a dynamic process where the objectives, goals, and sometimes even the mission can be adjusted over time.

Exercise 30.3: Developing goals and objectives

Refer back to Exercise 30.2. The administrator and director of nursing have several concerns about how they will implement the new dementia care unit at Lakeview. One of their concerns is ensuring investment in services and programmes that will most benefit persons with dementia and their families, while appropriately allocating resources across the entire home.

Try to identify a goal and objective around resource allocation on a new dementia care unit. Keep in mind that the goal and objective should be compatible with mission and values. Who should be involved in developing goals, objectives, and planning strategies to ensure the goal is met?

Systems thinking

Current leadership wisdom supports the need to focus on systems and how they operate in an organization (Sullivan and Decker 2001). Systems thinking is "a way of thinking that gives us the freedom to identify the root causes of problems and see new opportunities" (Meadows 2008). Systems thinking can lead to more sustainable, creative solutions that increase quality of life and quality of care. Through systems thinking, dementia care leaders also will find opportunities to identify necessary changes in policy at the organization, local, and national level.

All behaviour in organizations is affected by the system in which the behaviour occurs. For example, when staff are trying to be more responsive to patients who are wandering, there will be many "systems" factors that influence success of that effort. Safety measures, family involvement, fall prevention programmes, general staff knowledge, and the systems of accountability for responding to patients are only a few of the systems that influence wandering. Looking only at the responsiveness of a particular nurse, or the ability of a particular certified nurse assistant, to keep track of a resident will do little to address the problem. It might improve the situation for one resident at one time, but is unlikely to have any further impact. Implementing an accountability system for wander management will, on the other hand, affect many patients, influence all shifts and all levels of staff.

While it is ideal for staff to think about the system influences on care provision, leaders in the organization must take the lead. Leaders must respond (and must be seen to respond) to problems by looking at system contributors as well as other more local factors.

Case example 30.1: Albert Thorpe

Albert Thorpe is an 88-year-old with mild dementia who has just had particularly difficult cataract surgery and is staying overnight at the hospital. Consider the following scenario based on information gleaned from Albert and the staff's perspectives of his experience the following day.

Albert's perspective

Albert wakes up from his surgery and is not sure where he is. He needs to use the restroom but does not see one nearby. He tries to get up to find one and hears alarms sounding. Then there is pain in his arm where a plastic cord is taped. He continues to get up so he can locate a bathroom and knocks over a pole. More alarms start sounding. Albert is very confused about what is going on now. He heads to the door to find help, feels dizzy, and falls on the floor. He feels pain in his backside and now really needs to use the restroom. He tries to call for help, but cannot seem to find the right words. He sees two women coming to him, possibly to help and he tries to explain what happened but they did not seem to be listening. They keep telling him to go back to bed but he keeps trying to tell them he needs to use the restroom. He becomes angry and frustrated that they will not help him.

Staff perspective

The physician knows Albert also has very mild dementia. The morning after his surgery, a staff nurse comes to take Albert's vital signs and finds him on the floor in the doorway of his room. Albert starts to yell at the nurse, insisting he wants to leave and nobody is to touch him. The startled nurse goes to the door and calls for another nurse to help. Meanwhile, Albert's daughter happens to arrive for his discharge and is upset to find her father in such distress. Albert eventually calms down and they get him back into bed, as he appears to be unaffected by the fall. The charge nurse, recalling the note about dementia in his chart, informs Albert's daughter that hospitalizations and surgery can sometimes trigger more severe episodes of dementia. The staff nurse who took his vital signs is embarrassed, as she did not realize Albert had dementia, and might have approached him a bit differently had she known (although she does not really know how she would have done it differently, she just knows people with dementia have special care and communication needs). Albert's daughter is still upset, as she now has more than his vision to worry about when he gets home. She has only dealt with Albert's mild dementia and is now worried he will not know his family and accept their help.

Issues to be considered

How might hospital staff help understand the unique needs of, and communicate with, persons like Albert? What changes in the system could be implemented so that hospital stays could best address care from the perspective of persons with dementia (e.g. policies on use of bed alarms)?

How could hospital staff prepare Albert's daughter for discharge? Consider, in particular, the roles of the social worker, discharge nurse, physician, and pharmacist.

Not all staff knew the patient had dementia, and many seemed unprepared to work with dementia patients. What systems issues should be addressed to prevent similar problems in the future?

Supporting and empowering employees

66 I realize how important it is to demonstrate that I care and I am really listening to the staff and acting on their suggestions. There is an organizational, a scientific, and a psychological benefit to asking them what they want and then delivering on it. 99

—Nursing Home Administrator David Farrell (in Farrell *et al.* 2011: 48)

Every leader needs an effective team of employees to carry out the organization's mission and vision. When working with people with dementia, staff flexibility in responding to needs in person-centred ways is of paramount importance. To effectively respond, employees must be empowered to solve problems on the frontline. In the quote by David Farrell above, he was surprised at the simplicity of the first request he received from staff: bendable straws so that nursing home residents could drink more easily. The staff knew the answer to a problem, but were not empowered to change the supply ordering. Many leaders are unsure what constitutes empowering their staff. To some, verbal encouragement is the equivalent of empowerment. While verbal support is important, structures for decision-making and encouragement at all levels are necessary.

Consider the following example. Visiting home care aides are to provide basic health care needs to individuals, but they often observe other needs while in the homes. They might see a person suffering from social isolation, or a person unable to complete an activity he or she enjoys due to lack of adaptive equipment. This information is quite likely not shared with a health care provider, advocate or social worker because the aide has not been empowered with the training to recognize these as reportable problems or lacks the confidence, or authority, to directly contact these key persons with concerns outside their direct scope of practice. Consequently, important needs may continue to be unmet.

Empowerment comes from two primary sources: environment (Kanter 1993) and personal psychological state (Manojlovich 2007). Empowerment from one's environment is often referred to as "structural empowerment" (Laschinger and Havens 1996), and includes (Kanter 1993):

- access to resources, information, and support
- actual structures for advancement opportunities
- organizational awareness of worker contributions

Leaders can have a direct impact on structures to empower staff. Providing career ladders, mentor programmes, and adequate resources for staff are all leadership tasks, although this is not always simple. Leaders must look for ways to creatively maximize effectiveness of available resources. Some examples of providing resources to empower staff include:

- more/redesigned space for facility operations
- incentive programmes for employees
- career ladders for employees
- redesign of patient living and social environments
- staff training/education in primary areas of concern
- technology to help staff do jobs efficiently
- alternative staffing models that create efficiency

Leaders can work with internal teams to identify resource needs, anticipate future needs, and consider ways to address those needs.

Exercise 30.4: The power of words

In a literature review by Dwyer (2011), nurses in long-term care were found to associate the words "quality of care" with compliance and accreditation. Nurses felt increased motivation when the focus of management and staff was framed as "improving quality of life" for individuals (Dwyer 2011). When management's focus was on quality of care and regulatory compliance, nurses felt unrecognized for "what you did right" and only recognized for "what you did wrong". How can this finding influence what dementia care leaders do in an organization to support employees?

Debates and controversies

Leadership theories continue to evolve as technology, consumer preferences, and economic realities shift in the business world. Health care, particularly long-term care, has been a slow adopter of changes. While debates and controversies in leadership styles and methods continue, some important considerations include:

- How will education of leaders evolve and how will success be measured? Is it worthwhile to invest in developing a leader who does not have natural skills?
- Will established methods of strategic planning and assessment give way to more efficient methods, and how will that influence the work environment, consumer satisfaction, and long-term planning?
- How can leaders ensure consumer preferences are honoured in a tightly regulated environment?
- How can organizations provide modern, person-centred care given scarce financial and staff resources?

Research has demonstrated that engaged and supportive leadership is key to successful delivery and sustainability of person-centred care. Transforming dementia practices to be person-centred is a complex, ongoing process with unique challenges related to changing the fundamental values driving care. It is imperative that the field continues to articulate the leadership practices that are particularly relevant to achieve this goal.

Conclusion

Challenges to the delivery of person-centred dementia care have resulted in an environment in which staff are stressed, confused, and dissatisfied, influencing the continuity and quality of person-centred dementia care. Leadership is becoming recognized as a key factor in overcoming these challenges, although health care has been slow to adapt. In recent years, however, groups caring for persons with dementia have been focusing on instilling evidenced-based, person-centredness throughout their organizations. This creates a situation ripe for leaders to embrace strategic planning as a tool to enhance both the work and care environment.

Across varying approaches to leadership, different skills and abilities are emphasized as being important. However, the culture leaders create is pivotal in many environments and key skills and strategies that have been implicated in the success of creating this culture include a leader's ability to develop and implement a vision for the organization, create supportive staff relationships, and think at a system level. These essential ingredients, when present, can greatly enhance the delivery of person-centred care.

Further information

The Mind Tools web site provides management and leadership resources, including strategy tools [http://www.mindtools.com/index.html].

Loveday, B. (2012) *Leadership for Person-Centred Dementia Care.* London: Jessica Kingsley. One of the Bradford Dementia Group's Good Practice Guides [http://www.jkp.com/catalogue/book/9781849052290#.Uj2708ZJOAg].

References

Bryson, J.M. (2011) *Strategic Planning for Public and Nonprofit Organizations: A Guide to Strengthening and Sustaining Organizational Achievement* (4th edn.). New York: Wiley.

Cameron, K.S. and Quinn, R.E. (2011) *Diagnosing and Changing Organizational Culture* (3rd edn.). San Francisco, CA: Jossey-Bass.

Collins, J.C. and Hansen, M.T. (2011) *Great by Choice.* New York: Harper Business.

Dolak, D. (2001) *Creating and Communicating Vision: The Business Leader's Primary Responsibility* [http://www.davedolak.com/articles/dolak5.htm, accessed 19 January 2008].

Dwyer, D. (2011) Experiences of registered nurses as managers and leaders in residential aged care facilities: a systematic review, *International Journal of Evidence-Based Healthcare,* 9: 388–402.

Farrell, D., Brady, C. and Frank, B. (2011) *Meeting the Leadership Challenge in Long Term Care: What You Do Matters.* Baltimore, MD: Health Professions Press.

Gadiesh, O. and Gilbert, J.L. (2001) Transforming corner-office strategy into frontline action, *Harvard Business Review,* 79: 72–9.

Gershon, R.R.M., Stone, P.W., Bakken, S. and Larson, E. (2004) Measurement of organizational culture and climate in healthcare, *Journal of Nursing Administration,* 34: 33–40.

Helms, M.M. and Nixon, J. (2010) Exploring SWOT analysis – where are we now? A review of academic research from the last decade, *Journal of Strategy and Management,* 3: 215–51.

Kanter, R.M. (1993) *Men and Women of the Corporation.* New York: Basic Books.

Kaplan, R.S. and Norton, D.P. (1996) *The Balanced Scorecard: Translating Strategy into Action.* Boston, MA: Harvard Business School Press.

Langley, G.L., Nolan, K.M., Nolan, T.W., Norman, C.L. and Provost, L.P. (2009) *The Improvement Guide: A Practical Approach to Enhancing Organizational Performance* (2nd edn.). San Francisco, CA: Jossey-Bass.

Laschinger, H.K. and Havens, D.S. (1996) Staff nurse work empowerment and perceived control over nursing practice: conditions for work effectiveness, *Journal of Nursing Administration,* 26: 27–35.

Manojlovich, M. (2007) Power and empowerment in nursing: looking backward to inform the future, *Online Journal of Issues in Nursing,* 12(1): 2.

Meadows, D. (2008) *Thinking in Systems: A Primer.* White River Junction, VT: Chelsea Green.

Mintzberg, H. (2000) *The Rise and Fall of Strategic Planning.* Toronto: Prentice-Hall.

Morgan, D.G., Stewart, N.J., D'Arcy, C. and Cammer, A.L. (2005) Creating and sustaining dementia special care units in rural nursing homes: the critical role of nursing leadership, *Nursing Research,* 18: 74–99.

National Audit Office (2010) *Improving Dementia Services in England: An Interim Report.* London: TSO [http://www.nao.org.uk/report/improving-dementia-services-in-england-an-interim-report/, accessed 29 April 2014].

Neely, A., Adams, C. and Kennerley, M. (2002) *The Performance Prism: The Scorecard for Measuring and Managing Business Success.* New York: Pearson.

Paranjape, B., Rossiter, M. and Pantano, V. (2006) Performance measurement systems: successes, failures and future – a review, *Measuring Business Excellence*, 10: 4–14.

Prajogo, D.I. and McDermott, D.M. (2005) The relationship between total quality management practices and organizational culture, *International Journal of Operations and Production Management*, 25: 1101–22.

Sullivan, E.J. and Decker, P.J. (2001) *Effective Leadership and Management in Nursing*. Upper Saddle River, NJ: Prentice-Hall.

Yukl, G.A. (2006) *Leadership in Organizations*. New York: Prentice-Hall.

Zuckerman, A. (2006) *Raising the Bar: Best Practices for Healthcare Strategic Planning*. Philadelphia, PA: Health Strategies and Solutions, Inc. and SHSMD of the AHA.

Index

Locators shown in *italics* refer to figures, tables and boxes.